TRANSGENDER AND GENDER DIVERSE HEALTH CARE:
The Fenway Guide

Editors

Alex S. Keuroghlian, MD, MPH
Associate Professor of Psychiatry
Harvard Medical School
Director, Massachusetts General Hospital Psychiatry Gender Identity Program
Director, Division of Education and Training at The Fenway Institute
Boston, Massachusetts

Jennifer Potter, MD
Professor of Medicine and Advisory Dean
Harvard Medical School
Founding Director, Women's Health Center, Beth Israel Deaconess Medical Center
Co-Chair and Director of the LGBT Population Health Program at The Fenway Institute
Boston, Massachusetts

Sari L. Reisner, ScD
Assistant Professor of Medicine
Harvard Medical School
Assistant Professor of Epidemiology Harvard T.H. Chan School of Public Health
Director of Transgender Research
Brigham and Women's Hospital
Director of Transgender and Gender Diverse Health Research
The Fenway Institute
Boston, Massachusetts

Mc
Graw
Hill

New York   Chicago   San Francisco   Athens   London   Madrid   Mexico City
New Delhi   Milan   Singapore   Sydney   Toronto

Transgender and Gender Diverse Health Care: The Fenway Guide

1 2 3 4 5 6 7 8 9 LCR 26 25 24 23 22 21

ISBN 978-1-260-45993-7
MHID 1-260-45993-4

Notice

Medicine is an ever-changing science. As new research and clinical experience broaden our knowledge, changes in treatment and drug therapy are required. The authors and the publisher of this work have checked with sources believed to be reliable in their efforts to provide information that is complete and generally in accord with the standards accepted at the time of publication. However, in view of the possibility of human error or changes in medical sciences, neither the authors nor the publisher nor any other party who has been involved in the preparation or publication of this work warrants that the information contained herein is in every respect accurate or complete, and they disclaim all responsibility for any errors or omissions or for the results obtained from use of the information contained in this work. Readers are encouraged to confirm the information contained herein with other sources. For example and in particular, readers are advised to check the product information sheet included in the package of each drug they plan to administer to be certain that the information contained in this work is accurate and that changes have not been made in the recommended dose or in the contraindications for administration. This recommendation is of particular importance in connection with new or infrequently used drugs.

This book was set in Minion Pro by MPS Limited.
The editors were Jason Malley and Kim J. Davis.
The production supervisor was Catherine Saggese.
Project management was provided by Jyoti Shaw, MPS Limited.
The cover designer was Tess McKenney.
This book was printed on acid-free paper.

Library of Congress Cataloging-in-Publication Data

Names: Keuroghlian, Alex S., editor. | Potter, Jennifer (Physician) editor.
  | Reisner, Sari L., editor. | Fenway Institute.
Title: Transgender and gender diverse health care / editors, Alex S.
  Keuroghlian, Jennifer Potter, Sari L. Reisner.
Description: New York: McGraw Hill, [2022] | Includes bibliographical
  references and index. | Summary: "This book covers topics such as the
  history and background of transgender and gender-diverse health care,
  gender identity, primary, preventive, and specialty care, and
  community-building, advocacy, and partnership"—Provided by publisher.
Identifiers: LCCN 2021031256 (print) | LCCN 2021031257 (ebook) | ISBN
  9781260459937 (alk. paper) | ISBN 9781260459944 (ebook)
Subjects: MESH: Health Services for Transgender Persons | Sexual and Gender
  Minorities | Delivery of Health Care. | Preventive Health
  Services—methods. | United States.
Classification: LCC RA564.9.T73 (print) | LCC RA564.9.T73 (ebook) | NLM
  WA 300 AA1 | DDC 362.1086/7—dc23
LC record available at https://lccn.loc.gov/2021031256
LC ebook record available at https://lccn.loc.gov/2021031257

McGraw Hill books are available at special quantity discounts to use as premiums and sales promotions, or for use in corporate training programs. To contact a representative, please visit the Contact Us pages at www.mhprofessional.com.

Authors

Stefan Baral, MD, MPH, MBA
Department of Epidemiology
Johns Hopkins Bloomberg School of Public Health
Baltimore, Maryland
*Chapter 22: Health Needs and Service Delivery Models for
  Transgender Communities in Low- and Middle-Income
  Countries*

Sebastian Mitchell Barr, PhD
Cambridge Health Alliance / Harvard Medical School
Cambridge, Massachusetts
Chapter 12: Obtaining a Gender-Affirming Sexual History

S. Wilson Beckham, PhD, MPH/MA
Department of Health, Behavior and Society
Johns Hopkins Bloomberg School of Public Health
Baltimore, Maryland
*Chapter 22: Health Needs and Service Delivery Models for
  Transgender Communities in Low- and Middle-Income
  Countries*

Sarah Berman, MD
Psychiatry Resident
Cambridge Health Alliance
Cambridge, Massachusetts
*Chapter 11: Basic Principles of Trauma-Informed and
  Gender-Affirming Care*

Gaines Blasdel
Research Associate
New York University Grossman School of Medicine
New York, New York
Chapter 9: Surgical Gender Affirmation

Rachel Bluebond-Langner, MD
Laura and Isaac Perlmutter Associate Professor of
  Reconstructive Plastic Surgery
Co-Director, Transgender Reconstructive Surgery Program
NYU Langone Health System
New York University Grossman School of Medicine
New York, New York
Chapter 9: Surgical Gender Affirmation

Jack Bruno, BA
National LGBTQIA+ Health Education Center
The Fenway Institute
Boston, Massachusetts
*Chapter 21: Transgender and Gender Diverse People Who Are
  Black, Indigenous, and People of Color*

Sean Cahill, PhD
Director, Health Policy Research
The Fenway Institute
Affiliate Associate Clinical Professor
Bouve College of Health Sciences
Northeastern University
Adjunct Associate Professor of the Practice in Health Law
Policy and Management
Boston University School of Public Health
Boston, Massachusetts
*Chapter 27: Advocacy for Transgender and Gender Diverse
  Patients*

Kirsty A. Clark, PhD, MPH
Postdoctoral Research Fellow
Yale University School of Public Health
New Haven, Connecticut
*Chapter 23: Transgender and Gender Diverse People and
  Incarceration*

Katharine B. Dalke, MD, MBE
Director of the Office for Culturally Responsive Health
  Care Education
Assistant Professor of Psychiatry and Behavioral Health
Penn State College of Medicine
Hershey, Pennsylvania
Chapter 25: Affirming Care for People with Intersex Traits

Heidi J. Dalzell, PsyD
Licensed Psychologist
Private Practice
Newtown, Pennsylvania
Chapter 15: Eating Disorders, Body Image, and Body Positivity

Christine Darsney, PhD
Psychologist
Child Cognitive-Behavioral Therapy Program
Massachusetts General Hospital
Boston, Massachusetts
*Chapter 6: Behavioral Health Considerations for Transgender
  and Gender Diverse People*

Steph de Normand, BS, MA
Trans Health Program Manager
Fenway Health
Boston, Massachusetts
Chapter 8: Nonmedical, Nonsurgical Gender Affirmation

Flavia Vaz De Souza, BA
Clinical Research Coordinator
Massachusetts General Hospital
Boston, Massachusetts
*Chapter 6: Behavioral Health Considerations for Transgender
  and Gender Diverse People*

Mason J. Dunn, JD
Deputy Director
Division of Education and Training
The Fenway Institute
Boston, Massachusetts
Chapter 19: Reproductive Health, Obstetric Care, and Family Building

Katherine N. Elfer, PhD, MPH
Johns Hopkins Bloomberg School of Public Health
Baltimore, Maryland
Chapter 22: Health Needs and Service Delivery Models for Transgender Communities in Low- and Middle-Income Countries

Sadie Elisseou, MD
Clinical Instructor of Medicine
Boston VA Healthcare System/Boston
Boston, Massachusetts
Chapter 13: Performing a Trauma-Informed Physical Examination

Hilary Goldhammer, SM
Technical Writer
Division of Education and Training,
The Fenway Institute
Boston, Massachusetts
Chapter 6: Behavioral Health Considerations for Transgender and Gender Diverse People

Zil G. Goldstein, FNP-BC
Associate Medical Director for TGNB Health
Callen-Lorde Community Health Center
New York, New York
Chapter 16: Screening and Prevention of HIV and Sexually Transmitted Infections

Alex Gonzalez, MD, MPH
Medical Director
Fenway Health
Boston, Massachusetts
Chapter 18: Screening for Cancer and Cardiovascular Disease

Chris Grasso, MPH
Associate Vice President for Informatics and Data
Fenway Health
Boston, Massachusetts
Chapter 4: Harnessing Information Technology to Improve Clinical Care

Frances W. Grimstad, MD, MS
Division of Gynecology
Department of Surgery
Boston Children's Hospital
Harvard Medical School
Boston, Massachusetts
Chapter 25: Affirming Care for People with Intersex Traits

Samara Grossman, MSW, LICSW
Clinical Social Worker
Brigham and Women's Hospital
Boston, Massachusetts
Chapter 11: Basic Principles of Trauma-Informed and Gender-Affirming Care

Omar Harfouch, MD
Department of Infectious Disease
University of Maryland Medical Center
Baltimore, Maryland
Chapter 22: Health Needs and Service Delivery Models for Transgender Communities in Low- and Middle-Income Countries

Aude Henin, PhD
Co-Director, Child Cognitive-Behavioral Therapy Program
Director, Child Resiliency Programs, Benson Henry Institute
Massachusetts General Hospital
Assistant Professor of Psychology in the Department of Psychiatry Harvard Medical School
Boston, Massachusetts
Chapter 6: Behavioral Health Considerations for Transgender and Gender Diverse People

Jaclyn White Hughto, PhD, MPH
Assistant Professor
Departments of Behavioral and Social Sciences; and Epidemiology
Brown University School of Public Health
Center for Health Promotion and Health Equity
Brown University
Providence, Rhode Island
Chapter 23: Transgender and Gender Diverse People and Incarceration

Stacy K. Hunt, PhD
Licensed Clinical Psychologist, Managing Director
Bucks Support Services
Newtown, Pennsylvania
Chapter 15: Eating Disorders, Body Image, and Body Positivity

Michael R. Kauth, PhD
Director, VHA LGBT Health, Department of Veterans Affairs
Michael E. DeBakey VA Medical Center
Houston, Texas
Chapter 24: Caring for Transgender and Gender Diverse Veterans

JoAnne Keatley, MSW
Chair
IRGT: A Global Network of Trans Women and HIV
Chapter 21: Transgender and Gender Diverse People Who Are Black, Indigenous, and People of Color

Alex S. Keuroghlian, MD, MPH
Associate Professor of Psychiatry
Harvard Medical School
Director, Massachusetts General Hospital Psychiatry Gender
    Identity Program
Director, Division of Education and Training at The Fenway
    Institute
Boston, Massachusetts
*Chapter 2: Gender Identity: Terminology, Demographics, and
    Epidemiology; Chapter 4: Harnessing Information Technology
    to Improve Clinical Care; Chapter 6: Behavioral Health Con-
    siderations for Transgender and Gender Diverse People*

Farah Naz Khan, MD
Clinical Assistant Professor of Medicine
University of Washington
Seattle, Washington
*Chapter 1: A History of Transgender and Gender Diverse Health
    Care: From Medical Mistreatment to Gender-Affirmative
    Health Care*

Niki S. Khanna, MA, MFT
Therapist and Educator
San Francisco, California
Chapter 25: Affirming Care for People with Intersex Traits

Cei Lambert, MFA
CEO, Diversity Consulting, Inc
Owner and Artist, Meadowlark Tattoo
Fort Collins, Colorado
Chapter 26: Community Engagement and Outreach

Alex McDowell, PhD, MPH, MSN, RN
Research Fellow
Massachusetts General Hospital and Harvard Medical School
Boston, Massachusetts
Chapter 3: Health Disparities

Meghan McGrath, MSW, LICSW
Behavioral Health Specialist
Fenway Health
Boston, Massachusetts
Chapter 5: Gender Identity Emergence and Affirmation in Adults

Ami Multani, MD
Medical Director of Infectious Disease, Fenway Health
Clinical Instructor, Beth Israel Deaconess Medical Center,
    Harvard Medical School Boston, Massachusetts
*Chapter 17: Treatment of HIV and Sexually Transmitted
    Infections*

Danielle O'Banion, MD
Family Physician
Fenway Health
Boston, Massachusetts
Chapter 12: Obtaining a Gender-Affirming Sexual History

Samuel C. Pang, BSc, MD, FACOG, FRCS(C)
Medical Director
Third Party Reproduction Program
Boston IVF—The Lexington Center
Lexington, Massachusetts
*Chapter 19: Reproductive Health, Obstetric Care, and Family
    Building*

Jennifer Potter, MD
Professor of Medicine and Advisory Dean
Harvard Medical School
Founding Director, Women's Health Center, Beth Israel Dea-
    coness Medical Center
Co-Chair and Director of the LGBT Population Health Pro-
    gram at The Fenway Institute
Boston, Massachusetts
*Chapter 2: Gender Identity: Terminology, Demographics, and
    Epidemiology; Chapter 11: Basic Principles of Trauma-
    Informed and Gender-Affirming Care; Chapter 13: Performing
    a Trauma-Informed Physical Examination*

Kayti Protos, MSW, LCSW
Clinical Coordinator
Bucks LGBTQ Center
Newtown, Pennsylvania
Chapter 15: Eating Disorders, Body Image, and Body Positivity

Xavier Quinn, LICSW
Violence Recovery Program Manager
Fenway Health
Boston, Massachusetts
*Chapter 14: Recognizing and Addressing Intimate Partner
    Violence*

Asa Radix, MD, PhD, MPH
Senior Director of Research and Education
Callen-Lorde Community Health Center
New York, New York
*Chapter 16: Screening and Prevention of HIV and Sexually
    Transmitted Infections*

Jenna J. Rapues, MPH
Program Director
San Francisco Department of Public Health
San Francisco, California
*Chapter 21: Transgender and Gender Diverse People Who Are
    Black, Indigenous, and People of Color*

Sari L. Reisner, ScD
Assistant Professor of Medicine
Harvard Medical School
Assistant Professor of Epidemiology Harvard T.H. Chan School
    of Public Health
Director of Transgender Research
Brigham and Women's Hospital
Director of Transgender and Gender Diverse Health Research
The Fenway Institute
Boston, Massachusetts
*Chapter 2: Gender Identity: Terminology, Demographics, and
    Epidemiology*

Jennifer Reske-Nielsen, MD, MPH
Director of Medical Education
Fenway Health
Boston, Massachusetts
Chapter 10: Case Studies in Gender Emergence and Affirmation;
Chapter 20: Case Studies in Transgender and Gender Diverse
Primary Care

Eli Sauerwalt
Johns Hopkins Bloomberg School of Public Health
Baltimore, Maryland
Chapter 22: Health Needs and Service Delivery Models for
Transgender Communities in Low- and Middle-Income
Countries

Jillian C. Shipherd, PhD
Director
LGBT Health for the Veterans Health Administration
Washington, DC
Clinical Research Psychologist
Women's Health Sciences Division of the National Center for
PTSD
VA Boston Healthcare System
Professor of Psychiatry
Boston University School of Medicine
Boston, Massachusetts
Chapter 24: Caring for Transgender and Gender Diverse Veterans

Colleen A. Sloan, PhD
Clinical Psychologist
VA Boston Healthcare System & Boston University School of
Medicine
Boston, Massachusetts
Chapter 24: Caring for Transgender and Gender Diverse Veterans

Carl G. Streed, Jr., MD, MPH
Assistant Professor of Medicine, Research Lead
Center for Transgender Medicine & Surgery
Boston Medical Center
Boston University School of Medicine
Boston, Massachusetts
Chapter 3: Health Disparities

Julie Thompson, PA-C
Medical Director of Trans Health
Fenway Health
Boston, Massachusetts
Chapter 7: Gender-Affirming Hormone Therapy for Adults

Rebekah P. Viloria, MD, FACOG
Obstetrician-Gynecologist
Beth Israel Deaconess Medical Center
Boston, Massachusetts
Chapter 19: Reproductive Health, Obstetric Care, and Family
Building

Meredith Walker, MSW, LICSW
Clinical Supervisor and Psychotherapist
Fenway Health
Boston, Massachusetts
Chapter 5: Gender Identity Emergence and Affirmation in Adults

Vanessa Warri
Sociology & Civic Engagement
University of California
Los Angeles, California
Chapter 21: Transgender and Gender Diverse People Who Are
Black, Indigenous, and People of Color

Lee C. Zhao, MD, MS
Associate Professor of Urology
Director, Male Reconstructive Surgery, NYU Health System
Co-Director, Transgender Reconstructive Surgery Program,
NYU Langone Health System
New York University Grossman School of Medicine
New York, New York
Chapter 9: Surgical Gender Affirmation

Contents

Preface

Increasing social acceptance, service availability, and insurance reimbursement during the last decade are leading more and more transgender and gender diverse (TGD) people to seek gender-affirming health care. Consequently, health professionals are demanding education and training to fill critical gaps in their knowledge and skills. Rapid expansion of the field of TGD health across disciplines is generating groundbreaking innovations and evidence-informed best practices in gender-affirming health care.

This comprehensive textbook is a resource for health professionals at all levels of training and in diverse specialties. Our authors—leading clinicians, researchers, and advocates in the field—outline best practices you can utilize to optimize care for adult TGD patients, with the overarching goal of achieving health equity for TGD communities.

We intend this book to be used as a practical clinical reference. It contains useful tables and diagrams for clinical care (e.g., hormone therapy) and practice transformation (e.g., gender identity data collection in electronic health records). The book can also be used as a teaching tool, as each chapter contains at least one clinical case for self-study or discussion during facilitated group learning exercises. Lastly and perhaps most important given our overarching goal, the information in this book can be leveraged to support your advocacy efforts in implementing systemic changes within your own school, clinical practice, hospital, or community.

Our journey in creating this book has deepened our appreciation of the diversity and richness of TGD identities, expressions, and lived experiences. The fact that these pages took shape in the context of the #MeToo and #BlackLivesMatter movements and during the COVID-19 pandemic added intensity and immediacy to the work. It has been an incredible honor to work with and learn from each of our talented contributing authors and our extraordinary freelance editor, Kathleen H. Scogna.

With thanks to each one of you as we continue this journey.

Alex S. Keuroghlian
Jennifer Potter
Sari L. Reisner

Preface

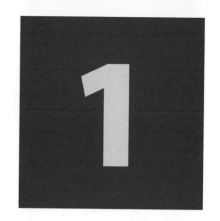

A History of Transgender and Gender Diverse Health Care: From Medical Mistreatment to Gender-Affirmative Health Care

Farah Naz Khan

INTRODUCTION

This chapter describes the history of **transgender and gender diverse (TGD)** health care in the United States (Figure 1-1). This historical context is essential to understanding both the progress made in the United States health care system and current gaps that need to be addressed in the clinical care of TGD populations.

KEY FIGURES IN THE HISTORY OF TRANSGENDER AND GENDER DIVERSE HEALTH CARE

The founder of transgender health care could easily be German physician Magnus Hirschfeld. Hirschfeld coined the now obsolete term "transvestite" in 1910 in his work, Die Transvestiten.[1] Although this term is no longer considered acceptable, Hirschfeld's definition of the term provided an initial framework for articulating the experience of gender diversity: "It is the urge to present and conduct oneself in the outer raiment of the sex to which a person does not belong—as regards the visible sexual organs."[2] In a time when his contemporaries aimed to "cure" gender diverse patients, Hirschfeld developed and implemented "adaptation therapy" at his Institute for Sexual Science in Berlin, to help patients live "according to their nature."[2] Hirschfeld even worked with the legal advisor of his institute to support name changes, something which is a struggle to achieve even in many modern medical records.[2] It would also not be a stretch to align Hirschfeld's pluralist sexual theory with the modern-day concepts of gender and sexual diversity. In his theory, Hirschfeld posited that there are a multitude of gender expressions, all of mixed "absolute male" and "absolute female" characteristics.[2]

Much of the institute's history was lost in the wake of Nazi book burnings in 1933,[3] but as far as history demonstrates, Hirschfeld likely was the first to offer **gender-affirming surgery** when he performed castration in 1922 on one of his employees who identified as a woman.[2] Perhaps the institute's most famous patient was Danish painter Lili Elbe (born Einar Wegener), whose life story was fictionalized for the Hollywood film The Danish Girl. Hirschfeld performed castration on Elbe before she sought other gender-affirming surgeries elsewhere in Germany.[4] After the institute's destruction, Hirschfeld was forced into exile, and very few additional advancements in TGD health care were made by his group.[2]

The 1940s saw the emergence of pioneering influences in America, particularly Alfred Kinsey, the biologist who founded the Institute for Sex Research at Indiana University in 1947 (now known as the Kinsey Institute).[5] Kinsey was one of the first to use the term "transsexual" in his gender studies, and he helped introduce America to this term that was to reflect a concept of an "intermediate sex."[6] To this day, the Kinsey Institute conducts research on sexual behavior and health and has contributed to the evolution of our understanding of gender and sex.

The first American to undergo a gender-affirming surgery was Christine Jorgensen. She brought significant attention to the transgender revolution in America when her story was featured in The New York Times' headlines in 1952.[7] Jorgensen's willingness to publicly tell her story gave a face to the growing transgender revolution in the United States. However, the lack of high-quality or even safe transgender health care in America at the time led to Jorgensen traveling to Denmark to receive treatment with surgeon Christian Hamburger.[8] Hamburger was an endocrinologist based in

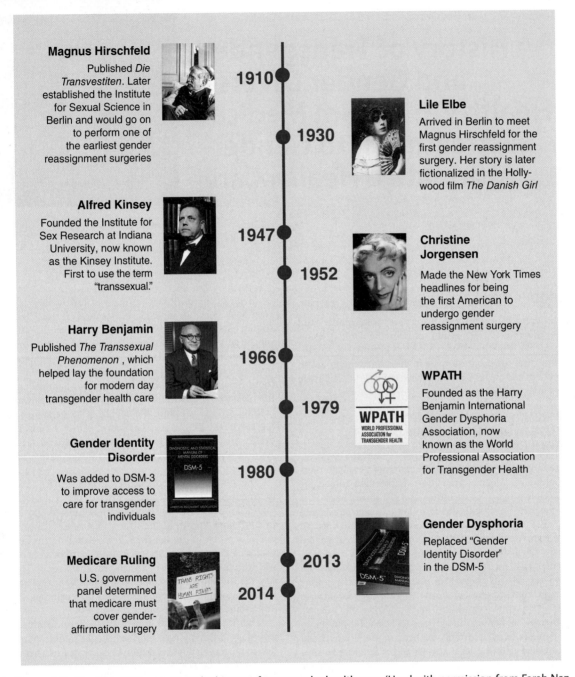

Magnus Hirschfeld

Published *Die Transvestiten*. Later established the Institute for Sexual Science in Berlin and would go on to perform one of the earliest gender reassignment surgeries

1910

1930

Lile Elbe

Arrived in Berlin to meet Magnus Hirschfeld for the first gender reassignment surgery. Her story is later fictionalized in the Hollywood film *The Danish Girl*

Alfred Kinsey

Founded the Institute for Sex Research at Indiana University, now known as the Kinsey Institute. First to use the term "transsexual."

1947

1952

Christine Jorgensen

Made the New York Times headlines for being the first American to undergo gender reassignment surgery

Harry Benjamin

Published *The Transsexual Phenomenon* , which helped lay the foundation for modern day transgender health care

1966

1979

WPATH

Founded as the Harry Benjamin International Gender Dysphoria Association, now known as the World Professional Association for Transgender Health

Gender Identity Disorder

Was added to DSM-3 to improve access to care for transgender individuals

1980

Gender Dysphoria

Replaced "Gender Identity Disorder" in the DSM-5

Medicare Ruling

U.S. government panel determined that medicare must cover gender-affirmation surgery

2013

2014

▲ **Figure 1-1.** Timeline of key events in the history of transgender health care. (Used with permission from Farah Naz Khan)

History and Background

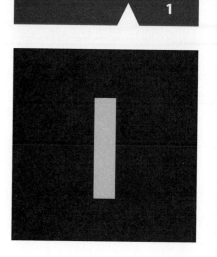

History and
Background

Copenhagen who supported a "wrong body theory" and performed surgery on patients who described having a female "personality" in a male body.[9]

Back in America, a new pioneer of TGD medicine was emerging in endocrinologist Harry Benjamin. Benjamin had been studying gender diversity since at least the 1950s,[10] but his 1966 book, *The Transsexual Phenomenon*, is what has left his most indelible impact on American TGD health care.[11] Benjamin spent time with Hirschfeld at his Berlin institute, so he espoused many of Hirschfeld's principles, namely that those who reported their sex assigned at birth to be discordant with their gender identity deserve treatment in the form of hormonal therapy and affirming surgeries and not psychotherapy for a "cure." Benjamin argued that preventing TGD people from obtaining hormones and surgical treatments was akin to withholding insulin from patients with diabetes.[9] *The Transsexual Phenomenon* laid the foundation for modern TGD health care by highlighting the fact that hormonal and surgical treatments are therapeutic and life-saving for this patient population.

HISTORY OF TREATMENTS IN TRANSGENDER AND GENDER DIVERSE HEALTH CARE

TGD health care should not be viewed as exclusively psychosocial, medical, or surgical, but rather as a combination of one or more of these approaches tailored for each person. For the purposes of this chapter, we will look at the history of each approach separately while acknowledging that the medical and surgical treatments evolved in tandem over time to improve gender-affirming health care.

Hirschfeld's Institute for Sexual Science performed the first known gender-affirming surgeries; it was, however, Jorgensen's successful surgery in Denmark with Hamburger that sparked increased demand for gender-affirming surgical care in the United States. The first surgical center for TGD people in the United States was established in the 1960s at Johns Hopkins University under the guidance of the same physicians and researchers working with intersex children. This clinic eventually closed amid the reactions to a controversial study that suggested there were no psychosocial differences in patients who had undergone surgical procedures for gender affirmation compared to those who went without these procedures.[12] This study has since been discredited, with several experts questioning its methods, and it has been criticized for having damaging effects on transgender health care in America. By the time the Hopkins center closed, several other institutions across America had established gender clinics for TGD patients.[13]

Gender-affirming hormone therapy for TGD people became an option after testosterone, progesterone, and estrogen were discovered in the 1930s.[14] Hamburger published one of the earliest known cases that discussed hormone use as part of gender-affirming therapy.[8] He would later go on to successfully use hormone therapy with Jorgensen as well. In America, the pioneer of gender-affirming hormone therapy was Benjamin, with his book *The Transsexual Phenomenon* outlining the use of hormonal therapy for gender affirmation.[11] The Harry Benjamin International Gender Dysphoria Association was formed in 1979 and is now known as the World Professional Association for Transgender Health (WPATH).[14] WPATH regularly publishes standards of care to help guide the management of care for TGD people across the world, the first of which published in 1979 and the most recent, Standards of Care Version 7, in 2012.[15]

TRANSGENDER AND GENDER DIVERSE HEALTH CARE TODAY

The concepts of **sex assigned at birth** (SAAB), **gender**, **gender identity**, and **sexual orientation** have often been difficult for even medical professionals to fully understand. The approach to transgender care has been heavily influenced by one's ability to understand the nuances and differences between these concepts without conflating them.[16]

With an increasingly streamlined and progressive approach to transgender health care that has developed over the past few decades, the American Psychiatric Association's 1980 addition of the diagnosis of "gender identity disorder" to the third *Diagnostic and Statistical Manual of Mental Disorders* (DSM-3) was dismaying.[17] While this addition may have been intended to help transgender people access care, it remains a controversial topic to this day. However, with time, gender identity was separated from the concept of a "disorder,"[18] and the DSM-5 replaced gender identity disorder with the diagnosis of "**gender dysphoria**" in 2013. Within the DSM-5, gender dysphoria has been moved out of the category of "sexual disorders" and into its own category, with distinctions made between gender dysphoria in adults, children, and otherwise unspecified or specified gender dysphoria.[19]

While this attempted step toward destigmatization does not remove the diagnosis from the DSM-5, it was viewed as a major milestone for transgender health care, and further strides were made in 2014 when it was ruled that Medicare must cover gender-affirming surgeries.[20] This historic event overturned a policy that had been in place since the 1980s and reflects that gender-affirming surgeries were no longer considered "experimental."[21] To further optimize care for TGD people, the Endocrine Society published its first set of clinical practice guidelines for gender-affirming medical care in 2009, and then released an updated set of guidelines in 2017.[22] These guidelines cover diagnosis, treatment, and preventive care needs for TGD people, while also discussing potential benefits and risks associated with gender-affirming therapies.

Despite the progress made over the past several years, there are parallel movements that seek to stifle further progress and potentially reverse much of what has been accomplished to date. Specifically, many antipediatric TGD health care bills have been introduced across the United States in the last year.[23] Given that more anti-TGD bills may be enacted, we will also see the growing importance of TGD activist groups in shaping the future of TGD health care. Going forward, it will be important for clinicians to understand the historical context of transgender health care. A proper understanding of this historical evolution can help clinicians better understand the stigmas faced by the TGD communities they serve.

SUMMARY

- Transgender health care has evolved from mismanagement and discriminatory practices to incrementally more standardized and progressive treatment regimens over the years.
- The field of TGD health care has evolved dramatically over the past century, as have the policies and laws that once restricted health care for TGD people.
- Current clinical practice guidelines strive to optimize care for TGD people while also touching on potential risks of treatment.
- Ongoing vigilance is needed to prevent implementation of recidivist policies that seek to limit universal access to gender-affirming care.

CASE STUDY

An 18-year-old trans woman **assigned male sex at birth (AMAB)** from South Dakota has been referred to you for advice regarding possible medical gender affirmation. This patient has questions about the evolution of transgender medicine and wonders how future changes might impact them.

▶ Discussion Questions

1. What particular aspects about the history of transgender health care may be of particular importance to this patient?
2. How might evolving standards in transgender health care affect this patient's future?

REFERENCES

1. Bullough VL. Magnus Hirschfeld, an often overlooked pioneer. *Sex Cult.* 2003;7(1):62-72.
2. Rimmele H. Society. http://www.hirschfeld.in-berlin.de/institut/en/theorie/theo_22.html.
3. May 6, 1933 80. Jahrestag der Zerschlagung des Instituts für Sexualwissenschaft. 80. Jahrestag der Zerschlagung des Instituts für Sexualwissenschaft. http://80jahre.mh-stiftung.de/.
4. Cox D. The Danish Girl and the sexologist: a story of sexual pioneers | Science | The Guardian. https://www.theguardian.com/science/blog/2016/jan/13/magnus-hirschfeld-groundbreaking-sexologist-the-danish-girl-lili-elbe.
5. Dr. Alfred C. Kinsey. https://kinseyinstitute.org/about/history/alfred-kinsey.php.
6. Ekins R, King D. Pioneers of transgendering: the popular sexology of David O. Cauldwell. Updated 2001. http://www.symposion.com/ijt/cauldwell/cauldwell_01.htm.
7. BRONX "BOY" IS NOW A GIRL; Danish treatments change sex of former army clerk. *The New York Times*; December 2, 1952. https://www.nytimes.com/1952/12/02/archives/bronx-boy-is-now-a-girl-danish-treatments-change-sex-of-former-army.html.
8. Hamburger C, Stürup GK, Dahl-Iversen E. Transvestism: hormonal, psychiatric, and surgical treatment. *JAMA.* 1953;152(5).
9. MacKenzie GO. *Transgender Nation.* Bowling Green State University Popular Press; 1994.
10. Benjamin H. Transsexualism and transvestism as psychosomatic and somatopsychic syndromes. *Am J Psychother.* 1954;8(2):219-230.
11. Benjamin H. The transsexual phenomenon. *Trans N Y Acad Sci.* 1967;29(4):428-430.
12. Meyer JK, Reter DJ. Sex reassignment: follow-up. *Arch Gen Psychiatry.* 1979;36(9):1010-1015.
13. Beemyn G. Transgender history in the United States. In: *Trans Bodies, Trans Selves*; 2011.
14. Shumer DE, Nokoff NJ, Spack NP. Advances in the care of transgender children and adolescents. *Adv Pediatr.* 2016;63(1):79-102.
15. Coleman E, Bockting W, Botzer M, et al. Standards of care for the health of transsexual, transgender, and gender-nonconforming people, Version 7. *Int J Transgenderism.* 2012; 13(4):165-232.
16. Beek TF, Cohen-Kettenis PT, Kreukels BPC. Gender incongruence/gender dysphoria and its classification history. *Int Rev Psychiatry Abingdon Engl.* 2016;28(1):5-12.
17. Glicksman E. Transgender today. https://www.apa.org. https://www.apa.org/monitor/2013/04/transgender.
18. Lev A. Disordering gender identity: Gender identity disorder in the DSM-IV-TR. *J Psychol Hum Sex.* 2006;17(3-4):35-69.
19. *Diagnostic and Statistical Manual of Mental Disorders* (DSM–5). Updated 2013. https://www.psychiatry.org/psychiatrists/practice/dsm.
20. Pierson B. UnitedHealth Medicare plan must cover U.S. sex reassignment surgery. *Reuters*; January 29, 2016. https://www.reuters.com/article/us-unitedhealth-grp-medicare-transgender-idUSKCN0V72R5.
21. Know your rights: Medicare. National Center for Transgender Equality. https://transequality.org/know-your-rights/medicare.
22. Hembree WC, Cohen-Kettenis PT, Gooren L, et al. Gender Dysphoria/Gender Incongruence Guideline Resources | Endocrine Society. https://www.endocrine.org/clinical-practice-guidelines/gender-dysphoria-gender-incongruence.
23. Murib Z. A new kind of anti-trans legislation is hitting the red states. *Washington Post*; February 25, 2020. https://www.washingtonpost.com/politics/2020/02/25/new-kind-anti-trans-legislation-is-hitting-red-states/.

Gender Identity: Terminology, Demographics, and Epidemiology

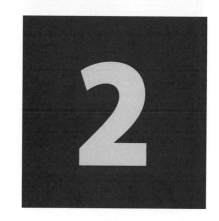

Sari L. Reisner

Alex S. Keuroghlian

Jennifer Potter

INTRODUCTION

This chapter introduces the most current terminology used to describe **sex**, **gender**, and **sexual orientation**; reviews key demographic and epidemiologic metrics of **transgender and gender diverse** (TGD) populations; describes some of the social and health inequities faced by these populations; and explores the critical need for **gender-affirming** health care for all patients. Depending on their level of experience in providing care for the TGD community, some readers may be unfamiliar with these basic concepts, while others may have some preexisting knowledge. Many of the definitions, concepts, and models introduced in this chapter are discussed in greater detail in subsequent chapters of the textbook, as are the practical aspects of delivering health care for these populations. References to the appropriate chapters are given where feasible.

TERMINOLOGY

Terminology is constantly changing. Terms that were acceptable 20 years ago (e.g., "transsexual") are considered offensive and are now no longer used. Likewise, what is acceptable terminology today will also continue to evolve and may one day become outdated. A simple way to avoid **misgendering** a patient (i.e., referring to a person by a pronoun or other gendered term, such as *Ms./Mr.*, that incorrectly indicates a person's gender identity or that is personally inappropriate or offensive) is for health care professionals to ask each patient specifically how they self-identify and what their pronouns are. Asking these questions is a basic first step in providing gender-affirming care.

Health care professionals should also familiarize themselves with the concepts of sex and gender which are core determinants of health and wellbeing. In addition to the biological differences of sex, which can have a profound impact on specific disease risks, pharmacological effects, and

screening recommendations for cancer and other illnesses, social and economic aspects of gender play important roles in access to quality health care, including mental health treatment and preventive services, that can lead to different health outcomes based on gender. To provide the best care for all patients, clinicians must recognize the ways in which both sex and gender influence health care access and outcomes and work to equalize inequities so that all patients receive respectful and responsive care.

▶ Sex

Although the terms "sex" and "gender" are often used interchangeably, these terms have distinct definitions. Sex refers to a person's physical characteristics—the anatomical, genetic, and biological traits that have traditionally been categorized as either female or male. The term **sex assigned at birth** specifies sex as defined by anatomical and other biological sex characteristics and designated at birth (Table 2-1). It is important to note that, contrary to traditional expectations, sex is not a binary variable—that is, many people are born with variations in sex development that are beyond traditional societal notions of binary female or male bodies. Acceptable terms used to describe these variations include **intersex** and **differences of sex development**.

▶ Gender

Gender encompasses the characteristics and roles of individuals according to social and cultural norms. Gender is multidimensional, with aspects that are psychological, social, and behavioral. A person's **gender identity** reflects their inner sense of themselves as girl/woman/feminine, boy/man/masculine, combinations of or beyond girl/woman/feminine or boy/man/masculine (such as having a **nonbinary** gender identity), or having no gender. An important concept associated with gender identity is

gender expression, the outward manifestation of how a person expresses their gender, for example, through behaviors, mannerisms, voice, gait, and clothing, which may be interpreted differently depending on culture, context, and historical period.

The term **transgender** describes a person whose gender identity and sex assigned at birth do not correspond based on traditional societal expectations. For example, a transgender man is a person assigned a female sex at birth who identifies as a man; a transgender woman is a person assigned a male sex at birth who identifies as a woman. In contrast, the term **cisgender** (from the Latin prefix *cis*, meaning "on the same side of") describes a person whose gender identity is consistent in a traditional sense with their sex assigned at birth, for example, a person assigned a female sex at birth whose gender identity is woman/female.

"Transgender" also includes those who are nonbinary, that is, people with gender identities that are a combination of or beyond the girl/woman and boy/man **binary** paradigm. For example, people assigned a male sex at birth and who identify with femininity to a greater extent than with masculinity may be described as **trans feminine.** People who were assigned a female sex at birth and who identify with masculinity to a greater extent than with femininity may be described as **trans masculine.** In addition, there is a diversity of nonbinary identities that describe people whose gender identities or expressions expand beyond traditional or expected gender notions. General terms used to comprehensively describe this constellation of gender identities include gender diverse (which is the term used in this textbook) or **gender expansive**. Gender diverse people may have more than one gender (**pangender**), some combination of genders (**genderqueer, genderfluid**), or no gender (**agender**).

Gender also has cultural connotations. Some cultures recognize unique gender identities with deep historical, social, and sometimes religious or spiritual roots. In the Indian subcontinent, for example, *hijra* is a specific gender identity that is neither completely female nor male. In Latin America, *travesti* are people assigned a male sex at birth but whose gender identity is expressed as feminine. Among Indigenous people in North America, Two-Spirit describes a person with both a feminine and masculine spirit who has a traditional ceremonial and social role in the culture. These cultural expressions of gender reflect the diversity within and across TGD communities worldwide and speak to the fact that there is no one way to be "transgender." Health care professionals should approach their TGD patients with the same sensitivity to and respect for cultural influences and underpinnings as they do with their cisgender patients and should recognize the multidimensional aspects of what TGD lived experience may mean to each person they serve and care for.

Table 2-1. Gender Identity Terminology

Term	Definition
Sex	A person's physical characteristics based on anatomical, genetic, and biological factors that are traditionally classified as female, male, or intersex.
Gender	A term that encompasses the multidimensional characteristics and roles of individuals, inclusive of but not limited to women and men, according to social and cultural norms in social, psychological, and behavioral domains.
Gender identity	A person's inner sense of themselves as girl/woman/feminine, boy/man/masculine, beyond girl/woman/feminine or boy/man/masculine (such as having a nonbinary gender identity), or having no gender.
Gender expression	The outward manifestation of how a person expresses their gender, for example, through behaviors, mannerisms, voice, gait, and clothing, which may be interpreted differently depending on culture, context, and historical period.
Cisgender man	A person assigned a male sex at birth who identifies as a man.
Cisgender woman	A person assigned a female sex at birth who identifies as a woman.
Transgender man	A person assigned a female sex at birth who identifies as a man.
Transgender woman	A person assigned a male sex at birth who identifies as a woman.
Nonbinary	Describes a person whose gender identity is a combination of or beyond traditional girl/woman/feminine and boy/man/masculine binary identities.
Trans masculine person	A person assigned a female sex at birth who identifies with masculinity to a greater extent than with femininity.
Trans feminine person	A person assigned a male sex at birth who identifies with femininity to a greater extent than with masculinity.
Genderfluid	Describes a person whose gender identity is not fixed. A person who is genderfluid may always feel like a mix of more than one gender, or may feel more aligned with a certain gender some of the time, another gender at other times, multiple genders sometimes, and sometimes no gender at all.
Genderqueer	An umbrella term that describes a person whose gender identity is beyond the traditional gender binary of girl/woman/feminine or boy/man/masculine.
Agender	Describes a person who identifies as having no gender, or who does not experience gender as a primary identity component.

▶ Sexual Orientation

Sexual orientation refers to how a person identifies in terms of their physical, emotional, and romantic attachments to other people. Sexual orientation should not be referred to as a "preference." Some terms for sexual orientation include straight, gay (an adjective, as in "gay man"), and lesbian (or gay woman) to refer to people who are primarily emotionally and physically attracted to people of the same gender as themselves; bisexual (not "bi") to describe people who are emotionally and physically attracted to more than one gender; and asexual to describe people who have little to no sexual attraction to others; asexual people may still engage in sexual activity. Pansexual is an expansive term that describes people who are emotionally and physically attracted to people of all genders, or whose attractions are not based on other people's genders. The term "homosexual" in English is mostly considered an offensive term with pejorative connotations and should be avoided.[1] "Heterosexual" is considered an acceptable term, although some people prefer the word "straight."

Like cisgender people, TGD people have diverse sexual orientations that include, but are not limited to, being gay, lesbian, bisexual, pansexual, or asexual. The term "queer" is used to describe people who think of their sexual orientation as outside of societal norms and often with greater inclusivity than traditional categories for sexual orientation. While queer was historically used in a derogatory manner as a slur, it has been reclaimed by many to embrace fluidity in sexual and romantic attraction that is not exclusively directed toward the same or other genders and that may change over time as a person explores their gender identity.[2] In a study of TGD adults in Massachusetts, more than 40% of respondents described their sexual orientation as "queer," 19% as "other nonbinary," and 16% as bisexual.[2] This study demonstrates the diversity in sexual and romantic attractions experienced by TGD people and the complex relationship between a person's gender identity and sexual orientation.

SEXUAL AND GENDER MINORITIES

The term **sexual and gender minorities** (SGM) was introduced in 2011 by the Institute of Medicine in its report "The Health of Lesbian, Gay, Bisexual, and Transgender People: Building a Foundation for Better Understanding." This report was commissioned by the National Institutes of Health (NIH) to review the existing research about the health needs of these populations and identify priority research areas for future study. In 2016, the National Institutes of Health (NIH) designated SGM populations, including transgender and nonbinary people, as a health disparity population for NIH research purposes. In making this designation, the NIH acknowledged that despite having unique health care challenges, SGM populations often have less access to health care services and bear higher burden of specific diseases and conditions, including HIV infection, suicidality and depression, and cancer (see Chapter 3, "Health Disparities").[3,4] While "SGM" is a convenient term to use when describing SGM populations for research and academic purposes, it is important to note that members of these communities do not typically refer to themselves as sexual and gender minorities.

GENDER AFFIRMATION

The term **gender affirmation** refers to the process of making social, legal, or medical changes to recognize, accept, and express one's gender identity. People pursue various means of affirming their gender to reduce **gender dysphoria**, the emotional distress experienced when there is a misalignment of one's physical body and perceived gender with the inner sense of self. Social changes can include changing one's pronouns, name, clothing, and hairstyle. Legal changes may entail changing one's name, sex designation, and gender markers on legal documents. Medical changes can include receiving gender-affirming hormonal therapy and surgeries. Although this process has sometimes been referred to as *transition*, the term *gender affirmation* is recommended. Gender affirmation is covered in detail in Chapter 7, "Gender-Affirming Hormone Therapy for Adults"; Chapter 8, "Nonmedical, Nonsurgical Gender Affirmation"; and Chapter 9, "Surgical Gender Affirmation."

People affirm their gender in different ways. Affirming one's gender identity is a highly individualized process, and there is no one particular path or timeline that all TGD people take toward affirmation. Some people do not make any of these changes, while others may choose some or all options. For example, a person may choose to affirm their gender only socially or legally but not be interested in medical affirmation. Another person may view medical affirmation as an integral part of their gender affirmation. It is important for health care professionals to avoid assumptions about how, when, and why a person accesses any particular type of affirmation or not.

Recent research exploring the mental health outcomes for people who pursue hormonal gender affirmation shows improvements in psychological functioning and quality of life.[5,6] A study evaluating the associations between gender-affirming surgical procedures and mental health outcomes found that participants who underwent one or more gender-affirming surgical procedure(s) reported lower past-month psychological distress, lower rates of smoking, and reduced suicidal ideation.[7] These results demonstrate the mental health benefits of gender affirmation and expand the existing evidence-base supporting gender-affirming medical and surgical care.

Pronouns are one way that a TGD person may socially affirm their gender. Stating one's pronouns has become more common; for example, many people state their pronouns at the end of email signatures or on name tags at professional meetings. Examples of pronouns are she/her/hers, he/him/his, and they/them/theirs. The English language has not always had a singular gender-inclusive pronoun; instead, the traditionally plural pronouns they/them/theirs are increasingly being used as non–gender-specific singular pronouns. Other gender-inclusive pronouns, sometimes called **neopronouns**, include zie/zim/zis, sie/sie/hir, and many others. Neopronouns are sets of pronouns created outside the officially recognized language that are intended to be gender-inclusive. Some neopronoun sets have been developed by activists, authors, and others to express additional aspects of gender not implied in traditional pronoun forms. For example, the Spivak pronouns were created by Michel Spivak in 1990 for use in Internet chat rooms; the fae pronouns are pagan-themed and are used by people who wish to express this particular dimension of their gender identity (Table 2-2).[8]

To avoid making mistakes in pronoun usage, health care professionals are encouraged to ask their patients about their personal pronouns. The appropriate phrasing is "What are your pronouns?" (not "What are your preferred pronouns?") when seeking this information.

INITIALISMS AND ACRONYMS

The initialism "LGBT" originated in the 1990s to refer to the community of people with nonheterosexual orientations and those who are not cisgender or who are transgender or gender diverse. LGBT stands for the following groups of people:

L-Lesbian

G- Gay

B-Bisexual

T-Transgender

In recent years, the LGBT initialism has been expanded to include additional groups. Common expansions are LGBTQ and LGBTQIA+, which include the following groups:

Q-Queer or questioning

I-Intersex (people who have variations in sex development beyond traditional notions of female and male bodies)

A-Asexual

+-Any and all sexual and gender minorities

Some newspapers and style guides specify the use of LGBT as the only acceptable initialism for this diverse community. This textbook uses the more inclusive initialism LGBTQIA+.

EPIDEMIOLOGY

As noted in Chapter 3, "Health Disparities," historical efforts to estimate the size of the TGD populations have been imperfect. Two methods by which estimates have been generated

Table 2-2. Pronouns

When used as the subject of a sentence (___ has the book.)	When used as an object in a sentence (Give the book to ___).	Possessive adjective (___ favorite book is unknown.)	Possessive pronoun (The book is ___).	Reflexive (<Subject pronoun> bought ___ a new book.)
He	Him	His	His	Himself
She	Her	Her	Hers	Herself
They	Them	Their	Theirs	themselves
Zie	Zim	Zir	Zis	Zieself
Sie	Sie	Hir	Hirs	Hirself

Data from University of Wisconsin-Milwaukee. Gender Pronouns. https://uwm.edu/lgbtrc/support/gender-pronouns/. Accessed May 23, 2021.

are through data collected from various surveys, which typically rely on self-report, and from research studies that used administrative or clinical data with various algorithms (e.g., surgical procedures, gender dysphoria codes) to serve as a proxy for gender identity. Population estimates of the number of adults (age 18 years or older) in the United States who identify as transgender or gender-nonconforming range from 0.58% to 0.87%,[9,10] with estimates higher in adolescents (1.8%). The 2015 U.S. Transgender Survey, which enrolled the largest sample of TGD populations in the United States (>27,000) to date, shows that about one-third (35%) of respondents identify as nonbinary. The youngest age group surveyed (18–24 years) comprises the highest proportion of those identifying as nonbinary; 61% of people in this group identify as nonbinary, while 35% of people in the 25–44 age group, 4% in the 45–64 age group, and 1% in the 65+ age group identify as nonbinary.[11] These data have implications for future health care; as TGD populations age, health care systems will need to adapt to the growing number of aging patients who also identify as TGD.

TGD people in the United States represent a diverse group of races and ethnicities. In 2014, The Centers for Disease Control and Prevention's Behavioral Risk Factor Surveillance System, a national survey that tracks and monitors the health of the U.S. population, released data from an optional module that states could add to their survey instruments regarding transgender adults in the United States. Although not all states participated in collecting this information, the data gathered give a clearer picture of the heterogeneity of U.S. transgender populations. In general, the population of adults who identify as transgender are more racially and ethnically diverse than the U.S. population as a whole[10]; overall, they are less likely to be non-Hispanic White compared with cisgender adults (Table 2-3).

Additional characteristics that emerged from the Behavioral Risk Factor Surveillance System survey show that, in general, TGD populations are subject to comparatively high levels of social and economic stressors leading to disenfranchisement and marginalization than their cisgender peers. For example, more TGD people than cisgender people are unemployed and uninsured, and they report lower incomes than cisgender adults. Social inequities, including homelessness, poverty, and incarceration, are also found at higher rates in TGD relative to cisgender respondents.[12] TGD people are less likely to have never been married and to have a minor child living in their household, and they are less likely to speak English. More TGD adults than cisgender respondents report having a medical need that has not been met due to the high cost of medical care in the last 12 months, as well as some type of cognitive or physical impairment.[13] This information highlights a key take-home message about the makeup of TGD populations: being a TGD person has intersections with other social identities, and the economic position of TGD people impacts their lived experiences and their health status across the life course.

HEALTH DEMOGRAPHICS AND OUTCOMES

A health disparity can be defined as a particular type of health difference that is closely linked to social, economic, or environmental disadvantage. Health disparities adversely affect groups of people who have systematically experienced greater obstacles to health based on race, ethnicity, religion, socioeconomic status, gender, age, and other characteristics historically linked to discrimination or exclusion.[14] Health disparities are remediable because they exist based on the conditions of societal structures. For TGD people, being a marginalized group confers additional stressors at the individual, interpersonal, and structural levels—stressors shared by other marginalized groups and TGD-specific stressors—and those stressors in turn produce and ultimately sustain the health disparities seen at the population level (see Figure 2-1). The **minority stress model** of health inequities, first introduced in 2003 in relation to sexual minorities, has been further elaborated by Hendricks and Testa in 2012 into a clinical framework that explores the unique experiences of TGD populations and incorporates the adverse events experienced by many TGD people related to their gender identities and expressions.[15] The minority stress model is discussed in more detail in Chapter 3, "Health Disparities," and referred to often throughout the textbook as an important basis for gender-affirming care.

Table 2-3. Percentage Estimates by Race and Ethnicity for the General U.S. Population and Adults Who Identify as Transgender[10]

	Adult General Population	Transgender-Identified Adults
	%	%
White, non-Hispanic	66	55
African-American or Black, non-Hispanic	12	16
Hispanic or Latino	15	21
Other Race or Ethnicity, non-Hispanic	8	8

Data from the Behavioral Risk Factor Surveillance System and the U.S. Transgender Survey give a general picture of the health inequities faced by TGD populations. Across all domains, these surveys reveal that TGD people commonly experience poor physical and mental health, poor health status, and lack of access to culturally responsive and gender-affirming care. In addition to poor self-rated general health, which is a high predictor of early mortality in any population, TGD respondents report high rates of HIV infection and other sexually transmitted infections and a variety of mental health challenges, such as depression, eating disorders, anxiety, suicidality, substance use disorders, and violence victimization. TGD participants also report delays in preventive care and lack of access to recommended preventive screening tests.

Several research studies have explored specific physical and mental health disparities affecting TGD populations using the Behavioral Risk Factor Surveillance System and other data sources to understand the interconnectedness of health disparities, social and economic stressors, and being transgender. Recent studies include comparisons of mental health disparities, such as depression, anxiety, and suicidal ideation and self-harm, affecting TGD and cisgender youth[16]; suicidality in gender minority versus cisgender Medicaid beneficiaries[17]; and self-reports of more frequent mentally and physically unhealthy days, poorer self-rated general health, and greater comorbid problems and impairments for sexual minority TGD adults vs. heterosexual TGD adults.[18] All of these studies point to elevated health risks and poorer health outcomes for TGD people; in some cases, the likelihood that a transgender person will have a poorer outcome is two, three, and sometimes four times higher than

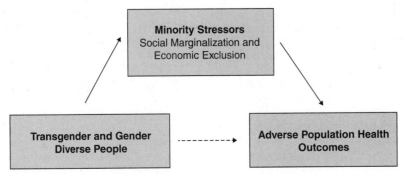

▲ Figure 2-1. Transgender and gender diverse population health disparities: gender minority stress pathways to poor health.

for a cisgender person. For instance, suicidal ideation is three times as likely in transgender youth versus cisgender youth, and attempting suicide twice as likely.[16]

HIV infection is one of the most burdensome health issues affecting TGD people, especially among Black and African American transgender women. Globally, the pooled prevalence of HIV infection in transgender women is extremely high—about one in five transgender women (19%) are living with HIV worldwide.[19] In the United States, about one-half (44–51%) of all transgender people with HIV are Black or African American.[20] These statistics demonstrate that a person's gender minority status is only one factor that places them at increased risk for HIV; other factors, such as race and gender identity, have a profound influence as well. Within transgender populations, Black and African American transgender women are disproportionately affected. More research is needed to understand the complexity of health disparities facing TGD populations as a whole and explore the differential risks that lead to the health disparities seen in these subgroups, including in gay, bisexual, queer, and other transgender men who have sex with men who are a subgroup at elevated risk of HIV exposure.

Bullying and victimization are also very common experiences for TGD communities. In a recent probability sample of the U.S. transgender population, almost one-half (46.2%) of transgender respondents report being bullied "often" before age 18 years compared with 14% of cisgender straight respondents.[21] Discrimination due to gender identity is common; 83% of TGD adults report discrimination that they attribute to gender identity, which is but one of approximately 14 additional reasons (e.g., sexual orientation, appearance as masculine or feminine, sex, age, and other appearance-related factors) that TGD adults cite as motivators of discriminatory treatment they incur.[22] A Massachusetts study reveals that transgender people experience unique forms of intimate partner violence (IPV) related to being transgender, for example, being forced to conform to an undesired gender presentation or stop gender-affirming practices and treatments, or being pressured to remain in an undesired relationship through coercion or threats of being "outed."[23] Almost 40% of TGD respondents said they have experienced this type of IPV, and 10% reported that they had experienced IPV in the past year. Mental health effects of IPV include posttraumatic stress disorder, depression, and psychological distress.[23,24]

Discrimination within the health care system toward TGD people—defined as mistreatment on the basis of gender identity or expression—is also common. Health care coverage for TGD-related care is often denied; 25% of respondents to the U.S. Transgender Survey report being denied insurance for gender-affirming hormone therapy, and more than half report insurance denial for gender-affirming surgery. About one-third of respondents said they had experienced verbal harassment or were refused treatment by a health care provider; in addition, respondents reported having to educate their health care providers about appropriate gender-affirming care.[11] The more visually nonconforming a TGD person's expression is, the more likely they are to experience discrimination: 22% of those with low visual nonconformity versus 44% of those with high visual nonconformity reported discrimination within the previous 12 months.[25] As a result of this discrimination, nearly one-quarter (23%) did not access health care services because of their fear of being mistreated: they postponed care when sick or injured or put off receiving routine preventive care.[11]

The toll that so-called "everyday" discrimination, as well as discrimination related to health care, can take on TGD people in the form of PTSD symptoms has been studied in relation to other potential contributors, including childhood sexual abuse, IPV, depression, use of two or more illicit drugs, unstable housing, and high visual nonconformity. Using a linear regression model, researchers found that everyday discrimination, combined with a higher number of reasons a person endorses for their discrimination experiences, was independently associated with PTSD symptoms, even after adjusting for prior trauma experiences and other covariates and confounders. The magnitude of the effect that these two combined factors have in their association with PTSD is very close to that of childhood sexual abuse ($\beta=0.25$ vs. 0.029, respectively). This study demonstrates the profound impact that discrimination can have on TGD people; when controlling for all other factors, discrimination by itself is a significant driver of PTSD symptoms.[22]

RESPONSIVE HEALTH CARE

This overview of appropriate terminology and brief snapshot of the health demographics and health outcomes of TGD communities summarize the many challenges facing TGD people, and the impact these challenges have on their health and wellbeing. Health care professionals need to become aware of these challenges and approach all of their patients with a heightened awareness of and sensitivity to the negative experiences that may have preceded their patients' encounters with the health care system. Clinicians must acknowledge that past experiences shape current experiences as they interact patients and think holistically about patients' lived experiences within the medical care setting.

The sensitive and respectful use of language is necessary for all patients and should include asking each patient their names and pronouns. It is important for health care professionals not to make assumptions about a person's gender identity or expression; asking respectful questions of all patients is a way to avoid making mistakes. Similarly, clinicians should not assume that all TGD people want to medically or surgically affirm their gender identity or prescribe pathways to gender affirmation that a person may or may not wish to have. Clinicians should recognize that a person's desire for gender affirmation in general or for a specific type of gender affirmation may likely change over time. Meeting patients "where they are" at the time of each health care visit is essential, along with acknowledging that no one path exists for everyone.

Another important aspect for clinicians to grasp is that a person's sexual orientation cannot be assumed based solely on gender identity. For example, a trans masculine person may have sex with both cisgender and transgender men, which can have implications for the types of health screening tests recommended for this person. Clinicians also should be aware of the stigma surrounding sexual orientation and gender identity and recognize that these constructs, while distinct, are often interrelated.

For all patients, assessment of social stressors is vital. Research confirms that in addition to vulnerabilities due to stigma, TGD populations experience economic marginalization and disenfranchisement due to a lower socioeconomic status, including homelessness, unemployment, and lack of health insurance. And because TGD people tend to be ethnically and racially diverse, racism and discrimination based on race and ethnicity may also be intersecting social stressors, all of which can impact a person's health and wellbeing.

In caring for TGD populations, health care professionals may find it useful to gain context and knowledge that is grounded in the lived experiences of TGD people. Clinicians and health care systems can work with other TGD people to inform care at all levels, from the individual clinician all the way to the institutional level. Whether through community advisory boards or other creative forms of meaningful community engagement, these interactions will help ensure that health care is patient-centered and gender-affirming. It will also help build trust with all patients, especially TGD communities who have not felt seen or heard in health care settings.

SUMMARY

- Clinicians should familiarize themselves with the most current terminology used to describe sex, gender, and sexual orientation.

- Clinicians must recognize the ways in which sex and gender influence health care access and outcomes and work to address health inequities so that all patients receive respectful and responsive care.

- Gender identity and sexual orientation are separate yet related constructs. A person's sexual orientation cannot be assumed from their gender identity.

- Gender may have cultural connotations. Some cultures recognize unique gender identities with deep historical, social, and sometimes religious or spiritual roots.

- TGD people in the United States have diverse races and ethnicities; in general, transgender people are more racially and ethnically diverse than the U.S. population as a whole and are less likely to be non-Hispanic White compared with cisgender adults.

- According to the U.S. Transgender Survey, one-third of transgender adults identify as nonbinary, with the highest proportion of nonbinary people in the 18–24 age group.

- Some, but not all, TGD people pursue social, medical, or surgical gender affirmation to express their gender identity, reduce gender dysphoria, and increase gender euphoria. There is no single pathway to affirm one's gender identity or a specific order in which gender affirmation should be pursued.

- TGD populations are subject to comparatively high levels of social and economic stressors leading to disenfranchisement and marginalization compared to their cisgender peers. As a result, TGD people face a number of health disparities that arise from various obstacles and stressors linked to discrimination or exclusion.

- Clinicians should acknowledge that past experiences shape current experiences as they interact with patients. Work with TGD communities to gain meaningful context around these lived experiences will help foster understanding and drive change in health care systems.

CASE STUDY: SAM

Sam Robinson is a 22-year-old person who was assigned a female sex at birth, whose pronouns are he/him/his, and who identifies as nonbinary. After thinking about it for a number of months, Sam recently made an appointment to see a gynecologist to see if there is a way to stop having monthly bleeding, which he finds highly distressing. Arriving at the gynecologist's office, Sam notices several people sitting in the waiting room, all of whom appear to be pregnant. The décor of the waiting room is pastel with prints of large flowers on the wall; the magazines in a wall rack include *Allure*, *Cosmopolitan*, and *Vanity Fair*. As he checks in, the staff member behind the desk says, "Good morning honey, how can I help you today?" After Sam hands over his insurance card and provides his copay, the staff person goes on to say, "So nice to meet you Ms. Robinson. Please take a seat and complete this intake form. The medical assistant will bring you back to meet with Dr. Porter shortly." Sam finds a seat and begins to complete the intake form, which includes questions such as, "Do you consider yourself: Straight? Gay/lesbian? Bisexual? Other?" "When was your last menstrual period?" "Are you pregnant?" "Do you have any of the following problems: Breast pain? Vaginal discharge?" Sam hesitates when he gets to the sexual orientation question because he identifies as asexual, and finally decides to leave it blank. After looking at the rest of the questions, he also leaves them blank because the idea of periods, pregnancy, breasts, and vaginas makes him feel uncomfortable. After a 10-minute wait, a medical assistant calls out "Samantha, Dr. Porter is ready to see you now." When Sam doesn't immediately respond, the medical assistant calls out again, "Samantha, we're ready for you now. Is Samantha here?" The receptionist points to Sam and says, "She's sitting right over there." As Sam gets up to go with the medical assistant, he notices several of the other patients in the waiting room looking at him curiously.

▶ Discussion Questions

1. Identify all of the ways in which Sam's experience at the gynecology office was not gender-affirming.
2. What could the office have done differently to create an environment that is welcoming to people of all genders?

REFERENCES

1. GLAAD. GLAAD Media Reference Guide. 10th ed. 2016. https://www.glaad.org/reference. Accessed May 30, 2021.
2. Katz-Wise SL, Reisner SL, Hughto JW, Keo-Meier CL. Differences in sexual orientation diversity and sexual fluidity in attractions among gender minority adults in Massachusetts. *J Sex Res*. 2016;53(1):74-84.
3. Institute of Medicine. The Health of Lesbian, Gay, Bisexual, and Transgender People: Building a Foundation for Better Understanding. Washington, DC; 2011.
4. National Institutes of Health. Sexual and Gender Minorities Formally Designated as a Health Disparity Population for Research Purposes. 2016. https://www.nimhd.nih.gov/about/directors-corner/messages/message_10-06-16.html. Accessed May 16, 2021.
5. White Hughto JM, Reisner SL. A systematic review of the effects of hormone therapy on psychological functioning and quality of life in transgender individuals. *Transgend Health*. 2016;1(1):21-31.
6. Murad MH, Elamin MB, Garcia MZ, et al. Hormonal therapy and sex reassignment: a systematic review and meta-analysis of quality of life and psychosocial outcomes. *Clin Endocrinol (Oxf)*. 2010;72(2):214-231.
7. Almazan AN, Keuroghlian AS. Association between gender-affirming surgeries and mental health outcomes. *JAMA Surg*. 2021.
8. LGBTA Wiki. Neopronouns. 2020. https://lgbta.wikia.org/wiki/Neopronouns. Accessed May 30, 2021.
9. Collin L, Reisner SL, Tangpricha V, Goodman M. Prevalence of transgender depends on the "case" definition: a systematic review. *J Sex Med*. 2016;13(4):613-626.
10. Flores AR. How many adults identify as transgender in the United States? 2016. https://williamsinstitute.law.ucla.edu/publications/trans-adults-united-states/. Accessed November 15, 2020.
11. James SE, Herman JL, Rankin S, Keisling M, Mottet L, Anafi M. The Report of the 2015 U.S. Transgender Survey. Washington, DC: National Center for Transgender Equality; 2016.
12. Meyer IH, Brown TN, Herman JL, Reisner SL, Bockting WO. Demographic characteristics and health status of transgender adults in select US regions: behavioral risk factor surveillance system, 2014. *Am J Public Health*. 2017;107(4):582-589.
13. Streed CGJr., McCarthy EP, Haas JS. Association between gender minority status and self-reported physical and mental health in the United States. *JAMA Intern Med*. 2017;177(8):1210-1212.
14. Braveman PA, Kumanyika S, Fielding J, et al. Health disparities and health equity: the issue is justice. *Am J Public Health*. 2011;101(Suppl 1):S149-S155.
15. Hendricks M, Testa R. A conceptual framework for clinical work with transgender and gender nonconforming clients: an adaptation of the Minority Stress Model. *Prof Psychol Res Practice*. 2012;43(5):460-467.
16. Reisner SL, Vetters R, Leclerc M, et al. Mental health of transgender youth in care at an adolescent urban community health center: a matched retrospective cohort study. *J Adolesc Health*. 2015;56(3):274-279.
17. Progovac AM, Mullin BO, Dunham E, et al. Disparities in suicidality by gender identity among Medicare beneficiaries. *Am J Prev Med*. 2020;58(6):789-798.

18. Cicero EC, Reisner SL, Merwin EI, Humphreys JC, Silva SG. The health status of transgender and gender nonbinary adults in the United States. *PLoS One*. 2020;15(2):e0228765.

19. Baral SD, Poteat T, Strömdahl S, Wirtz AL, Guadamuz TE, Beyrer C. Worldwide burden of HIV in transgender women: a systematic review and meta-analysis. *Lancet Infect Dis*. 2013;13(3):214-222.

20. Clark H, Babu AS, Wiewel EW, Opoku J, Crepaz N. Diagnosed HIV infection in transgender adults and adolescents: results from the National HIV Surveillance System, 2009-2014. *AIDS Behav*. 2017;21(9):2774-2783.

21. Meyer IH, Reisner S, Herman J, Feldman J, Poteat T, Bockting W. National Study of the US Trans Population USPATH. Washington, DC; 2019.

22. Reisner SL, White Hughto JM, Gamarel KE, Keuroghlian AS, Mizock L, Pachankis JE. Discriminatory experiences associated with posttraumatic stress disorder symptoms among transgender adults. *J Couns Psychol*. 2016;63(5):509-519.

23. Peitzmeier SM, Hughto JMW, Potter J, Deutsch MB, Reisner SL. Development of a novel tool to assess intimate partner violence against transgender individuals. *J Interpers Violence*. 2019;34(11):2376-2397.

24. Peitzmeier SM, Malik M, Kattari SK, et al. Intimate partner violence in transgender populations: systematic review and meta-analysis of prevalence and correlates. *Am J Public Health*. 2020;110(9):e1-e14.

25. Reisner SL, Hughto JM, Dunham EE, et al. Legal protections in public accommodations settings: a critical public health issue for transgender and gender-nonconforming people. *Milbank Q*. 2015;93(3):484-515.

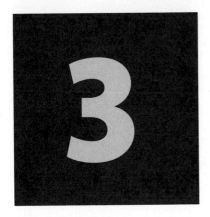

16

Health Disparities

Alex McDowell
Carl G. Streed, Jr.

INTRODUCTION

Increasing evidence suggests that **transgender and gender diverse (TGD)** people experience disproportionately high rates of several mental and physical health problems compared with cisgender people. Many researchers attribute these health disparities among TGD populations, including high rates of psychiatric and substance use disorders, to minority stress, a social and public health framework describing how the long-term effects of stigma, prejudice, and discrimination create a hostile environment that impacts a person's health and well-being. An important corollary of this model is the concept of resilience—the coping strategies that enable minority populations to thrive amid adversity on both the individual and community levels. This chapter explores the health disparities experienced by TGD populations, and delineates the minority stress model and multilevel interventions that address individual, institutional, organizational, and societal/public policy issues.

DEFINING THE PROBLEM OF HEALTH INEQUITIES IN TGD COMMUNITIES

Health inequities experienced by TGD people gained increasing attention between 2010 and 2020. In 2011, the Institute of Medicine released a landmark report acknowledging extensive gaps in research on the health of LGBT populations.[1] In the same year, the US Department of Health and Human Services published its first annual report on LGBT health, outlining policy objectives for reducing discrimination against sexual and gender minorities (SGM) in health care and social services.[2] Both reports pointed to the lack of information on gender identity in nationally representative data as a critical barrier to studying the health of TGD populations. Additionally, in 2016, the National Institutes of Health formally designated SGM as a health disparity population to advance research in this

area.[3] More recently, increases in the volume of research on TGD populations, improvements in the quality of data inclusive of gender identity, and advancements in methodology for identifying TGD individuals in existing dataset have amplified evidence of significant inequities in health. New evidence suggests that TGD people experience higher rates of several mental and physical health conditions. Collective knowledge, however, about how these inequities vary across specific communities within the overall TGD population (e.g., by race, ethnicity, immigration status, socioeconomic position, geography, age, ability, or gender identity) remains limited.

DATA SOURCES FOR STUDYING HEALTH INEQUITIES AMONG TGD PEOPLE

Typically, researchers study rates of health conditions among subpopulations in the United States using survey and administrative data that are representative of a larger population (e.g., the population of the United States, the population of Nevada, or the population of individuals enrolled in Medicare). Representative data are generated using random or probability sampling techniques, through which researchers collect or have access to data on a subset of individuals who were randomly selected from the larger population. With these data sources, researchers can make broad inferences about the health of the entire subpopulation and assess how health varies within this subpopulation based on other important characteristics. Until recently, evidence of health inequities experienced by TGD communities came largely from studies that used nonrepresentative data. Examples include surveys at community centers or distributed through various internet forums and focus groups conducted with students and teachers participating in gay–straight alliances at schools. Research that uses nonrepresentative data can be tailored to explore or address issues that are specific to TGD communities and often provides more relevant detail on characteristics of interest. For example, using nonrandom or nonprobability sampling techniques, researchers are better able to study the experiences of marginalized populations (e.g., TGD people who engage in sex work, are undocumented, or live in institutionalized settings). Nonrepresentative data can also provide critical insight into the needs of or interventions tailored for specific communities within TGD populations.

Research using representative data is important because it provides information on the true size of a given health inequity (e.g., the number of TGD people with a substance use disorder living in the United States) and thus informs policymakers and advocates in the allocation of resources. In order to characterize health inequities at the population level, researchers must first know how many TGD people live in the United States (or within a city or state of interest). For example, if a clinician, researcher, policymaker, or advocate wants to know if the rate of hypertension among TGD older adults living in the South is higher than that of cisgender older adults living in the South, it is first important to know how many TGD older adults are living in the South.

Historically, estimation of the size of the TGD population in the United States has been imperfect. A 2016 meta-analysis of 27 studies found that estimates varied widely based on how the study defined the TGD population and which data source was used, particularly because not all data sources were nationally representative.[4] Research in this meta-analysis defined TGD populations using self-report (typically in surveys) or, when self-report was not available, using other measures that could serve as a proxy for gender identity (typically in administrative or clinical data). The prevalence of self-reported transgender identity (identified using survey data) was 355 per 100,000. The prevalences, however, of TGD identities using an affirmation surgery/hormone therapy definition and a transgender-related diagnosis definition (both identified using various forms of administrative and clinical data) were estimated to be 9.2 per 100,000 and 6.8 per 100,000, respectively.[4,5]

New studies using representative survey data have advanced our collective knowledge of health inequities among TGD communities. In a 2017 review, Meerwijk and Sevelius[6] cited five surveys that randomly sampled participants from a larger population and included self-reported data on gender identity. These five surveys comprise the Behavioral Risk Factor Surveillance System (BRFSS), the National College Health Assessment, the National Adult Tobacco Survey, the National Health Interview Study, and the National Inmate Study, though many of these surveys only collected gender identity data for select years between 2006 and 2016.[6] Additionally, existing survey data remain imperfect due to inconsistent approaches to assessing gender identity, limited evidence on willingness to disclose one's gender identity among TGD communities, and undersampling of TGD people.[7]

In addition to increased availability of representative survey data, research on health inequities has been expanded through studies that use large databases of insurance claims and electronic health records.[8–17] In these studies, researchers use diagnostic codes (and sometimes clinician notes) to identify TGD people. Such studies, however, fail to capture a significant subset of TGD people who do not have diagnostic codes or clinician notes related to gender identity or gender-affirming health care services. For example, TGD people may be excluded from these samples because their health insurance did not cover gender-affirming services, their clinician was unaware of their TGD identity or did not record their TGD identity, or they did not have access to health care services. With this limitation in mind, such studies still provide important insight into the health status of a specific subset of the TGD population.

GENDER MINORITY STRESS AND RESILIENCE MODEL

Health disparities among TGD populations, including high rates of psychiatric and substance use disorders, have been attributed to **gender minority stress**.[18] Meyer[2,3,19,20] proposed the Minority Stress model to describe how experiences of social stress (e.g., stigma, discrimination, and violence) lead to higher rates of psychiatric and substance use disorders among sexual minority people (e.g., those who identify as lesbian, gay, or bisexual). Extending Meyer's Minority Stress model to gender minority people, Testa et al.[21] proposed the Gender Minority Stress and Resilience (GMSR) model outlining a clear pathway from experiences of gender minority stress to negative health outcomes (Figure 3-1).

Broadly, models of minority stress have three key assumptions. First, minority stress is unique to the stigmatized group and adds to general social stress experienced by all groups, as well as to stress associated with other minority identities. As a result of this additional stress, the minority group must adapt to stress beyond what is typically needed among nonstigmatized groups. Second, minority stress is chronic, given its relationship to persistent social and cultural norms. Third, minority stress is socially based, meaning that it is rooted in broader social processes and institutional structures, rather than in any unique genetic or biological characteristics of the individual or the stigmatized group.[20]

The GMSR model distinguishes between distal and proximal gender minority stressors (Table 3-1). **Distal stressors** are external, stress-inducing events that occur due to an individual's gender minority identity. These stressors include gender-related discrimination, rejection, victimization, and identity nonaffirmation.[22,23] Rates of distal minority stressors are alarmingly high among gender minorities. For example, among a national sample of transgender adults reflecting on their experiences in kindergarten through 12th grade, 54% were verbally harassed, 24% were physically assaulted, and

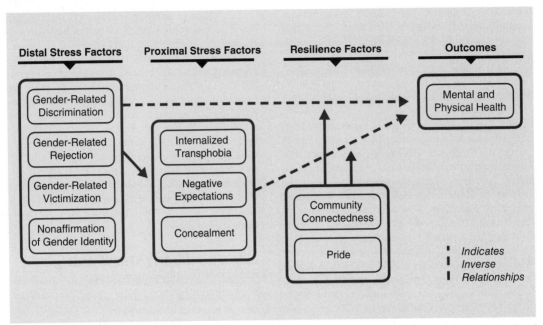

▲ **Figure 3-1.** Gender Minority Stress and Resilience (GMSR) Model. This model outlines how stressors (both distal and proximal) and resilience factors affect mental and physical health outcomes in transgender and gender diverse people. *Dashed line* indicates inverse relationship. (Data from permission from Hendricks ML, Testa RJ. A conceptual framework for clinical work with transgender and gender nonconforming clients: An adaptation of the Minority Stress Model, *Prof Psychol Res Pr* 2012 Aug;43(5):460-467.)

13% were sexually assaulted because they were transgender. In the same study, 15% of adults had been verbally, physically, or sexually assaulted in their workplace in the past year because of their gender identity or expression. Another 33% of adults experienced mistreatment in health care settings due to their gender identity or expression.[24]

Proximal stressors describe gender minority individuals' internal reactions to distal stressors, including expectations of violence or discrimination, and nondisclosure of one's gender identity to avoid mistreatment.[23] For example, 59% of transgender adults reported that they avoided using a public restroom in the past year due to fear of mistreatment, and 23% avoided a necessary medical appointment in the past year due to fear of mistreatment.[24] Internalized transphobia, a process in which a gender minority person adopts society's negative views about gender minority people as their own, is also a proximal stressor. The persistent presence of proximal stressors can weaken psychological coping resources, resulting in worsened mental health.[22]

The GMSR model outlines the relationships between distal stressors, proximal stressors, resilience, and health outcomes. Specifically, both distal and proximal stressors may directly induce negative health outcomes. Distal stressors may also work through proximal stressors to reduce health.

Resilience, a phenomenon that may emerge in the face of minority stress, is a buffering process that can counteract the detrimental effects of both distal and proximal stressors.[23,25] For example, a proximal or distal stressor could trigger community connectedness or pride regarding one's gender identity, two resilience factors that could mitigate the effect of that stressor on health outcomes.[25]

HEALTH DISPARITIES

▶ General Health

TGD adult respondents to the BRFSS in 2014–2017 reported worse physical and mental health compared with their cisgender peers,[26] including higher rates of reporting poor or fair health, no physical exercise, severe mental distress, cigarette use, alcohol use, and ever being diagnosed with depression. TGD respondents also experienced more days of poor physical and mental health compared with cisgender respondents.[26] Table 3-2 summarizes the disparities revealed by the BRFSS, which are discussed in more detail below.

Unfortunately, few studies examine how these inequities vary among important subgroups of the TGD population (e.g., by race, ethnicity, or gender identity). One study,

Table 3-1. Gender Minority Stress Model Stressors

Type of Stressor	Definition	Example
Distal Stressors		
Gender-based victimization	Physical or verbal actions perpetrated against a TGD person or their belongings due to their gender identity/ expression	A trans masculine high school student is pushed down the stairs as a peer shouts transphobic slurs at him.
Gender-based rejection	Any form of rejection based on the person's gender identity/expression, including from individuals, communities, or institutions	The son of a trans feminine adult refuses to speak to his parent after learning his parent is transgender. Additionally, he refuses to bring the grandchildren around her.
Gender-based discrimination	Experiencing discrimination in housing, medical care, employment, or legal documentation due to their gender identity/expression	A gender-fluid college student is denied on-campus housing as the dorms are all-female or all-male. They are asked to pick one gender, or live off campus.
Identity nonaffirmation	Challenges associated with the person's gender identity/expression being rejected or unacknowledged by others	A teacher refuses to change the name of their trans masculine student in the gradebook and uses feminine pronouns for this student.
Proximal Stressors		
Negative expectations for future events	Believing they will likely experience discrimination, prejudice, and rejection in the future due to their gender identity/expression	A gender nonbinary person does not apply for a job within the local school district as they hope to avoid discrimination from the parents and administrators.
Internalized transphobia	Internalizing the negative societal attitudes about TGD individuals and adopting them as their own beliefs	A trans feminine person stays in a toxic relationship because she doubts her ability to find someone who would love her and treat her with respect.
Nondisclosure of one's identity	Trying to conceal their gender identity/expression to protect themselves or others from perceived harm	A trans masculine construction worker avoids questions about his childhood to prevent colleagues from learning about his history.
Resiliency Factors		
Community connectedness	Sense of belonging and kinship with other TGD individuals	A gender-fluid adolescent describes feeling most comfortable attending a support group with other gender expansive teenagers.
Pride	Internal sense of esteem associated with one's TGD identity	A trans masculine adult posts a YouTube video demonstrating the effect of hormones on his voice.

Source: Data from Hendricks ML, Testa RJ. A conceptual framework for clinical work with transgender and gender nonconforming clients: An adaptation of the Minority Stress Model. Professional Psychology: Research and Practice. 2012;43(5):460-467 and Testa RJ, Michaels MS, Bliss W, Rogers ML, Balsam KF, Joiner T. Suicidal ideation in transgender people: Gender minority stress and interpersonal theory factors. *J Abnorm Psychol.* 2017;126(1):125-136 by Heidi J. Dalzell, PsyD; Kayti Protos, MSW, LCSW; and Stacy K. Hunt, PhD.

however, which compared the BRFSS responses of binary transgender and nonbinary respondents, observed that non-binary respondents were more likely than binary transgender respondents to describe their health as poor or fair and to experience activity limitation due to physical, mental, or emotional problems.[27] Another study found that TGD veterans do not experience the same health inequities as TGD civilians. While TGD veterans were more likely than their cisgender peers to experience at least one disability, they were not more likely to experience any other negative health outcomes.[28]

▶ Mental Health and Substance Use Disorders

Evidence suggests that TGD populations tend to experience higher rates of some psychiatric and substance use disorders compared to cisgender populations. The magnitude of this health inequity and the degree to which this inequity is consistent across communities within the broader TGD population (e.g., by race, ethnicity, age, or gender identity) is less certain. Additional research is also needed to better understand the role of gender minority stress and gender-affirming

Table 3-2. Summary of Health Disparities in TGD Populations

General health	• Higher odds of reporting poor or fair health. • More days of poor physical and mental health.
Mental health	• Higher likelihood of being diagnosed with any psychiatric disorder, depression, anxiety, or psychosis. • Gender nonbinary persons more likely to have recent depressive distress and hazardous alcohol use.
Physical health	• Gender-affirmation therapy with testosterone is associated with elevated blood pressure, insulin resistance, and lipid derangements. • Gender-affirmation therapy with estrogen is associated with a higher cardiovascular disease mortality rate compared with cisgender women.
Sexually transmitted infections/HIV	• Transgender women experience some of the highest rates of HIV infection. • Transgender women have higher rates of HPV.
Health care access	• Less likely to report having health insurance and more likely to report financial barriers to care. • TGD persons more likely to report difficulty finding competent and welcoming clinicians.

health care services in psychiatric and substance use disorder inequities.

Using a nationally representative sample of all community hospital discharges in the United States from 2007 to 2014, Hanna et al.[29] found that TGD patients (identified using diagnosis codes, rather than self-report) were more likely than cisgender patients to have diagnoses for any psychiatric disorder, depression, anxiety, and psychosis. Similarly, Wanta et al.[17] identified TGD individuals in electronic health record data for 60 million patients from across the United States and found that they had a higher prevalence of diagnoses for all psychiatric and substance use disorders listed in the *Diagnostic and Statistical Manual of Mental Disorders*, Fifth Edition (DSM-5). In both studies, however, the sample included only TGD people with diagnosis codes related to gender identity or gender-affirming services, meaning that experiences of many TGD individuals are not represented in these results. Additionally, the common health insurance requirement to have a mental health visit prior to coverage of certain gender-affirming services[30] might result in higher rates of diagnosis of mental health and substance use disorders in these samples.[17,29]

Whereas transgender and cisgender adult respondents to the 2014 BRFSS reported similar rates of risky drinking and any unhealthy alcohol use, TGD respondents were more likely to report ever being diagnosed with depression.[26,31] Using an online nonprobability survey, Thoma et al.[32] found that TGD adolescents had higher odds than cisgender adolescents of reporting lifetime suicidality and nonsuicidal self-injury. In a nonprobability sample of adult TGD survey respondents in Massachusetts, nonbinary individuals were less likely than binary individuals to report a diagnosis of anxiety or history of self-harm. Nonbinary respondents, however, were more likely to have recent depressive distress and hazardous alcohol use, compared to binary respondents.[33] Additionally, among TGD veterans, non-Hispanic Black veterans had more diagnoses for serious mental illness, tobacco use, and alcohol use disorder, but fewer diagnoses for depression, compared to non-Hispanic White veterans.[34]

▶ Physical Health Conditions

Using data from the 2015 BRFSS, Nokoff et al.[35] observed that TGD respondents did not report higher prevalence than cisgender respondents for several important health conditions: hypertension, myocardial infarction, angina or coronary heart disease, stroke, diabetes, and obesity. For transgender men, however, current research has demonstrated an association between exogenous testosterone and elevated blood pressure, insulin resistance, and lipid derangements.[36,37] For transgender women, current research suggests a higher CVD mortality rate than cisgender women,[38,39] but the potential relationship to exogenous feminizing hormone therapy and experiences of minority stress remain unclear.[40] (see https://www.ahajournals.org/doi/10.1161/CIR.0000000000000914)

Among TG veterans (identified using diagnoses codes in administrative data), non-Hispanic Black individuals were more likely than non-Hispanic White individuals to have diagnoses for benign prostatic hyperplasia, congestive heart failure, HIV/AIDS, hypertension, and end-stage renal disease. Non-Hispanic Black veterans were less likely to be diagnosed with hypercholesterolemia and obesity.[34]

▶ Sexually Transmitted Infections and HIV

Sexually transmitted infections (STIs) and HIV have been extensively studied in gay, bisexual, and other men who have sex with men (see Chapter 16, "Screening and Prevention of HIV and Sexually Transmitted Infections"). Transgender women have often been grouped in this category based on the assumption of sexual behavior and risk of HIV infection. More recently, efforts have been made to study transgender women and transgender men separately from cisgender gay, bisexual, and other men who have sex with men, to better understand their unique risk of STIs and HIV.[41–45] A systematic review by Poteat et al.[46] found that estimates of HIV infection varied by location and subpopulation globally, but that transgender women experience some of the highest rates of HIV infection (up to 40%). They noted that data were sparse regarding transgender men, but that there may be increased rates of HIV among transgender men who have sex with men.

▶ Health Care Access

TGD adult respondents to the BRFSS in 2014–2017 were less likely to report having health insurance and more likely to report financial barriers to care compared with cisgender respondents.[26,27] Further, nonbinary respondents were less likely than binary transgender respondents to be up-to-date on their annual wellness visit. Nonbinary respondents were also less likely to report receiving any mental health care in the past year.[33]

Adult TGD respondents to the 2014 BRFSS were just as likely as cisgender respondents to be screened by a health care professional for alcohol use disorder.[31] Similarly, Narayan et al.[47] found that TGD adults were just as likely as cisgender adults to undergo breast cancer screening with mammography.

RESILIENCE

Research on health inequities has revealed the unique ways TGD populations experience health and well-being compared with their cisgender peers. More research has begun to explore how TGD populations thrive despite a myriad of adversities, with a particular focus on the factors that facilitate resilience. Resilience describes the ability to bounce back or to cope successfully in the setting of minority stress and can occur at the individual and community-level.[25,48,49] Community-level resilience often comes in the form of access to resources or social values specific to TGD populations, such as protective policies, community centers, knowledgeable health care professionals, peer support, and role models.[25]

Resilience has been the subject of research among LGBTQIA+ youth and, more recently, among TGD populations.[18,22,50–61] In a systematic review of minority stress and mental health among TGD populations, Valentine and Shipherd[18] cite recent research that describes the cross-sectional relationship between various measures of resilience and mental health outcomes. For example, using an online sample of TGD adults, Bockting et al.[62] found that peer support from other TGD people moderated the association between social stigma and mental health problems. Puckett et al.[56] measured social support and assessed anxiety and depressive symptoms in a sample of transgender youth. They found that greater than one half of participants reported moderate to severe levels of anxious and depressive symptoms. They found that family social support had the strongest correlations with symptoms of anxiety and depression

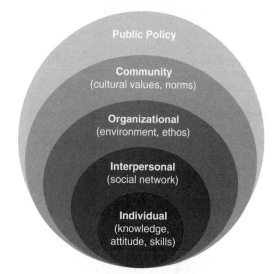

▲ **Figure 3-2.** Ecological Framework for Health Research.

and was the only form of support associated with resilience when controlling for other forms of support. Similarly, Ryan et al.[63] found that family acceptance predicts greater self-esteem, social support, and general health status and also protects against depression, substance use disorders, and suicidal ideation and behaviors among TGD youth. Early support of TGD identities likely engenders resilience.

INTERVENTIONS

Reducing the various inequities and barriers to health and well-being for TGD populations requires multilevel interventions that address individual, institutional, organizational, and societal/public policy issues. This **ecological or eco-social framework** has been applied to LGBTQIA+ population research to both understand and intervene on health disparities (Figure 3-2).[64–67]

An ecological framework for understanding and addressing health disparities posits that no individual factor alone can predict health and well-being, because each person is impacted by others close to them, the communities in which they live, the institutions with which they interact, and dominant societal level discourses, laws, and policies. Further, factors across this sociocultural trajectory may support or prevent resilience development. Consequently, the policy and societal levels of the ecological framework are particularly critical in fostering health equity. If there were no societal stigma created by dominant discourses of law, medicine, media, education, and religion, there would be little-to-no impetus for subsequent levels of stigma and discrimination and the resulting gender minority stress for TGD persons. If a society and culture valued the diversity of gender as experienced by TGD persons, hatred would not be experienced at the interpersonal and individual level. Primary prevention of stigma is a priority.

Examples of meaningful changes at the public policy level that have the potential to affect individual experiences of health and well-being include nondiscrimination policies, identity document policies, access to health care and housing, protective policies within the criminal justice system, comprehensive education in schools, antibullying programs that explicitly address gender identity, and changes in responses to religious doctrines and dogma regarding TGD persons. The upsurge of "religious" or "conscious" laws that allow for discrimination in health care settings is a threat to the safety and equality of TGD communities, as these proposed rules and regulations allow health care professionals and health care institutions to actively discriminate against people with diverse sexual orientations and gender identities.

Despite recent efforts to promote marriage equality and its positive effects on health and well-being,[68,69] including access to health care services via insurance, TGD people can still be denied housing based on their gender identity in some states.[70] National policies explicitly including gender identity as a protected class are necessary to ensure equitable treatment across jurisdictions.

Community and organizational initiatives involve not only the continued support of existing TGD communities but also cultural change across various demographics. Because cultural and community change is slow, exposure to TGD persons via daily interactions (whether interpersonal or via media) helps foster broader acceptance of gender diversity.[60,71] Interpersonal interactions have the potential to contribute to change at higher levels of the ecological model.[72] Interpersonal and individual-level interventions have been well-studied among families[73,74] and youth experiencing bullying.[75–77] What is most necessary is the creation of a safe environment in which an individual may disclose their gender identity.

The creation of a safe environment to facilitate TGD persons disclosing their gender identity and moving toward a healing interaction are best rooted in the principles of trauma-informed care: safety, trustworthiness and transparency, peer support, collaboration and mutuality, empowerment and choice, and acknowledgment of cultural, historical, and gender issues affecting the well-being of a person. Trauma-informed care for TGD persons is discussed in detail in Chapter 11, "Basic Principles of Trauma-Informed and Gender-Affirming Care."

CASE STUDY: Eli

Eli is a 23-year-old gender diverse adult assigned female sex at birth currently completing their final year of college. They have demonstrated significant resilience in attending college despite having been kicked out of their home by their parents for being gender diverse. Having identified community support online and later in-person through their student center, they have managed to create a family of choice. Nevertheless, they still experience stress when they are misgendered. They have started smoking to manage these stressful episodes. They would like to appear more masculine and are considering top surgery and hormone therapy to appear less feminine. They have, however, delayed seeking gender-affirming medical care, as their student insurance explicitly denied coverage until recently. They are concerned about seeking medical care as they have heard from other students that the physicians at the college health service are not responsive in providing gender-affirming care. Eli is considering seeking care outside their insurance coverage as a result.

▶ Discussion Questions

1. What are the distal stress factors affecting Eli's health and well-being?

2. What are the proximal stress factors affecting Eli's health and well-being?

3. What are the resilience factors affecting Eli's health and well-being?

SUMMARY

- Current evidence suggests that TGD people experience higher rates of several mental and physical health conditions than cisgender people. Despite this evidence, research into how these inequities vary across important communities within the overall TGD population (e.g., by race, ethnicity, immigration status, socioeconomic position, geography, age, ability, or gender identity) remains limited.

- Research on health inequities affecting TGD populations in the United States is hampered by a lack of accurate data on population size. New research studies based on survey instruments such as the Behavioral Risk Factor Surveillance System (BRFSS) address this limitation by using representative data to advance our collective knowledge of health inequities among TGD individuals.

- TGD respondents to the BRFSS report considerable health disparities, including those related to general health, mental health, substance use disorders, and STIs/HIV. TGD people report multiple barriers to health care access, including lack of health insurance and insufficient numbers of affirming and skilled health care professionals.

- In the Minority Stress Model, proximal and distal stressors based on one's identity have downstream effects on health outcomes and are a driver of health inequities. Resilience is the ability to thrive despite adversity and exerts a buffering effect against these stressors. Key factors in resilience include family, community, and social support.

- Interventions cannot focus only on the individual. The ecological model posits that successful interventions must be multilevel to eliminate disparities and achieve equitable outcomes.

REFERENCES

1. Institute of Medicine (US) Committee on Lesbian, Gay, Bisexual, and Transgender Health Issues and Research Gaps and Opportunities. *The Health of Lesbian, Gay, Bisexual, and Transgender People: Building a Foundation for Better Understanding.* National Academies Press; 2011. http://www.ncbi.nlm.nih.gov/books/NBK64806/.
2. U.S. Department of Health and Human ServicesHealth (ASH). Recommended Actions to Improve the Health and Well-Being of Lesbian, Gay, Bisexual, and Transgender Communities. HHS.gov. Published May 22, 2014. https://www.hhs.gov/programs/topic-sites/lgbt/enhanced-resources/reports/health-objectives-2011/index.html.
3. Pérez-Stable EJ. Director's Message for October 6, 2016. National Institute on Minority Health and Disparities. Published 2016. https://www.nimhd.nih.gov/about/directors-corner/messages/message_10-06-16.html.
4. Collin L, Reisner SL, Tangpricha V, Goodman M. Prevalence of transgender depends on the "case" definition: a systematic review. *J Sex Med.* 2016;13(4):613-626.
5. Bockting W, Reisner S, Herman J, Meyer I, Feldman J, Poteat T. Findings from the U.S. transgender population survey. Presented at the: USPATH2019; Washington, DC, USA.
6. Meerwijk EL, Sevelius JM. Transgender population size in the United States: a meta-regression of population-based probability samples. *Am J Public Health.* 2017;107(2):e1-e8.
7. Henderson ER, Blosnich JR, Herman JL, Meyer IH. Considerations on sampling in transgender health disparities research. *LGBT Health.* 2019;6(6):267-270.
8. Dragon CN, Guerino P, Ewald E, Laffan AM. Transgender Medicare beneficiaries and chronic conditions: exploring fee-for-service claims data. *LGBT Health.* 2017;4(6):404-411.
9. Brown GR, Jones KT. Mental health and medical health disparities in 5135 transgender veterans receiving healthcare in the Veterans Health Administration: a case-control study. *LGBT Health.* 2016;3(2):122-131.
10. Brown GR, Jones KT. Incidence of breast cancer in a cohort of 5,135 transgender veterans. *Breast Cancer Res Treat.* 2015;149(1):191-198.
11. Ehrenfeld JM, Gottlieb KG, Beach LB, Monahan SE, Fabbri D. Development of a natural language processing algorithm to identify and evaluate transgender patients in electronic health record systems. *Ethn Dis.* 2019;29(suppl 2):441-450.
12. Roblin D, Barzilay J, Tolsma D. A novel method for estimating transgender status using electronic medical records. Abstract. Europe PMC. https://europepmc.org/article/med/26907539.
13. Progovac AM, Cook BL, Mullin BO, et al. Identifying gender minority patients' health and health care needs in administrative claims data. *Health Aff (Millwood).* 2018;37(3):413-420.
14. Progovac AM, Mullin BO, Creedon TB, et al. Trends in mental health care use in Medicare from 2009 to 2014 by gender minority and disability status. *LGBT Health.* 2019;6(6):297-305.
15. Progovac AM, Mullin BO, Dunham E, et al. Disparities in suicidality by gender identity among Medicare beneficiaries. *Am J Prev Med.* 2020;58(6):789-798.
16. Blosnich JR, Brown GR, Wojcio S, Jones KT, Bossarte RM. Mortality among veterans with transgender-related diagnoses in the Veterans Health Administration, FY2000–2009. *LGBT Health.* 2014;1(4):269-276.
17. Wanta JW, Niforatos JD, Durbak E, Viguera A, Altinay M. Mental health diagnoses among transgender patients in the clinical setting: an all-payer electronic health record study. *Transgend Health.* 2019;4(1):313-315.
18. Valentine SE, Shipherd JC. A systematic review of social stress and mental health among transgender and gender nonconforming people in the United States. *Clin Psychol Rev.* 2018;66:24-38.
19. Meyer IH. Minority stress and mental health in gay men. *J Health Soc Behav.* 1995;36(1):38-56.
20. Meyer IH. Prejudice, social stress, and mental health in lesbian, gay, and bisexual populations: conceptual issues and research evidence. *Psychol Bull.* 2003;129(5):674-697.
21. Testa RJ, Habarth J, Peta J, Balsam K, Bockting W. Development of the gender minority stress and resilience measure. *Psychol Sex Orient Gend Divers.* 2015;2(1):65-77.
22. Hendricks ML, Testa RJ. A conceptual framework for clinical work with transgender and gender nonconforming clients: an adaptation of the Minority Stress Model. *Professional Psychology: Research and Practice.* 2012;43(5):460-467.
23. Testa RJ, Michaels MS, Bliss W, Rogers ML, Balsam KF, Joiner T. Suicidal ideation in transgender people: gender minority stress and interpersonal theory factors. *J Abnorm Psychol.* 2017;126(1):125-136.
24. James SE, Herman JL, Rankin S, Keisling M, Mottet L, Anafi M. The Report of the 2015 U.S. Transgender Survey. *National Center for Transgender Equality.* Published online 2016.
25. Meyer IH. Resilience in the study of minority stress and health of sexual and gender minorities. *Psychol Sex Orient Gend Divers.* 2015;2(3):209-213.
26. Baker KE. Findings from the behavioral risk factor surveillance system on health-related quality of life among US transgender adults, 2014-2017. *JAMA Intern Med.* Published online April 22, 2019.
27. Streed CG, McCarthy EP, Haas JS. Self-reported physical and mental health of gender nonconforming transgender adults in the United States. *LGBT Health.* 2018;5(7):443-448.
28. Downing J, Conron K, Herman JL, Blosnich JR. Transgender and cisgender US veterans have few health differences. *Health Aff (Millwood).* 2018;37(7):1160-1168.
29. Hanna B, Desai R, Parekh T, Guirguis E, Kumar G, Sachdeva R. Psychiatric disorders in the U.S. transgender population. *Ann Epidemiol.* 2019;39:1-7.e1.
30. Streed CG, Arroyo H, Goldstein Z. Gender minority patients' mental health care. *Health Aff (Millwood).* 2018;37(6):1014. doi:10.1377/hlthaff.2018.0548
31. Blosnich JR, Lehavot K, Glass JE, Williams EC. Differences in alcohol use and alcohol-related health care among transgender and nontransgender adults: findings from the 2014 Behavioral Risk Factor Surveillance System. *J Stud Alcohol Drugs.* 2017;78(6):861-866.

32. Thoma BC, Salk RH, Choukas-Bradley S, Goldstein TR, Levine MD, Marshal MP. Suicidality disparities between transgender and cisgender adolescents. *Pediatrics*. 2019;144(5).

33. Reisner SL, Hughto JMW. Comparing the health of non-binary and binary transgender adults in a statewide non-probability sample. *PLoS One*. 2019;14(8).

34. Brown GR, Jones KT. Racial health disparities in a cohort of 5,135 transgender veterans. *J Racial Ethnic Health Disparities*. 2014;1(4):257-266.

35. Nokoff NJ, Scarbro S, Juarez-Colunga E, Moreau KL, Kempe A. Health and cardiometabolic disease in transgender adults in the United States: Behavioral Risk Factor Surveillance System 2015. *J Endocr Soc*. 2018;2(4):349-360.

36. White Hughto JM, Reisner SL. A systematic review of the effects of hormone therapy on psychological functioning and quality of life in transgender individuals. *Transgend Health*. 2016;1(1):21-31.

37. Gooren LJ, Wierckx K, Giltay EJ. Cardiovascular disease in transsexual persons treated with cross-sex hormones: reversal of the traditional sex difference in cardiovascular disease pattern. *Eur J Endocrinol*. 2014;170(6):809-819.

38. Nota NM, Wiepjes CM, de Blok CJM, Gooren LJG, Kreukels BPC, den Heijer M. Occurrence of acute cardiovascular events in transgender individuals receiving hormone therapy. *Circulation*. 2019;139(11):1461-1462.

39. Getahun D, Nash R, Flanders WD, et al. Cross-sex hormones and acute cardiovascular events in transgender persons: a cohort study. *Ann Intern Med*. 2018;169(4):205-213.

40. Streed CG, Harfouch O, Marvel F, Blumenthal RS, Martin SS, Mukherjee M. Cardiovascular disease among transgender adults receiving hormone therapy: a narrative review. *Ann Intern Med*. 2017;167(4):256-267.

41. Reisner SL, Hughto JMW, Pardee D, Sevelius J. Syndemics and gender affirmation: HIV sexual risk in female-to-male trans masculine adults reporting sexual contact with cisgender males. *Int J STD AIDS*. 2016;27(11):955-966.

42. Reisner SL, Radix A, Deutsch MB. Integrated and gender-affirming transgender clinical care and research. *J Acquir Immune Defic Syndr*. 2016;72(suppl 3):S235-S242.

43. Reisner SL, Poteat T, Keatley J, et al. Global health burden and needs of transgender populations: a review. *Lancet*. 2016;388(10042):412-436.

44. Reisner SL, Murchison GR. A global research synthesis of HIV and STI biobehavioural risks in female-to-male transgender adults. *Glob Public Health*. 2016;11(7-8):866-887.

45. Baral SD, Poteat T, Strömdahl S, Wirtz AL, Guadamuz TE, Beyrer C. Worldwide burden of HIV in transgender women: a systematic review and meta-analysis. *Lancet Infect Dis*. 2013;13(3):214-222.

46. Poteat T, Scheim A, Xavier J, Reisner S, Baral S. Global epidemiology of HIV infection and related syndemics affecting transgender people. *J Acquir Immune Defic Syndr*. 2016;72(suppl 3):S210-S219.

47. Narayan A, Lebron-Zapata L, Morris E. Breast cancer screening in transgender patients: findings from the 2014 BRFSS survey. *Breast Cancer Res Treat*. 2017;166(3):875-879.

48. Rutter M. Developing concepts in developmental psychopathology. In: Hudziak JJ, ed. *Developmental Psychopathology and Wellness: Genetic and Environmental Influences*. Arlington, VA: American Psychiatric Association; 2008: 3-22.

49. Zautra AJ, Hall JS, Murray KE. Resilience: a new definition of health for people and communities. *Handbook of Adult Resilience*. Published online January 1, 2010.

50. Scourfield J, Roen K, McDermott L. Lesbian, gay, bisexual and transgender young people's experiences of distress: resilience, ambivalence and self-destructive behaviour. *Health Soc Care Community*. 2008;16(3):329-336.

51. Mustanski B, Liu RT. A longitudinal study of predictors of suicide attempts among lesbian, gay, bisexual, and transgender youth. *Arch Sex Behav*. 2013;42(3):437-448.

52. Cortes J, Fletcher TL, Latini DM, Kauth MR. Mental health differences between older and younger lesbian, gay, bisexual, and transgender veterans: evidence of resilience. *Clin Gerontol*. 2019;42(2):162-171.

53. Logie CH, Wang Y, Marcus N, et al. Syndemic experiences, protective factors, and HIV vulnerabilities among lesbian, gay, bisexual and transgender persons in Jamaica. *AIDS Behav*. 2019;23(6):1530-1540.

54. Todd K, Peitzmeier SM, Kattari SK, Miller-Perusse M, Sharma A, Stephenson R. Demographic and behavioral profiles of nonbinary and binary transgender youth. *Transgend Health*. 2019;4(1):254-261.

55. Edwards LL, Bernal AT, Hanley SM, Martin S. Resilience factors and suicide risk for a sample of transgender clients. *Family Process*. n/a(n/a). https://onlinelibrary.wiley.com/doi/abs/10.1111/famp.12479.

56. Puckett JA, Matsuno E, Dyar C, Mustanski B, Newcomb ME. Mental health and resilience in transgender individuals: what type of support makes a difference? *J Fam Psychol*. 2019;33(8):954-964.

57. Eliason MJ, Streed C, Henne M. Coping with stress as an LGBTQ+ health care professional. *J Homosex*. 2018;65(5):561-578.

58. Arayasirikul S, Pomart WA, Raymond HF, Wilson EC. Unevenness in health at the intersection of gender and sexuality: sexual minority disparities in alcohol and drug use among transwomen in the San Francisco Bay Area. *J Homosex*. 2018;65(1):66-79.

59. Byne W. Resilience and action in a challenging time for LGBT rights. *LGBT Health*. 2018;5(1):1-5.

60. Flores AR, Hatzenbuehler ML, Gates GJ. Identifying psychological responses of stigmatized groups to referendums. *Proc Natl Acad Sci USA*. 2018;115(15):3816-3821.

61. McConnell EA, Janulis P, Phillips G, Truong R, Birkett M. Multiple minority stress and LGBT community resilience among sexual minority men. *Psychol Sex Orient Gend Divers*. 2018;5(1):1-12.

62. Bockting WO, Miner MH, Swinburne Romine RE, Hamilton A, Coleman E. Stigma, mental health, and resilience in an online sample of the US transgender population. *Am J Public Health*. 2013;103(5):943-951.

63. Ryan C, Russell ST, Huebner D, Diaz R, Sanchez J. Family acceptance in adolescence and the health of LGBT young adults. *J Child Adolesc Psychiatr Nurs*. 2010;23(4):205-213.

64. Eliason MJ, Fogel SC. An ecological framework for sexual minority women's health: factors associated with greater body mass. *J Homosex*. 2015;62(7):845-882.

65. Boehmer U, Ozonoff A, Miao X. An ecological approach to examine lung cancer disparities due to sexual orientation. *Public Health*. 2012;126(7):605-612.

66. Gibbs JJ, Rice E. The social context of depression symptomology in sexual minority male youth: determinants of depression in a sample of Grindr users. *J Homosex.* 2016;63(2):278-299.

67. White Hughto JM, Reisner SL, Pachankis JE. Transgender stigma and health: a critical review of stigma determinants, mechanisms, and interventions. *Soc Sci Med.* 2015;147:222-231.

68. Raifman J, Moscoe E, Austin SB. Legalization of same-sex marriage and drop in adolescent suicide rates: association but not causation—reply. *JAMA Pediatr.* 2017;171(9):915-916.

69. Raifman J, Moscoe E, Austin SB, McConnell M. Difference-in-differences analysis of the association between state same-sex marriage policies and adolescent suicide attempts. *JAMA Pediatr.* 2017;171(4):350-356.

70. Movement Advancement Project | Nondiscrimination Laws. https://www.lgbtmap.org//equality-maps/non_discrimination_laws.

71. Flores AR, Haider-Markel DP, Lewis DC, Miller PR, Tadlock BL, Taylor JK. Transgender prejudice reduction and opinions on transgender rights: results from a mediation analysis on experimental data. *Res Politics.* 2018;5(1):1-7.

72. Flores AR, Haider-Markel DP, Lewis DC, Miller PR, Tadlock BL, Taylor JK. Challenged expectations: mere exposure effects on attitudes about transgender people and rights. *Political Psychol.* 2018;39(1):197-216.

73. Forcier M, Johnson M. Screening, identification, and support of gender non-conforming children and families. https://europepmc.org/article/med/23159349.

74. Ryan C, Huebner D, Diaz RM, Sanchez J. Family rejection as a predictor of negative health outcomes in white and Latino lesbian, gay, and bisexual young adults. *Pediatrics.* 2009;123(1):346-352.

75. Gower AL, Rider GN, Coleman E, Brown C, McMorris BJ, Eisenberg ME. Perceived gender presentation among transgender and gender diverse youth: approaches to analysis and associations with bullying victimization and emotional distress. *LGBT Health.* 2018;5(5):312-319.

76. Huebner DM, Thoma BC, Neilands TB. School victimization and substance use among lesbian, gay, bisexual, and transgender adolescents. *Prev Sci.* 2015;16(5):734-743.

77. McConnell EA, Birkett MA, Mustanski B. Typologies of social support and associations with mental health outcomes among LGBT youth. *LGBT Health.* 2015;2(1):55-61.

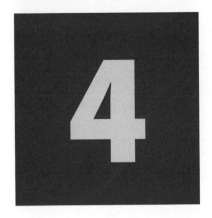

Harnessing Information Technology to Improve Clinical Care

Chris Grasso

Alex S. Keuroghlian

INTRODUCTION

This chapter discusses the use of **health information technology (HIT)**, including **electronic health records (EHRs)**, to improve care for **transgender and gender diverse (TGD)** patients. It also addresses the policy changes that led to the requirement of data collection fields for gender identity in EHRs and the US Health Resources and Services Administration's Bureau of Primary Health Care (HRSA/BPHC) annual data reporting for Federally Qualified Health Centers (FQHCs).

THE IMPORTANCE OF COLLECTING GENDER IDENTITY DATA

Sexual and gender minority (SGM) people face significant barriers to adequate and culturally responsive health care, leading to numerous health disparities. Ongoing efforts supported by both federal and other funding agencies are responding to the need to reduce these health inequities by increasing SGM visibility through data collection in health care. In 2015, the Office of the National Coordinator for Health Information Technology (ONC) officially made patient sexual orientation and gender identity (SOGI) data collection a requirement for the Base EHR Meaningful Use certification. The requirement mandated that by January 2018, all certified EHRs were required to have a place to document SOGI using standard definitions and value sets. In 2016, HRSA/BPHC mandated the collection of SOGI demographic information by all FQHCs, a necessary step for improving FCHQs' ability to identify and better serve their SGM patients.

Health care organizations are often reluctant to ask gender identity questions, believing that patients will become offended or will refuse to answer the questions. It is important, however, to understand both patient and staff perspectives. Several studies have evaluated the feasibility of collecting gender identity data in health care organizations. These various studies came to similar conclusions: that patients will answer the questions when asked.[1-3] Providing patients with informational pamphlets about gender identity data collection can alleviate confusion and reduce staff concerns (Figure 4-1).

Collecting gender identity data for patients is critical for health care organizations to provide a welcoming, inclusive environment and allow health care professionals to better understand their patients. Routine gender identity data collection within the EHR can be used to measure and track health outcomes at the individual and population levels. EHRs have the potential to improve quality of care, provide timely clinical information, and improve communication among patients and members of the health care team, creating a more patient-centered care experience. HIT is an important tool for increasing quality, monitoring reports, and managing the health of a population. For example, the use of a transgender health "dashboard" that tracks a set of health measures within the practice's TGD patient population can help reduce health disparities. Experiences and processes of implementing changes within the EHR and workflows can be shared, including approaches to significantly reduce and eliminate the occurrence of errors such as incorrect names, **pronouns**, and **gender markers**.

Health care is increasingly turning to technology to help improve systems and processes to benefit patients and their health. EHRs have greatly improved the ability to track clinical markers and health outcomes by collecting and storing data in a standardized, structured format that can be used to evaluate activities. The goal of HIT is to improve data capture to reduce health disparities and create more patient-centered care. TGD patients comprise an underserved population largely invisible in health care systems. Identifying both technology- and workflow-related needs and capacities in

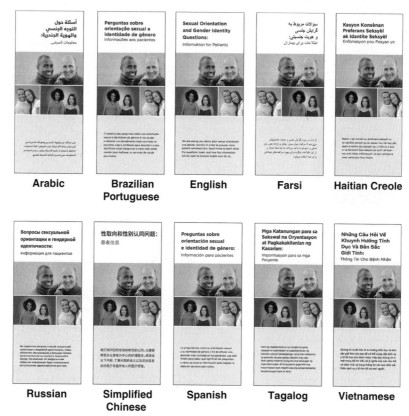

▲ **Figure 4-1.** Patient education pamphlets about sexual orientation and gender identity (SOGI) data collection. Informational pamphlets are available in many languages to help educate patients about why gender identity data collection is important. The pamphlets shown here are available from the National LGBTQIA+ Health Education Center at The Fenway Institute (Reproduced with permission from Ready, Set, Go! A Guide for Collecting Data on Sexual Orientation and Gender Identity. Updated 2020. National LGBT Health Education Center. A Program of the Fenway Institute.)

EHRs is a collaborative effort among the following key staff: senior leadership/management, clinical care team members (including physicians, nurses, medical assistants, and behavioral health clinicians), front-line staff (including front-desk and registration staff), EHR and HIT vendors, and informatics/data staff (Figure 4-2).

USE OF ELECTRONIC HEALTH RECORDS IN DATA COLLECTION

An EHR system is an electronic version of a patient's medical chart and includes key elements, such as demographics, insurance, appointments, diagnoses, medications, laboratory values, and visit notes. EHRs are required to meet a minimum set of expectations to receive certification through ONC. A certified EHR has a designated field to capture a patient's gender identity.

▶ Recommended Data Fields in Certified EHRs

Key recommended data fields that should be included in EHRs to provide optimal care include **name used**, pronouns, current **gender identity**, and **sex assigned at birth**, as well as an **anatomical inventory** (Table 4-1). A patient's gender identity cannot be assumed based on how they look or sound; therefore, name used and pronouns should be collected for all patients. Collecting name used and pronouns allows for effective and respectful communication and the delivery of culturally responsive care. When designed correctly, these data fields should be visible, interconnected, and harnessed throughout the EHR and integrated HIT systems. As an example, Figures 4-3 and 4-4 demonstrate the use of color blocks with pronoun text that are used in the EHR patient banner at Fenway Health to display the patient's pronouns.

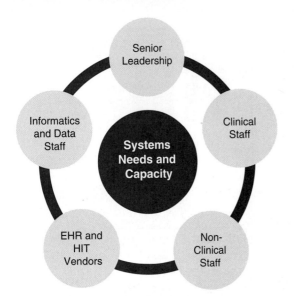

▲ **Figure 4-2.** Stakeholder involvement to meet systems needs and optimize capacity for gender identity data collection. Key stakeholders for sensitive and effective gender identity data collection and utilization include clinical staff, nonclinical staff, EHR and HIT vendors, informatics and data staff, and senior leadership.

The use of the word "preferred" in prefacing the data block for name and pronouns is strongly discouraged, as this creates the false impression that use of the patient's name used and pronouns is optional. Thus, the best practice in health care settings is to ask: "What name do you go by?" "What is the name listed on your insurance?" and "What are your pronouns?"

Because gender identity concepts and pronouns are continually evolving, new terminology is frequently introduced within TGD communities. Terminology that no longer accurately reflects current pronoun and gender identity concepts is outdated or archaic. Systems must be able to accommodate the expansion of new terminology as these changes occur. The Systematized Nomenclature of Medicine (SNOMED), an international coding system used in HIT, currently has a limited number of standard codes for gender identities. Value sets, which are lists of codes and corresponding terminology from standard clinical vocabularies, such as the International Statistical Classification of Diseases and Related Health Problems (ICD-10), Current Procedural Terminology (CPT), SNOMED, and Logical Observation Identifiers Names and Codes (LOINC), should be updated to support standardization in systems and interoperable health information exchange. Robust and culturally responsive value sets also prevent downstream billing issues.

Table 4-1. Key Recommended Fields for Electronic Health Records, Their Importance, and Suggested Language for Data Collection with Patients

Recommended Data Field	Necessity	Suggested Language for Data Collection with Patients
Name used	For addressing patient in an affirming manner	*What name do you go by?*
Pronouns	For addressing the patient in an affirming manner	*What are your pronouns? Some people's pronouns are she/hers, or he/him, or they/them, or something else.*
Name listed in electronic health record, on health insurance, and on official documents	For documenting in the correct chart, ensuring insurance reimbursement, and when writing certain letters	*What is the name listed on your chart/health insurance/official documents?*
Current gender identity	For clinical decision-making and care	*What is your current gender identity?*
Sex assigned at birth	For population health management	*What was your sex assigned at birth?*
Anatomical inventory (see Figure 4-5 for more details)	For clinical decision-making and care	*In order to provide you good clinical care, I will need to know if you have certain body parts. Is it OK if we talk through a list of body parts, and you can let me know whether you have these, and also what language you use to describe these for yourself?*

▶ Gender Identity, Sex Assigned at Birth, and Administrative Sex Fields

Virtually all current EHR systems include a patient demographic section where sex is recorded. This sex field is also referred to as "**administrative sex**" and is reported for administrative use (e.g., for billing and claims). The administrative sex may be different from the sex assigned at birth and current gender identity. Along with the patient's name used and pronouns, a

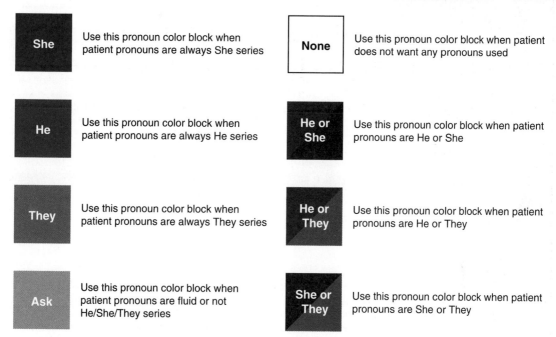

▲ **Figure 4-3.** Sample color blocks with pronoun text for use within EHR patient banners.

patient's administrative sex, current gender identity, and sex assigned at birth should be collected at registration. Asking about a patient's sex assigned at birth is important because some gender-minority people do not identify as transgender or gender diverse, and identify simply as woman/female or man/male. Collecting data about a patient's current gender identity and sex assigned at birth helps minimize assumptions.

An increasing number of states and municipalities have expanded the sex options available on birth certificates. Unfortunately, many EHR and insurance company systems have not yet developed systems that accommodate sex fields beyond the binary options of either female or male. In these circumstances, it is critical to communicate with the patient to understand which sex designation they have recorded with their insurance provider. Asking the patient specifically how they would like the practice to record this designation in the sex field can help minimize billing claim denials.

EHR templates often generate questions, clinical prompts, and visibility regions based on the sex field in the registration section. Default EHR system clinical prompts and visibility regions based on a sex field alone can result in barriers to providing optimal care. For example, EHR fields that are prepopulated (i.e., automatically filled out) based on a sex field alone may prevent clinicians from entering gynecological history and physical exam findings. In contrast, EHR algorithms that are inclusive of current gender identity, sex assigned at birth, and, as discussed in the next section, an anatomical inventory, should be integrated to determine questions, clinical prompts, and field visibility on EHR forms.

Because patients typically review and update all demographic information at registration, updating gender identity at this point in the workflow ensures that this information is routinely reviewed and updated with each patient. Asking these questions as standard demographic variables helps to ensure the collection of these data in health care. Patients should be informed that this information will help health care professionals deliver appropriate prevention, screening, and treatment services and be assured that this information will remain confidential.

Patients may leave gender identity questions blank at intake or registration because they missed the questions, they did not understand the questions, or because they understood the questions and do not want to answer them at this time. If gender identity questions are left blank at registration, the clinician can follow up during the visit and ask, "I see you left these questions blank at registration. We have begun asking all patients about gender identity to provide affirming care for everyone. I was wondering if you had questions and whether we might take a few minutes to talk about how you think about yourself in this regard?"[4]

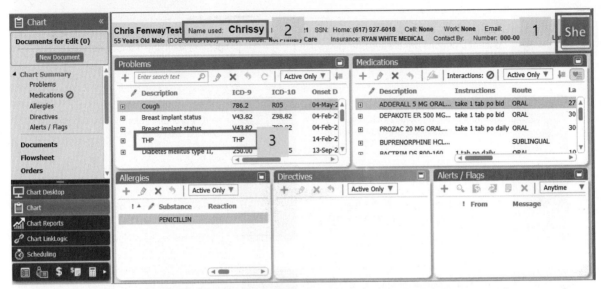

▲ **Figure 4-4.** Gender identity-related features in a sample EHR patient chart interface. This image is from a sample test patient in Fenway Health's Centricity-based EHR. The patient's pronoun color block is displayed (1), and a pop-up alert can also be used to notify staff of the patient's pronouns. The patient's name used is shown in the banner. Optimally, the name used can be made more visually prominent by bolding or increasing the font beyond that of the patient's name used for insurance purposes (2). The entry "THP" in the Problems List indicates that the patient receives care in the Transgender Health Program (3).

Staff Training

As members of the extended care team, registration staff must be able to collect and use patient names and pronouns to provide respectful care.[5,6] Staff members may need additional coaching and reassurance that, with appropriate training, they will be capable of conducting sensitive and effective gender identity data collection. Supervisors can explain to front-line staff that the health care organization is collecting this information to provide the best possible care for all patients, and that staff do not need to change their personal values or religious beliefs to collect these data and meet the organization's expectations. Regular check-ins with staff members can help identify and address their concerns and also serve as a source of front-line input for continuous quality improvement and iterative refinement of the gender identity data collection process.[4,5]

An important aspect of training is to teach care teams, front-line staff, and all personnel within the organization that a patient's gender identity, correct name, and pronouns cannot be determined based on how the patient looks or sounds. Staff can learn to apologize and correct themselves if they make a mistake and use the wrong name or pronouns, by saying, "I'm sorry, I did not mean to be disrespectful," and then promptly using the correct name and pronouns.[4,7] Staff can also learn to

address their own implicit bias toward TGD people as a means of reducing the likelihood of **misgendering** patients. These efforts may also increase their comfort, confidence, and competence in engaging in sensitive and effective communication to collect patient gender identity information.[8]

As noted above, this information should be available to clinicians when reviewing the patient's clinical chart. By having access to this information, health care professionals are better equipped to serve their patients. Addressing a patient's gender identity during a clinical visit, which is a best practice for all patients, can facilitate discussions of preventive screenings, risk reduction, family and social support, behavioral health concerns, and other topics critically important for patient-centered care.

Anatomical Inventory

Review of Systems (ROS) forms are standard in EHRs and used in medical care to gather comprehensive health information about a patient to develop the plan of care. Although most ROS forms are organized by organ systems, they typically do not include a detailed **anatomical inventory** (also referred to as **organ inventory**). An anatomical inventory allows documentation of sex-related and other organs (e.g., prostate) in a patient's EHR (Figure 4-5). An anatomical

Breasts/Chest

Chest Reconstruction ☐

Bilateral Mastectomy ☐

Unilateral Mastectomy, R ☐

Unilateral Mastectomy, L ☐

Breast Augment/Implant(s) ☐

Uterus

Hysterectomy - Cervix Removed ☐

Hysterectomy - Cervix Remains ☐

Ovaries

Bilateral Salpingo-Oophorectomy ☐

Unilateral Salpingo-Oophorectomy, R ☐

Unilateral Salpingo-Oophorectomy, L ☐

Cervix

Congenital Absence ☐

Vagina

Colpocleisis - Closure of the Vagina ☐

Vaginoplasty ☐

Penis

Phalloplasty/Penile Implant ☐

Erectile Device ☐

Urethra

Urethral Lengthening ☐

Testes

Testicular Implant(s) ☐

Bilateral Orchiectomy ☐

Unilateral Orchiectomy, R ☐

Unilateral Orchiectomy, L ☐

Prostate

Prostatectomy ☐

▲ **Figure 4-5.** Sample EHR anatomical inventory. This image is taken from Fenway Health's Centricity-based EHR. (Reproduced with permission from Fenway Health's Centricity-based HER.)

inventory does not make anatomical assumptions based on an individual's sex or gender. Instead, it eliminates the need to make such assumptions by providing a structured format to document organs that are present or absent. Currently, the availability of an anatomical inventory as a standardized

form varies by EHR vendor. If an anatomical inventory form is unavailable, some EHR systems permit the use of custom forms or templates that allow an organization to develop its own organ inventory form.

The anatomical inventory should include the following organs: breasts/chest, cervix, ovaries, penis, prostate, testes, urethra, uterus, and vagina. A detailed list of conditions and surgeries is provided for each organ with a corresponding checkbox for each option. Ideally, each of these conditions and surgeries is associated with a code from the 10th revision of the International Statistical Classification of Diseases and Related Health Problems (ICD-10). Using the ICD-10's comprehensive, systematized, and widely understood documentation method and value sets in the anatomical inventory process contributes to the consistency of information and helps maintain quality in clinical practice.

Ideally, anatomical inventory data are captured in discreet data fields that are stored in problem lists and surgical histories. Conveniently, data stored in problem lists can be used in clinical decision support tools and for billing or coding purposes. Using these data in billing claims can justify why a procedure was or was not done for a patient. Using these data in clinical decision support allows for more accurate recommendations regarding screening interventions or procedures a patient may need.

Anatomical inventories should be updated as necessary to ensure that each patient receives all recommended preventive screening tests. For example, a **trans masculine** person may retain a cervix and need cervical cancer screening. Cultural sensitivity to unique barriers to these screenings is important, such as adopting a trauma-informed and gender-affirming approach during conversations about cervical cancer screening with trans masculine patients (as discussed in Chapter 11, "Basic Principles of Trauma-Informed Care") while emphasizing the importance of regular screening based on a current anatomical inventory.

▶ Clinical Decision Support Tools

Clinical decision support (CDS) is a function within EHRs that uses available data to alert care teams about potential health risks, provide recommendations to the clinical team and patients on services that are due, and suggest ways to reduce costs. The goal of these tools is to improve health outcomes. Historically, individual health care organizations have maintained CDS by building rules manually within each of their EHRs as evidence-based guidelines evolve or new guidelines are added. This manual process requires expertise, time, and resources, which may hamper the standardized and timely implementation of CDS and decrease adherence to clinical guidelines. Currently, a variety of CDS tools are available from vendors that can be integrated into existing EHRs. These tools provide care teams with timely recommendations to improve health outcomes based on various patient-level criteria, which typically include age, sex, and health history. A technical challenge related to CDS tools is the required manual oversight of alert mismatches, which increases the burden on both network and clinical site staff due to the extra time needed to review and resolve alert mismatches identified by the system. Increasingly, EHR vendors are providing more routine updates to CDS systems so that individual health care organizations do not need to maintain these alert and recommendation triggering systems in-house.

CDS systems do not typically include gender identity, sex assigned at birth, or anatomical inventory data within their clinical decision algorithms. One of the reasons that TGD patients may not receive the correct procedures is that CDS systems base recommendations on the administrative sex field only. When anatomical inventory information is integrated into CDS systems, the accuracy of recommendations increases dramatically (Figure 4-6). Systems that can automate this process have a significant benefit for clinicians, and ultimately for patient outcomes. Although large-scale studies of the impact on health outcomes of incorporating gender identity data into CDS tools do not yet exist, our health center's experience is that these systems can lead to improved quality of care, reduced clinician and data utilization burden, and decreased fragmentation of patient information within the EHR system.

DATA QUALITY AND REPORTING

Maintaining updated patient information is critical in providing the most culturally responsive care. Routine and standardized collection of information in EHRs help assess access to, satisfaction with, and quality of care; inform the delivery of appropriate health services; and begin to address health inequities. Updating of name used, pronouns, current gender identity, and sex assigned at birth should be done at least annually, as these are dynamic demographic variables that may change over time. Optimally, gender identity data should be collected and stored in the EHR, similar to a vital sign for which data are tracked over time and not overwritten. Health care organizations should also translate questions for patients best served in a language other than English and should add or change categories to ensure culturally and linguistically tailored terminology.

High-quality data are necessary to conduct population health management and address health inequities. Data quality is evaluated based on validity, completeness, accuracy, and timeliness. Validity is the degree of correctness and reasonableness of the data. Completeness is the measure of how many recorded responses are in a given EHR field. Evaluating accuracy involves checking for abnormal values. Timeliness is the degree to which EHR information is kept current. Differentiating between questions not being asked, responses not being entered, and patients choosing not to

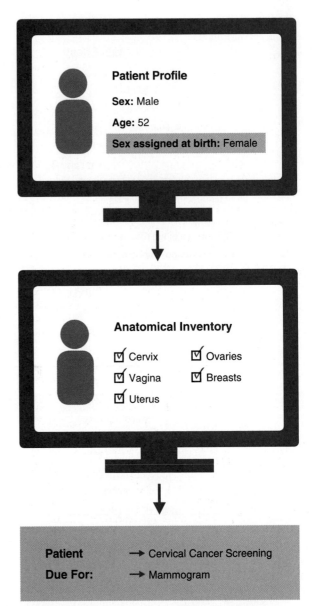

▲ **Figure 4-6.** Clinical decision support. Collection of current gender identity, sex assigned at birth, and anatomical inventory data to generate clinical decision support related to cervical cancer screening and mammogram for a trans masculine patient.

disclose information allows health care organizations to determine why specific data may be missing. Understanding patterns of missing data reveals both staff training issues and data integrity issues. Limited studies suggest that health care professionals do not routinely ask gender identity questions.[1]

Listed below are some sample questions to examine the data quality in your organization:

- Are you able to differentiate between refused and not entered values?

- Are staff entering the data into the correct fields? Are there response categories that do not belong in that field? For example, are current gender identity and sex assigned at birth responses being entered incorrectly in the same field?

- How does the accuracy of gender identity data compare with the accuracy of other data being collected at the same visit (e.g., race, ethnicity, income)?

- Are you observing trends in missing data relative to other demographic factors (e.g., age, country of birth, gender, race, ethnicity, language, facility location)?

- How does data completeness compare across different clinic locations or health care professionals?

- What is the frequency of gender identity data updates at the health care organization?

- Are there varying trends in gender identity data collection over time? Is there a sudden drop or spike at specific time points?

A common mistake in querying and reporting patient data is to rely on gender identity alone to identify TGD patients. As discussed in previous chapters, not all people whose sex assigned at birth and current gender identity are not aligned based on traditional expectations identify with the term *transgender*. Asking patients about both sex assigned at birth and current gender identity increases the accuracy of TGD patient data.

Health care organizations and EHRs must also consider the intersecting identities and experiences of TGD patients to understand the cumulative discrimination and nuanced health inequities these diverse communities face (see Chapter 21, "Transgender and Gender Diverse People Who Are Black, Indigenous, and People of Color"). When data are combined, it may be difficult to identify problem areas. Stratifying TGD identities based on other demographic data (e.g., race, ethnicity) can be used to evaluate service utilization and health outcomes for patient subpopulations. An example of this method would be evaluating differences in response rates between TGD patients born in the United States and those who are not.

Routine reporting of TGD patient data to senior leadership and department directors is essential to enlist support in maintaining or addressing gaps in care. Opportunities for reporting can include summary reports, incorporating into existing reports or workgroups (e.g., a diabetes working group), presentations to senior management or all-staff meetings, and development of transgender dashboards. Integration of these data into existing workgroups reinforces the importance of evaluating health outcomes and contributes to ongoing meaningful utilization of these data. Additionally, comparing health outcomes of **cisgender** patients with those of TGD patients can identify disparities in the overall patient population. For example, comparing the rates of prostate-specific antigen (PSA) testing in cisgender patients with a prostate versus TGD patients with a prostate may reveal important disparities.

POPULATION HEALTH MANAGEMENT

Pay-for-performance (P4P) or value-based (VB) program policies provide financial incentives to health care organizations based on quality and cost measures. The expectation is that the P4P/VB improves quality and reduces cost. P4P/VB programs are based on nationally recognized quality measures, such as the Healthcare Effectiveness Data and Information Set (HEDIS). Many of these measures exclude TGD people because they are currently sex-based, not anatomy-based. For example, the cervical cancer screening measure defines the cohort as "women 21–64 years of age"; however, a trans masculine person may still retain a cervix and would effectively be excluded from this measure.

As a result of increasing demands from various federal initiatives, P4P, and global contracts, it is becoming difficult for clinicians to keep track of the specifics of each measure to meet these requirements. As a result, care teams are relying increasingly on population health management tools to advise them. Frequently, individuals are grouped based on specific health conditions or preventive screening needs. These tools are utilized by clinical teams to monitor outcomes and provide actionable insights for care delivery. Population health management tools are developed to align with P4P/VB measures and therefore use the same national measures that currently exclude TGD people.

Similar to CDS, most off-the-shelf population health management tools do not incorporate essential data fields such as gender identity, sex assigned at birth, or an anatomical inventory. Some vendors of these tools allow customizations to incorporate these fields into their tools in order to identify and serve TGD patients more accurately. Accuracy of information is critical for categorizing patients correctly. An alert that recommends a procedure for a patient that is not appropriate for them may be just as detrimental as an alert that fails to recommend a needed procedure. For example, while patients with a retained cervix require cervical cancer screening, if a patient does not have a cervix, it would at best be irrelevant and at worst, offensive to contact them regarding an overdue cervical Pap test. Using both anatomical inventories (e.g., indicating that a cervix is not retained) and ICD-10 code data (e.g., for "agenesis of cervix") can assist in identifying patients correctly.

Additionally, some systems integrate features that automate secure email or text outreach to patients when necessary. When outreaching to patients, a key principle is to be cognizant of the name and pronouns the patient goes by outside the health care organization within their broader community, which may differ from the patient's chosen name and pronouns within the health care organization. This consideration also applies when receiving or sending health records externally. It is critical to ask the patient and not assume that their name and pronouns are necessarily the same in all settings. Because most EHR systems do not have a designated field to indicate this contextual variability in name and pronouns for a given patient, organizations need to develop a notification system, such as using alerts, to store this contextual information for each patient. Ideally, this information should be saved in a separate field that can be automatically queried for retrieval.

Accurate gender identity data can be used to measure and track health outcomes at the population level and give organizations more significant insights into the needs and disparities of the TGD communities they serve. Since population health management tools do not have modules specific to TGD health outcomes, the development of additional dashboards can address this gap. Developing a transgender health dashboard provides a condensed and comprehensive analytical tool that can include aggregate data and visual reports of key performance indicators. Executives, managers, and clinicians within health systems rely on dashboards to provide critical information to support data-driven decisions. Presenting metrics in a dashboard makes the information easier to understand, allows viewers to track progress and barriers, and offers a high-level snapshot of how an organization is meeting the health needs of TGD communities. Suggested metrics include the number of new and returning patients; demographics (e.g., age categories, race, ethnicity); number of patients by service and clinician panel; number of patients on gender-affirming hormones; rate of behavioral health screenings (e.g., depression, anxiety, substance use, tobacco); common comorbidities (e.g., diabetes, hypertension, HIV); and preventative screenings (e.g., cervical cancer, breast/chest cancer, colon cancer) (Figure 4-7).

Routine preventative care can significantly reduce health disparities. Health care is increasingly turning to technology to improve systems and processes to benefit patients and their health. EHRs and HIT tools have greatly improved the ability to track clinical markers for patients and improve health outcomes by collecting and storing data in standardized, structured formats that can be combined with data sources and used to evaluate clinical activities. Despite these advancements, there continue to be gaps and opportunities for improvement to develop systems for managing clinical information and ensuring that patients get the care and screening tests they need. Systems that can inclusively process expanded gender identity and anatomical

	Previous Year: 2018	YTD: 2019	Q1 (JAN-MAR)	Q2 (APR-JUN)
HORMONES by Insurance Sex				
Sex listed as male				
% on hormones				
Sex listed as female				
% on hormones				
Sex listed as unknown				
% on hormones				
HORMONES by type				
# on any hormones				
% on testosterone				
% on estradiol/progesterone				
% on antiandrogens				
% on puberty blockers				
PAP Tests				
# Patients 23 and older				
Anal or Cervical PAP within last 3 years				
Anal PAP within last 3 years				
Cervical PAP within last 3 years				
COMORBIDITIES				
HIV+				
Diabetes				
Depression/Mood Disorders				
Anxiety disorders including PTSD				
SMOKING				
Patients who are current smokers				
Current smokers who received smoking cessation counseling				

▲ **Figure 4-7.** Sample transgender health dashboard from Fenway Health showing performance on key primary care measures pertaining to transgender and gender diverse health.

inventory fields, track outcomes, and automate recommendations can have a major positive impact on clinical decisions, and ultimately, patient outcomes within TGD communities. These improvements allow care teams to accurately determine patients' health needs and thus allow patients to receive tailored care that is more gender-affirming, timely, and cost-effective.

SUMMARY

- Electronic health records (EHRs) and health information technology (HIT) are important tools for managing quality of care, particularly for invisible/hidden populations.

- Routine and standardized collection of patient information regarding name used, pronouns, current gender identity, and sex assigned at birth in EHRs enhances assessment of, access to, and satisfaction with quality of care. Collection of these data informs the delivery of appropriate health services and helps address health disparities. These elements should be included as standard demographic variables and collected at least annually.

- An anatomical inventory is imperative to document a person's organs and improves health outcomes by more accurately identifying appropriate types and timing of routine screening tests and procedures for each patient.

- Clinical decision support (CDS) tools can improve clinical care by determining when patients should receive recommended preventive screening tests. These tools should be reviewed periodically and can be customized within the EHR.

- Transgender patient dashboards provide an overview of important patient metrics as a way to engage in longitudinal population health management and continuous quality improvement for TGD populations.

CASE STUDY: Rodrigo

Rodrigo scheduled an appointment and presented at the clinic with pain. Since Rodrigo was a new patient for Dr. Becks, the physician assistant reviewed the patient's chart in advance of the appointment and noticed that Rodrigo was listed as a 40-year-old male. Rodrigo was brought back to the exam room by the medical assistant, who proceeded to obtain his vital signs and enter this information into the EHR. The medical assistant asked Rodrigo to provide more specific details about the location of the pain. Rodrigo explained that the pain was in the lower abdominal area but declined to provide any more details. The medical assistant entered the information and said that Dr. Becks would be in shortly.

Upon entering the exam room, Dr. Becks greeted Rodrigo and began completing the clinical review of systems. Dr. Becks asked, "Can you describe the pain and any additional symptoms?" Rodrigo replied reluctantly, "I've been having

pain in my pelvic area and am bleeding there." Dr. Becks noticed that the current gender identity and sex assigned at birth questions were not answered. She asked, "I noticed that you didn't answer the current gender identity or sex assigned at birth questions. Would you tell me what your gender identity is?" Rodrigo replied, "I'm a trans man." Dr. Becks replied, "Thank you. And can you tell me what your sex assigned at birth was?" Rodrigo hesitantly replied, "Female." Dr. Becks thanked the patient and asked if she could perform a pelvic exam. She performed a trauma-informed exam, which revealed that Rodrigo retained a cervix. Dr. Becks documented this physical exam finding in the anatomical inventory form in Rodrigo's chart. Cervical cancer screening was performed; cytology revealed a high-grade intraepithelial lesion and human papillomavirus testing was positive for high-risk HPV. Rodrigo subsequently underwent a colposcopy and biopsy, which revealed that he had cervical cancer.

▶ Discussion Questions

- Why might Rodrigo have been hesitant to provide specific details about his pain when making the appointment? When talking with the medical assistant?

- Why was it important for Dr. Becks to ask Rodrigo about his current gender identity and sex assigned at birth?

- Why might past clinicians never have recommended cervical cancer screening for Rodrigo?

- How could a clinical decision support tool prevent this from happening with other patients?

- How is the use of an anatomical inventory form useful in this situation?

REFERENCES

1. Haider A, Adler RR, Schneider E, et al. Assessment of patient-centered approaches to collect sexual orientation and gender identity information in the Emergency Department: the EQUALITY study. *JAMA Netw Open.* 2018;1(8):e186506.
2. Cahill S, Singal R, Grasso C, et al. Do ask, do tell: high levels of acceptability by patients of routine collection of sexual orientation and gender identity data in four diverse American community health centers. *PLoS One.* 2014;9(9):e107104.
3. Rullo JE, Foxen JL, Griffin JM, et al. Patient acceptance of sexual orientation and gender identity questions on intake forms in outpatient clinics: a pragmatic randomized multisite trial. *Health Serv Res.* 2018;53(5):3790-3808.
4. Ready, Set, Go! Guidelines and Tips For Collecting Patient Data on Sexual Orientation and Gender Identity (SOGI)—2020 Update. Published June 26, 2020. LGBTQIA+ Health Education Center. LGBTQIA+ Health Education Center. https://www.lgbtqiahealtheducation.org/publication/ready-set-go-guidelines-tips-collecting-patient-data-sexual-orientation-gender-identity/.

5. Grasso C, McDowell MJ, Goldhammer H, Keuroghlian AS. Planning and implementing sexual orientation and gender identity data collection in electronic health records. *J Am Med Inform Assoc.* 2019;26(1):66-70.

6. Grasso C, Goldhammer H, Funk D, et al. Required Sexual Orientation and Gender Identity Reporting by US Health Centers: First-Year Data. *Am J Public Health.* 2019;109(8):1111-1118.

7. Goldhammer H, Malina S, Keuroghlian AS. Communicating with patients who have nonbinary gender identities. *Ann Fam Med.* 2018;16(6):559-562.

8. McDowell MJ, Goldhammer H, Potter JE, Keuroghlian AS. Strategies to mitigate clinician implicit bias against sexual and gender minority patients. *Psychosomatics.* 2020;61(6):655-661.

Gender Identity Emergence and Affirmation in Adults

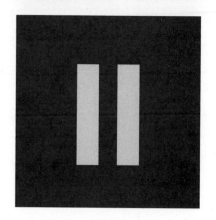

Gender Identity Emergence and Affirmation in Adults

Meredith Walker

Meghan McGrath

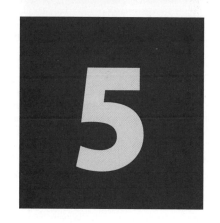

INTRODUCTION

Among those who are transgender or gender diverse, the process of **gender emergence,** or "coming out," is defined as the experience of becoming self-aware or the act of disclosing to others that one is **transgender or gender diverse (TGD).** This developmental process involves both recognizing and accepting one's identity as a transgender or gender diverse person and achieving a state of readiness to present this identity to others both publicly and privately.

Health care professionals can play a supportive role in the lives of their patients who identify or are beginning to identify as TGD in multiple ways. This chapter explores the nuance of **gender identity** emergence in adulthood, addresses various pathways toward **gender affirmation,** and speaks to relevant clinical considerations for practitioners. In caring for this population, health care professionals must confront their own unconscious and conscious biases. Such biases may affect clinicians' interactions with TGD CLIENTS? therefore steps must be taken to overcome these internalized assumptions. It is also important for health care professionals to recognize that their TGD patients are unique individuals, with varied histories, experiences, and backgrounds. No one pathway for coming out fits all people.

OVERVIEW OF TRAUMA-INFORMED CARE

Given the history of pathologizing gender diversity and gatekeeping of gender-affirming care within the medical and behavioral health fields, many TGD people will present to care with a history of previous unsatisfactory or outright traumatic experiences.[1] Such experiences can cause patients to feel trepidation, anger, sadness, or other emotions about not only the clinician but also the health care system as a whole. In addition, experiences in which the patient has had to educate their clinicians can be a consideration in their access to care, as "many [TGD] people are forced into

the role of educating their clinicians about the medical and emotional needs of [TGD] individuals, while also correcting misinformation and combating stigma and bias."[1] It can be exhausting and may drive people away from care when they have to educate a medical or mental health professional about gender identity and care. Further, it can negatively impact clients' ability to trust clinicians, engage in treatment, and can detract from time spent delivering key therapeutic interventions.

To provide the best care for their patients, clinicians must appreciate the adverse historical impact of medical and behavioral health professions on adult TGD patients and demonstrate accountability in current interactions with adult TGD patients. Chapter 11, "Principles of Trauma-Informed and Gender-Affirming Care," reviews the basic principles of offering care that acknowledges the burden of trauma that many TGD patients bring to health care encounters, but also acknowledges the inherent strengths and resilience that allow people to recover and heal. **Trauma-informed care** involves asking for and using a patient's correct pronouns and names, respecting their right to self-determination with regard to identifying as TGD, and supporting them in exploring their gender identity and expression, such as facilitating them coming to clinical sessions dressed to reflect a new gender expression (or even changing upon arrival). It is assumed throughout this chapter on gender emergence that readers are familiar with trauma-informed care; if not, Chapter 11 offers a thorough introduction to the topic.

CONSIDERATIONS SPECIFIC TO GENDER IDENTITY EMERGENCE IN ADULTHOOD

Coming out as a transgender person not only involves revealing one's inner sense of self, but may also entail changes in appearance, social and personal roles, and, sometimes, physical anatomy.[2] Many people think of coming out as a linear process that starts with self-questioning and culminates in the assimilation of a specific gender identity. However, coming out is seldom so straightforward. It more often proceeds as a series of steps or tasks toward self-acceptance and growth as new life events trigger a re-examination of one's identity and one's place in the world.[3] For TGD people, coming out may involve experimentation with a spectrum of gender expressions to find one that accurately expresses their inner experience of gender identity.

The process by which a person becomes self-aware of their gender identity is as varied as each individual. Many influences shape the coming out process (Figure 5-1), resulting in a wide variety of experiences for both the person coming out and those in whom the person confides. Health care professionals can help their patients clarify the reasons they want to come out, the ways in which coming out can be accomplished, and how to anticipate and respond to the possible reactions to their disclosure by the people to whom they chose to come out.[2]

For some, gender emergence in adulthood (for the purposes of this chapter, defined as age 25 years and older) can seem like a welcome unveiling of an aspect of themselves that was hidden or repressed yet ever-present.

Phoebe, a 52-year-old trans woman, comes out as her youngest child prepares to enter college. Although internally she identified as a girl from childhood on, she married her high school sweetheart and had a family. Phoebe explains, "I've always known, but I do love my wife, and I honestly never imagined I could come out."

For others, it is akin to learning a new language and finally being able to express what had not been tangible or identified before.

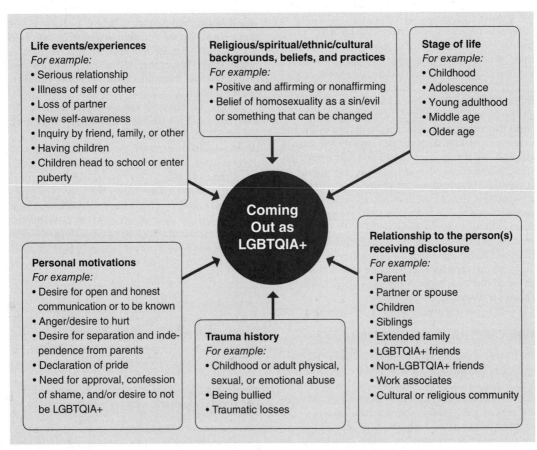

▲ **Figure 5-1.** Influences on the coming out experience. (Reproduced with permission from Makadon HJ, Mayer KH, Potter J, et al: *The Fenway Guide to Lesbian, Gay, Bisexual, and Transgender Health*, 2nd ed. Philadelphia, PA: The American College of Physicians; 2015.)

River, a 38-year-old, comes out after seeing a **nonbinary** character on a TV show their niece was watching. After searching online and finding terms, narratives, and community, they feel they have finally found an experience that resonates with their own. When asked to describe their gender identity, River states, "I am both masculine and feminine and it is super liberating to realize I don't have to force or contort myself into being one or the other."

Awareness can build on both physical and emotional levels, prompted by social interactions, personal reflection, media/cultural exposure, spiritual exploration, or physical experiences and sensations. In some cases, awareness leads to a sense of urgency and eagerness to proceed with various pathways to gender affirmation; in others, it prompts an exploration into the potential ramifications of these revelations, which can be fraught with fear and uncertainty.

Annie, a 43-year-old trans woman with a **cisgender** wife and 13-year-old son has just come out to her family and wants to come out rapidly in other spaces as well. She notes, "I am so excited and want to move forward as quickly as I can. I want to be me, the real me." She asks to schedule multiple appointments as soon as possible to discuss next steps.

Miriam, a 39-year-old divorced trans woman, cries as she describes the intense loneliness she experiences, difficulty she has been having with dating, and her fears about being alone as she ages. She mourns what she believes is the loss of her chance to have a biological family in her 20s or 30s, or to parent in her affirmed gender. Miriam reports, "Coming out has been scary at times and, though I truly want and need to be honest with myself and those I love, it is hard sometimes."

Feelings of regret or longing may appear when people consider what could have been had they been able to come out sooner in life or have different options available to them earlier.

The previous descriptions of the coming out process assume that the person is making these changes of their own volition and has chosen the timing for acknowledging their gender identity. However, some TGD people are forced "out" by their nontraditional gender presentation or during the affirmation process.[2]

Tucker, a 40-year-old trans masculine person, has started gender-affirming hormone therapy (GAHT) and begun to experience the growth of facial hair and the deepening of his voice. He both attends and volunteers at a church where other members have begun to notice the changes. He recently overheard a fellow church member laughing at a transphobic joke told by another member who then looked to Tucker and insulted his manhood. Tucker notes, "I'm proud of who I am and who I am becoming but I am still struggling. If I'm being honest, I'm not sure I know how to keep living like this or if I want to."

Being "**outed**" is a violation of privacy and consent, and it can have profound detrimental effects on a person, including harassment, discrimination, violence, and self-harm.[4] Health care professionals should be aware of the possibility of forced outing and help their patients by offering referrals and support. Practitioners should also be alert to the risk of suicide in such patients and provide comprehensive assessment and management of this risk.

▶ Implications of Coming Out for Adults

Many TGD individuals who come out as adults may have considered the daunting implications in the past and rejected affirmation because it seemed too overwhelming. Many fear the loss of existing support, which can have a negative impact on the quality of life while and after a person comes out.[5] A person who comes out in adulthood contends not only with their own personal identity but also with the prospect of introducing this new identity to others in their lives. For example, how will one's friends and family feel about one's affirming pronouns or a new name?

Vaughn, a 34-year-old trans man who recently changed his name and began using male pronouns, worries about coming out to his politically and religiously conservative grandfather. Vaughn shares that he "put a lot of time and thought into finding a name that really feels like it fits me." Additionally, he worries about confusing his grandmother, who has dementia.

For partners, what does gender affirmation mean for sexual orientation identity and sexual intimacy within the relationship?

Joia, a 25-year-old cisgender lesbian woman, uses individual therapy and a partner support group to explore the struggles she has been having with physical intimacy as she adjusts to the changes in her partner Jason's body. She struggles with how to name her sexual identity—wanting to honor both herself individually and be respectful to her partner—and wonders, "I've been an out and proud lesbian since adolescence but Jason is a man, and I love him, so where does that leave me?"

In addition to wondering about their own sexual orientation, "partners may also be overwhelmed by a host of other affirmation-related factors, which may include trying to see their partner in a new way, using different names and pronouns with their partners, and navigating new gender roles, expectations, and/or sexual repertoires."[6]

Uli, a 29-year-old nonbinary individual, is using **neopronouns**, while zir partner uses they/them. Uli names some sadness that zir dysphoria has been intense lately, while zir partner's libido has increased, leading to difficult conversations about physical intimacy, expectations, and the consideration of polyamory. Zi presents asking, "Can our relationship actually survive us both affirming our genders?

Having to consider some or all of these aspects of life change can bring up feelings of resentment, longing, and wonder about "what could have been" had patients been cisgender or had access to gender-affirming care earlier in life. It can also lead to feelings of excitement, a sense of urgency or desire for validation, and gratification related to a life goal long sought, consciously or otherwise.

Clinicians who hold space for and explore the multitude of options and potential affective reactions of patients coming out in adulthood are best positioned to support adjustment and improvement in mental health. Maintaining up-to-date knowledge of best practices is crucial, as is remaining humble, which allows patients to be the experts on their own experiences, free to share openly about their needs and desired path forward. Referral to a mental health professional with expertise in providing therapeutic support for TGD individuals contemplating coming out, while not something that should be mandated, can be invaluable. Psychotherapy can help TGD individuals clarify their gender identity, explore how stigma and trauma have impacted their mental health, and provide practical guidance about the coming out process. Mental health professionals can also collaborate with the patient's primary care provider to assess and treat mental health concerns, such as anxiety and depression.[7]

▶ Coping Mechanisms

Most people, whether they are transgender or **cisgender**, are subject to socially constructed internal and external pressures and narratives about gender, something especially true for those considering or experiencing gender affirmation in adulthood. Societal and personal expectations can lead to people concealing their gender identity out of concern for how coming out might impact them and those around them; "issues of stigma, rejection, and discrimination force many to live lives of inauthentic gender expression."[8]

Sami, 68, a trans woman, reports her awareness of her gender identity throughout her life though notes she feared acknowledging it. Her wife of 40 years passed away two years ago and since that time she has bought and worn more feminine clothing at home though she has not spoken of this to her two adult children. She presents to care with internal conflict between her lifelong dysphoria and worry about the further impact

coming out could have on her family life. Sami shares, "I want to move forward but I don't know if I could survive if my children don't accept me."

The stress of hiding one's gender identity and the sense of being "different" can lead to unhealthy behaviors, such as misuse of alcohol and drugs, overeating, sexual promiscuity, or other self-destructive behaviors.

Laverne, 63, internally identified as a woman from an early age but, due to her religious beliefs, worries about social stigma, and lack of access, did not pursue gender-affirming care until her mid-50s. For decades, she presented femme only when traveling for work, out at bars at night after conferences. Over the years, her drinking spiraled and she presents for care just after receiving a third DUI and acknowledges, "I've been using alcohol to not feel, to not have to face all this."

Another common coping strategy is social isolation, in which a person restricts their interactions with others, often out of fear that revealing their true selves will result in discrimination and victimization by family members, peers, and others. Self-isolation is often used by teenagers and young adults who lack affirming support, but it can contribute to anxiety, depression, or suicidal ideation.

Eli, a 27yo trans man, lives in the Northeast and has just moved in with three cisgender male roommates. GAHT has dropped his voice to a low register, broadened his shoulders, and led to a full beard, but he still wonders what to say when asked where he got his undergraduate degree, as he attended a women's college pre-gender-affirmation. As such, he finds himself staying in his room and avoiding conversations entirely. Eli adds, "I'm so proud of who I am but I don't necessarily want to have such a personal conversation with everyone who asks, which happens a lot around here."

In coming out, many adults who used such coping mechanisms during adolescence may feel a sense of deprivation or loss about the time they spent being isolated, confused, or hidden.

My'qel, a 26yo trans masculine person, feels sadness looking back at his youth and adolescence, stating "I never got to be the little boy I actually was. I was always feeling outside of things." He wonders what high school and college might have felt like had he been able to engage more authentically with peers at the time.

As Greenfield states, "health professionals should recognize that many [LGBTQIA+] clients require a 'catch-up period' in which to experience what was missed earlier." For

TGD people, this "catch-up" may include not only reclaiming an authentic gender expression but also experiences such as dating, sexual exploration, and connecting with the LGBTQIA+ community.

GENDER AFFIRMATION

Gender affirmation (formerly known as "transition") is the process of making social, legal, medical, or surgical changes to recognize, accept, and express one's gender identity. Current thinking related to gender affirmation, and the possible steps considered necessary for this option within health care, has evolved significantly over the years as the field has come to recognize that one size does not, indeed, fit all. The World Professional Association for Transgender Health,[7] an international, multidisciplinary, professional association dedicated to transgender health, has developed the now widely accepted Standards of Care (SOC). The overall goal of these standards is to provide clinical guidance for health professionals to assist transgender and gender-nonconforming people "with safe and effective pathways to achieving lasting personal comfort with their gendered selves, in order to maximize their overall health, psychological well-being, and self-fulfillment."[7]

The increasing prioritization of transgender health care has led to a broader range of gender-affirming interventions available to TGD individuals.[1] It is important to work with each individual, free of preconceived notions. People have different goals for gender affirmation. "Blending" means wanting not to be seen as transgender; this term is preferred by some over the term "passing," which implies deception.

Jamal, 34, says he's tired of feeling hypervigilant about how others might be perceiving him, reading their eye movements as they try to "figure me out." He dreams of a time when he blends "and no one gives me a second glance—when I'm not a trans man, just a man."

Others seek relief from **gender dysphoria**, defined as distress experienced by some people whose gender identity does not correspond with their sex assigned at birth.

Access to gender-affirming health care is critical for TGD individuals and can be not only affirming but life-saving. Gender dysphoria is common among TGD people. It is not a static state; rather, it can shift in focus and intensity over time. According to Lapinski et al, "Current medical, psychological, and social research has increasingly shown that, while being transgender is not a mental disorder or medical condition, gender dysphoria can be treated."[1] Treatment involves helping patients recognize their symptoms as separate from their identity and facilitating their path toward gender affirmation. If a patient can work toward affirming their gender identity, it can help resolve emotional distress. Despite the many barriers to accessing desired gender-affirmative health care, these options are crucial for TGD patients.

PATHWAYS TO GENDER AFFIRMATION

The three major categories of gender affirmation are non-medical/nonsurgical (reversible), hormonal (partially reversible), and surgical (irreversible). Within these broad categories are multiple pathways on the journey toward affirmation, which can, and should, be tailored to individual needs and desires. Moving toward gender affirmation is a highly personal and nuanced process for each individual.[8]

Historically, the path to gender affirmation was defined as a three-step process, or "triadic therapy," that began with real-life experience, followed by hormone therapy, and culminating in gender-confirming surgery.[9] This historical approach to the gender-affirmation timeline has likely impacted adult patients seeking care and may inform how they present their needs and wants. On their own or in some combination with each other, "all of these treatments can be used in an effort to relieve gender dysphoria by helping to align one's body with one's gender identity, allowing the individual to live and present in the world as the gender they authentically feel themselves to be."[10] Again, there is no universal treatment path that can, nor should, be applied to all TGD persons.

Some clinicians new to working within TGD health care default to thinking immediately of hormonal and surgical interventions when considering gender affirmation. However, it is important to validate each person's experience and to recognize that not all gender affirmation will necessarily require access to hormones or surgical procedures. "Health care professionals need to connect with their patients on an individual level regarding what (if any) medical interventions they desire, rather than making assumptions about what their patients desire as part of their transition [sic]."[1] Discussions focused on the specific goals a patient wishes to achieve with gender affirmation and their expectations can clarify the patient's needs. Clinicians also need to educate themselves about all of the options that are available and recognize that surgery does not necessarily need to be a part of a gender affirmation plan.

Hez, 37, identifies as trans and nonbinary and states, "I want to go on a dose of T just high enough to stop getting my period; that is the worst time for me with my dysphoria." They're comfortable with their voice dropping, but feel apathetic about other bodily changes.

Ines, 44, is a trans woman who has recently come out and notes she is "Really excited for my boobs to grow and for my skin and hair to get softer." She also shares of her hope to eventually access both facial feminization surgery and bottom surgery.

Kenzie, 63, is trans feminine and notes she is pleased with the way the fat has redistributed in her cheeks and body, her breast development, and the way she's able to style her hair. She states "that's all people react to, for me, and I like the rest of my parts so I don't need to do anything else for now."

Shazad, 49, initially came out as nonbinary and underwent top surgery after sharing with his provider his dysphoria was focused mostly on his chest and that binding was no longer feasible given his lengthy work days. About a year later he came in to discuss the possibility of starting hormones sharing, "I'm interested in the impacts T might have on the rest of my body" and acknowledging his gender identity has evolved toward trans masculine.

Finally, clinicians should be aware that there are a multitude of possible nonbinary gender identities and expressions.[9] Ultimately, the clinician and patient should work together to decide on a gender affirmation plan that improves a patient's quality of life and decreases gender dysphoria. Helping patients clarify their goals and expectations are integral to this decision process.

Gender affirmation on an individual level does not address the widespread discrimination, stigma, and health disparities that the TGD communities continue to experience.[10] Clinicians can help patients recognize their existing strengths and develop the skills necessary to cope with the social stigma and discrimination they experience as they pursue their authentic selves.

> Dal, a 39 year old trans man, has been on GAHT for almost a decade and had top surgery; he's socially out and pursues a job at a local agency as a trans advocate. He shares that he is "surprised at how much I want this job given the visibility of the role. Before that would have been way too much for me." He shares that he now feels confident about handling whatever comes his way and expresses passion about working with others in their gender-affirmation process.

Social Gender Affirmation

Nonmedical and nonsurgical steps toward social affirmation are often undertaken first, as individuals can make significant changes without accessing medical care or coming out. Further, such steps are generally reversible, which can help to ease or assuage possible initial ambivalence and fears. Social affirmation can include name and pronoun changes, legal sex/gender marker changes, changes in mode of dress, use of accessories, hairstyle changes, body hair removal, exercise or weightlifting, use of make-up and prosthetics, and chest binding (see Chapter 8, "Nonmedical, Nonsurgical Gender Affirmation").

> Stephen, 47, starts growing his hair and shaving his beard and has come out as trans feminine to his partner, around whom he feminizes other aspects of his presentation when they are together at home. As he further explores his gender identity, he asks his medical team to use female pronouns and the name "Marie" to see how it feels. A few months later, she decides to start a testosterone blocker.

As individuals consider making such initial changes toward presenting in a way that aligns their physical presentation with their gender identity, it can be useful for them to have access to behavioral health supports. In fact, according to the U.S. Transgender Survey, "more than three-quarters (77%) of respondents said they wanted counseling or therapy for their gender identity or gender transition [sic] at some point in their life."[11] Clinicians can provide support and serve as sources of information, guidance, and help when patients begin to consider the many elements of gender affirmation, including coming out in the workplace or navigating the shift in gender dynamics associated with intimate relationships.

Hormonal Gender Affirmation

Hormonal gender affirmation involves the use of GAHT as a means of altering an individual's physical presentation and secondary sex characteristics[10] (see Chapter 7, "Hormonal Gender Affirmation in Adults"). GAHT is generally considered partially reversible. GAHT often informs patients' or clients' choices related to social gender affirmation as physical changes progress and become noticeable. Access to behavioral health support when starting GAHT can be quite helpful, although it should not be mandated. Often as an individual begins to see increased alignment of their body with their gender identity, they experience relief from previously reported symptoms of depression, anxiety, and other mental health concerns.[10]

> Nic, a 36 year old trans man, notices his shoulders broadening and his musculature changing as he continues taking testosterone. He reports "feeling more comfortable in my own skin and I've realized I'm feeling less self-conscious in social situations which is a relief." He further shares of a decrease in hypervigilance, an increase in confidence talking to peers, and the cessation of self-injurious behavior.

Of note, shifts in individual sexual orientation, behaviors, and partner choice can also occur with the addition of GAHT.

Access to GAHT does not match the reported demand by TGD communities. According to the U.S. Transgender Survey, 78% of respondents want to receive hormone therapy at some point in their lives, but only 49% of respondents have ever received it. Ninety-two percent of those who have ever received hormone therapy are currently still receiving it, representing 44% of all respondents.[11]

▶ Surgical Affirmation

Surgical options are generally considered irreversible and encompass multiple procedures aimed at the "surgical augmentation of internal and external hormone and sex-related organs."[10] Many procedures are available, and it is important to remember that patients may choose to access some, none, or all according to their individual goals and comfort levels (see Chapter 9, "Surgical Gender Affirmation in Adults"). Options for feminizing procedures include nongenital, nonbreast procedures, such as thyroid cartilage reduction, facial feminization, and gluteal augmentation; breast augmentation; and genital surgery, including penectomy, orchiectomy, clitoroplasty, vulvoplasty, and vaginoplasty. Options for masculinizing procedures include breast procedures (mastectomy); genital procedures, including hysterectomy, salpingo-oophorectomy, metoidioplasty, and phalloplasty; and nongenital, nonbreast procedures, such as liposuction, pectoral implants, and other aesthetic procedures.[7] According to the U.S. Transgender Survey, 25% of respondents reported having had some form of gender-affirmation surgery, with transgender men (42%) being more likely to have had any kind of surgery than transgender women (28%) or nonbinary respondents (9%).[7]

▶ Counseling Patients about Hormonal and Surgical Gender Affirmation

For patients who are accessing GAHT, the role of the clinician can be significant as they begin experiencing the physical changes and mood fluctuations associated with this therapy and can also be helpful as they navigate shifts or changes in sexual orientation. Clinicians should appreciate each patient's unique experience with GAHT and serve as a source of support, information, and validation.

Starting GAHT or accessing other gender-affirming medical and surgical procedures in adulthood also has a different physical impact than when it is started earlier in life. In adulthood, TGD people have likely progressed through puberty, and gender-affirming interventions may take longer or be more numerous than if this person had not undergone endogenous puberty.

Medical conditions a person may have developed in adulthood, such as high blood pressure and obesity, can increase the risk of complications when starting GAHT or impact a person's readiness for surgery. Many surgeons have specific requirements due to the need for general anesthesia, specific recovery needs, and the known risks of undergoing surgery with certain comorbid medical diagnoses. Most of these things are not barriers proceeding with affirming care and procedures, but their presence may necessitate increased monitoring by care teams along the way. For example, it is recommended that patients stop smoking prior to starting GAHT and before pursuing surgery because of the known possible correlation with higher-risk medical comorbidities.[10]

With patients considering surgical interventions, the role of the clinician can involve providing psychoeducation, support, and, if the decision is to access surgery, surgical referral letters. As with any other surgical procedure in an adult person, clinicians should provide presurgical counseling about the likely physical and psychological effects of the surgery. In addition, given the known data related to isolation in the TGD community, clinicians should discuss with adult patients pursuing gender-affirming surgery the need for personal and community support during recovery[10,12] and help patients plan for recovery and aftercare.

Behavioral health clinicians may be required to speak to these topics when drafting surgical referral letters; however, it is important for clinicians to attend to these considerations throughout treatment, as they can impact a patient's experience of the world and of their body. One might use therapy to both explore the motivations for gender affirmation while also weighing the motivations in relation to other health concerns. A patient can work with a therapist to determine what changes are possible, what changes they're ready for, the right pace at which to make those changes, and how to adjust expectations accordingly. If everything a patient hopes for is not possible, the therapeutic work can involve radical acceptance of what is possible, strengths-based framing around what is accessible, and an exploration of how to move forward most vibrantly with whatever amount of affirmation is feasible. Additionally, if someone is of an age or health status where it is determined that affirming care is not an option, feelings of grief may be expected, and often a mourning process is necessary.

HELPING PATIENTS NAVIGATE THE COMING OUT PROCESS

Gender identity emergence in adulthood presents unique challenges. Many people have forged friendships, are in intimate relationships, and have established themselves professionally. The trappings of an adult life are understandably impacted by gender, and it is important for those who are coming out to anticipate and adapt to the many changes they might expect to navigate. Unlike most youth and young adults, adults coming to terms with gender identity emergence may have existing structures, supports, and systems to which they answer, potentially including a professional career or job, family, friends, children, and other social supports who know them a certain way. Coming out when one has established social relationships and obligations is very different than coming out prior to establishing these bonds. As patients consider the impact of their emerging gender identity on other aspects of their identity, including sexual orientation and practices, gender presentation, and nomenclature (names and pronouns), it is important for health care professionals to consider how this emergence may affect a patient's family, friendships, and professional life.

Reed, a 29 year old agender individual, comes from a relatively conservative family of Italian heritage who live in New Hampshire. Reed's parents have been struggling to avoid the use of pronouns when Reed visits home, and Reed's mom, specifically, gets really defensive when Reed tries to remind her.

Heaven, a 36 year old trans woman, is thrilled when her teenage daughter wants to bond with her by going to get pedicures. Her younger daughter sees her toenails later that week and gets upset, saying, "Other dads don't do that!!"

Miguel, 41, and his partner go to their usual trivia night with their friends, a group of cisgender, queer- and lesbian-identified women. On the way in the bouncer takes them to be a straight couple and says something casually denigrating about their group of friends. Miguel and his partner have a heated discussion later about what it feels like to be perceived to be "straight passing" and the impact on them as individuals as well as their community.

▶ Dating

Intimate relationships can pose a particular conundrum for TGD people coming out later in life (whether partnered previously or not). Numerous social norms are associated with dating practices, most of them gendered, and adapting to these can feel like learning a new language. Navigating one's relationship with one's own body and then inviting another person, or persons, to navigate these changes can lead to anxiety or excitement. Dysphoria can be triggered that sometimes interferes with one's ability to be physically intimate.

Erik, a 47 year old trans man, has been on GAHT for 10 years, underwent both a hysterectomy and top surgery, and is currently readying for bottom surgery. He still becomes overwhelmed by dysphoria when his partner touches him intimately and shares, "I can't really be touched like that pretty much anywhere on my body. I end up wondering what he's thinking and wishing my body could be different, and then, a lot of times I dissociate." He notes that, as a result, he and his partner haven't had sex in 8 months.

Flora, 63, hasn't dated since before she married her now ex-wife. She goes on dating Apps for the first time and isn't sure how much to disclose about herself and when, or even how to define herself to others. She feels anxious about whether she'll find someone.

The pressure dating adds to disclosing how one relates to their body—and subsequently one's medical and surgical history—can sometimes lead to a sense of resentment at having to think about gender and physical intimacy at all. Research has shown that "throughout different components of transitioning [sic], sexual orientation can change."[10] Not only is a person experiencing new dating issues with regard to gender, they must also contend with sexual orientation and all the social mores that come along with it.

Gray, 43, a trans man, notices his libido surge as he continues on testosterone, which he notes is "both distracting and exciting."

Naomi, 51, a trans woman, notices a decrease in libido as she continues on estrogen and testosterone blockers; it takes her longer to orgasm, and the sensations in her body are different. She remarks, "I'm not sure about sex right now because I'm not as clear about how my body will react."

As a result of these pressures, "rejection is a common outcome… it can lead the trans person to feel shame, unworthiness, depression, and anxiety."[6]

Lo, 47, has recently reentered the world of online dating and finds himself reeling upon receipt of a harsh and rejecting message on Grindr after he discloses his transgender identity. He starts to notice profiles which name types of people the profile owner is not interested in meeting.

A clinician's task is to bear witness to, affirm, and validate a person's identity exploration as they develop confidence in asserting newly identified facets of themselves in the world.

▶ The Workplace

Many adult TGD patients already have a professional career and identity, which means another forum in which to consider the implications of coming out and the impact of gender affirmation. Some plan to come out and stay in their current job and industry and therefore need to consider what it will mean to be around people who knew them before.

Willow, 49, a trans woman, works with the human resources department to determine a timeline for coming out at her tech company. She holds a meeting with direct reports, sends an email to others more far-reaching, and changes her name and pronouns, along with all usernames and other identifiers in the system. She expresses concern about her upcoming meetings with outside clients and wonders, "Will I need to remind people again and again?"

Others consider what it will be like to apply for jobs—an already often intimidating process—and what it may feel like to establish new professional relationships.

Shaun, 37, wonders what to do as far as updating his resume and, specifically his references—some of whom he hasn't been in touch with since before he came out as a trans man. He worries his publications will no longer be easily located by employers looking him up in advance of an interview. Shaun also expresses frustration that "due to the articles and chapters I've published I can't just leave the old name and identity in the past."

For some, coming out professionally can entail a level of objectification, which is unwelcome or feels overly scrutinizing. There can be uncertainty about supportiveness among colleagues, particularly if there are many staff in the workplace, and this can create anticipatory anxiety about job security, having to navigate the coming out process on logistical and emotional levels, and maintaining or losing a connection to one's prior work product. The latter is an issue for creative professionals, especially for those who have been published or known for certain work under a former name. For example, Hollywood director and writer Lilly Wachowski, who came out along with her sister after making a series of well-known films, has stated, "There's a critical eye being cast back on Lana and I's work through the lens of our transness. This is a cool thing because it's an excellent reminder that art is never static."[13] The reaction and receptivity of a human resources department and gender-inclusiveness of facilities at work are important considerations for those who have such supports. It can be helpful for clinicians to think through with patients whether they have access to private space at work to attend to postsurgical aftercare needs, such as dilation after vaginoplasty, or to help devise an alternate plan if they do not. Before coming out at work, it is important to determine whether a workplace has an antidiscrimination policy that includes gender, and if not, whether advocating for one is a possibility. For some, making gradual changes to appearance offers a way to test the waters of acceptance, whereas others may prefer to come out over an abbreviated timeframe. In the clinical realm, as with any major change in a person's life, therapy ought to entail thoughtful consideration of the anticipated change, motivation, preparation, and processing of associated affect. A clinician can help patients "skillfully facilitate disclosure planning... [and] determine [patients'] readiness to come out, as well as how safe it is to inform others of their transgender status and/or the decision to begin a medical or gender role transition [sic] process."[14] Many feelings can arise, including excitement, fear, and anticipated loss, and it is helpful to co-create space with patients to fully explore, if possible, these aspects of the decision to pursue gender affirmation.

▶ Generational Differences

Generational differences can also impact the timing of gender affirmation. Those from a generation taught to repress feelings or deprioritize one's own needs in the face of the responsibilities associated with one's gender assigned at birth might believe gender affirmation at an older age is "selfish" or "indulgent." Others may ask "what is the point?" of engaging in affirming care later in life. Patients may have endured negative prior experiences with medical professionals in a time or place that was less affirming of gender diversity and other aspects of identity, including race and socioeconomic status. Such experiences can impact how patients present currently and may have deterred them from pursuing care or added to anxiety about the kind of care they may receive if they are forthcoming about their identity. Research supports anecdotal experience that patients delay seeking health care—which is associated with poorer health outcomes—because of the fear of discrimination and cost barriers.[15]

> Max, 77, whose husband of 45 years passed away 10 years ago, began to pursue gender-affirming care within the last year. He notes that he has always dressed androgynously and "allowed everyone to think I was a tomboy because getting married and having babies was just what was expected." He reports feeling that he has lived his life according to expectations but that now it's "time for me to take care of me."

Clinicians should be aware of their own potential generational bias and also explore how a patient's age might impact the patient's experience and view. Engaging with a patient to understand what has influenced their life prior to pursuing gender affirmation can be validating for the patient and help the clinician build context for how they may be approaching decisions about care.

▶ Family Structure

Reproductive options are different for people whose gender identity emerges in adulthood. They may have already had biological children while living in, as opposed to identifying in, their gender assigned at birth, which can be associated with a variety of feelings and responsibilities. Their children can be expected to have their own feelings about a parent's gender affirmation, as can their child's other caretakers.

> Zayn, 50, didn't come out until after his kids were in college, having worried earlier in his life that having a trans dad would be too difficult for their family to navigate in addition to his single parent status and the various forms of related discrimination. It was difficult for him to manage his dysphoria throughout the years but he notices of his children, as he feels more affirmed, "Our relationships are improving and our connections feel deeper, genuine on both sides."

If the person has decided not to have children, the start of gender-affirming hormone therapy may feel challenging, as a discussion of reproduction and ways to preserve fertility are a part of the informed consent process.

Multiple resources are available for partners and family members of TGD people. These resources include peer support groups, meet-ups, readings, activities, political involvement, and more:

GenderSpectrum.org
HRC.org
LGBTMap.org
PFLAG.org
SAMHSA.gov
Transequality.org
Transgenderpartners.com

CJ, 28, a **genderqueer** individual using he-series pronouns, feels ready to start testosterone but wants to complete egg harvestation first "just in case" he ever wants to have access to having a biological child. He talks with his parents about how to pay for the storage fees, as that would be the most prohibitive factor for him. He names some feelings of resentment at "having to make these decisions now," and incurring the associated financial fees.

Much of the work for clinicians and patients specific to reproduction focuses on a combination of acceptance and adjustment. A therapeutic dyad might focus on adjustments to the pacing of gender affirmation to give a family member time to accept and adjust to gender affirmation–related changes and assess how it impacts them. Clinicians could focus on communication, constructive feedback, working through affective reactions to how others react to their gender affirmation process, and aspects of identity relating to family structure—nomenclature and familiar nicknames that may be gendered, for example. Anticipating these issues can help patients navigate them in real time in other relationships (Box 5-1).

▶ Financial Considerations

Financial resources and support are often a determining factor for gender affirmation, as many elements of social, medical, and surgical gender affirmation are predicated on access to care, which is often contingent upon finances and socioeconomic status. Meier et al notes, "common stressors… that may be sources of depression and anxiety include losing one's job… not having access to medically necessary transition [sic]-related medical interventions or routine health care, and financial strain."[6] Adults are sometimes better positioned to access affirmative care either by having insurance or the ability to pay out-of-pocket. However, some adults do not have adequate financial resources and may face

a longer timeline before they can access care, which may feel challenging if "blending" or "passing" is an immediate goal. Some adults may opt to wait "until [they] have everything figured out," and it can be important to explore these expectations with them.

Brent, a 52 year old trans man, wants to wait until he has saved enough money to pay for top surgery out of pocket as his insurance plan doesn't cover it. He delays starting HRT, though, since he wants to come out to his family "all at once" and worries that they might challenge him if they started to notice any changes.

Waiting to acquire the financial resources to afford medical or surgical gender affirmation can be frustrating. Clinicians can work with patients to build frustration tolerance (i.e., the ability to wait and to endure suboptimal conditions by making them manageable with smaller adjustments or steps forward), and even, potentially, to process grief. Highlighting existing strengths, resources, and capacities with patients can provide a constructive focus that enables them to determine what can be done and achieved despite existing barriers to accessing gender-affirming care. Health care professionals can also help patients look forward by identifying realistic future goals and delineating the next steps that are needed to take place in order to achieve these.

SUMMARY

- "Coming out," also called gender emergence, is defined as the experience of becoming self-aware or the act of disclosing to others that one is transgender or gender diverse (TGD). Health care professionals can play a supportive role in the lives of their patients who identify or are beginning to identify as TGD in many ways.

- Primary care providers should recognize that many TGD patients have experienced trauma and stigma during past encounters with medical and mental health care. Clinicians should demonstrate accountability and incorporate the principles of trauma-informed care in their interactions with TGD patients.

- There is no one pathway to coming out that fits all TGD people. The journey to self-acceptance and gender affirmation varies by individual. Primary care providers should also acknowledge that TGD patients may identify as one gender or may have a nonbinary identity. Clinicians should be prepared to explore the multitude of options and potential affective reactions of patients coming out in adulthood.

- Psychotherapy can help individuals clarify their gender identity, explore their symptoms of gender dysphoria, and help them to access reserves of strength and resilience. Mental health professionals can also collaborate with the primary care provider to assess and treat a patient's mental health conditions.

- Gender affirmation is the process of making social, legal, medical, or surgical changes to recognize, accept, and express one's gender identity. Primary care providers can play key roles in facilitating access to gender-affirmation services by providing education, guidance, counseling, and referrals.

- Primary care providers can help their TGD patients navigate the coming out process and offer support in many areas, such as dating, sexual relationships, and familial relationships.

CASE STUDY: OMID

Omid has just met with her primary care physician to discuss the start of gender-affirming hormone therapy and asks to use a feminine name and pronouns in appointments, though she hasn't started doing so in other areas of her life. Given her symptoms of anxiety and desire for more support in exploring the process of gender affirmation, her primary care practitioner refers her to the behavioral health specialist affiliated with the office. Able-bodied, in her mid-40s, of Middle Eastern descent but having lived in Europe and the United States for most of her adolescence and adult life, Omid is married to a cisgender woman with whom she has two teenagers. She endorses 1 year of sobriety from alcohol dependence after being arrested for driving under the influence. She states that her identity as a woman has recently "just clicked," but describes earlier feelings about gender identity as existing since childhood. Omid notes such earlier feelings were "compartmentalized" and something "to visit" on occasion, often under the influence; "I thought the only way I could be [me] was with alcohol." She reports memories as early as 6 years old of wanting to dress in her mother's clothing and a sense that something "wasn't quite right." She says, "I married a woman at about 22 and did my best to keep busy so I could forget about my identity." She tells you that she and her wife have a supportive relationship, though she titrated coming out carefully out of a sense of wanting "to have more of the answers first." She reported a change in self-acceptance, however, noting, "I'm feeling great, but I'm doing therapy to be sure I stay okay as I face all the change."

A couple years later, in a subsequent visit, Omid has undergone facial feminization surgery and requests another letter in support of vaginoplasty in the near future. She had come out to her children, parents, and siblings within a year of starting GAHT. At times, her children's initial discomfort slowed her planned timeline for change due to her desire to proceed with their support, which she described with frustration as "almost like they're thinking 'if I hold the covers over my head maybe it won't be true.'" In this appointment, Omid confides that she and her wife no longer have a sexual relationship, but she describes feeling closer to her than ever due to the increased honesty in communication as they have navigated her gender affirmation. She continues to wrestle with her shift in gender role and related privilege; for example, she notices she isn't always given space to speak in settings where she was previously afforded it, and wonders if this is due to societal sexism and privileging of maleness. She is currently sober and her anxious symptoms are well managed. Omid notes a sense that "being trans is a part of things but not my entire identity anymore—it's more in the background now."

▶ Discussion Questions

1. How do intersections of identity impact a person's recognition of their gender identity?

2. What are some of the challenges an adult endeavoring to affirm their gender may face?

3. What strategies can practitioners utilize to provide empowering experiences for people as they explore and accept their gender identities?

4. What community resources are available to support people who are experiencing gender identity emergence in adulthood?

REFERENCES

1. Kattari SK, Atteberry-Ash B, Kinney MK, Walls NE, Kattari L. One size does not fit all: differential transgender health experiences. *Soc Work Health Care.* 2019;58(9):899-917.

2. Greenfield J. Coming out: the process of forming a positive identity. In: Makadon HJ, Mayer KH, Potter J, Goldhammer H, eds. *The Fenway Guide to Lesbian, Gay, Bisexual, and Transgender Health.* 2nd ed. Philadelphia, PA: The American College of Physicians; 2015.

3. Weick A. A growth-task model of human development. *Social Casework.* 1983;64:131-137.

4. Schwartz AP, Fellow HL, National LGBTQ Task Force. Why outing can be deadly. https://www.thetaskforce.org/why-outing-can-be-deadly/. Accessed November 24, 2020.

5. Wylie K, Knudson G, Khan SI, Bonierbale M, Watanyusakul S, Baral S. Serving transgender people: clinical care considerations and service delivery models in transgender health. *Lancet.* 2016;388(10042):401-411.

6. Meier SC, Sharp C, Michonski J, Babcock JC, Fitzgerald K. Romantic relationships of female-to-male trans men: a descriptive study. *Int J Transgend.* 2013;14:75-85.

7. Coleman E, Bockting W, Botzer M, et al. Standards of care for the health of transsexual, transgender, and gender-nonconforming people. 7th ed. *Int J Transgend.* 2012; 13(4):165-232.

8. Alegria CA, Ballard-Reisch D. Gender expression as a reflection of identity reformation in couple partners following disclosure of male-to female transsexualism. *Int J Transgend.* 2013;14:49-65.

9. deMonteflores C. Notes on the management of difference. In: Stein TS, Cohen CJ, eds. *Contemporary Perspectives on Psychotherapy with Lesbians and Gay Men.* New York, NY: Plenum; 1986.

10. Lapinski J, Covas T, Perkins JM, et al. Best practices in transgender health: a clinician's guide. *Prim Care*. 2018;45(4):687-703.

11. James SE, Herman JL, Rankin S, Keisling M, Mottet L, Anafi M. The Report of the 2015 U.S. Transgender Survey. Washington, DC: National Center for Transgender Equality; 2016.

12. Amodeo AL, Vitelli R, Scandurra C, Picariello S, Valerio P. Adult attachment and transgender identity in the Italian context: clinical implications and suggestions for further research. *Int J Transgend*. 2015;16(1):49-61.

13. Lachenal J. Lilly Wachowski Acknowledges Re-Examination of The Matrix With Lens Focused on Transness. *The Marysue*. April 5, 2016. https://www.themarysue.com/the-matrix-trans-lens/.

14. Collazo A, Austin A, Craig SL. Facilitating transition among transgender clients: components of effective clinical practice. *Clin Soc Work J*. 2013; 41:228-237.

15. Reisner SL, White JM, Bradford JB, Mimiaga MJ. Transgender health disparities: comparing full cohort and nested matched-pair study designs in a community health center. *LGBT Health*. 2014;1(3):177-184.

Behavioral Health Considerations for Transgender and Gender Diverse People

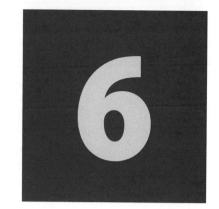

Aude Henin

Christine Darsney

Flavia Vaz De Souza

Hilary Goldhammer

Alex S. Keuroghlian

INTRODUCTION

There is increasing recognition that **transgender and gender diverse (TGD)** people have specific health care needs, including gender-affirming, evidence-based behavioral health care offered by trained, culturally responsive clinicians. Although TGD youth and adults experience a range of stressors related to their gender minority status and are at increased risk for various associated psychiatric and behavioral health problems, they experience numerous barriers to receiving appropriate behavioral health care.[1,2] This inequity is one reason for the disproportionate rates of mental health disorders, suicidality, substance use disorders, and functional impairments often reported in this population.

Historically, the field of psychiatry has often adopted a pathologizing stance toward TGD communities.[3-5] The 5th Edition of the *Diagnostic and Statistical Manual of Mental Disorders* (DSM-5) marked a diagnostic shift from "gender identity disorder" toward the relatively more affirming construct of **gender dysphoria.** However, this diagnostic evolution fell short of completely disentangling gender diversity from classification as a psychiatric disorder, which many TGD community advocates argue carries inherent pathologization, stigmatization, and an often false assumption of distress.[5]

Recent studies suggest that approximately 50% of gender minority adults meet diagnostic criteria for a psychiatric diagnosis, with more than one-fourth experiencing an anxiety disorder, more than one-third meeting criteria for major depression, 14–40% reporting a history of a suicide attempt, and 20% reporting a lifetime history of substance use disorder.[6-9] A large population survey of college students found that transgender people were more than twice as likely as their cisgender peers to have depression and anxiety diagnoses, self-injurious behaviors, suicidal ideation, and suicide attempts.[8] Thus, there remains a great need for evidence-based behavioral health interventions that are culturally sensitive to and tailored for TGD people.

The purpose of this chapter is to contextualize behavioral health inequities and needs among TGD people across diagnostic categories within a gender minority stress framework; propose culturally responsive tailoring of evidence-based behavioral health clinical practices; and offer strategies for building responsive, affirming, and effective behavioral health services for TGD communities, in order to optimize mental health outcomes.

GENDER IDENTITY CHANGE EFFORTS

Gender identity change efforts are psychological approaches that aim to change a person's **gender identity** to align with societal expectations based on their **sex assigned at birth.**[10] While these efforts are often referred to as "conversion therapy," we intentionally avoid this term as it falsely implies that these efforts constitute a legitimate clinical practice rather than a form of harmful discrimination rooted in societal stigma and transphobia. Approximately 13.5% of TGD people in the United States report a lifetime exposure to these efforts, amounting to an estimated 188,000 TGD U.S. adults.[10] One study with a large national sample of U.S. TGD adults found that recalled lifetime exposure to gender identity change efforts is associated with more than twofold increased odds of a lifetime suicide attempt.[11] In the same study, recalled exposure to gender identity change efforts before age 10 was associated with more than fourfold increased odds of lifetime suicide attempts. Interestingly, there was no significant difference in the odds of attempting suicide when comparing exposure to gender identity change efforts by secular professionals with exposure to change efforts by religious advisors. Several U.S. states have passed legislation banning gender identity change efforts, and several health professional organizations, such as the American Academy of Child & Adolescent Psychiatry, the American Academy of Pediatrics, the American Medical Association, and the American Psychiatric Association, have declared these practices ineffective and harmful to TGD people.[11]

MISINTERPRETING GENDER MINORITY STRESS AS PERSONALITY DISORDER: A COMMON ERROR

As behavioral health clinicians become increasingly aware of TGD communities seeking clinical services, there is more demand for affirming frameworks to help with diagnostic formulation and clinical management that effectively meet the needs of these patients. In the absence of adequate training for behavioral health clinicians in gender-affirming care, these clinicians may be unequipped to adopt a **gender minority stress** framework for their diagnostic formulation and a gender-affirming care lens for clinical management of behavioral health needs. Based on their traditional clinical training and frame of reference, behavioral health clinicians may incorrectly conclude that a TGD identity is merely a manifestation of identity diffusion in the context of borderline personality traits.[12] In this situation, the behavioral health clinician risks adopting an invalidating and dismissive stance toward TGD patients rather than therapeutically supporting TGD patients' strong need for gender identity affirmation.

In reality, rather than being an indicator of identity diffusion, a gender minority identity is typically the result of the TGD person's deliberative gender identity exploration, discovery, and consolidation.[12] Through thoughtful and sensitive elicitation of a patient's gender identity development history, behavioral health clinicians can better understand and appreciate the patient's TGD identity. Chronic exposure to gender minority stressors can produce signs mimicking certain symptoms and characteristics traditionally associated with borderline personality disorder, such as challenges with coping skills, interpersonal relationships, and emotion dysregulation. Rather than interpreting these byproducts of gender minority stress as internal psychopathology within the TGD person, behavioral health clinicians must appreciate that the fundamental problem lies in the TGD person's stigmatizing social environment and therefore prioritize a clinical focus on cultivating resilience and adaptive coping skills.

SUBSTANCE USE DISORDERS AMONG TGD PEOPLE

This section reviews epidemiological data regarding substance use disorders among TGD people, with a specific focus on alcohol and opioid use disorders as important illustrative examples. It also presents relevant guiding principles for affirming and effective clinical care using a gender minority stress framework.

▶ Opioid Use Disorders Among TGD People

An analysis of data from the 2013–2015 California Healthy Kids Survey revealed that TGD students in middle and high school are twice as likely as their cisgender counterparts to report recently using prescription pain medication.[13] Prevalence of opioid use among transgender women has been estimated at as high as 3.0% in San Francisco and 3.5% in New York City.[14,15] TGD adult Medicare recipients have more prevalent chronic pain, a risk factor for opioid misuse, than cisgender adults on Medicare.[16] With expanding access to gender-affirming surgery for TGD people, estimated to have increased by 20% from 2015 to 2016 by the American Society of Plastic Surgeons,[17] the near-ubiquitousness of opioid prescriptions for postoperative pain may place TGD people who undergo gender-affirming procedures at heightened risk of developing an opioid use disorder.[18,19] Moreover, TGD people are more likely than the general population to be living with HIV,[19,20] which is associated with a 54–83% increased likelihood of moderate or severe chronic pain.[21] Thus, there is a need for judiciousness in starting and attentively monitoring the use of opioids with TGD patients.[22]

Medication-assisted therapy (MAT), combined with tailored gender-affirming **cognitive-behavioral therapies**, as described later in this chapter, is the primary clinical intervention for TGD people with opioid use disorders.[23] Although opioid agonists like methadone and buprenorphine may interact with some medications commonly prescribed as gender-affirming hormone therapies, such as spironolactone, it is important for patients and clinicians to appreciate that these pharmacological treatments for opioid use disorders can save lives, and that, with routine monitoring, these treatments are both safe and effective to prescribe alongside gender-affirming hormone therapy.

▶ Alcohol Use Disorders Among TGD People

Research on alcohol use disorders among TGD people has historically been limited by methodological problems, including conflation of participants' sex and gender, imprecise and gender-exclusionary definitions of at-risk alcohol consumption, and a lack of both probability sampling methods and longitudinal study designs.[24] Recommendations for future studies include the rigorous operationalization of sex- and gender-related variables relevant to study hypotheses; development of measures for at-risk alcohol use that do not falsely assume only cisgender and binary gender identities; and validation of existing alcohol use screening tools with TGD populations.

The National Institute on Alcohol Abuse and Alcoholism (NIAAA)[25] and the Dietary Guidelines for Americans from the U.S. Department of Health and Human Services and U.S. Department of Agriculture (HHS and USDA)[26] define heavy alcohol use only for presumed cisgender women and men, which presents a challenge for behavioral health clinicians who aim to conduct patient-centered alcohol screening and counseling with TGD patients.[27]

The NIAAA provides gendered cutoffs for healthy alcohol use, and also specifies binge drinking as "a pattern of drinking that brings blood alcohol concentration (BAC) to 0.08 gram percent or above."[28] In the absence of TGD-inclusive alcohol use guidelines, clinicians may more crudely consider body fat and muscle composition as factors relevant to ethanol metabolism, with broad variability based on natal sex-based physiology, age of gender-affirming hormone therapy initiation, and the specific gender-affirming hormone therapies a TGD patient has received.[27] While a nuanced history of gender-affirming medical care for TGD patients may seem relevant to clinicians attempting to estimate parameters for healthy alcohol use with TGD patients, minimal evidence exists to inform clinical decision-making based on this approach.

Although patterns of social drinking are gendered with regard to women and men who are presumed to be cisgender, social drinking patterns, including the differential impact of sex- and gender-related factors on alcohol consumption, remain understudied for TGD communities.[24,27] Some differences in alcohol use between TGD and cisgender populations include a higher frequency of binge drinking among TGD adults compared with cisgender adults,[29] and lower odds of recent alcohol use among nonbinary teenagers assigned male sex at birth compared to cisgender teenagers.[30]

Beyond the lack of evidence-based tools to support identifying unhealthy alcohol use with TGD people, evidence-based guidelines are also lacking for alcohol-related clinical counseling and care with TGD communities.[27] Clinicians can discuss existing alcohol-related tools and guidelines with TGD patients, naming how these tools and guidelines are based on research that falsely assumed everyone has a cisgender and binary gender identity, and then propose to collaboratively develop a personalized plan for healthy alcohol use through shared decision-making. The TGD patient and their clinician may weigh the possible influence of past and current gender-affirming medical and surgical care on the patient's alcohol metabolism, as well as the specific psychosocial circumstances influencing the TGD patient's alcohol use. This shared decision-making process should also intersectionally prioritize the patient's own expressed considerations regarding race and ethnicity.[27]

Affirming psychoeducation by clinicians about alcohol use also centers experiences of gender minority stress and how these experiences can trigger a TGD patient's cravings to use alcohol. A gender-affirming framework can help tailor motivational enhancement strategies and guide careful referrals to specialized harm reduction, addictions treatment, and sobriety programs in community settings.[27]

SERIOUS MENTAL ILLNESS

TGD people, like the general population, can experience serious mental illness (SMI), including bipolar disorder, **posttraumatic stress disorder**, schizophrenia, and other persistent and debilitating psychiatric problems with significant adverse impacts on social, educational, and occupational functioning.[31] Although SMI can be well managed with comprehensively employed evidence-informed strategies to achieve psychosocial recovery based on personal life goals, those unable to access the full range of needed services can experience more pronounced stigma and ostracism.[32,33] This situation may be even worse for TGD people with SMI, who may already face societal stigma, isolation, and difficulty securing standard gender-affirming medical care. The dual stigma associated with having a gender minority identity and mental illness may predispose TGD people with SMI to even more severe psychiatric morbidity and adverse mental health outcomes.[34,35]

Evidence is lacking concerning tailored interventions for affirming gender identity, specifically in the context of SMI. Based on case reports, World Professional Association for Transgender Health Standards of Care, and clinical experience serving TGD patients, we can infer certain reasonable practices as suggestions, pending more research.[31,36-39]

Some clinicians with limited experience serving TGD patients with SMI may doubt whether a patient truly has a TGD identity and instead default to suspecting that the patient is experiencing gender-related delusions in the context of psychosis.[31,37,38] Clinicians often have a reflexive bias toward gatekeeping gender-affirming medical interventions with patients experiencing psychosis, believing that if they misdiagnose gender dysphoria, they may cause harm via partially or fully irreversible physical changes that aim to affirm the patient's gender identity. However, published reports indicate that TGD identities are distinct from psychosis and developmentally often emerge prior to the first psychotic episode. While a TGD person may initially articulate their gender identity to other people during acute psychosis, they may be doing so as a result of lowered social inhibitions during the psychotic episode, unconstrained by anti-TGD stigma and the usual concern for approval and acceptance by mainstream society. Moreover, TGD people often initiate social affirmation processes as older teenagers or young adults, when first-episode mania or psychosis occurs. In fact, rather than leading to premature or faulty gender affirmation, psychosis may derail timely gender affirmation within behavioral health care contexts.

To differentiate TGD identities from delusions, clinicians should consider the patient's history of gender identity development and distinguish the bizarre beliefs typically expressed in delusional states from the disclosure of a gender identity that defies society's expectations based on the person's sex assigned at birth.[31,37,38] Some published reports point toward the apparent amelioration of psychosis with gender-affirming medical care. Thus, TGD patients who possess medical decision-making capacity to provide informed consent should have facilitated access to gender-affirming medical and surgical care, with intentional minimization of psychiatric gatekeeping whenever possible. Since full remission of psychiatric symptoms is often not realistic, clinicians who seek this standard for a TGD patient with SMI in advance of granting referrals to gender-affirming medical and surgical care are likely to exacerbate mental health symptoms secondary to inappropriate gatekeeping, and to undermine the patient's autonomy and self-determination.

COGNITIVE BEHAVIORAL THERAPY: AN EVIDENCE-BASED PRACTICE

Although numerous psychological interventions have shown efficacy in treating a range of psychiatric disorders across the lifespan, one of the most widely assessed and implemented treatments is **cognitive behavioral therapy (CBT)**.[40] Therefore, we focus a significant portion of our discussion of evidence-based psychotherapy on this treatment approach and its use with TGD people, although we recognize that other therapeutic approaches may also be efficacious in addressing the needs of this vulnerable population.

CBT is a time-limited, problem-focused approach, emphasizing manualized or standardized interventions that implement empirically supported techniques in an individualized manner. CBT requires active collaboration between the therapist and the patient; active practice of skills between sessions; problem-focused, time-limited treatment; and ongoing evaluation of progress toward measurable goals. CBT includes many individual-, family-, and group-based protocols and interventions that address a range of problems, including anxiety, mood, substance use, attentional, eating, and personality disorders.[40] Significant empirical evidence supports the effectiveness of CBT approaches for children, adolescents, and adults.[41,42]

The CBT model underlying these approaches theorizes that symptoms can be divided into physiologic, cognitive, and behavioral components. CBT models also identify antecedents to symptoms, individual predispositions, consequences to particular behaviors (that may serve to increase or decrease the frequency of the behavior), and environmental factors that are both current and historical (e.g., learning histories, family environment, and cultural factors). These components are integrated into an individualized treatment plan, with specific techniques to address each component. Examples of these techniques include the following:

- Relaxation and mindfulness techniques aimed at reducing physiologic arousal associated with intense negative emotions
- Cognitive restructuring, in which unhelpful, maladaptive, or unduly negative thinking patterns are identified and replaced by positive and adaptive self-talk
- Behavioral approaches, such as progressive exposure, behavioral activation, and coping/self-care plans, to address the unhealthy behaviors that accompany psychiatric disorders (e.g., avoidance in anxiety disorders, withdrawal from meaningful/pleasant activities in depression, and self-destructive behaviors in personality, mood, and substance use disorders)

CBT interventions also focus on altering external factors to reduce modifiable triggers for negative emotions, improve the quantity and quality of relationships with others, and reinforce desired behaviors.

▶ Adapting CBT Interventions for TGD People

The minority stress model (as described in Chapter 3, "Health Disparities") is a useful framework for understanding not only the physical and mental health impact of particular stressors experienced by TGD people but also additional targets for treatment and adaptations of existing interventions. Although research on the most effective interventions for TGD people is very limited, we can draw from the literature on interventions for **sexual and gender minority (SGM)** people more generally to inform the development and implementation of gender-affirming, evidence-informed interventions.[43]

As detailed in the minority stress model,[44] individuals who are members of minority groups, such as TGD people, frequently experience serious stressors related to their minority status, including discrimination, bias, violence, and rejection. These stressors increase the risk for psychological and other health problems. In addition, psychological factors mediate the impact of these stressors, either by augmenting them via negative cognitions (e.g., internalized transphobia, expectations of rejection) or by mitigating their impact and enhancing resilience (e.g., social support, positive attributions toward minority group membership).

Based on recommendations from leading professional organizations, such as the American Psychological Association,[45] several CBT interventions have been developed specifically for SGM people. Common features of these approaches are described below.

Psychoeducation about the Nature and Impact of Minority Stress

Early in treatment, most culturally tailored interventions include explicit discussion about stressors experienced by

SGM people, the impact of these stressors on health, and strategies to mitigate these stressors. Many interventions include discussion of the impact of anti-LGBTQIA+ attitudes as well as individual, institutional, and cultural homophobia and transphobia. One common goal is to normalize anxiety and depression as natural, understandable reactions to ongoing stressors and to help correct attributions about the cause of these symptoms. Accurate recognition of psychosocial stressors and their impact on the individual is a pillar of culturally sensitive, trauma-informed care.[45]

Identifying and Restructuring Negative Cognitions about Minority Status

Most interventions offer explicit discussion of negative self-talk about gender identity, as well as strategies to challenge this self-talk. In addition, cognitive strategies focus on proximal gender minority stressors such as internalized transphobia, expectations of rejection, and rumination. Given that these proximal stressors are suggested as mediating factors for the impact of distal stressors on mental health outcomes,[46] they are important targets for intervention. Patients can understand how previous experiences have shaped negative core beliefs about themselves, their gender, and their relationships to others, recognize automatic thoughts that arise from these core beliefs, and adopt more adaptive self-talk. Some approaches with LGBTQIA+ people also incorporate compassion-focused cognitive and experiential techniques to decrease shame and internalized stigma, foster self-compassion and empathy, and cultivate a nonjudgmental perspective toward one's experiences.[47]

Addressing Hypervigilance

One of the consequences of repeated gender minority stress experiences with discrimination, violence, rejection, and abuse is chronic hypervigilance to potential threats.[48] This hypervigilance is associated with increased physiologic arousal, cognitive distortions, avoidance behaviors, and decreased self-regulation capacity.[48,49] Drawing from cognitive-behavioral interventions for posttraumatic stress disorders, which include hypervigilance as a core symptom, CBT helps people recognize triggers for hypervigilance, implement relaxation and mindfulness strategies to reduce physiologic symptoms of stress, challenge inaccurate threat-related cognitions, and differentiate safe versus unsafe situations.[50]

Facilitating Emotion Regulation

Because gender identity starts to develop early in life, repeated denigration or dismissal of TGD identities beginning in early childhood may teach the individual to ignore their internal sense of self or instincts, ignore or suppress gender-related emotions and thoughts, and conceal gender-expansive behaviors and expression to conform to cisgender societal norms and expectations. Growing up and existing in persistently invalidating environments increases the risk for emotion dysregulation, by decreasing awareness of internal states and emotion recognition, limiting the development of coping tools for managing negative emotional states, and increasing experiential avoidance. Gender dysphoria may further exacerbate these difficulties and increase associated risks for depression, anxiety, suicidality, and nonsuicidal self-injurious behaviors.

Clinicians may also draw upon and tailor components of **Dialectical Behavioral Therapy** (DBT), which integrates traditional CBT techniques with approaches from contemplative meditative practice shown to improve distress tolerance, awareness, and acceptance.[51] Emotion regulation and distress tolerance skills from DBT allow the individual to recognize and label various emotional states (including physiologic, affective, cognitive, and behavioral aspects of emotions), their triggers, and their consequences. To develop a range of skills to manage and tolerate intense negative emotional states in a nondestructive manner, TGD people can learn to implement strategies to tolerate intense negative emotions, including mindfulness, distraction, and self-soothing techniques. Strategies to enhance overall well-being (e.g., exercise, sleep hygiene, activity scheduling) may also reduce vulnerability to negative mood states and enhance resilience.

Using Exposure Techniques to Address Avoidance Behaviors

Progressive exposure techniques are among the best-established interventions to address anxiety-based avoidance, with demonstrated effectiveness for all anxiety disorders, trauma-related disorders, and obsessive-compulsive disorders.[52] Based on classical (extinction learning) and operant conditioning models, patients are asked to gradually confront anxiety-provoking situations without engaging in avoidance or safety-seeking behaviors. With repeated exposure practice, patients experience reduced anxiety in previously feared situations, an enhanced sense of mastery and control, and skills to cope with anxiety symptoms. Whenever appropriate, exposure exercises should incorporate issues of relevance to TGD people (e.g., identity disclosure when necessary, using the bathroom that accords with their gender identity, etc.). Many interventions also include a focus on assertiveness skills, both directly (e.g., correcting others when being misgendered) and indirectly (e.g., initiating a new relationship).[53] These may be important in addressing difficulty in interpersonal relationships and enhancing health-related behaviors (e.g., substance refusal skills, sexual health negotiations).

Identifying Sources of Resilience

In any discussion of behavioral health, it is essential to highlight known sources of resilience in TGD people, both to avoid pathologizing gender diversity and to offer targets for behavioral health interventions that can enhance well-being and positive outcomes. There is evidence that social support, especially parental and familial support and affirmation, is a powerful protective factor for TGD people, especially youth. Several studies emphasize the mental health benefits of parental acceptance and support, with increased self-esteem and decreased substance use, suicidal thoughts, and depression.[54,55] Conversely, family rejection or maltreatment is associated with increased risks for depression, suicidal ideation and behaviors, substance use disorders, and homelessness.[55] In addition, having community supports improves mental health outcomes among TGD people. For example, among youth, having an effective Gender-Sexuality Alliance in school enhances well-being and positive mental health outcomes in young adulthood and buffers young people against the negative effects of anti-LGBTQIA+ school victimization on well-being.[56] Finally, focusing on the unique strengths of TGD people, including enhancing pride in TGD identities and supporting community building and social activities, further enhances resilience.[48] Helping clients identify TGD role models and community champions and increasing positive representation of TGD people in media, literature, and education may also foster self-esteem, pride, and hope for the future.

▶ Examples of Adapted CBT-based Interventions for SGM People

The following CBT-based interventions serve as examples of approaches that can be modified to serve the unique needs of TGD people. Some of these projects are currently being evaluated in randomized clinical trials; others are undergoing initial feasibility evaluation.

- Compassion-Focused Therapy for Sexual Minority Young Adults is an eight-session CBT intervention that focuses on mindfulness and compassionate self-care to reduce shame and self-criticism and enhance resiliency to stress. A randomized controlled trial of this intervention, with young adults age 18–25 years who identify as gay or bisexual and have elevated depressive symptoms, is ongoing.[47]

- Project ESTEEM is a 10-session CBT intervention to enhance mental health and sexual health.[48] The goals of ESTEEM are to normalize the adverse impact of minority stress to increase emotional awareness, regulation, and acceptance, reduce emotional and behavioral avoidance, empower assertiveness, restructure maladaptive cognitions related to minority status, validate SGM young adults' unique strengths, foster supportive relationships, and affirm healthy, rewarding expressions of sexuality. This intervention is currently being evaluated using a three-arm randomized controlled trial.

- Project Youth AFFIRM is an eight-session group CBT intervention that integrates a focus on understanding the impact of anti-LGBTQIA+ attitudes and behaviors on stress and social relationships with more traditional cognitive restructuring, assertiveness training, and LGBTQIA+-affirming activities.[57] The intervention is currently being evaluated with LGBTQIA+ youth and young adults (ages 14–29 years) via a randomized controlled trial.

- Being Out with Strength (BOWS) is a small-group intervention that focuses on recognizing and modifying negative cognitions stemming from internalized oppression (heterosexism and cisgenderism).[58] An early feasibility study suggested that there is demand from both youth and providers for this intervention and that the intervention is feasible and acceptable.

- Resilience Against Depression Disparities (RADD). This protocol features a CBT-based resilience class called Building Resilience and Increasing Community Hope (B-RICH), which includes a seven-session psychoeducational intervention and a CBT-based manual to address mood and anxiety symptoms.[59] It has been adapted for SGM people, including finding affirming social support and using cognitive restructuring to cope with discrimination. Classes are led by community health workers who are both SGM and Black, Indigenous, and People of Color (BIPOC), and these classes are supplemented by text messages to reinforce basic concepts and remind participants of appointments.

INTEGRATION OF BEHAVIORAL HEALTH SERVICES WITH PRIMARY MEDICAL CARE FOR TGD PEOPLE

Models for integration of culturally responsive behavioral health services with gender-affirming primary medical care hold promise for meeting the combined physical and mental health needs of TGD communities. The basis of behavioral health integration is a comprehensive, interdisciplinary, and interprofessional approach to patient-centered care that serves the whole person, including needs related to mental health and substance use.[60,61] The Center for Integrated Health Services in the U.S. Substance Abuse and Health Services Administration (SAMHSA) has delineated how behavioral health integration exists along a continuum across health systems: level 1, coordinated care (minimal-to-some collaboration across behavioral and primary care providers in separate locations); level 2, colocated care (minimal-to-some systems-level integration across providers in the same location); and level 3, integrated care (extensive-to-full collaboration across providers in a single cohesive practice).[62]

Behavioral health integration offers the advantages of improved wait times, streamlined paperwork, efficient workflows, and ease of communication within a practice to foster more responsive and patient-centered clinical care.[63] Behavioral health integration for TGD people can also reduce the dual stigma of a TGD identity combined with a behavioral health or substance use problem, which may in turn promote more engagement in both primary and behavioral health care. Gender-affirming primary care clinicians may not always have the training or availability to treat complex behavioral health problems that can interfere with their focus on addressing patients' physical health concerns.[64] Integrated behavioral health clinicians can deliver evidence-informed interventions to enhance TGD patients' self-care practices, and psychiatric prescribers within integrated care models can scale up psychopharmacology consultation and management across a large panel of TGD patients. Primary care clinicians themselves can also build personal capacity to effectively deliver behavioral health therapies for TGD patients within their own practice, including buprenorphine/naloxone for maintenance of sobriety from opioids or motivational enhancement strategies for substance use disorders. Below we describe two common examples of systems-level behavioral health integration: (1) psychiatric collaborative care and (2) screening, brief intervention, and referral to treatment.

▶ Psychiatric Collaborative Care

Psychiatric collaborative care models facilitate addressing behavioral health problems in primary care settings by obviating the need for patients to visit directly with a psychiatrist and by avoiding overwhelming primary care clinicians with patients behavioral health needs.[65,66] The primary care clinician, a consultant psychiatrist or psychiatric prescriber, and a behavioral health care manager (e.g., a nurse or clinical social worker) all function as a collaborative team along with the patient to delineate the behavioral health treatment plan. The behavioral health care manager leads engagement of the patient and coordinates care across the treatment team, including monitoring treatment effectiveness and tolerance, providing psychoeducation and self-management counseling, and overseeing referrals as needed. Collaborative care models employ measurement-based psychopharmacology regimen modifications based on symptom scores on standard instruments, such as the Patient Health Questionnaire 9-item tool (PHQ-9), until treatment goals are achieved. Psychiatric consultants review case information and provide recommendations to team members, usually without engaging with patients themselves. The primary care clinician ultimately makes behavioral health treatment decisions with the patient. Collaborative care models monitor patients' treatment progress over time with a registry system that is available online.[65,66] These models have been studied extensively and found to improve common behavioral health problems across diverse patient populations.

▶ Screening, Brief Intervention, and Referral to Treatment

Screening, Brief Intervention, and Referral to Treatment (SBIRT) is a systems-level intervention increasingly adopted by health care organizations serving a broad range of patient populations as a means to identify and address at-risk use of alcohol and drugs.[67-69] The first step in SBIRT is the screening of all patients for substance use; subsequently, care teams can more extensively assess substance use among patients who have positive screens.[70] Clinicians positively reinforce those patients with low-risk scores, while patients with moderate-risk scores benefit from a brief clinician intervention that often applies: motivational enhancement strategies that focus on making patients more aware of their own substance use; goal-setting; and substance use reduction counseling. Patients with higher-risk scores may benefit from more intensive brief therapy in the primary care setting. Patients with a probable substance use disorder require treatment referrals to clinicians with addictions specialization.[69,71,72]

SUMMARY

- Transgender and gender diverse (TGD) people have unique behavioral health needs in the context of pervasive gender minority stress, as well as historical pathologization of TGD identities within the field of psychiatry, including ineffective and harmful gender identity change efforts.

- A gender affirmation framework helps guide clinicians in effective and culturally responsive screening, assessment, formulation, counseling, and treatment across a variety of diagnostic categories and considerations, including personality, substance use, and psychosis.

- CBT is evidence-based and can be tailored for TGD patients based on a gender minority stress framework to treat depression, anxiety, and other mental health problems by providing psychoeducation, restructuring minority stress cognitions, addressing hypervigilance, decreasing avoidance, and enhancing resilience.

- Systems-level behavioral health strategies within gender-affirming primary medical care settings may include psychiatric collaborative care for mental health problems, as well as Screening, Brief Intervention, and Referral to Treatment (SBIRT) for substance use.

CASE STUDY

L.P. is a 20-year-old Latinx, transgender man (he/him pronouns) who is currently attending community college. He recently sought CBT to address his social anxiety and depression, as well as provide a safe, affirming space to further explore and discuss his gender identity. He has attended six sessions of CBT and appears to have a strong relationship with Dr. Smith. During previous sessions, they have worked on identifying negative and self-critical thinking patterns and building positive coping skills. He has been implementing breathing and mindfulness techniques to manage stress from school and social relationships.

L.P. comes to today's session looking more down and withdrawn. Dr. Smith points this out and L.P. reports that over the past few days he has been feeling more distressed and worthless and has been experiencing more gender dysphoria. L.P. has been missing some classes and sleeping more during the day. Dr. Smith asks L.P. about triggers for this recent symptom exacerbation. L.P. states "I've had a rough week. My parents are kind of supportive but this week I got into an argument with my mom about going on T. She doesn't believe that I should do anything to change my body and doesn't understand why I need to do this." Dr. Smith asks L.P. about his relationship with his parents and previous experiences with invalidation of his gender identity. She also explores the impact of this (both recently and historically) on L.P.'s mood, self-esteem, and gender dysphoria. L.P. describes the stress of these experiences; "It's unbearable when my parents don't understand me. I feel like I have to choose between who I really am and my family. What am I supposed to do?" Dr. Smith helps L.P. to differentiate his parents' beliefs from his own and to develop more positive self-talk around his gender identity and his decision to move forward with gender-affirming treatment, "It's hard to separate your thoughts and feelings from those of your parents, but I would bet that you have a better sense of what you need around your gender journey. I wonder how you might coach yourself in a more compassionate manner when these difficult interactions occur?" Dr. Smith also encourages L.P. to increase self-care activities such as playing his guitar and reaching out to friends, and to join a young-adult group for transgender people to increase support. Finally, they work together to think about and practice more effective ways of asserting himself and setting appropriate limits in difficult interactions with his parents.

▶ Discussion Questions

1. Dr. Smith focused on several concrete steps to help L.P. cope with the family stress he is experiencing. What alternative approaches could be helpful to L.P.? Could Dr. Smith have focused on alternative aspects of L.P.'s experience in therapy?

2. In the case example, L.P. was described as Latinx. How might his cultural background impact his experiences as a transgender man and his interactions with his family? How might this be considered in his treatment plan?

3. As a young adult, L.P. is in a unique developmental stage with regard to several aspects of self-regulation, identity development, and individuation from parents. How might this developmental stage shape treatment goals and approaches? Can you think of ways in which treatment would differ with adults who are in different developmental stages?

4. Dr. Smith suggested a group intervention as an adjunctive treatment approach. Which other interventions (e.g., psychopharmacologic treatment, family therapy) or collaborations (e.g., conversation with his endocrinologist) might you consider?

REFERENCES

1. Romanelli M, Lu W, Lindsey MA. Examining mechanisms and moderators of the relationship between discriminatory health care encounters and attempted suicide among U.S. transgender help-seekers. *Adm Policy Ment Health*. 2018;45(6):831-849.
2. White BP, Fontenot HB. Transgender and non-conforming persons' mental healthcare experiences: an integrative review. *Arch Psychiatr Nurs*. 2019;33(2):203-210.
3. Beek TF, Cohen-Kettenis PT, Bouman WP, et al. Gender incongruence of adolescence and adulthood: acceptability and clinical utility of the World Health Organization's proposed ICD-11 criteria. *PLoS One*. 2016;11(10):e0160066.
4. Suess Schwend A, Winter S, Chiam Z, Smiley A, Cabral Grinspan M. Depathologising gender diversity in childhood in the process of ICD revision and reform. *Glob Public Health*. 2018;13(11):1585-1598.
5. Perlson JE, Walters OC, Keuroghlian AS. Envisioning a future for transgender and gender-diverse people beyond the DSM. *Br J Psychiatry*. 2020:1-2.
6. Beckwith N, McDowell MJ, Reisner SL, et al. Psychiatric epidemiology of transgender and nonbinary adult patients at an urban health center. *LGBT Health*. 2019;6(2):51-61.
7. Schulman JK, Erickson-Schroth L. Mental health in sexual minority transgender women. *Psychiatr Clin North Am*. 2017;40(2):309-319.
8. Liu CH, Stevens C, Wong SHM, Yasui M, Chen JA. The prevalence and predictors of mental health diagnoses and suicide among U.S. college students: implications for addressing disparities in service use. *Depress Anxiety*. 2019;36(1):8-17.
9. Witcomb GL, Bouman WP, Claes L, Brewin N, Crawford JR, Arcelus J. Levels of depression in transgender people and its predictors: results of a large matched control study with transgender people accessing clinical services. *J Affect Disord*. 2018;235:308-315.
10. Turban JL, King D, Reisner SL, Keuroghlian AS. Psychological attempts to change a person's gender identity from transgender to cisgender: estimated prevalence across US states, 2015. *Am J Public Health*. 2019;109(10):1452-1454.
11. Turban JL, Beckwith N, Reisner SL, Keuroghlian AS. Association between recalled exposure to gender identity conversion efforts and psychological distress and suicide attempts among transgender adults. *JAMA Psychiatry*. 2020;77(1):68-76.
12. Goldhammer H, Crall C, Keuroghlian AS. Distinguishing and addressing gender minority stress and borderline personality symptoms. *Harv Rev Psychiatry*. 2019;27(5):317-325.
13. De Pedro KT, Gilreath TD, Jackson C, Esqueda MC. Substance use among transgender students in California Public Middle and High Schools. *J Sch Health*. 2017;87(5):303-309.

14. Rowe C, Santos GM, McFarland W, Wilson EC. Prevalence and correlates of substance use among trans female youth ages 16-24 years in the San Francisco Bay Area. *Drug Alcohol Depend.* 2015;147:160-166.

15. Nuttbrock L, Bockting W, Rosenblum A, et al. Gender abuse, depressive symptoms, and substance use among transgender women: a 3-year prospective study. *Am J Public Health.* 2014;104(11):2199-2206.

16. Dragon CN, Guerino P, Ewald E, Laffan AM. Transgender Medicare beneficiaries and chronic conditions: exploring fee-for-service claims data. *LGBT Health.* 2017;4(6):404-411.

17. American Society of Plastic Surgeons. Plastic Surgery Statistics Report. Arlington Heights, IL: American Society of Plastic Surgeons; May 2017. www.plasticsurgery.org/documents/News/Statistics/2016/plastic-surgery-statistics-full-report-2016.pdf.

18. Edlund MJ, Martin BC, Russo JE, DeVries A, Braden JB, Sullivan MD. The role of opioid prescription in incident opioid abuse and dependence among individuals with chronic noncancer pain: the role of opioid prescription. *Clin J Pain.* 2014;30(7):557-564.

19. Centers for Disease Control and Prevention (CDC). HIV Surveillance Report, 2016; vol. 28. Atlanta; 2017.

20. Baral SD, Poteat T, Stromdahl S, Wirtz AL, Guadamuz TE, Beyrer C. Worldwide burden of HIV in transgender women: a systematic review and meta-analysis. *Lancet Infect Dis.* 2013;13(3):214-222.

21. Parker R, Stein DJ, Jelsma J. Pain in people living with HIV/AIDS: a systematic review. *J Int AIDS Soc.* 2014;17:18719.

22. Uebelacker LA, Weisberg RB, Herman DS, Bailey GL, Pinkston-Camp MM, Stein MD. Chronic pain in HIV-infected patients: relationship to depression, substance use, and mental health and pain treatment. *Pain Med.* 2015;16(10):1870-1881.

23. Girouard MP, Goldhammer H, Keuroghlian AS. Understanding and treating opioid use disorders in lesbian, gay, bisexual, transgender, and queer populations. *Subst Abus.* 2019;40(3):335-339.

24. Gilbert PA, Pass LE, Keuroghlian AS, Greenfield TK, Reisner SL. Alcohol research with transgender populations: a systematic review and recommendations to strengthen future studies. *Drug Alcohol Depend.* 2018;186:138-146.

25. National Institute on Alcohol Abuse and Alcoholism. Helping patients who drink too much: a clinician's guide. 2005. https://pubs.niaaa.nih.gov/publications/practitioner/cliniciansguide2005/guide.pdf.

26. U.S. Department of Health and Human Services and U.S. Department of Agriculture. 2015–2020 Dietary Guidelines for Americans. 8th ed. Washington, DC; 2015. https://health.gov/sites/default/files/2019-09/2015-2020_Dietary_Guidelines.pdf.

27. Arellano-Anderson J, Keuroghlian AS. Screening, counseling, and shared decision making for alcohol use with transgender and gender-diverse populations. *LGBT Health.* 2020;7(8):402-406.

28. National Institute on Alcohol Abuse and Alcoholism. NIAAA council approves definition of binge drinking. *NIAAA Newslett* 2004;3:3. https://pubs.niaaa.nih.gov/publications/Newsletter/winter2004/Newsletter_Number3.pdf.

29. Coulter RW, Blosnich JR, Bukowski LA, Herrick AL, Siconolfi DE, Stall RD. Differences in alcohol use and alcohol-related problems between transgender- and nontransgender-identified young adults. *Drug Alcohol Depend.* 2015;154:251-259.

30. Watson RJ, Fish JN, McKay T, Allen SH, Eaton L, Puhl RM. Substance use among a national sample of sexual and gender minority adolescents: intersections of sex assigned at birth and gender identity. *LGBT Health.* 2020;7(1):37-46.

31. Smith WB, Goldhammer H, Keuroghlian AS. Affirming gender identity of patients with serious mental illness. *Psychiatr Serv.* 2019;70(1):65-67.

32. The Division of Psychologists in Public Service and the APA Task Force on Serious Mental Illness and Severe Emotional Disturbance. *Proficiency in Psychology Assessment and Treatment of Serious Mental Illness.* Washington, DC: American Psychological Association; 2009. www.apa.org/practice/resources/smi-proficiency.pdf.

33. Health care reform for Americans with severe mental illnesses: report of the National Advisory Mental Health Council. *Am J Psychiatry.* 1993;150(10):1447-1465.

34. Kidd SA, Howison M, Pilling M, Ross LE, McKenzie K. Severe mental illness in LGBT populations: a scoping review. *Psychiatr Serv.* 2016;67(7):779-783.

35. Cole CM, O'Boyle M, Emory LE, Meyer WJIII. Comorbidity of gender dysphoria and other major psychiatric diagnoses. *Arch Sex Behav.* 1997;26(1):13-26.

36. Coleman E, Bockting W, Botzer M, et al. Standards of care for the health of transsexual, transgender, and gender-nonconforming people, version 7. *Int J Transgend.* 2012;13:165-232.

37. Meijer JH, Eeckhout GM, van Vlerken RH, de Vries AL. Gender dysphoria and co-existing psychosis: review and four case examples of successful gender affirmative treatment. *LGBT Health.* 2017;4(2):106-114.

38. Gerken AT, McGahee S, Keuroghlian AS, Freudenreich O. Consideration of clozapine and gender-affirming medical care for an HIV-positive person with schizophrenia and fluctuating gender identity. *Harv Rev Psychiatry.* 2016;24(6):406-415.

39. Reisner SL, Bradford J, Hopwood R, et al. Comprehensive transgender healthcare: the gender affirming clinical and public health model of Fenway Health. *J Urban Health.* 2015;92(3):584-592.

40. Hofmann SG, Asnaani A, Vonk IJ, Sawyer AT, Fang A. The efficacy of cognitive behavioral therapy: a review of meta-analyses. *Cognit Ther Res.* 2012;36(5):427-440.

41. Butler AC, Chapman JE, Forman EM, Beck AT. The empirical status of cognitive-behavioral therapy: a review of meta-analyses. *Clin Psychol Rev.* 2006;26(1):17-31.

42. de Arellano MA, Lyman DR, Jobe-Shields L, et al. Trauma-focused cognitive-behavioral therapy for children and adolescents: assessing the evidence. *Psychiatr Serv.* 2014;65(5):591-602.

43. Janssen A, Busa S, Wernick J. The complexities of treatment planning for transgender youth with co-occurring severe mental illness: a literature review and case study. *Arch Sex Behav.* 2019;48(7):2003-2009.

44. Hendricks ML, Testa RJ. A conceptual framework for clinical work with transgender and gender nonconforming clients: an adaptation of the Minority Stress Model. *Prof Psychol Res Practice.* 2012;43(5):460.

45. American Psychological Association. Guidelines for psychological practice with transgender and gender nonconforming people. *Am Psychologist.* 2015;70(9):832-864.

46. Hatzenbuehler ML. How does sexual minority stigma "get under the skin"? A psychological mediation framework. *Psychol Bull.* 2009;135(5):707-730.

47. Pepping CA, Lyons A, McNair R, Kirby JN, Petrocchi N, Gilbert P. A tailored compassion-focused therapy program for sexual minority young adults with depressive symotomatology: study protocol for a randomized controlled trial. *BMC Psychol.* 2017;5(1):5.

48. Pachankis JE, McConocha EM, Reynolds JS, et al. Project ESTEEM protocol: a randomized controlled trial of an LGBTQ-affirmative treatment for young adult sexual minority men's mental and sexual health. *BMC Public Health.* 2019;19(1):1086.

49. Goldbach JT, Gibbs JJ. Strategies employed by sexual minority adolescents to cope with minority stress. *Psychol Sex Orientat Gend Divers.* 2015;2(3):297-306.

50. Rothbaum BO, Meadows EA, Resick P, Foy DW. Cognitive-behavioral therapy. In: Foa EB, Keane TM, Friedman MJ, eds. *Effective Treatments for PTSD: Practice Guidelines from the International Society for Traumatic Stress Studies.* New York: Guilford Press; 2000:320-325.

51. McKay M, Wood JC, Brantley J. *The Dialectical Behavior Therapy Skills Workbook: Practical DBT Exercises for Learning Mindfulness, Interpersonal Effectiveness, Emotion Regulation, and Distress Tolerance.* Oakland, CA: New Harbinger Publications; 2019.

52. Abramowitz JS, Deacon BJ, Whiteside SP. *Exposure Therapy for Anxiety: Principles and Practice.* New York: Guilford Publications; 2019 Apr 9.

53. Speed BC, Goldstein BL, Goldfried MR. Assertiveness training: a forgotten evidence-based treatment. *Clin Psychol Sci Practice.* 2018;25(1):e12216.

54. Simons L, Schrager SM, Clark LF, Belzer M, Olson J. Parental support and mental health among transgender adolescents. *J Adolesc Health.* 2013;53(6):791-793.

55. Seibel BL, de Brito Silva B, Fontanari AMV, et al. The impact of the parental support on risk factors in the process of gender affirmation of transgender and gender diverse people. *Front Psychol.* 2018;9:399.

56. Toomey RB, Ryan C, Diaz RM, Russell ST. High School Gay-Straight Alliances (GSAs) and young adult well-being: an examination of GSA presence, participation, and perceived effectiveness. *Appl Dev Sci.* 2011;15(4):175-185.

57. Craig SL, McInroy LB, Eaton AD, et al. An affirmative coping skills intervention to improve the mental and sexual health of sexual and gender minority youth (Project Youth AFFIRM): protocol for an implementation study. *JMIR Res Protoc.* 2019;8(6):e13462.

58. Hall WJ, Rosado BR, Chapman MV. Findings from a feasibility study of an adapted cognitive behavioral therapy group intervention to reduce depression among LGBTQ (Lesbian, Gay, Bisexual, Transgender, or Queer) young people. *J Clin Med.* 2019;8(7):949.

59. Vargas SM, Wennerstrom A, Alfaro N, et al. Resilience against depression disparities (RADD): a protocol for a randomised comparative effectiveness trial for depression among predominantly low-income, racial/ethnic, sexual and gender minorities. *BMJ Open.* 2019;9(10):e031099.

60. Sandoval BE, Bell J, Khatri P, Robinson PJ. Toward a unified integration approach: uniting diverse primary care strategies under the primary care behavioral health (PCBH) model. *J Clin Psychol Med Settings.* 2018;25(2):187-196.

61. Sanchez K, Ybarra R, Chapa T, Martinez ON. Eliminating behavioral health disparities and improving outcomes for racial and ethnic minority populations. *Psychiatr Serv.* 2016;67(1):13-15.

62. Heath B, Wise R, Reynolds K. *Standard Framework for Levels of Integrated Healthcare.* Washington, DC: SAMHSA-HRSA Center for Integrated Health Solutions; 2013.

63. Ward MC, Miller BF, Marconi VC, Kaslow NJ, Farber EW. The role of behavioral health in optimizing care for complex patients in the primary care setting. *J Gen Intern Med.* 2016;31(3):265-267.

64. Curran GM, Pyne J, Fortney JC, et al. Development and implementation of collaborative care for depression in HIV clinics. *AIDS Care.* 2011;23(12):1626-1636.

65. Unutzer J, Katon W, Callahan CM, et al. Collaborative care management of late-life depression in the primary care setting: a randomized controlled trial. *JAMA.* 2002;288(22):2836-2845.

66. Archer J, Bower P, Gilbody S, et al. Collaborative care for depression and anxiety problems. *Cochrane Database Syst Rev.* 2012;10:CD006525.

67. Aldridge A, Linford R, Bray J. Substance use outcomes of patients served by a large US implementation of Screening, Brief Intervention and Referral to Treatment (SBIRT). *Addiction.* 2017;112(Suppl 2):43-53.

68. Barata IA, Shandro JR, Montgomery M, et al. Effectiveness of SBIRT for alcohol use disorders in the emergency department: a systematic review. *West J Emerg Med.* 2017;18(6):1143-1152.

69. Bray JW, Del Boca FK, McRee BG, Hayashi SW, Babor TF. Screening, Brief Intervention and Referral to Treatment (SBIRT): rationale, program overview, and cross-site evaluation. *Addiction.* 2017;112(Suppl 2):3-11.

70. Knox J, Hasin DS, Larson FRR, Kranzler HR. Prevention, screening, and treatment for heavy drinking and alcohol use disorder. *Lancet Psychiatry.* 2019;6(12):1054-1067.

71. Babor TF, Del Boca F, Bray JW. Screening, Brief Intervention and Referral to Treatment: implications of SAMHSA's SBIRT initiative for substance abuse policy and practice. *Addiction.* 2017;112(Suppl 2):110-117.

72. Agerwala SM, McCance-Katz EF. Integrating screening, brief intervention, and referral to treatment (SBIRT) into clinical practice settings: a brief review. *J Psychoactive Drugs.* 2012;44(4):307-317.

Gender-Affirming Hormone Therapy for Adults

Julie Thompson

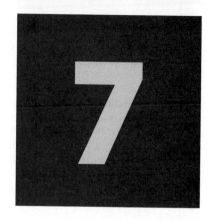

INTRODUCTION

This chapter focuses on the recommended approach to prescribing **gender-affirming hormone therapy (GAHT)**. It includes guidance for the health care professional in recognizing an individual's appropriateness for hormone therapy, providing informed consent, and developing a patient-centered, individualized approach to treatment. Various hormone therapy options are discussed, as is the rationale for decision making in choosing specific medications. Additionally, this chapter provides information on the importance of understanding patient goals and providing education on expectations, the wide-ranging effects of GAHT, and guidelines for monitoring treatment. Hormonal gender affirmation is still a relatively new field of study, with data on health outcomes and medication safety being actively researched, and recommendations for best practices modified frequently. The dynamic nature of this field is both exciting and challenging; this chapter presents current guidelines.

BACKGROUND AND DEFINITION

Gender affirmation for many **transgender and gender diverse (TGD)** individuals is a multidimensional process involving aspects of social, emotional, and physical affirmation to reduce gender dysphoria. **Gender dysphoria** refers to the range of emotional distress experienced when there is a misalignment of one's physical body and perceived gender with the internal sense of self. GAHT refers to **sex steroids** (mainly **testosterone** or **estrogen**) administered in various forms to produce or enhance **secondary sex characteristics** that promote physical affirmation. Using GAHT can reduce the internal stress of gender dysphoria as one's physical body begins to align with the desired sense of self. Physical affirmation may also allow some people to move more comfortably or safely through the world as their affirmed and authentic self. Several studies have shown significant reductions in mental health comorbidities (depression, suicidality, substance use) and an overall improvement in quality of life with the ability to access GAHT.[1-4] As such, for many individuals, access to GAHT is an important and necessary part of their self-actualization process.

The goal of GAHT is to create the internal hormone environment that best aligns with one's gender identity, with the aim of achieving physical characteristics that are culturally accepted and expected as a presentation of that gender. GAHT often involves taking hormone medications (**exogenous hormones**) that are affirming and suppressing the body's production of hormones (**endogenous hormones**) that do not align with one's gender identity. GAHT therapy is most often focused on increasing or decreasing estrogen and testosterone with various medication options to produce a combination of reversible and permanent changes to the body. Not all TGD-identified individuals seek hormonal therapy as part of their affirmation. There is a great diversity of gender identities and expressions, and health care professionals must assess each individual's goal for accessing care in a nonjudgmental and supportive way. According to the 2015 U.S. Transgender Survey, 79% of TGD respondents desired hormone therapy as part of their gender affirmation (which corresponded to 95% of transgender men and women respondents and 49% of nonbinary respondents).[5] The TGD population is a diverse group of individuals, and therefore creating a low-barrier, welcoming environment to discuss patients' needs and goals for gender-affirming care can allow for an individualized approach to treatment, health education, and support.

ESTABLISHING THE GOALS FOR HORMONE THERAPY

For many individuals, the aim of initiating hormones is to achieve the maximum changes to their bodies that culturally represent a feminine or masculine identity. However, some people with **nonbinary** or **genderqueer** identities may desire a nuanced hormonal makeup to achieve a more androgynous appearance to decrease gender dysphoria. Understanding a patient's goals prior to starting on hormone therapy can ensure proper expectation setting and allow for tailoring of individual treatment regimens to achieve these desired goals whenever possible and safe. Hormones can affect external appearance, leading to secondary sex characteristics of the affirmed gender—for example, testosterone can cause a deeper voice and facial hair growth, whereas estrogen may induce breast development. Additionally, GAHT can promote affirming changes in body function by suppressing endogenous hormones, for example, cessation of menses with testosterone or decreased spontaneous erections with estrogen. Hormones do have limitations. In individuals who have already experienced natal puberty, hormones do not alter bone structure, height, and other changes that have occurred over time due to endogenous hormones.

To reject the rigid concepts of binary identities, clinicians should consider moving away from classifying hormones as "feminizing" or "masculinizing" and referring to hormones by their generic names—testosterone, estrogen, androgen-blocker—and known physical effects. In this way, clinicians can be specific about the effects of the hormones without tying physical traits or body characteristics to a gender.

INFORMED CONSENT

Often, individual clinicians and health institutions have established protocols for evaluating appropriateness for initiating hormone therapy. The most commonly adopted and referenced guidelines were developed by the World Professional Association of Transgender Health (WPATH), an international, multidisciplinary organization comprised of medical and mental health care professionals, researchers, advocates, and policymakers with expertise in transgender health and policy. WPATH sets international standards of care for transgender health practices and health equity. WPATH recommends an informed consent approach before starting GAHT for assessment and education with the patient.[6] The informed consent process can be performed by either a medical or mental health clinician experienced in transgender health.

Informed consent refers to the conversation between a health care professional and patient that thoroughly explains the benefits and risks of and realistic expectations for the full range of treatment options available for that patient. It also includes the process of assessing the patient's capacity to understand this explanation. There is no one structured or prescribed way to provide informed consent; rather, it should be individualized to a patient's cognitive and emotional needs, age, and cultural context. It is critical to set clear expectations with patients regarding unknowns due to gaps in research, limitations of medications, and the long-term health outcomes of therapy. Patients should be given the opportunity to discuss how these limitations and outcomes may align with their current and future goals and expectations.[7] Throughout this process, the individual's sense of self and agency should be promoted and supported.[8]

For some patients, assessment for appropriateness of hormone therapy is straightforward, while for others, more time may be needed to understand goals or to ensure support for ongoing medical, behavioral health, or social issues. WPATH recommends consideration of the following four criteria during the assessment:

1. Persistent, well-documented gender dysphoria (of at least 6 months as assessed by either a medical or behavioral health professional).

2. Capacity to make a fully informed decision and consent to treatment.

3. Age of majority in a given country.

4. If significant medical or mental health concerns are present, they should be reasonably well controlled.[6]

The presence of co-occurring medical or mental health conditions should not necessarily contraindicate or delay access to GAHT. If an underlying medical or mental health condition is both poorly controlled and presents a risk specifically in the setting of GAHT, it is recommended that the condition is stabilized before initiating hormone therapy. This recommendation requires nuanced decision-making and an individualized approach, which should include assessment of the patient's health history, baseline level of functioning, and current level of functioning. Finally, the role of the patient's gender dysphoria or the impact of hormone therapy use on this health condition should be assessed to determine the potential positive or negative impact of starting or continuing hormone therapy.

The decision to deny or delay care should not be taken lightly. In most cases, GAHT has significant positive protective mental health benefits, and denial of hormone therapy can worsen depression, anxiety, and suicidality. Additionally, blocking access to gender-affirming treatment can lead to procurement of nonmedically supervised hormones and disengagement from medical care.[3,9,10] Therefore, practicing gender-affirming care with a harm reduction philosophy should be the standard of care. **Harm reduction** aims to minimize negative health, social, or legal impacts of a potential high-risk behavior without requiring the individual to stop the behavior or blaming them for engaging in the behavior.[11,12] Whenever possible, an attempt to stabilize a condition should be made while initiating GAHT.

GUIDING EXPECTATIONS

Before starting GAHT, patients should be able to demonstrate clear and realistic expectations of hormone therapy, while also understanding the unique and largely unpredictable responses of each individual to hormone therapy. The age at which therapy is started, body habitus, and genetics likely play a role in the degree and speed at which changes may occur. These aspects also tend to influence the potential for risk factors from GAHT. The clinician and patient should review the physical and behavioral changes that are expected, limitations of hormone therapy, and the general timeline of these changes to guide patient expectations. It is also necessary to discuss the potential risks of hormone therapy on the body that are known, as well as the unknowns that still exist in this field regarding these medications and their outcomes. This information should be discussed in the context of the individual's goals and how these may, or may not, affirm their gender and meet their needs.

Effects of Testosterone Therapy

Testosterone therapy can cause lowering of the pitch of the voice, fat redistribution from the buttocks and hips to the abdomen, increased muscle mass, and growth of facial and body hair. For most individuals, testosterone also causes cessation of menses[13,14] (Table 7-1). Testosterone is generally safe. Although testosterone has been associated with a negative effect on lipids (specifically an increase in low-density lipoprotein and decrease in high-density lipoprotein), elevation in hematocrit, and a small increase in blood pressure, research has not shown an increase in cardiovascular events in those taking gender-affirming testosterone when compared with the general population. However, longer-term follow-up studies are still lacking. More data on cardiovascular outcomes in older (65 years of age or older) individuals will be helpful to better understand this risk with longer use of testosterone and as individuals age.[13,14] Additionally, testosterone does not appear to increase the risk of breast or other reproductive cancers.[14-16]

Effects of Estrogen and Antiandrogen Therapy

Estrogen and **antiandrogen therapy** (medications that suppress the body's production or response to testosterone and allow the effects of estrogen to be more apparent) often lead to breast growth, fat redistribution from the abdomen to the buttocks and hips, slowing of facial and body hair growth, and softening of skin. These medications may also decrease spontaneous erections, testicular size, and libido[14,17] (Table 7-2). Estradiol therapy has been associated with an increase in cardiovascular events, such as venous thromboembolism and stroke.[18,19] It is unclear about the extent to which the type of estrogen and other comorbidities (hyperlipidemia, tobacco use, hypertension) increases the likelihood of these events. However, it remains imperative to proactively manage cardiovascular health in anyone starting estrogen therapy. Estrogen and antiandrogens are not associated with an increased risk of breast cancer in transgender women compared with

Table 7-1. Expected Effects of Testosterone Therapy

Effect	Onset (months)	Maximum (years)
Acne and skin oiliness	1–6	1–2
Fat redistribution	1–6	2–5
Cessation of menses	2–6	
Clitoral/phallus enlargement	3–6	1–2
Atrophy of frontal canal/vagina	3–6	1–2
Deepening of voice	3–12	1–2
Increased sex drive	Variable	
Emotional changes	Variable	
Facial/body hair growth	6–12	4–5
Scalp hair loss	Variable	Variable
Increased muscle mass and strength	6–12	2–5
Coarser skin/increased sweating	3–12	
Weight gain/fluid retention	Variable	
Tendon injury	Variable; may be more likely with heavyweight training exercise	

Adapted with permission from Hembree WC, Cohen-Kettenis PT, Gooren L, et al: Endocrine Treatment of Gender-Dysphoric/Gender-Incongruent Persons: An Endocrine Society Clinical Practice Guideline, *J Clin Endocrinol Metab* 2017 Nov 1;102(11):3869-3903.

cisgender women.[16,20,21] Finally, estradiol appears to protect bone, and data indicate decreased bone turnover markers in individuals on estradiol therapy. Additionally, there does not appear to be an increased fracture risk in those using gender-affirming estrogen therapy.[22-24]

Because GAHT suppresses endogenous hormone production, fertility may be affected. It remains unclear if these effects on the reproductive system are fully reversible in all adults who have undergone their natal puberty. Several studies suggest that stopping GAHT and allowing endogenous hormones to return to their prior physiologic levels may restore fertility; however, the age of the individual must be considered.[25,26] Additional research is needed to counsel patients with more confidence and predictability about the effects of GAHT on fertility. At this time, it is still recommended to encourage individuals to consider cryopreservation of their gametes before starting hormone therapy if

Table 7–2. Expected Effects of Estrogen and Antiandrogen Therapy

Effect	Onset (months)	Maximum (years)
Decreased libido	1–3	0.25–0.5
Decreased spontaneous erections	3–6	
Decreased testicular volume	3–6	2–3
Decreased sperm production	Variable	Variable
Breast growth/breast tenderness	3–6	2–3
Redistribution of body fat	6–12	2–3
Decreased muscle mass	3–6	1–2
Softening of skin	3–6	2–3
Decreased or slower growth of facial and body hair	6–12	>3

Adapted with permission from Hembree WC, Cohen-Kettenis PT, Gooren L, et al: Endocrine Treatment of Gender-Dysphoric/Gender-Incongruent Persons: An Endocrine Society Clinical Practice Guideline, *J Clin Endocrinol Metab* 2017 Nov 1;102(11):3869-3903.

biological children are desired.[27] It can also be beneficial to discuss family planning on an ongoing basis for those whose family planning goals are evolving or for whom cryopreservation before initiation of GAHT is not an option.

TAKING AN APPROPRIATE HISTORY

The clinician must attain relevant medical, behavioral health, and social history from the individual to guide safe and effective care.[28] Assessment for medical safety should occur in the setting of underlying medical issues and family health history. Before initiating hormone therapy, baseline laboratory tests and a physical exam may also be warranted depending on the individual's underlying medical conditions, age, and family medical history. A behavioral health history should also be performed to assess the patient's need for supportive referrals as well as to ensure that any mental health conditions are relatively stable and that the individual can consent to treatment. Additionally, a social history can illuminate safety issues and support needs that the patient may have and experience throughout their affirmation.

Finally, it can be helpful to obtain a **gender narrative**, which is a history of experienced gender awareness and includes the development, exploration, acceptance or rejection, identification, and persistence of one's gender, as well as any symptoms of gender dysphoria. There is no one "right" story. Gender narratives often vary and may be nuanced and influenced by the intersectionality of identities

and experiences of an individual.[29] A gender narrative can help contextualize a patient's experience and goals to help guide treatment and create a clearer understanding between the patient and clinician on how to provide individualized, affirming care for that patient. See Table 7-3 for a review of the various components of medical, behavioral health, family, and social histories that should be obtained before starting GAHT.

TESTOSTERONE THERAPY

There are several options for the administration of testosterone, including injectables, topical gels or patches, and implantable long-acting pellets. Choosing which formulation is best depends on patient preference, ability to self-inject, risks of medication transfer to others, response to hormone therapy, insurance coverage, and cost.

▶ Injectable Testosterone Formulations

The most common form of testosterone is injectable due to its low cost and ability to increase testosterone levels quickly and efficiently. Testosterone can be injected subcutaneously (SC) or intramuscularly (IM).

Injectable Testosterone Formulations

Medication name	Testosterone cypionate (cottonseed oil) Or Testosterone enanthate (sesame seed oil)
Frequency	Injected weekly or every 2 weeks, IM or SC
Additional comments	Dose recommendations are the same whether using IM or SC injections. SC injections use smaller needles than IM and tend to be less painful. IM injections may be preferred or necessary for larger volumes.[30-33] Biweekly dosing reduces the number of injections but leads to greater fluctuations in testosterone levels that can be uncomfortable for some patients. Weekly dosing may be a better choice for those concerned about the impact of fluctuating hormone levels on mood or other medical conditions.

IM, intramuscular; SC, subcutaneous.

▶ Transdermal Testosterone Formulations

Because it is dosed daily, the effects of transdermal testosterone more closely parallel the natural physiologic fluctuations of testosterone than is true with other forms of testosterone. Transdermal formulations can be considered if there are concerns about the effects of significant fluctuations in hormone levels, if more gradual changes are desired, or both.

Table 7–3. Components of the Medical History

Component	Description
Gender narrative	History of experienced gender awareness and the development, exploration, acceptance/rejection, identification, and persistence of that gender Any symptoms of gender dysphoria Goals for nonmedical affirmation of gender, GAHT, or other gender-affirming medical care
Medical history	Personal history of coronary artery or cerebrovascular disease, arterial or venous thromboembolism, hypertension, diabetes, hormone-sensitive cancer, polycythemia, pituitary adenoma, liver disease, HIV infection, and other sexually transmitted infections Current specialists for any underlying medical issues Use of current or past prescribed and unprescribed hormone use, as well as any history of surgical procedures, including body modifications or injectable silicone use
Behavioral health history	History of major depression or bipolar disorder, psychosis, suicidality, impulse control disorder, disordered eating patterns, and substance use and abuse Current behavioral health care professionals and any past or present psychiatric medications Psychiatric hospitalizations Past or present sexual, physical, or emotional abuse or trauma (although it may not be necessary or possible to explore this fully in the initial assessment—see Chapter 11, "Basic Principles of Trauma-Informed Care") Current or previous suicidality or self-injurious behavior
Family history	Family history of any cancer, cardiovascular disease, diabetes, or blood clotting disorders
Social history	Biological family, chosen family, friend support, rejection, acceptance Cultural influences that may affect access to care or acceptance by community—religion, ethnicity, age, race, socioeconomic status, etc. Supports at work or school Community involvement, TGD peer support Sexual history, sexual orientation, safety

Transdermal Testosterone Formulations

Gels	
Medication names	Testosterone gel
Frequency	Applied daily
Additional comments	Patients must use caution to avoid skin-to-skin contact at application area(s) with partners, children, or pets until the medication is completely absorbed. Hands should be washed immediately after application. If skin-to-skin contact is anticipated, the area should be washed with soap and water or covered. The majority of the dose is absorbed within 4 hours of application.[34] Recommended application site is the upper arms.[35]

Transdermal Testosterone Formulations

Patches	
Medication name	2 mg or 4 mg testosterone transdermal system
Frequency	New patch(es) applied daily
Additional comments	Patches commonly cause skin irritation. They are not recommended for patients known to have sensitive skin.

▶ Long-Acting Testosterone Formulations

Long-acting formulations can be good options for people who find regular injections difficult and who are not candidates for transdermal formulations. These injections and implantable pellets may provide more consistent levels of testosterone over longer periods. They tend to be more expensive and must be administered by a medical professional in the clinic. Typically, long-acting formulations are only recommended after other methods have been tried.

Long-Acting Testosterone Formulations

Implantable Pellets	
Medication name	Testosterone pellets
Frequency	Implanted every 3–4 months
Additional notes	Requires minor surgical procedure to implant pellets under the skin in the upper, outer area of the buttock
	It is recommended that individuals initiate therapy with another form of testosterone prior to initiating testosterone pellets to ensure testosterone is tolerable and affirming.

Long-Acting Injectables	
Medication name	Testosterone undecanoate
Frequency	Initial injection
	Injection at 4 weeks
	Injections every 10 weeks thereafter
Additional notes	Potential for rare, adverse side effect of pulmonary oil microembolism, anaphylaxis, or both following injection. Therefore, patients must remain in the clinic for 30 minutes following injections for observation.
	Due to these unique risks, the FDA has approved this medication only under a restricted prescribing scheme.

FDA, US Food and Drug Administration.

Additional or Alternative Hormone Therapy

Some **trans masculine** or nonbinary individuals may desire or require additional medications to reduce symptoms of dysphoria. For example, cessation of menses may be critical to gender affirmation, but testosterone and its effects may not be desired. In these cases, hormonal contraceptives can be used to reduce or stop menstrual bleeding. Additionally, these medications may also be used to prevent pregnancy when requested and warranted, as testosterone alone does not reliably prevent pregnancy.[30]

ESTROGEN AND ANTIANDROGEN THERAPY

17β-estradiol, more commonly known as estradiol, is the recommended medication for GAHT. It is molecularly identical to the estrogen that circulates in the body and is observed to have the lowest risk profile, while also being quite effective.[31,32] Estrogen can suppress testosterone and its effects, but estrogen alone may not be enough to suppress testosterone sufficiently for some individuals. Antiandrogen therapy may be needed to allow the effects of estrogen to be more apparent.

Estrogen Therapy

Like testosterone, there are several options for administration. The choice is typically based on patient preference, accessibility, effectiveness, cost, and individual safety considerations.

Oral Estrogen Formulations

Oral estradiol is dosed daily and therefore provides steady levels of estrogen in the body. This formulation is relatively cheap, accessible, and easy to administer.

Oral Estrogen Formulations

Medication names	Estradiol tablets
Frequency	By mouth daily
Additional comments	Dissolving these tablets under the tongue, called sublingual (SL) dosing, may decrease the potential for estradiol affecting the liver (and the liver affecting the medication). However, there are no data to support that SL dosing is any safer or more beneficial than swallowing the tablets. The amount absorbed under the tongue is likely to be variable and unpredictable. The benefits versus risks of this dosing method are largely unknown.
	There may be pharmacokinetic differences in serum levels produced by oral vs. sublingual dosing of the estradiol, but the average serum levels throughout the day are likely the same.[39]

Transdermal Estrogen Formulations

Transdermal estradiol appears to be the safest formulation from a cardiovascular standpoint, showing little impact on lipids and a decreased risk of thromboembolic events (blood clots) compared with other formulations.[33-36] Transdermal formulations may be more appropriate for those with a higher than average cardiovascular risk, such as patients who are hypertensive, diabetic, or smokers. Like oral formations, transdermal formulations also provide the benefit of steady estrogen levels as well as ease of use.

Transdermal Estrogen Formulations

Patches	
Medication names	Estradiol transdermal system
Frequency	Patch(es) applied once or twice a week, depending on the brand
Additional comments	Patches formulated for twice-weekly use may be preferable for patients for whom adhesiveness is an issue.

Gels	
Medication names	Estradiol gel
Frequency	Applied daily
Additional comments	May be more expensive than other formulations. Less likely to cause a skin reaction (no adhesive as with the patch).

Injectable Estrogen Formulations

Injectable estradiol is typically dosed intramuscularly (IM) every 2 weeks, although weekly dosing with smaller amounts is possible, with the benefit of decreasing the fluctuations between doses. Some patients believe that injectable dosing produces changes more rapidly than transdermal preparations; however, there is no evidence to support this contention. Some avoid injectable formulations due to needle phobia, the inconvenience and timing of injections (whether self-injecting or by a medical professional), and the wider fluctuations in hormone levels from dose to dose.

Injectable Estrogen Formulations

Medication name	Estradiol valerate
Frequency	Injected every week or every 2 weeks IM
Additional comments	Injectable estrogens have few applications outside of their use in gender affirmation, resulting in periodic shortages from the manufacturer and/or difficulty obtaining injectable estradiol. These shortages are likely to continue, and those with concerns about this may consider topical or oral formulations instead.
Medication name	Estradiol cypionate
Frequency	Injection every 2 weeks IM
Additional comments	If switching from the valerate to the cypionate formulation, dosage adjustment is needed. The dosage of estradiol cypionate should be lowered to about 1/3 to 1/4 of the valerate dose. Estradiol cypionate tends to produce a lower, later, and longer peak level when compared to estradiol valerate, but the average levels in the blood, and effects on the body, should be the same.

IM, intramuscularly.

▶ Antiandrogen Therapy

For many, androgen-blocker medications are needed or desired to decrease endogenous production of and response to testosterone, allowing the effects of estrogen to be more apparent. Estrogen alone can suppress testosterone, but for some patients, estrogen alone may not be enough to suppress testosterone sufficiently.

Antiandrogen Formulations

Medication name	Spironolactone
Frequency	By mouth once or twice daily
Additional Comments	Spironolactone is a potassium-sparing diuretic that can directly inhibit testosterone production and its effects, as well as potentially having its own small estrogenic effect. Those who are smaller and thinner, have lower blood pressure, are on certain blood pressure medications, or have underlying kidney disease may be at increased risk of experiencing adverse side effects. It is currently the antiandrogen of choice in the United States.
Medication name	Finasteride, dutasteride
Frequency	By mouth once daily
Additional comments	These medications block the conversion of testosterone to its more potent form, DHT. They do not inhibit the production of testosterone and therefore will not lower blood testosterone levels. May be most effective for those with androgenic hair loss/baldness, significant facial hair, or those who are unable to tolerate higher doses of spironolactone.
Medication name	Leuprolide
Frequency	Injected monthly or every 3 months, depending on the formulation. This injection is done by a medical professional.
Additional comments	Decreases endogenous production of sex hormones and is used to block gonadal (testicular or ovarian) function. In prepubertal individuals, it can also reversibly block pubertal development prior to starting on gender-affirming hormone therapy. Leuprolide can be an option for some adults as part of a hormone therapy regimen, but it may be cost-prohibitive and therefore is not a first-line therapy.

The most common antiandrogen medication used in the United States is spironolactone, a potassium-sparing diuretic. At high doses, it directly inhibits both the production and binding of testosterone to the testosterone receptor and may also exert a small estrogenic effect of its own.[37-39] Spironolactone is inexpensive and generally well tolerated.

Recently, some have challenged the safety and effectiveness of spironolactone. One study questioned the effectiveness of spironolactone and its actual mechanism of action in the setting of estrogen therapy.[40] Anecdotal reports from patients and clinicians have raised concerns about possible long-term effects on endogenous corticosteroid production and mental health.[41,42] None of these issues has been explored in depth, and there is no proven clinical significance or relevance to these theories at this time. Despite these challenges, spironolactone remains one of the most studied, affordable, and safest antiandrogen medications available. As additional medications are evaluated for their effectiveness and safety in the context of gender-affirming care, these recommendations may change, and more desirable alternatives for testosterone suppression may emerge.

Some individuals are able to achieve testosterone suppression without an antiandrogen, either with estrogen alone or post-post-gonadectomy. In these cases, no additional medication is indicated for the suppression of endogenous testosterone. Antiandrogens should be discontinued after a patient undergoes orchiectomy.

▶ Progesterone Therapy

The benefit of progestins for gender affirmation is not well established. Some patients and medical professionals report that progesterone may help improve breast development, promote improvement in mood and libido, and have other positive benefits. However, progesterone has also been known to cause weight gain, fatigue, irritability, and negative mood changes in other individuals. Progesterone is part of a cisgender female's hormonal makeup and may be desired on this basis as part of a patient's gender-affirming hormone therapy. It is important to weigh the benefits vs. potential risks of starting progesterone.

In a few studies, progesterone has been shown to play a role in suppressing testosterone production, which supports its use as supplemental, or alternative, antiandrogen medication when needed.[43] Progesterone may be considered if estrogen alone or estrogen and spironolactone are not effective in adequately suppressing testosterone. Micronized progesterone (Prometrium) is the formulation that is molecularly identical to the progesterone produced in the body. It appears to be the safest option in terms of cardiovascular health.

Progesterone Formulations

Medication name	Micronized progesterone
Frequency	By mouth once daily, or cyclical dosing (10 days every month)
Additional comments	Some patients may prefer cyclic dosing as its effects may mimic a menstrual cycle, which can be affirming for some. However, others may find the hormonal fluctuations with cyclic dosing troubling and may prefer to take this medication daily. Progesterone's role in breast development has yet to be proven. Reported increases in breast size seem most likely due to general weight gain and fat deposition in the breasts as caused by progesterone and estrogen, and not the direct effect of progesterone on the breast tissue itself. So far, there is no evidence to show any specific benefit (or lack of benefit) regarding progesterone's effect on breast development.[44]
Medication name	Depot medroxyprogesterone acetate (DMPA or Depo Provera)
Frequency	Injected every 3 months
Additional comments	DMPA has been shown to have a slightly higher risk of side effects than micronized progesterone. DMPA is associated with bone loss in cisgender women and mood changes (irritability, depression). DMPA may also pose an increased risk of blood clotting events compared with the micronized progesterone, but this association needs to be studied further.[45] The benefit may be in the 3-month injectable dosing, but the risks may outweigh the benefits in many individuals.

GAHT FOR NONBINARY/GENDERQUEER INDIVIDUALS

Some nonbinary or genderqueer individuals may desire sex hormone levels in a range midway between the physiologic cisgender male and female ranges or to use gender-affirming hormones for a limited amount of time. The decision to prescribe GAHT and the dosages used should be based on a discussion with the patient. A clear understanding of patient goals and ensuring realistic expectations are necessary, given the unique and often unpredictable responses of each individual to hormone therapy.

"Microdosing" is a term that is sometimes used to describe using low doses or limited doses of testosterone or estrogen to affirm a gender identity. Most often, microdosing

Table 7–4. Laboratory Monitoring for Individuals on Testosterone Therapy

Laboratory test	Baseline	3 months	6 months	12 months	Yearly	As needed	Additional comments
Total testosterone		X	X	X	X	X	
Estradiol						X	
Hematocrit	X		X	X	X	X	
Lipids						X	Only as recommended by current USPSTF guidelines
Glucose or A1c						X	Only as recommended by current USPSTF guidelines

USPSTF, United States Preventive Services Task Force.

is requested by individuals identifying as nonbinary or gen-derqueer, but it may be requested by anyone for whom these alternative dosing options affirm their nuanced identity.

There is no one way to "microdose"; rather, microdosing should be viewed as another example of an individualized approach to prescribing hormone therapy. Patients are often started on low doses, and changes are closely monitored to ensure that the medication continues to affirm their identity and that changes that are not desired do not occur. Patients should be counseled that it is not possible to predict the changes that may occur as a result of hormone therapy or how fast they may occur. It is imperative to discuss changes that may be permanent and that it may not be possible to tailor hormone regimens to allow for some changes and not others. Patients should be given the option to stop hormone therapy whenever they feel the medication is no longer affirming or desired.

Some patients may wish to start on lower-than-usual doses and slowly increase their dosage over time. Giving the option for slowly experiencing the effects of hormones may provide relief from dysphoria, decreased anxiety, and autonomy over the process. A safe but flexible approach to dosing should be presented during the informed consent process for all patients when initiating hormone therapy.

FOLLOW-UP AND MONITORING

The important aspects of monitoring include gender affirmation and safety of GAHT. Despite premedication assessment and expectation setting, a person will not know whether the effects of GAHT will feel affirming to their gender until they start GAHT. It is important to follow up with patients to assess their experience and satisfaction with treatment. Additionally, a person's goals, gender, safety profile, and support can change over time, which may require individualized adjustments in medication or supportive referrals. Follow-up office visits are recommended regularly within the first year and semiregularly

thereafter to ensure that GAHT is meeting their needs and expectations. Follow-up visits also provide an opportunity to reassess behavioral health, social supports, and stability to provide holistic care for general health and well-being.

Another aspect of follow-up care may include laboratory monitoring to determine if hormone levels are within expected or therapeutic safe ranges. It may also be important to monitor underlying medical conditions, organ systems, or other aspects of the body that may be affected by GAHT and pose a potential health risk to the patient. As with other aspects of gender-affirming care, these recommendations can be individualized to a patient's specific risks and ability to access care (such as insurance coverage or distance from the clinic). A patient-centered, harm-reduction approach is encouraged. Requiring regular laboratory testing in order to continue on GAHT can pose unnecessary risk and harm to certain patients who require lower barriers to care to remain engaged. Medical professionals should thoughtfully assess risks versus benefits of the lab studies ordered before recommending them to patients. Suggestions for follow-up laboratory testing are presented in Tables 7-4 and 7-5.

SUMMARY

- GAHT is one aspect of gender affirmation. It is sought out by TGD individuals to reduce gender dysphoria. GAHT is known to be generally safe, effective, and life-saving for many TGD individuals. A flexible, patient-centered approach to initiation and maintenance of care is strongly encouraged.

- GAHT has been shown to decrease depression, anxiety, and suicidality, while improving overall health outcomes, making accessibility to gender-affirming medical care important in the overall well-being of TGD individuals.

Table 7–5. Laboratory Monitoring for Individuals on Estradiol and Antiandrogen Therapy

Laboratory test	Baseline	3 months	6 months	12 months	Yearly	As needed	Additional comments
Estradiol		X	X	X	X	X	
Total testosterone		X	X	X	X	X	Monitoring no longer necessary following gonadectomy
BUN, Cr, Potassium	X	X	X	X	X	X	Only necessary at baseline and monitoring if taking spironolactone
Lipids						X	Only as recommended by current USPSTF guidelines
Glucose or A1c						X	Only as recommended by current USPSTF guidelines
Prolactin						X	Only if symptoms of prolactinemia or on medications known to cause prolactinemia (i.e., antipsychotics)

BUN, blood urea nitrogen; Cr, creatinine; USPSTF, United States Preventive Services Task Force.

- Providing low-barrier access to GAHT through the informed consent process promotes engagement of the patient with the health care professional to discuss expectations, potential risks, and all available options for treatment—both medical and nonmedical.

- Clinicians should know about medication options and their associated risks, benefits, and limitations in order to best educate and guide patients in joint decision-making that best meets their goals. Creating an environment that empowers patients to discuss individual needs as they develop over time is an important aspect of guiding care and providing management as it may relate to physical changes, adverse side effects, family planning, or safety over months to years.

- Follow-up monitoring to assess for affirmation and reduction in dysphoria, as well as social and medical safety, are also important aspects of care. Regular check-ins within the first years can provide support during a dynamic time in an individual's physical, emotional, and social life. Laboratory monitoring may also be recommended depending on individual risks, medication, and access to care.

CASE STUDY 1: CH

CH is a 65-year-old, self-identified Caribbean-American trans woman who presents to Dr. York's office for the first time seeking estrogen and antiandrogen hormone therapy. As her new primary care physician, Dr. York welcomes her to the practice, "I'm so happy that you came in. Please share with me how you have experienced your gender over time and how you came to the decision to medically affirm your gender at this point in your life." CH responds that she has known she is a woman most of her life, but never had the language to define these thoughts, nor did she have any role models to show her it was a possibility. She married a woman when she was in her early 20s and had two children with this partner. She reports that her life has been fulfilling, but she has always suffered from depression, which she associates with her gender dysphoria. In her 30s, she attempted suicide and was admitted to the hospital for a week because she felt hopeless about never being able to socially or physically affirm her female identity. However, due to fear of rejection at the time, she told her family and medical professionals that her depression was caused by extreme work stress.

She goes on to say that her wife of 40 years passed away 2 years ago, and since then, she has been researching hormone therapy options and becoming more interested in pursuing gender-affirming care. She has bought "female clothes" and wears them at home but has not yet felt safe wearing them in public. She is close to her children and active in her church, and is very concerned about what gender affirmation will mean in terms of her relationship with her family and community, but feels she can no longer wait to affirm her female gender identity. When she broached the topic briefly with her children, they were shocked, marginally supportive, and said they needed time to process the news.

Dr. York reviews CH's medical history. She has hypertension and diabetes, for which she is taking lisinopril 20 mg daily, amlodipine 10 mg, metformin 1000 mg ER, and Lantus 60 U daily. Both conditions are moderately well-controlled: current blood pressure is 130/80 and hemoglobin A1c is 7.5%.

Her goals today are clear: she would like to affirm her female identity with estradiol and decrease her testosterone. She is also interested in connecting with the TGD community for peer support, as she is worried about rejection from her current family and friends.

▶ Discussion Questions

1. Dr. York asks CH what brings her in to affirm her gender at the age of 65. How can understanding an individual's gender narrative and gender history help you as their health care professional?

2. What identities—besides her trans identity—may have impacted CH's choices to start hormone therapy, and how may these intersecting identities continue to impact her sense of self and community acceptance?

3. CH discloses a history of chronic depression and a suicide attempt. How might this history, and the context in which it occurred, influence Dr. York's assessment of CH's behavioral health stability and appropriateness to start on GAHT, if at all? If the suicide attempt were more recent, how might a harm reduction approach to care be applied?

4. What aspects of CH's medical history might impact Dr. York's discussion of feminizing hormone therapy? Might Dr. York consider a certain type of estradiol or dosing considerations?

5. What laboratory tests might Dr. York want to monitor for CH based on her medical history and risks? How often should they be monitored?

6. CH is 65 years old, and a cisgender woman of this age would likely be postmenopausal with very low estrogen levels. Would you consider not starting CH on estrogen for this reason or starting on a very low dose of estradiol? What could be the physical and emotional benefits vs. the risks of not offering her estrogen? How do you think CH would feel or respond to Dr. York if estradiol were not offered?

CASE STUDY 2: XB

XB is a 19-year-old self-identified Latinx, nonbinary individual who was assigned female sex at birth and has been in care with physician assistant (PA) Ruiz-Marquez since they were 11 years old. XB has been using they/them pronouns since age 15, feels very comfortable talking to their PA about their gender, and has had good support from their friends and school. Both PA Ruiz-Marquez and XB speak Spanish as their first language, but now mostly speak English in their daily lives and speak English with each other.

XB scheduled an appointment with PA Ruiz-Marquez to discuss starting on gender-affirming testosterone therapy to further affirm their nonbinary identity. They are able to clearly describe aspects of themselves they do not identify with and that cause them dysphoria—menses, their chest (breasts), and voice. However, they are equally clear that they

have no interest in growing a beard, losing their hair, or having big muscles; none of those things would feel affirming. XB is asking about options to affirm their identity.

When PA Ruiz-Marquez asks about social and family support, XB acknowledges that their friends continue to be very supportive, but they have been struggling more and more with their family. XB is quite close to their parents and siblings, as well as their large extended family. Initially, XB was forgiving with their family when they did not use their affirmed name and pronouns, but they now feel increasingly frustrated and irritated by their lack of understanding. XB speaks Spanish at home with family and has modified their Spanish to make it less gendered but has received negative feedback from their parents that XB is not respecting the Spanish language and culture. XB asks PA Ruiz-Marquez for suggestions and support.

▶ Discussion Questions

1. XB is requesting support to further affirm their nonbinary identity with testosterone. Besides testosterone, what other medical or nonmedical options are available that might affirm XB's identity and meet their goals?

2. Would XB be a good candidate for testosterone? If so, what recommendations for testosterone might PA Ruiz-Marquez discuss with XB in regards to formulations and dosing? In what ways might the idea of "microdosing" meet or not meet XB's goals? If Dr. Ruiz-Marquez were going to prescribe testosterone for XB, what aspects of informed consent might be key in setting expectations?

3. How might a shared language or culture positively or negatively impact the formation of a productive relationship between XB and PA Ruiz-Marquez? XB feels very comfortable with PA Ruiz-Marquez, but can you envision a situation where a shared culture, identity, or religion might make it harder to disclose identity?

4. What supportive resources can you think of for XB? Are there any resources to support gender identity, gender-affirming language, or nongendered language in non-English speaking, nonwestern cultures that you can think of? How can we work to create these?

CASE STUDY 3: DG

DG is a 31-year-old self-identified white transgender male who has been engaged in care with nurse practitioner (NP) Hwang for the past 8 years. DG has a history significant for cerebral palsy (CP), and he also sees a neurologist, physiatrist, and physical therapist at a nearby medical facility. DG is on oxcarbazepine for his CP and muscle contractions. He has never been on testosterone therapy but had gender-affirming chest reconstruction 3 years ago. DG is quite healthy and is very active in adaptive sports (sled hockey, skiing, wheelchair basketball, rock climbing, etc.), which is where he gets his social supports and connections, as well as self-esteem and empowerment.

DG was referred to NP Hwang by his neurologist after he asked his neurology team what the impacts of testosterone therapy might be on his CP if he were to start gender-affirming hormones. DG comes into NP Hwang's office today looking for some answers to this question. DG reports to NP Hwang that he has been quite dysphoric due to being often misgendered, and very much wants to start on testosterone. However, he is worried about any negative impact testosterone might have on his CP and whether it could compromise his activity level and engagement in sports.

Since there are multiple causes of cerebral palsy, a paucity of information about sex-linked or hormonal influences on CP, and no current research on how exogenous testosterone might impact CP (in either cisgender or transgender individuals), answers to these questions are difficult. NP Hwang can discuss the known effects of testosterone on bone and muscle in individuals without CP but it is unclear if these effects will be the same in those with CP and how testosterone might specifically affect DG's function.

▶ Discussion Questions

1. As a medical professional, how do you provide informed consent in the setting of unknowns? How does this make you feel as a medical professional? As a patient, how would you feel hearing that "the expert" does not have the answers?

2. What are some of the changes that are expected when starting testosterone therapy that might be relevant to DG?

3. What might be some of the benefits of starting testosterone therapy? What might be the risks? Can you speculate how these benefits and risks might impact DG both physically and emotionally?

4. If NP Hwang and DG decided together that the benefits of testosterone likely outweighed the risks, what would be the best way to monitor DG's response to therapy? How might you engage DG's medical specialists in this process?

REFERENCES

1. Nguyen HB, Chavez AM, Lipner E, et al. Gender-affirming hormone use in transgender individuals: impact on behavioral health and cognition. *Curr Psychiatry Rep.* 2018;20(12):110.

2. Dhejne C, Van Vlerken R, Heylens G, Arcelus J. Mental health and gender dysphoria: a review of the literature. *Int Rev Psychiatry.* 2016;28(1):44-57.

3. Witcomb GL, Bouman WP, Claes L, Brewin N, Crawford J, Arcelus J. Levels of depression in transgender people and its predictors: Results of a large matched control study with transgender people accessing clinical services. *J Affect Disord.* 2018;235:308-315.

4. Defreyne J, Motmans J, T'Sjoen G. Healthcare costs and quality of life outcomes following gender affirming surgery in trans men: a review. *Expert Rev Pharmacoecon Outcomes Res.* 2017;17(6):543-556.

5. James SE, Herman JL, Rankin S, Keisling M, Mottet L, Anafi M. *The Report of the 2015 U.S. Transgender Survey.* Washington, DC: National Center for Transgender Equality; 2016.

6. Coleman E, Bockting W, Botzer M, et al. Standards of care for the health of transsexual, transgender, and gender-nonconforming people, Version 7. *Int J Transgenderism.* 2011;13(4):165-232.

7. Cocanour CS. Informed consent: it's more than a signature on a piece of paper. *Am J Surg.* 2017;214(6):993-997.

8. Cavanaugh T, Hopwood R, Lambert C. Informed consent in the medical care of transgender and gender-nonconforming patients. *AMA J Ethics.* 2016;18(11):1147-1155.

9. Tomson A. Gender-affirming care in the context of medical ethics: gatekeeping v. informed consent. *Afr J Bioethics Law.* 2018;11(1):24-28.

10. White Hughto JM, Reisner SL. A systematic review of the effects of hormone therapy on psychological functioning and quality of life in transgender individuals. *Transgender Health.* 2016;1(1):21-31.

11. Hawk M, Coulter RW, Egan JE, et al. Harm reduction principles for healthcare settings. *Harm Reduct J.* 2017; 14(1):70.

12. Aitken S. The primary health care of transgender adults. *Sex Health.* 2017;14(5):477-483.

13. Defreyne J, T'Sjoen G. Transmasculine hormone therapy. *Endocrinol Metab Clin North Am.* 2019;48(2):357-375.

14. T'Sjoen G, Arcelus J, Gooren L, Klink DT, Tangpricha V. Endocrinology of transgender medicine. *Endocr Rev.* 2019;40(1):97-117.

15. Irwig M. Testosterone therapy for transgender men. *Lancet Diabetes Endocrinol.* 2017;5(4)301-311.

16. de Blok CJM, Dreijerink KMA, den Heijer M. Cancer risk in transgender people. *Endocrinol Metab Clin.* 2019;48(2):441-452.

17. Unger CA. Hormone therapy for transgender patients. *Transl Androl Urol.* 2016;5(6):877-884.

18. Getahun D, Nash R, Flanders WD, et al. Cross-sex hormones and acute cardiovascular events in transgender persons: a cohort study. *Ann Intern Med.* 2018;169(4):205-213.

19. Nota NM, Wiepjes CM, de Blok CJM, Gooren LJG, Kreukels BPC, den Heier M. Occurrence of acute cardiovascular events in transgender individuals receiving hormone therapy. *Circulation.* 2019;139(11):1461-1462.

20. de Blok CJM, Wiepjes CM, Nota NM, et al. Breast cancer risk in transgender people receiving hormone treatment: nationwide cohort study in the Netherlands. *BMJ.* 2019;365:l1652.

21. Gooren LJ, van Trotsenburg MAA, Giltay EJ, van Diest PJ. Breast cancer development in transsexual subjects receiving cross-sex hormone treatment. *Sex Med.* 2013;10(12): 3129-3134.

22. Van Caenegem E, Taes Y, Wierckx K, et al. Low bone mass is prevalent in male-to-female transsexual persons before the start of cross-sex hormonal therapy and gonadectomy. *Bone.* 2013;54(1):92-97.

23. Wiepjes CM, Vlot MC, de Blok CJM, Nota NM, de Jongh RT, den Heijer M. Bone geometry and trabecular bone score in transgender people before and after short- and long-term hormonal treatment. *Bone.* 2019;127:280-286.

24. Wiepjes CM den Heijer M, T'Sjoen GG. Bone health in adult trans persons: an update of the literature. *Curr Opin Endocrinol Diabetes Obes.* 2019;26(6):296-300.

25. Light AD, Obedin-Maliver J, Sevelius JM, Kerns JL. Transgender men who experienced pregnancy after female-to-male gender transitioning. *Obstet Gynecol.* 2014;124(6):1120-1127.

26. Leung A, Sakkas D, Pang S, Thornton K, Resetkova N. Assisted reproductive technology outcomes in female-to-male transgender patients compared with cisgender patients: a new frontier in reproductive medicine. *Fertil Steril.* 2019;112(5):858-865.

27. De Roo C, Tilleman K, T'Sjoen G, De Sutter P. Fertility options in transgender people. *Int Rev Psychiatry.* 2016;28(1):112-119.

28. Radix A. Hormone therapy for transgender adults. *Urol Clin North Am.* 2019;46(4):467-473.

29. Wilson Y, White A, Jefferson A, Danis M. Intersectionality in clinical medicine: the need for a conceptual framework. *Am J Bioeth.* 2019;19(2):8-19.

30. Krempasky C, Harris M, Abern L, Grimstad F. Contraception across the transmasculine spectrum. *Am J Obstet Gynecol.* 2020;222(2):134-143.

31. Asscheman H, Giltay EJ, Megens JAJ, Pim de Ronde W, van Trotsenburg MAA, Gooren LJG. A long-term follow-up study of mortality in transsexuals receiving treatment with cross-sex hormones. *Eur J Endocrinol.* 2011;164(4):635-642.

32. Tangpricha V, den Heijer M. Oestrogen and anti-androgen therapy for transgender women. *Lancet Diabetes Endocrinol.* 2017;5(4):291-300.

33. Olson J, Schrager SM, Clark LF, Dunlap SL, Belzer M. Subcutaneous testosterone: an effective delivery mechanism for masculinizing young transgender men. *LGBT Health.* 2014;1(3):165-167.

34. Canonico M, Oger E, Plu-Bureau G, et al. Hormone therapy and venous thromboembolism among postmenopausal women: Impact of the route of estrogen administration and progestogens: The ESTHER Study. *Circulation.* 2007;115(7):840-845.

35. Straczek C, Oger E, Yon de Jonage-Canonico MB, et al. Prothrombotic mutations, hormone therapy, and venous thromboembolism among postmenopausal women: Impact of the route of estrogen administration. *Circulation.* 2005;112(22):3495-3500.

36. Shufelt CL, Merz CNB, Prentice RL, et al. Hormone therapy dose, formulation, route of delivery, and risk of cardiovascular events in women: Findings from the WHI Observational Study. *Menopause.* 2014;21(3):260-266.

37. Sinclair R, Patel M, Dawson TL, et al. Hair loss in women: medical and cosmetic approaches to increase scalp hair fullness: approaches to increase scalp hair fullness. *Br J Dermatol.* 2011;165:12-18.

38. Liang JJ, Jolly D, Chan KJ, Safer JD. Testosterone levels achieved by medically treated transgender women in a United States endocrinology clinic cohort. *Endocr Pract.* 2018;24(2):135-142.

39. Prior JC, Vigna YM, Watson D. Spironolactone with physiological female steroids for presurgical therapy of male-to-female transsexualism. *Arch Sex Behav.* 1989;18(1):49-57.

40. Leaning MC, Feustel PJ, Joseph J. Hormonal treatment of transgender women with oral estradiol. *Transgender Health.* 2018;3(1):74-81.

41. Verman A. Spironolactone, a controversial drug used in hormone replacement therapy, is not right for all trans women. Slate Magazine. 2019. https://slate.com/technology/2019/06/spironolactone-hormone-trans-women-side-effects.html. Accessed December 19, 2019.

42. Cosgrove B. The case against spironolactone. MTF Trans Hormonal Therapy. 2018. https://moderntranshormones.com/2018/01/01/whats-wrong-with-spironolactone/. Accessed December 19, 2019.

43. Jain J, Kwan D, Forcier M. Medroxyprogesterone acetate in gender-affirming therapy for transwomen: results from a retrospective study. *J Clin Endo Metab.* 2019;104(11): 5148-5156.

44. Wierckx K, Gooren L, T'Sjoen G. Clinical review: Breast development in trans women receiving cross-sex hormones. *J Sex Med.* 2014;11(5):1240-1247. doi:10.1111/jsm.12487

45. Mueck AO. Postmenopausal hormone replacement therapy and cardiovascular disease: the MEDICAL CARE OF TRANS AND GENDER DIVERSE ADULTS 53 value of transdermal estradiol and micronized progesterone. *Climacteric.* 2012;15(Suppl 1): 11-17. doi:10.3109/13697137.2012.669624

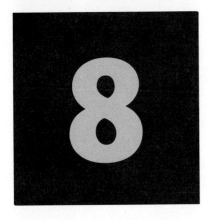

8

Nonmedical, Nonsurgical Gender Affirmation

Steph DeNormand

INTRODUCTION

It is essential for those who care for and about **transgender and gender diverse (TGD)** people to continue to learn about what **gender affirmation** means for the people they are engaging with, as well as to understand some of the more common ways TGD people pursue gender affirmation outside of a medical context. This chapter uses TGD to indicate all people who were assigned a sex at birth that is not in line with their gender identity, as well as anyone who is affirmed by aspects of gender expression that are not typically associated with someone of the same sex they were assigned at birth. A specific transgender or gender diverse identity is not necessary to benefit from the techniques and tools outlined in this chapter, and individual consideration is necessary when discussing any aspect of gender with a person, including gender affirmation.

This chapter is by no means an exhaustive list of affirming practices; it serves to introduce a variety of potential options and ideas outside of medically or surgically altering the body that TGD people may engage in. There is still a large gap in medical and academic literature describing the spectrum of strategies TGD people use to affirm their gender and sparse information addressing the medical, mental, and emotional impact of these behaviors. Therefore, this chapter includes a mixture of medical and academic sources and content created by and for TGD communities to describe their own bodies and experiences.

CONCEPTS OF GENDER AFFIRMATION

For most people, gender roles and gendered expectations are integral to how they choose to express their gender. Concepts and expectations of gendered expression are heavily based on a person's cultural and social background. As one impact of cultural colonialism, predominantly white, Eurocentric ideals of femininity and masculinity are typically privileged over

all others as the expected norms. Gender expression and gender affirmation are deeply personal; therefore, it is up to each individual to define what is right for them. Regardless of our personal perspectives and beliefs about what is feminine or masculine, what aspects of gender expression "go together," or what is the most important aspect of gender affirmation to pursue, service providers must listen to the expressed needs of each individual and do whatever is possible to assist them in achieving their goals.

The gender-affirmation concepts, tools, and techniques described in this chapter are often viewed as assisting TGD people to "pass," defined here as appearing in the world as a cisgender person, and is most often used in reference to a person being consistently seen by others as their affirmed gender. This use of gender-affirmation tools and techniques may also be described as addressing social **gender dysphoria**, in which individuals experience a marked and distressing incongruence between the way their gender is perceived by others and the way they see or understand themselves. It is also important to consider the impact of gender expression on safety. Given the high frequency of harassment and violence against TGD people—especially **trans** women and **trans feminine** people of color—blending in with cisgender peers may be necessary to remain safe.[1] However, while blending in with cisgender peers may be a high priority for some TGD people, others may be more affirmed by being "visibly" trans, nonbinary, or gender-nonconforming. Given that individual aims for social perception vary widely, it is essential that each person is considered the expert on their own needs and experiences and that their expressed needs and priorities serve as the driving force behind gender-affirmation conversations.

The majority of the options described in this chapter are not permanent and can be removed or reversed with relative ease. For those people who are unsure about which gender expression(s) are most affirming or whose gender identity or expression fluctuates, a removable or reversible option that mimics the effect of a more permanent intervention can be an ideal way to try different options at different points in time. A removable or reversible option may also be optimal when medical intervention is not feasible or when the effect is not desired at all times. In addition, some options may be selected because they result in more subtle effects or augment physical changes beyond what is possible with medical interventions alone.

Gender-affirmation tools and techniques may also be able to address gender dysphoria that is specific to an individual's unique perception of their body or its function. Working to create an authentic representation of how one sees themselves is another common reason to pursue any gender affirmation. While individuals may pursue gender affirmation as a way to combat gender dysphoria as described above, they may also be striving for gender euphoric experiences of the self. Within dominant academic literature, the majority of discussion regarding TGD experiences revolves around distress, dysphoria, discrimination, complications, and functional impairments. This focus often misses or underrepresents the relief and joy many TGD people feel when they are seen as who they are or are able to find a sense of alignment between themselves and their bodies. Gender affirmation can be emotional and complicated but can also be a space for exploration, joy, excitement, and play. Without acknowledging both dysphoria and euphoria with gender affirmation, it is impossible to build a cohesive picture of the experiences of TGD people.

NAMES, PRONOUNS, AND SEX/GENDER MARKERS

Most names and pronouns carry gendered assumptions. Since names and pronouns are used constantly for most people in everyday life, using more affirming names and pronouns are some of the most common ways people affirm their gender. This discussion of names and pronouns is specific to the English language. While some of this content applies to those who are not speaking English, it is important to maintain a culturally specific approach to conversations about names and gendered references. Language used to refer to the self and others is specific to an individual's personal background, language, and cultural conceptions, and it is essential that these nuances are always considered when addressing a concept as socioculturally complex as gender.

In a 2015 survey of the transgender population in the United States, 84% of those surveyed reported using a different set of pronouns than those typically associated with the sex they were assigned at birth, while only 11% reported that all of their identity documents listed the correct name and gender marker.[2] Legally updating names and sex/gender

markers[A] can be an essential part of someone's gender affirmation, with research indicating a lower prevalence of psychological distress and suicidal ideation in those with affirming documentation.[3] Given the frequency with which requirements for changing names and sex/gender markers on identification documents changes, those who are interested in pursuing this should consult the most updated local legal resources for accurate information. In the United States, legal advocacy and activist organizations often have free legal assistance or consultation to support TGD people in this process, and many reputable websites can provide guidance with this process.[4] Some state and federal identification documents require the person to have accessed specific forms of gender-affirming care, which makes obtaining affirming identification documents impossible for those who are not pursuing or do not have access to the relevant medical or surgical intervention(s). The majority of these documents also do not have sex/gender markers other than M (male) and F (female), and many TGD people are not reflected in those options.

Regardless of the name and sex/gender marker reflected on legal documents, it is necessary for those interacting with TGD people to use their affirmed name, pronouns, and appropriately gendered terms when communicating with or about them. This necessity may include the use of pronouns that are not typically used by cisgender people or using alternating combinations of pronouns when referring to the person. There is now significant evidence to support this necessity, including improved mental health and decreased suicidality.[5] Creating space in both clinical and social settings for TGD people to try out, use, or change their name or pronouns can be instrumental in helping to find what best fits how they would like to be referred to in other spaces. The use of affirmed names and pronouns can be especially helpful for those who are unable to use these names or pronouns in other aspects of their life and is one of the most concrete ways for any person to express support for TGD people.

BODY MODIFICATION

Medical and surgical gender affirmation are not the only ways for people to modify their bodies in an affirming way. There is a wide variety of permanent and semipermanent techniques people may use to change the way their body looks and feels. Some TGD people find that tattoos, piercings, and

---

[A] The phrasing "sex/gender markers" is used throughout this section in acknowledgment of the lack of standardization of language used by various state/federal agencies in describing these markers. In some cases, it is unclear whether the document is intended to record the sex, gender, or sex that was assigned at birth for the individual, which may create additional confusion for TGD individuals attempting to obtain affirming documentation.

other similar body modifications can be gender-affirming ways to change their appearance or experience of their body. Many people of all gender identities have described these methods as a way of reclaiming the body by creating a more aesthetically pleasing or more comfortable physical form. Certain tattoo and piercing locations and styles may be considered more feminine or masculine, or have the ability to accentuate or obscure particular features, creating an overall more gender-affirming experience of the body. Piercings, in particular, are also used by some people to adjust the appearance and functionality of the genitals, creating opportunities for different sensations and experiences of these body parts.[6]

Tattoos and piercings following gender-affirming surgery are also somewhat common. For example, someone who has had a gender-affirming chest reconstruction surgery may pursue medical tattooing for their nipples and areolas or have their nipples pierced. These body modifications can be useful techniques to conceal scars or divert attention away from the appearance of a surgical modification of the body, or accentuate affirming surgical results. The person's relevant surgeon can provide guidance as to how long after surgery pursuing a tattoo or piercing is best, taking into account the individual person's healing process.

Genital pumping (sometimes referred to as pumping or clitoral pumping) is a practice of mechanically applying suction to the phallus of an individual who was assigned female at birth, typically with the intention of enlarging this tissue or enhancing the effect of exogenous testosterone on this part of the body. While there are limited data on the effectiveness of this practice in creating permanent growth, some genital surgeons recommend particular pumping protocols prior to **metoidioplasty** or **phalloplasty**.[7] This practice may require coaching from a medical provider, as serious damage can occur if done incorrectly.[8] Genital pumping is typically performed with a cylinder surrounding the phallus and a device to create suction within the cylinder. Pump set-ups with a quick-release valve are preferred, as they allow for faster removal if needed. Some of these devices may have a pumping apparatus that is removable. This allows the cylinder to maintain suction without the pump. Users can then wear the cylinder for longer periods of time or use it during sexual activity. Some people interested in pumping may need assistance in determining appropriate cylinder size or coaching in identifying potential hazards or warning signs of tissue damage.

Exercise and weightlifting can also provide gender-affirming body modification. While not traditionally included in this category, different forms of exercise and strength training can have a significant impact on the shape of the body. A person who desires wider shoulders and narrower hips may spend more time and focus on building shoulder, back, and chest muscles, and less in other areas of the body. A person for whom larger visible muscles would be less affirming might opt for more aerobic exercise to maintain leaner muscles without significantly increasing muscle size. It is worth noting that gyms and other fitness facilities can be a fraught topic for TGD people. There is typically a heavy focus on body appearance, in addition to contending with showers and locker rooms. This atmosphere may prevent some TGD people from being able to pursue the exercise they desire, opting for at-home options to avoid these concerns. Other gender-affirmation products such as binders may also make exercise more difficult or dangerous while using them, adding further complications. While exercise is an important part of every person's health, it can be used as a tool to modify the body in unhealthy ways as well. Additional information about body image, disordered eating, and excessive exercise can be found in Chapter 15, "Eating Disorders, Body Image, and Body Positivity."

FACIAL AND BODY HAIR REMOVAL

Hair removal, particularly facial hair removal, can be an essential aspect of gender affirmation. In the United States, there is often no insurance coverage for semipermanent and permanent hair removal for gender affirmation,[B] with some limited exceptions. To maintain a seemingly hairless face, many people who have had prolonged exposure to testosterone require shaving multiple times a day or frequent use of other hair-removal products, such as waxing or chemical hair removal. This repeated exposure can result in skin irritation or a variety of other skin concerns, in addition to being time consuming, expensive, and requiring frequent attention to a typically gendered aspect of the body.

Permanent and semipermanent options include **laser hair removal** and **electrolysis**. Advantages of these options include less skin irritation and less frequent need to engage with a dysphoric aspect of the body; they also provide a more consistent result that may increase a person's safety or ability to be seen as their affirmed gender.[9] Laser hair removal is often faster and considered less painful than electrolysis. However, it is also less permanent and requires particular skin and hair characteristics in order to be effective with minimal skin irritation and damage. Electrolysis is considered more permanent and effective for most people, but it requires more time, is more expensive, and is less readily accessible than laser hair removal. While electrolysis is the more expensive option of the two, both are often prohibitively expensive and rarely covered by health insurance.[10]

[B] Hair removal at surgical sites for genital surgery is often required, and a prerequisite for surgery (see Chapter 9, "Surgical Gender Affirmation"). This is generally covered by insurance companies within the United States; however, it can be difficult to find a provider who is able and willing to work with insurance coverage. This section is exclusively discussing hair removal on the face and body for gender affirmation, and not the hair removal required prior to surgery.

SILICONE PUMPING

While many body modification methods are very safe when done correctly, a few practices pose significant adverse health risks. One such practice is silicone pumping, in which nonmedical professionals inject free silicone into the body or face to create drastic and immediate physical changes. This procedure has been illegal within the cosmetic industry for several years due to safety concerns[11] but continues to be practiced without medical supervision for cosmetic or gender-affirmation purposes. Often the silicone is mixed with other substances or of unknown quality, such as silicone industrial lubricant.[12] "Pumping parties," in which multiple people gather to be injected with silicone sequentially,[11] are common venues in which this practice takes place. There is a high risk of contracting HIV or hepatitis C with this practice, especially when needles and syringes are shared.

Silicone pumping is more prevalent in communities with less access to gender-affirming resources, particularly communities facing multiple layers of oppression and disenfranchisement. In following with harm reduction models of care, health care providers should refrain from shaming patients for taking part in silicone pumping and assist the person in accessing safer forms of gender affirmation. While silicone pumping is typically used to create more feminine features, anyone may attempt it if looking for immediate, visible results at a low cost. Clinicians working with TGD communities should be screening for this practice in their patient populations, understanding of the reasons TGD people may seek out this body modification, and familiar with the potential complications of silicone pumping that may necessitate current or future medical follow-up.

NONPERMANENT AND REMOVABLE GENDER-AFFIRMATION TECHNIQUES

In addition to the permanent and semipermanent physical changes to the body described above, there are many other ways that TGD people may alter their appearance in gender-affirming ways. The items described below may be used to change the appearance of gendered aspects of the body that cannot otherwise be changed or when a more permanent option is not currently available or accessible. These approaches may also be used long-term by people who are not seeking permanent bodily changes. Those who only feel safe, comfortable, or affirmed with particular gendered presentations at some times and not others may also employ these nonpermanent techniques. The following discussion is organized anatomically.

▶ Face and Voice

The face is often the first part of one's body others see and often one's most recognizable physical aspect. There are a wide variety of ways people modify the appearance of their face, including facial hair, grooming, makeup, and hairstyle.

For those who desire it, facial hair can be a notable feature for cultivating individuality, creativity, and gender euphoria. Since most facial hair changes are impermanent, people can try many different styles or expressions over a comparatively short period. The practice of shaving itself may also be a source of affirmation, particularly for those who begin growing significant facial hair as a result of gender-affirming hormones.

Makeup can also be a great source of gender affirmation. Similar to shaving facial hair, applying makeup is a traditionally gendered behavior for which the ritual of application itself may also be affirming, separate from the intended results. Makeup can be an effective way to accentuate or de-emphasize aspects of the face in an affirming manner. Most children who were assigned male at birth were not taught how to apply makeup if not explicitly forbidden from doing so, which may present a challenge as they begin exploring its potential benefits. There are, however, a growing number of cosmetic companies that are expressing specific interest in helping TGD people develop these skills, with some even holding classes specifically for TGD clients.

Hair and hairstyling are other areas in which personality and creativity can be displayed. Finding an affirming haircut or hairstyle can have a significant impact on the way someone feels about their appearance, as well as how they are perceived by others. For those who have had a significant amount of testosterone-induced balding, wigs may also be a helpful option. Wigs are available in a variety of styles and hair types, with a wide range of options with regard to quality and cost. A variety of resources are available online for TGD people interested in purchasing a wig, and often conferences for TGD people have wig vendors who can provide guidance as well. Wigs may also be used by people who would like to present with or who would be affirmed by a given hairstyle only part of the time.

Voice therapy is also a semimedical intervention that can have a significant impact on day-to-day life for TGD people. The effects of testosterone on the voice are permanent: whether endogenous or administered, the deepening of the voice that occurs with testosterone exposure cannot be reversed with decreased exposure to testosterone or with subsequent exposure to estrogen. Voice therapy, however, can have a significant impact on the tone and timbre of a person's voice and allow for more control over one's vocal patterns and has a high satisfaction rate among TGD patients.[13] Typically under the supervision of a speech-language pathologist, this voice therapy focuses on the ways in which not only vocal patterns, but also vocal mannerisms and conversation styles are socially interpreted in gendered ways, and assists TGD people in understanding and using a more affirming voice. While certainly a more common need for those who were assigned male at birth, people of all genders and assigned sexes can see benefits from voice therapy.

▶ Chest and Breasts

The presence of breasts on a person's chest is one of the most visible and socioculturally recognized markers of being female. As a result, those who do not want to be read as women may experience significant discomfort with having this social marker visible, and those who want to be read as women may desire this visibility. This section addresses the ways people may affirm their gender with regard to modifying the size and shape of their breasts or chest.

People with significant amounts of breast tissue may choose to bind their chest to reduce its appearance or prominence, and create a flatter and more masculine or androgynous appearance. There are many methods a person can use to bind their chest, often depending on what they can access or afford. As with many of the gender-affirmation options discussed throughout this chapter, there are both commercial and do-it-yourself methods. Commercial chest binders for TGD people have become much more freely available since the mid-2010s and are now made by a variety of companies, some of which are also owned and operated by TGD people. There are both off-the-rack and custom-made products and options, with ranges of skin tones, and some more fun and fashionable styles (Figure 8-1). Binder exchanges are an option for people who cannot otherwise afford to purchase a binder, including programs that are mostly sourced from TGD people who have already had chest reconstruction surgery. Appropriate sizing and level of compression are essential to maintain both the safety and efficacy of binding.

Other than commercial binders, there are a variety of ways people may bind their chests. Athletic tape, medical tape, and tape specially made for binding are some more popular choices (Figure 8-2). Depending on the size of the person's chest, their skin characteristics, and the tape used, some people find they are able to exercise, shower, and even swim with these options. Tapes are more likely to cause skin breakdown and other skin concerns than binders but may be a suitable option for some people with appropriate accompanying skincare and "off days" with no binder. Tapes are typically less compressing than binders as they do not wrap around the entire body, often allowing for a greater range of motion and less breathing concerns. Using tapes to bind tends to be more successful for people with smaller chests. Other craft or industrial tapes, such as duct tape, are more likely to cause damage and skin concerns, as these tapes are not designed to be applied to the skin.

Elastic bandages are another relatively accessible and low-cost option some people may use to bind. There has been a significant amount of intracommunity education, particularly on the internet, regarding the specific risks of using these bandages. Since this type of bandage or wrap is

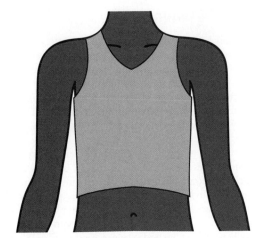

▲ **Figure 8-1.** Example of a binder.

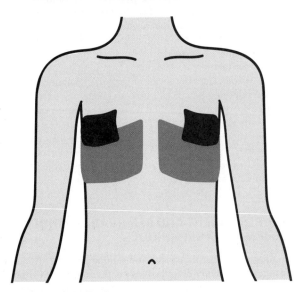

▲ **Figure 8-2.** Taping.

designed to compress swelling and injuries, it can be quite stiff and constricting when wrapped around the chest, potentially making both breathing and other movements more difficult.

Sports bras are also used by some people to bind their chest. Certain cuts and designs may work better than others, and some people find success in layering multiple sports bras on top of each other. Layering of these garments may also create significant chest compression similar to that of a binder and may cause damage if not sized appropriately and used with caution.

All methods of binding have some potential risk, depending on the method, frequency, and duration of binding. Some of the most common experiences include overheating, short-ness of breath, back and shoulder pain, skin damage, and infection.[14] People who find binding to be especially affirming may find it prohibitively distressing to not wear a binder for any duration, including to sleep, take breaks for the skin to heal, or even to wash the binder or binding material. This distress makes washing binders a particularly arduous task for some people, especially if they only own one binder. Regardless of the method, those who bind should be encouraged to pay attention to their body's needs, take breaks when possible, and consult their health care provider if they are experiencing pain or other negative effects of binding.

For other people, the absence of visible breasts can be a significant source of dysphoria. The intense focus and attention on breasts within the dominant Western culture as a sexualized marker of womanhood may cause problems for TGD people with a more feminine presentation, as both the presence and absence of these markers have the potential to attract unwanted attention. The absence of breasts in someone who otherwise presents or is read as a woman is not always overtly outing, as many cisgender women have little breast tissue. However, in combination with other information about a person's appearance or presentation, a lack of breast tissue may be used to make assumptions about the sex a person was assigned at birth. In those who were assigned male at birth and are taking estrogen, most people do not achieve mature Tanner 5 breasts with hormones alone. In these cases, surgery may be the only way to permanently create the appearance of mature breasts in a manner that is satisfactory for the TGD person.

Breast forms can be one way to manage this need, both in addressing the person's dysphoria and providing a socially and culturally identifiable marker of being female. These can be used by any person who would be affirmed by the presence of visible breasts, even in addition to any medical gender affirmation they may or may not have pursued. Hyper-realistic custom prosthetics made from high-quality materials are prohibitively expensive, but there are many moderate-to-low cost options as well. Bra fillers designed to augment the chest of cisgender women can also be used by people with little or no breast tissue. Do-it-yourself options may include hand-knit or hand-sewn pads or forms, which may have a less realistic appearance on their own, but can be a successful and low-cost option for filling out a bra or other undergarment.

Many people with breasts, regardless of gender identity, do not know how to size a bra for their body appropriately. People who were assigned male at birth may face the additional disadvantage of not having been taught or socially expected to size or wear a bra during adolescence and may be fearful of asking for help in traditional retail spaces. In general, those with a larger, wider chest cavity are more likely to find that larger forms look or feel more natural for their body habitus—this, however, is not true for every person, and the size of a breast form or amount of padding added to existing breasts is a personal choice. Having knowledge of retailers or community members within the local community who can assist TGD people in appropriately sizing bras can be an invaluable resource.

▶ Waist, Hips, and Silhouettes

TGD people may also find that their silhouette or general body shape causes them distress or causes them to be misgendered or identified as TGD in public spaces. A straighter line from shoulders to buttocks is generally seen as more masculine, whereas narrower waists and wider hips are typically seen as more feminine. While those who pursue hormone therapy may experience a change in their body shape with muscle and fat distribution changes, for some people, hormone therapy alone may not adequately create an affirming representation of the self.

Compression wear, corsets, and shapewear are all commercially available clothing items that may be able to assist in modifying the appearance of the waist and hips. These garments may also be combined with any combination of hip or buttock padding to accentuate the effect if desired. These compression garments may also assist people in fitting into or filling out clothing in a way that is more gender-affirming.

▶ Genitals

Similar to the way that breasts are considered a distinct social and cultural marker of being female, the presence of a penis or otherwise large, visible external genitalia is a social and cultural marker of being male. For some people, the presence of a "bulge" in one's pants may not only cause that person to experience heightened dysphoria, but it may also create a real safety risk with the potential of being visibly read as TGD. Creating the appearance of a flatter genital area, therefore, can be a matter of both comfort and safety.

The most common method of creating a flatter genital region is **tucking** (Figure 8-3). This typically involves tucking the testicles into the inguinal canals and securing the phallus tucked backward between the legs.[15] There are a variety of ways individuals may secure their tuck, including any combination of tapes, glues, and compression wear. One of the most common ways to secure a tuck includes using a combination of sports or medical tape and gauze to secure the phallus, and tight underwear or a compression garment to maintain secure placement. Specialized tapes designed for use while tucking have also been released and include guides for application. Compression garments or tapes can be used on their own; however, this method may be or feel less secure for some people, and a combination of both is often preferred.

Health care providers should be aware of the relative safety of the different tuck-securing methods as well as the potential medical implications of tucking. Online

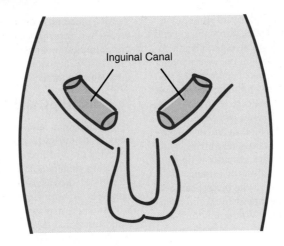

Inguinal Canal

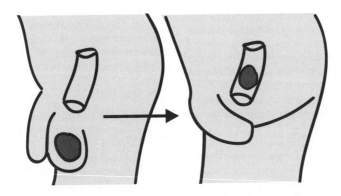

▲ **Figure 8-3.** Tucking.

recommendations for people interested in tucking may suggest using duct tape, crazy glue, or any variety of adhesives. These methods, especially when used repeatedly or for long periods, have the potential to cause serious skin and tissue damage. Any adhesive applied repeatedly to the skin may cause skin irritation or damage, and the use of gauze to protect especially sensitive or delicate skin can be effective in reducing this complication.[15] If someone is experiencing skin damage as a result of the use of tapes or adhesives, it may be helpful to use compression garments only or to alternate the method they use to secure their tuck.

Most methods of tucking make it impossible to urinate while tucked. In order to maintain appropriate urinary health, people who plan to tuck for extended periods of time or all of the time should make sure they are able to safely untuck and retuck to urinate. Damage to the internal structures is also possible, and those who frequently tuck should consult with

a health care provider if they notice any concerns, including unusual swelling or pain.[16] The effect of tucking on the testicles and spermatogenesis has not yet been fully defined, although tucking does appear to reduce the quality of a person's sperm.[17] For those interested in procreation with their own gametes, consultation with a fertility clinic may be helpful to best understand the available options, depending on the person's individual goals and what (if any) medical affirmation they have pursued.

In addition to tape and gauze, compression shapewear used to modify the appearance of someone's hips and waist may be able to securely maintain a tuck. Specialized garments are also available specifically for this purpose. **Gaffs** were initially created for use in theater[15] but can also be an effective tool to maintain a tuck. These garments are designed to be especially tight-fitting in the genital area, and in their most basic form have the outward appearance of underwear or a

G-string. Some gaffs may also have hip or buttock padding or padding in the genital area to create the appearance of a vulva. Having a secure method of creating a flatter genital appearance can greatly reduce gender dysphoria and may help make some "women's"-style clothing fit in more comfortable ways.

For those who would be affirmed by the presence of a penis, there are a variety of options for accomplishing this goal. **Packers** are prosthetic devices creating the appearance of a penis and testicles or large external genitalia (Figure 8-4). They are typically worn in the underwear or some form of harness, although there is a small selection of high-end models that are designed to be glued to the skin. Commercially available options come in a variety of materials, quality, and realism, each with their own benefits and disadvantages. The material is particularly important to be aware of, as some packers are made from porous materials and therefore may be able to harbor moisture and bacteria more easily than nonporous packers. Each commercial packer typically comes with care instructions, which should be followed carefully to prevent potential illness or complications.

Free and homemade options for creating the appearance of a penis are also widely discussed in TGD communities, and there are many tutorials for making packers online. Materials may include rolled-up socks and rubber bands, rice or sand-filled pouches, athletic cups, or any variety of other objects that can be appropriately shaped and sized. Given a packer's proximity to the genitals, it is important for the wearer to either wash or regularly replace their packer regardless of the material, and regularly inspect it for cleanliness and integrity.

While packers are typically sufficient in most situations to create the public appearance of having a penis, men's restrooms may still present a challenge. The social expectation or personal desire to use a urinal or urinate while standing may necessitate the use of Stand-To-Pee devices (STPs) (Figure 8-5). These devices typically have some type of wider-mouthed cup for the person to hold securely to the genitals surrounding the urethra, and a narrower tube or funnel through which the urine flows away from the body. Commercial STPs come in a wide variety of shapes, sizes, and styles, and can vary quite widely in cost depending on their quality, realism, and desired functionality. Available models range from hyper-realistic, custom-made prosthetics to products branded for cisgender women to use while hiking or camping that have no resemblance to a penis. Some STPs can also be used as a packer, while others are not appropriately shaped or sized to accomplish both purposes.

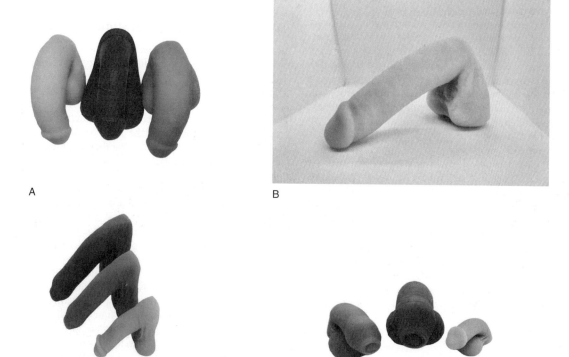

A

B

C

D

▲ **Figure 8-4.** Packers. (Used with permission from M. Massaquoi.)

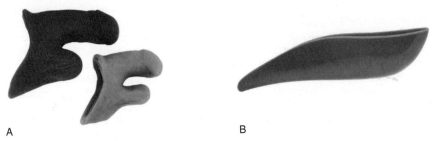

A   B

▲ **Figure 8-5.** Stand-to-pee devices. (Used with permission from M. Massaquoi.)

In addition to the commercially available options, there are a number of do-it-yourself tools individuals may use to accomplish the goal of standing to urinate. As an STP device is effectively a funnel or cup and tube, many household items can be adapted for this purpose. Tutorials are available on social media platforms with instructions for creating an STP using a commercial packer and plastic tubing. These lower-cost options may be more accessible for many TGD people and are effective in achieving urination while standing and easing dysphoria.

In addition to differences in aesthetic appearance, the design and function of these devices vary widely. Different shapes and sizes work better with a given person's anatomy, and it is difficult to know in advance the type that works best for a particular individual. The majority of STPs also require a significant amount of bladder control to prevent backflow or filling the mouth of the STP faster than the urine is able to flow out. It is highly recommended that people practice using any new STP at home before attempting to do so in public, to avoid encountering difficulties in a public restroom.

Regardless of the model, careful care and cleaning of packers and STPs are necessary to avoid potential genitourinary complications. Most commercial STPs come with care instructions, including recommended cleaning methods. Regular cleaning with soap and water is often sufficient to maintain appropriate hygiene, but many commercial STPs can even be boiled or washed in a dishwasher occasionally for a deeper clean or if sharing with another person. Similar to packers, STPs can also be powdered with cornstarch after cleaning to reduce stickiness and maintain a more skin-like texture on the exterior of the device. If the STP was adapted or created from materials that cannot be sterilized, it is even more important that the device is disassembled (if applicable) and cleaned regularly.

For some people who would be affirmed by having a penis, the use of a packer or STP may exacerbate dysphoria rather than ease it. While these tools can be used effectively to create the appearance of having a penis to others, the use of a prosthetic may also remind the person of their own lack of a penis, rather than affirming them. Any form of genital prosthetic has the potential to become displaced or unsecured, leading to potentially undesirable situations that may vary from embarrassing to dangerous for the wearer. STPs in particular frequently require the user to hold the opening against their existing genitals and directly surrounding the urethra, which may necessitate more physical engagement with one's own anatomy than some people are able to manage. For other people, using a packer or STP daily may be a logistical burden and not worth the bother on a day-to-day basis.

▶ Clothing, Shoes, and Style

Some people experience a significant amount of anxiety with their first attempts to dress differently or when trying a new clothing style. It may be helpful for professionals who serve TGD people to specifically name and address this concern, making it clear that they can dress or present in whatever way they are most comfortable during their time working together. Restrooms should be made available to anyone who may be interested in changing their clothing before or after a visit. Not only will this allow anyone to dress in a way that is most comfortable for them, but it may also allow some people to avoid public harassment and discrimination while being afforded access to a space in which it is safe to affirm their gender.

Finding clothing that fits and is gender affirming can be an especially difficult challenge. In popular outlets, clothing and shoes are available in highly gendered sections and a limited size range that is often not inclusive of the needs of TGD people. Traditionally feminine shoes in large sizes are often only available online, and people with smaller feet may need to shop for youth sizes to find masculine shoes that fit. Although there is a growing number of online retailers catering to TGD customers, selections available at these venues are often higher cost than a similar item would be elsewhere. A gender-affirming tailor can be a particularly useful resource, although having a significant amount of clothing that needs to be tailored can also become expensive quickly. Clothing swaps are a common and useful practice within the TGD community and can be an effective way to both build community and expand one's closet.

▶ Sex, Sexuality, and Sexual Behavior

Sex is a complicated subject for many and can be a source of affirmation, distress, or both for TGD people. This section briefly addresses ways some TGD people relate to and engage in sexuality and sexual behavior. While this section outlines some commonly affirming sexual practices, it is not meant to be an exhaustive overview of the variations in sexual practices in which TGD people take part. Overall, the sexual needs of TGD people are the same as those of their cisgender peers: to achieve mutual understanding and consent and to have their needs understood and met. These needs may include not engaging with or using particular body parts, keeping clothing or affirming prosthetics on during sex, or any variety of needs specific to the individual. Having a partner or partners who listen to these needs and respond to them in affirming ways can set the tone for all other aspects of sexual experiences.[8]

The use of language regarding sex and sex acts is an important aspect of communicating someone's sexual needs. Much of this language is laden with gendered implications, if not explicitly gendering. Using the language for body parts that a person finds most affirming can have a large impact, regardless of whether it is the anatomically correct language by other people's standards.

Many toys and tools are now being made specifically for TGD people to use during sex. For those without penises, genital pumps with penis extenders and some packers can be used for penetration. People can also use traditionally marketed strap-ons and vibrators, regardless of their gender identity or genital configuration. Anal sex may be appealing for many TGD people, since everyone has an anus and there are no genital requirements to engage in this form of sex. **Kink** and **BDSM**[C] can similarly be affirming and require little to no engagement with the genitals if this is not desired. The penetration of the inguinal canals through invagination

of the scrotal skin often results in sexual stimulation. The term muffing has been coined to describe this, and it can be particularly affirming for those who are not otherwise able to be penetrated in the front of their body.

For those without a partner or partners to engage in sexual behaviors with, or who engage in sexual acts alone, many of the techniques, tools, and toys described above can also be used on one's own body. There are also toys created specifically for personal use by TGD people, including items like masturbation sleeves (devices designed for masturbation, for those who have a phallus) available for a wide range of phallus sizes. It may be helpful for anyone to become familiar with what feels good for their body to improve their own experience as well as coach others, should the occasion arise.

MANAGEMENT OF MONTHLY BLEEDING

Menstruation[D] is an experience that many TGD people who were assigned female at birth may find distressing. While therapeutic levels of testosterone often stop monthly bleeding, this is not true for everyone.[18] In addition, many TGD people experience gender dysphoria with monthly bleeding but who do not have access to or would not otherwise be affirmed by taking testosterone. Menstruation can be a significantly distressing experience in and of itself, given the highly female-coded cultural norms and expectations of menstruation, but it can also present practical and social concerns. Purchasing menstrual products can be a very difficult social experience if not explicitly outing or unsafe, and often men's restrooms do not have sufficient receptacles to dispose of menstrual management products and their packaging.[19]

As a result, TGD people who menstruate may want to pursue other management options. Medical suppression of monthly bleeding through the use of hormonal contraceptives can be effective for some people, yet for others adding more estrogen or progesterone to the body is more distressing than menstruation.[19] Menstrual cups are another potential option, as they require no disposable elements (therefore reducing practical concerns) and may also be more cost-effective. However, menstrual cups require regularly and extensively engaging with one's genitals, which may cause more distress than other forms of disposable menstrual management, such as pads and tampons.

"Period-proof underwear" recently has also become more available and accessible, and some types are designed

---

[C] In this context, the word "kink" is used to indicate any sex or sexual practice that is considered unconventional. This creates significantly more flexibility for the person and any partner(s) to engage in practices that are affirming and pleasurable, and refrain from those which are not. The initialism BDSM represents the words bondage and discipline, dominance and submission, and sadism and masochism. The abbreviation is used in this context to describe a host of sexual, recreational, and relationship practices in which there is a consensual power exchange. Some people seek out particular sensations or experiences through kink and BDSM that are erotic or otherwise pleasurable for them, but which may not culminate an another form of sexual intimacy or orgasm.

[D] Menstruation and monthly bleeding are used interchangeably throughout this section. Commonly used language for the cyclic shedding of the uterine lining, such as period and menstruation, often carry gendered assumptions and can exacerbate dysphoria. Some TGD people are more affirmed by other language, such as monthly bleeding. Health care providers should be prepared to use the language patients feel most comfortable using when discussing the patient's body and its functions.

specifically as gender-affirming options for TGD people. This underwear typically comes in a selection of styles with varying absorbency and may be an option for someone who would benefit from having additional protection combined with another menstrual management method, or for those who find the absorbency of the underwear alone sufficient to meet their needs. Care instructions vary by brand, and some products may require additional care to maintain absorbency and efficacy. Although using this method may be cost-effective in the long-term, it is initially costly to purchase these garments, and therefore it may not be an accessible option for everyone.

DISCREET OR PERSONAL AFFIRMATION

Much of this chapter has described gender affirmation that is overtly visible or perceived by others; often, this is the intended focus of nonmedical gender-affirmation strategies. For some TGD people, however, publicly visible or perceivable gender affirmation is not safe, possible, or desired. Finding ways to affirm one's gender in a more personal realm can also be affirming, even if the TGD person is the only one who knows. Some examples include wearing undergarments more in line with one's affirmed gender, using affirming names and pronouns in online spaces, or attending private events in an affirmed presentation. Video games, role-playing games, and cosplay[E] are other opportunities for affirming experiences, in which people can play, create, or act as a character closer to their affirmed gender, and have the experience of being referred to as that character. These less overt or outwardly perceivable forms of gender affirmation can be beneficial, especially when it is not possible to be affirmed in other aspects of life.

SUMMARY

- TGD people may use a variety of potential options outside of medically or surgically altering the bodies to affirm their identities.
- Gender-affirmation tools and techniques are used in different ways by different people. Some use gender affirmation to increase their visibility as trans, nonbinary, or gender-nonconforming; others use gender affirmation to "blend" with their cisgender peers. Gender-affirmation techniques can be used to address gender dysphoria specific to an individual's perception of their body or function as well as a means of joyful exploration and play.

[E] Cosplaying describes the act of dressing as and emulating a character, typically done at conventions or other large events, or for online audiences. It is common practice within these spaces to refer to the cosplayer by the name, pronouns, and gendered references of the character being emulated, regardless of the actual or perceived gender of the person themselves.

- Nonmedical and nonsurgical gender-affirmation techniques include use of names, pronouns, and sex/gender markers; body modification such as tattoos and piercings; genital pumping; exercise and weight modification; body hair removal; and use of nonpermanent and removable items to alter appearance of gendered aspects of the body (such as binders, taping, tucking, and packers).
- Several options are available for TGD people to manage monthly bleeding that do not involve the use of hormonal contraception or testosterone.
- Care teams providing services for TGD people must be able to discuss each person's tailored needs and goals for gender affirmation and offer advice about any potential adverse health risks. They should also be knowledgeable about the services and resources that are available in their area to assist people with gender affirmation.

CASE STUDY 1: MARY

Mary is a 62-year-old trans woman who has come to understand her trans identity within the past 6 months and is making steps toward affirmation. She began attending a local trans support group for a few months before telling anyone else in her life, as she was particularly nervous about coming out to her wife. During this time, she also began growing her hair, with the intention to slowly build a more feminine appearance. Although disclosure of her trans identity to her wife did ultimately result in a divorce, her now ex-wife has begun using the correct name and pronouns when referring to Mary with other family members. Recently, Mary started gender-affirming hormones through her medical provider, and she is "not interested in any of those big surgeries" at this time.

Mary is gradually buying and collecting more feminine clothes but remains hesitant to wear them when interacting with her family. She feels strongly about wanting to maintain a positive relationship with her children and grandchildren and is unsure how they might react to this change. Mary has experimented with different clothing alone in public and at support groups, and found that wearing a bra and breast forms was affirming. She mentions a friend from her support group told her about tucking, but that it "hurt too much and was too much work." She doesn't anticipate wearing clothing that is especially form-fitting, but she is still looking for more ways to reduce the visibility of her genitals when wearing certain clothing. Despite the tumultuous year she has had and still seeing herself as "a beginner" when it comes to gender affirmation, she reports being the happiest she has been for as long as she can remember.

▶ Discussion Questions

1. Mary describes herself as a "beginner" when it comes to affirming her gender, and is not always familiar with the

tools and techniques available for TGD people to affirm their gender. What are some questions you might ask to further investigate her knowledge of available options and interest in additional information?

2. While Mary has expressed interest in having less visible external genitalia, she has had trouble finding a way to accomplish this. What might you ask about what she has tried, and what would you suggest as alternative options?

3. Are there additional conversations or recommendations you would have for Mary?

CASE STUDY 2: CARTER

Carter is a 19-year-old trans masculine nonbinary person. He describes his style and personality in high school as "super masculine," and he would only wear men's clothing and in multiple layers to mask the shape of his body. They were always very focused on passing and say they were "usually fine on the street, but at school everyone already knew me." Since Carter's parents weren't willing to consent to any medical treatment, he was unable to access any medical affirmation other than menstrual suppression using hormonal contraceptives. In their junior year Carter began using he pronouns, and would often borrow a binder from a friend to wear at school.

Once Carter turned 18 and left home for college, he immediately started taking testosterone. At the time, they had a detailed conversation with their health care provider about their goals for gender affirmation, and together decided a low dose would be the best course of action. As he noticed affirming body changes with testosterone and entered an accepting environment while at college, he felt less pressured to always dress and act in an inauthentically hypermasculine way, and began using both he and they pronouns interchangeably.

They only recently found a company that sells affordable packers in their skin tone, but often don't pack after having had some "awkward situations and an uncomfortable side effect" with the packer. They plan to still use the packer they bought "on special occasions" or when going out to clubs, but not daily. While dating has been difficult for Carter, he has found that experiences in which he is the anal receptive partner ("bottoming") with other queer, masculine people have been some of the most affirming. They continue to report being attracted to "just about everyone" and aren't interested in having a monogamous partner.

A few weeks ago, Carter contacted his health care provider and let her know that he is planning to stop taking testosterone. When they came in for their visit, they had been off of testosterone for about two weeks. He does not regret starting this medication and was affirmed by many of the changes he experienced, but was starting to have continued changes that were not desirable. They continue to be happy

with the decision to microdose testosterone for the past year, as well as the decision to stop this medication. He is somewhat worried about having a more feminine body shape return, but has been working out with a trainer and is excited about how affirming this experience has been.

They now continue to bind on a daily basis and find it difficult to take breaks given their active social life and living in a dormitory with a roommate. He has had some back and rib pain and shortness of breath while binding, but shrugs and states "I guess this is just how it'll be until I get top surgery." They have selected a surgeon for chest reconstruction, but are still working on meeting the documentation and insurance requirements to schedule their consultation.

▶ Discussion Questions

1. What follow-up questions might you ask about Carter's experiences with packing, and what would your recommendations be if they were interested in packing more frequently?

2. What would you recommend for Carter to be aware of regarding binding safety? Are there other ways he could maintain a flatter chest while taking a break from binding?

3. What other conversations would you have with Carter about their recent affirming experiences?

CASE STUDY 3: SKY

Sky is a 32-year-old genderqueer person who has been open about hir genderqueer identity since the age of 23. Ze has always been a gender-nonconforming person, and since a young age, Sky has enjoyed a variety of activities, including those that are traditionally considered feminine and masculine. Sky has been on multiple different hormone regimens while trying to find the right fit and regularly has conversations with hir doctor about the effects of the medication and whether it is affirming. Sky presents hir gender differently every day, depending on what feels most affirming at that time. Ze describes enjoying combining feminine and masculine attributes in hir appearance and finds that confusing the general public with hir gender expression is both exciting and affirming.

The combination of visible facial hair, bright makeup, and freshly manicured nails are the most consistent aspects of hir gender expression, but hir choices in clothing, hairstyle, and the visible appearance of having breasts differ from one day to the next. Sky doesn't have much of a connection with hir family anymore but is deeply immersed in the local queer and trans community.

Sky has been having frequent sinus infections and hir provider has decided to refer hir to an otolaryngologist. Ze seems hesitant during the visit, but follows through with the care plan and schedules hir appointment with the specialist. A few weeks later hir provider receives an email from Sky, in which ze explains hir concerns with seeing the specialist. Ze mentions that ze has not had a health care provider outside of hir primary care provider's office since ze changed hir name, and that the information on hir health insurance record does not match hir driver's license. Sky noted that ze understood ze would likely get misgendered throughout hir interaction with the specialist, but was concerned the office would not even accept hir insurance card without another form of identification that matched. Ze has not been sleeping well ever since ze scheduled hir appointment, and wants to know whether hir primary care provider has any ideas on how to get through the visit quickly and uneventfully.

▶ Discussion Questions

1. As Sky's primary care provider, what options can you offer to hir to assist in creating an affirming experience with the specialist?

2. What information, resources, or suggestions might you share with Sky to assist hir in having a successful visit?

3. During hir initial visit, how could the primary care provider have better addressed Sky's need for the referral, and assisted hir in navigating the medical system?

REFERENCES

1. Bockting WO, Miner MH, Swinburne Romine RE, Hamilton A, Coleman E. Stigma, mental health, and resilience in an online sample of the US transgender population. *Am J Public Health.* 2013;103(5):943-951.

2. James SE, Herman JL, Rankin S, Keisling M, Mottet L, Anafi M. The Report of the 2015 U.S. Transgender Survey. *National Center for Transgender Equality.* Published online 2016.

3. Scheim AI, Perez-Brumer AG, Bauer GR. Gender-concordant identity documents and mental health among transgender adults in the USA: a cross-sectional study. *Lancet Public Health.* 2020;5(4):e196-e203.

4. ID Documents Center. National Center for Transgender Equality. Published February 5, 2015. https://transequality.org/documents. Accessed October 18, 2020.

5. Russell ST, Pollitt AM, Li G, Grossman AH. Chosen name use is linked to reduced depressive symptoms, suicidal ideation and behavior among transgender youth. *J Adolesc Health.* 2018;63(4):503-505.

6. Nelius T, Armstrong ML, Rinard K, Young C, Hogan L, Angel E. Genital piercings: diagnostic and therapeutic implications for urologists. *Urology.* 2011;78(5):998-1007.

7. Chyten-Brennan J. Surgical transition. In: Erickson-Schroth L, ed. *Trans Bodies, Trans Selves: A Resource for the Transgender Community.* New York, NY: Oxford University Press; 2014:265.

8. Hill-Meyer T, Scarborough D. Sexuality. In: Erickson-Schroth L, ed. *Trans Bodies, Trans Selves: A Resource for the Transgender Community.* New York, NY: Oxford University Press; 2014:355.

9. Bradford NJ, Rider GN, Spencer KG. Hair removal and psychological well-being in transfeminine adults: associations with gender dysphoria and gender euphoria. *J Dermatol Treat.* 2019:1-8. Online ahead of print.

10. Thoreson N, Marks DH, Peebles JK, King DS, Dommasch E. Health insurance coverage of permanent hair removal in transgender and gender-minority patients. *JAMA Dermatol.* 2020;156(5):561-565.

11. Bartsich S, Wu JK. Silicon emboli syndrome: a sequela of clandestine liquid silicone injections. A case report and review of the literature. *J Plast Reconstr Aesthet Surg.* 2010;63(1):e1-3.

12. Bertin C, Abbas R, Andrieu V, et al. Illicit massive silicone injections always induce chronic and definitive silicone blood diffusion with dermatologic complications. *Medicine (Baltimore).* 2019;98(4):e14143.

13. Nolan IT, Morrison SD, Arowojolu O, et al. The role of voice therapy and phonosurgery in transgender vocal feminization. *J Craniofac Surg.* 2019;30(5):1368-1375.

14. Peitzmeier S, Gardner I, Weinand J, Corbet A, Acevedo K. Health impact of chest binding among transgender adults: a community-engaged, cross-sectional study. *Cult Health Sex.* 2017;19(1):64-75.

15. Reynolds H, Goldstein Z. Social transition. In: Erickson-Schroth L, ed. *Trans Bodies, Trans Selves: A Resource for the Transgender Community.* Oxford University Press; 2014:124.

16. Poteat T, Malik M, Cooney E. 2148 Understanding the health effects of binding and tucking for gender affirmation. *J Clin Transl Sci.* 2018;2(S1):76-76.

17. McCracken M, Nangia AK, Roby K, McLaren H, Gray M, Marsh CA. Total motile sperm in transgender women seeking hormone therapy: a case-control study. *Fertil Steril.* 2018;110(4):e22.

18. Kanj RV, Conard LAE, Trotman GE. Menstrual suppression and contraceptive choices in a transgender adolescent and young adult population. *J Pediatr Adolesc Gynecol.* 2016;29(2):201-202.

19. Chrisler JC, Gorman JA, Manion J, et al. Queer periods: attitudes toward and experiences with menstruation in the masculine of centre and transgender community. *Cult Health Sex.* 2016;18(11):1238-1250.

Surgical Gender Affirmation

Gaines Blasdel
Lee C. Zhao
Rachel Bluebond-Langner

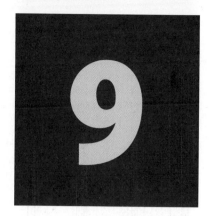

INTRODUCTION

Surgical interventions to affirm cultural and gendered roles in society, such as testicle removal, predate the Western conception of the gender binary and contemporary medical models of gender identity. The first gender-affirming surgical program in Western medical practice is considered to have been Magnus Hirschfield's Institute for Sexual Science, commencing gender-affirming procedures in 1922.[1] Early conceptions of the goal of gender-affirming surgery were to "correct" the external form to a discrete female or male appearance. Surgical intervention was treated as a required aspect of gender affirmation in many contexts, a legacy that continues today as jurisdictions require sterilization or other surgery for name or gender marker changes on official government-issued documentation. Simultaneously, surgery was withheld from the majority of treatment-seeking patients who were deemed poor surgical candidates for reasons that would now be considered inappropriate, such as not being heterosexual in their identified gender. Assessment for gender-affirming surgery has been explored in transgender studies, a field of inquiry whose foundational texts describe the social and medicolegal impact of power relations between medical professionals and **transgender and gender diverse (TGD)** patients seeking surgery.[2]

As the etiology of **gender dysphoria** has evolved, we now understand that a process of medical gender affirmation is personalized to the individuals' needs rather than approximating a singular ideal of "female" or "male" bodies. In turn, this evolving clinical understanding has impacted the clinical framework of gender-affirming surgery, in which the goal is to alleviate the specific source of incongruence for the individual patient rather than correct the body to a **cisnormative** form.[3] In addition to genital surgical procedures, gender-affirming surgery is now available for primary and secondary sex characteristics throughout the body. Meanwhile, expanding funding through health coverage mechanisms

has increased access to gender-affirming surgery for populations who seek it.[4] A diverse set of surgical interventions is becoming more widely available to an increasingly heterogeneous group of patients. Supporting TGD patients before and throughout the lifespan after surgery in this evolving landscape is an interdisciplinary practice we explore in this chapter.

TIMING AND CHOICE OF SURGERY

Although overall improvement in the quality of life has been demonstrated in TGD patients undergoing surgery, there is no inherent need to include surgical interventions as an aspect of gender affirmation.[5] In the absence of measures that would plausibly identify specific characteristics of patients who derive greater benefit from surgery, patient request is the ultimate surgical indication.[6] **Gatekeeping** is a term used in TGD care to describe an overly stringent approval process that withholds interventions from patients who do not conform to sanctioned care access pathways or personal gender narratives. The Standards of Care (SOC) put forth by the World Professional Association for Transgender Health (WPATH) state that certain once-commonplace approval processes, such as requiring a minimal time in psychotherapy before receiving biomedical treatment, could inhibit meaningful engagement in care and be counterproductive.[7] Gatekeeping has led to mistrust of care providers, patient disengagement from clinically indicated follow-up, and even risky, self-, or lay-practitioner attempts at surgical intervention.[8] Gatekeeping is best avoided by focusing on the patient's understanding of and ability to consent to the known risks and benefits of any specific intervention. Although fully informed consent is an ideal goal, many important questions patients have about surgery are not answerable with the current literature.[9]

By centralizing informed consent to the greatest extent possible and reducing gatekeeping, clinicians promote patient autonomy. Another important aspect of patient autonomy is the modular nature of gender-affirming surgery.[10] Just as there is no inherent need to include gender-affirming surgery in any individual's gender-affirmation process, there is also no inherent order of surgical interventions that should be undertaken. Interventions such as genital surgery are not one procedure but instead comprise many subprocedures that can be customized to treat an individual patient's source of gender incongruence while minimizing surgical risk. Additionally, techniques are involving and improving, and different methods, such as robotic assistance in pelvic surgery, may offer unique advantages. However, because certain surgical choices may interfere with future desired procedures, the extent to which surgeries can be customized is limited.

▶ Intersectionality and Surgical Decision-Making

Patients exist within families, societies, and cultures that may be important factors in their decision-making processes about surgery. These factors can facilitate autonomy in decision making; for example, a patient's family members may provide the material and emotional support needed to remove barriers to exploring surgical options. They can also passively or actively inhibit an individual's decision making. A patient's community, for example, may harbor misconceptions about surgery or may expect that surgery is the only means by which someone can fully inhabit their identified gender. Additionally, for TGD patients most affected by violence and harassment, such as TGD women of color, surgery can ease public persecution and increase safety and well-being.

Race and ethnicity profoundly impact TGD people, especially in their interactions with medical professionals and experiences with TGD health care.[11] Although reconstructive surgery broadly aims to restore "normal" form and function, anthropomorphic averages vary in different races and ethnicities, and notions of normative bodily function are created through sociocultural experiences. TGD patients who request surgical intervention that also affirms their racialized experience of gender should be treated in a culturally responsive manner that acknowledges their experience of race, ethnicity, or culture when undergoing gender-affirming surgery.

▶ Managing Surgical Expectations

Empowering patients by promoting autonomy and patient-centered decision making must work in tandem with setting appropriate expectations for the risk of adverse outcomes. Although gender-affirming surgery has high satisfaction and low morbidity generally, there are risks with any surgical intervention.[5] Particularly in patients who have not had previous intensive surgical interventions or illness, the impact

of complications on quality of life and well-being should be explored and reiterated. Because American academic surgical centers have been largely silent regarding gender-affirming surgery until recently, specific gaps in the literature exist about the outcomes of these interventions. These shortcomings should be acknowledged while also recognizing that all medical interventions are being continually improved. Ongoing work to improve available data about gender-affirming surgical outcomes should not delay necessary surgical care for individual patients, who have been demonstrated to have improved mental health outcomes after surgery.[12] Patients may need space to express a sense of grief or frustration with compromises attendant to decision making in gender-affirming surgery to arrive at the best treatment plan, given the resources and interventions available.

Additionally, no surgery can be expected to provide the "ideal" body part or body. The goal of surgery is to create structure and function such that the patient can begin to experience gender euphoria in their body. Surgery is used to reduce gender incongruence and cannot be expected to resolve all struggles with body image and mental health. Even after the most technically successful and visually ideal surgery, patients may still have symptomatic expressions of gender incongruence as they integrate a new bodily schema. Working with multidisciplinary care team members throughout the perioperative period, not just prior to surgical approval, can help patients experience optimal outcomes. Case 1 discusses these issues in further detail.

PREPARING PATIENTS FOR SURGERY

Setting patient expectations and obtaining informed consent is a continual process that should occur throughout the preoperative period. Given the heterogeneity of surgical techniques, it is expected that patients will experience a cyclical process of research, prioritizing, and decision making as they consult with surgeons. Patients should not hesitate to request a second informational consult to clarify or ask further questions prior to selecting a surgeon. Information can also be delivered in the form of surgery education classes, administered through the surgical center or primary care setting, some of which include narratives from recovered patients about their experiences.[13]

Peer education is a powerful tool to inform decision making in the absence of standardized patient-reported outcomes.[6] Patients may find peer education, including discussions about the postoperative experience and "show-and-tell" events, at community conferences. Online social media platforms frequently have TGD surgery discussion groups, and several independent websites purport to offer unmoderated anonymous reviews of transgender surgical offerings. Patients seeking information online should consider the "Yelp effect," wherein only very positive or very negative experiences are shared. In general, selecting a surgeon based only on others' reviews or selected surgical outcome pictures available online is ill-advised. Rapport and individualized counseling, as well as a surgeon's photos shared in the consultation, are important factors that should be considered when selecting a surgeon.

Chronic Health Conditions and Surgery

Surgery is a stressor on the body, and operative planning and healing are impacted by personal health history. Metabolic conditions, including diabetes and excess adipose tissue, place patients in differing risk categories per surgical society guidelines. Weight-loss counseling is intended to optimize metabolic health and is often administered using body mass index (BMI) limits for specific surgical interventions. We support screening all patients for **eating disorders** if weight loss or gain is advised before surgery, regardless of perceived history or current weight. If eating disorders are present, weight management strategies should be carefully considered and suggested while working in concert with a patient's mental health clinician. Smoking cessation and cessation of all nicotine products are required prior to any surgery, as nicotine constricts blood vessels and impairs wound healing. Patients with substance use disorder, including alcohol use disorder, should receive stabilizing treatment, which may include medically assisted therapy, and continue treatment for the duration of recovery. Those with bleeding and clotting disorders should be cleared for surgery by hematologists. Exogenous hormones have been associated with an increased risk for clotting, and many surgeons have asked patients to withhold their hormones in the perioperative period, although evidence is lacking for this practice in TGD populations.[14] Currently, our practice is to continue exogenous testosterone and to reduce but not suspend dosing of estrogen preoperatively. Table 9-1 lists additional medical conditions that may impact the operative experience and includes suggestions for surgical modifications, preoperative management, and postoperative care.

Mental Health Conditions and Surgery

In patients who are legally unable to consent to surgical care, consent may be provided on the patient's behalf by legal guardians, while multidisciplinary specialists ascertain the patient's informed assent. Mental health conditions also affect patients' recovery from surgical interventions. While acknowledging that a history of gatekeeping has incentivized patients to leave their mental health history undisclosed, in our practice, we welcome patients to discuss trauma history and mental health conditions. In particular, we are proactive in engaging with patients around the concept of **medical trauma** and its impact on the operative experience. This trauma is ongoing negative psychological consequences of a specific event in which a patient experienced abuse in a medical setting, or can result from a traumatizing event which involved interaction with the medical system. Hospitalization (being dependent on others, bedrest), opiate pain medication, and drugs used during anesthesia can have a depressant effect on mood. Postoperative wound care can exacerbate anxiety. For these reasons, we encourage patients with a history of depression or anxiety, which has previously impacted activities of daily living, to engage in psychotherapeutic support throughout the perioperative period, although it is not an absolute requirement.

For those with a history of medical mistreatment and other trauma related to TGD status, the hospital setting can trigger symptoms of distress related to this prior trauma. Genital surgery has a complex interaction with prior sexual trauma specifically, which can manifest during vaginal dilation or medical staff interactions with genitals as part of ongoing care provision. For this reason, we screen patients for sexual trauma and have forthright discussions about expectations for postoperative care. Case 1 explores such screening in further detail. Depression, anxiety, and prior trauma are not contraindications to surgery, and we stress this with patients when screening. We encourage patients to receive mental health letters of support from trusted referral partners of ours or their primary care clinicians, such that psychosocial preparedness and trauma-informed care practices can be focused on and optimized, and patients are adequately reassured that the letter writer can serve as a source of postoperative support if issues arise.

Psychosocial Preparedness

Financial toxicity is an emerging concept in the surgical literature, which is meant to incorporate direct and indirect costs of undergoing treatment experienced by the patient. It is particularly relevant in TGD surgery, as many patients undergo multiple gender-affirming surgeries and frequently require access to health care that is not covered by health insurance. Even when gender-affirming surgery benefits are covered, patients frequently receive discriminatory denials for "cosmetic" procedures.[15] *Pro-bono* legal services may aid qualifying patients in appealing unlawful care denials. Patients may also choose specific employment to access insurance coverage of gender-affirming medical care, weighing this aspect over location, reimbursement, or job satisfaction.

Because many patients travel for surgery, housing and travel expenses for the patient and caregivers must also be considered. Patients are often advised to stay in an area close to their surgeon for a week or longer following surgery, although complications and other factors could delay this timeline. For this reason, financial planning and care coordination are essential to alleviate stress during recovery. We encourage patients to have a caregiver accompany them for surgery to act as a supportive advocate in the hospital setting, an emotional confidant, and assist with activities of daily living after discharge. After returning home, patients

Table 9–1. Additional Medical Conditions and Their Impact on Gender-affirming Surgery

Condition	Potential Contraindication	Ideal Presurgical Management	Potential Surgical Adjustment[a]	Postoperative Considerations
Prior radical prostatectomy, pelvic radiation, or major bowel surgery	Pelvic surgery (vaginoplasty, vaginectomy)	Oncology clearance; imaging to determine the extent of alteration to the pelvic anatomy	- Zero-depth vaginoplasty - Robotic assistance in pelvic surgery	Oncologic surveillance with awareness and competency to account for new anatomy
Contraindication to hormone therapy or patient does not desire hormone therapy	Gonad removal (oophorectomy, orchiectomy)	Trial postoperative hormone milieu with GnRH agonists and patient selected postoperative hormonal regime	Ovarian-sparing hysterectomy	Patient no longer has endogenous hormone source
Diabetes mellitus	Multiple; wound-healing difficulty	- Hemoglobin A1c $\leq$ 7 - Acceptance of possibility for worsened outcomes and decreased nerve regeneration	Delay for stabilization of hemoglobin A1C	Ongoing glucose management
Feeding and eating disorders	Weight management counseling	- Patients should be able to consume enough calories to sustain healing in the postoperative period - Treatment to stabilize weight and allow patient to safely participate in metabolic optimization	Approaches to metabolic health which involve mental health treatment team	Consider dietary support and counseling in postoperative period
Herpes simplex virus	Genital surgery	Valaciclovir or alternate herpesvirus inhibitor	Delay for management of herpes outbreak	Continue herpesvirus inhibitor through postoperative period

[a]These adjustments are suggestions and may not be beneficial or necessary for every patient requesting surgery with the conditions listed. These adjustments may also be insufficient to provide safe-and-effective surgery, and patients may not be able to undergo the requested surgery.
GnRH, gonadotropin-releasing hormone.

should also have a plan for care duties, such as dog walking, childcare, and eldercare, that may be too physically demanding immediately following surgery. While delaying surgery in the setting of gender incongruence is not a neutral choice, doing so may be advisable while interventions are undertaken for patients whose postoperative course would benefit from additional supports. Psychosocial support and timing of surgery are addressed in **Case 2**.

SURGICAL OPTIONS

The following sections detail the most common surgical procedures used in gender affirmation. Table 9-2 lists each of these options as well as eligibility criteria and perioperative recommendations.

▶ Facial Reduction and Augmentation Procedures

Facial gender-affirming surgery applies both craniofacial and aesthetic techniques to gender-affirming reconstruction. Because it has historically been used to address the needs of transgender women, it is also known as **facial feminization surgery.** The specific visual goals of the surgery and the procedures selected depend on the patient's individual goals and preoperative anatomy. Specialized fellowship training in craniofacial reconstruction allows a surgeon to offer the full complement of surgical options.[16]

Frontal bossing (a prominent frontal bone) is frequently addressed with osteotomy and repositioning of the frontal bone. The frontal bone overlying the frontal sinus is removed, contoured to reduce the projection, and put back in place. The angle of the mandible and the chin can be reduced and reshaped. Angle reduction narrows the width of the lower face, and genioplasty reduces the height projection and overall shape of the chin.[16] Chin implants or other augmenting strategies can also be utilized.

Many individuals seek increased malar projection, which can be achieved with either implants or soft tissue fillers, fat being the most durable material. Rhinoplasty is utilized to reduce the length and projection of the nose and increase facial harmony. These surgical techniques of bone and soft tissue contouring can be applied to both feminizing or

Table 9–2. Surgical Options, Eligibility, and Perioperative Recommendations

	WPATH SOC v. 7 Criteria[7]	Specific Procedure	Eligibility and Preparation	Recovery
Head and neck	None described	Osteotomies and implants	Consultation with surgeons able to offer both reduction and augmentation techniques	- Several weeks of facial swelling - If oral or jaw surgery, postoperative liquid diet
		Vocal fold surgery	Preoperative work with voice therapist to understand role of pitch in vocal gender incongruence	- Complete vocal rest (silence) for a period of weeks - Continued work with voice therapist to appropriately use postoperative vocal range
		Dermatological interventions	- Electrolysis: Several millimeters of hair growth - Permanent hair removal: Engagement in many sessions over months to years - Hairline lowering: acceptance of scar in front of hairline	- Outpatient interventions have short recovery, with temporary swelling or redness
Chest surgery	- One mental health letter - Hormones NOT a prerequisite - One year hormone therapy suggested prior to breast augmentation	Double-incision mastectomy	- Any size chest - Accepts likelihood of nipple sensation loss and scarring	- Restrictions on utilizing arms and other physical activity in the months after surgery
		Periareolar mastectomy	- Smaller chest size, minimal redundant skin - Accepts potential for revision surgery to improve contour	- Restrictions on utilizing arms and other physical activity in the months after surgery
		Breast augmentation	- One year of hormone therapy to ascertain final size and tissue distribution - Understanding that implants should be replaced every 10–15 years	- Restrictions on utilizing arms and other physical activity in the months after surgery
Gonadectomy	- Two mental health letters - One year on hormone therapy unless contraindicated	Orchiectomy	- Presurgical fertility counseling should be offered	- Restricted physical activity in the weeks following surgery
		Hysterectomy and bilateral salpingo-oophorectomy	- Presurgical fertility counseling should be offered - Patient-centered decision making regarding oophorectomy	- Restricted physical activity in the weeks to months following surgery
Genital surgery	- Two mental health letters - One year on hormone therapy unless contraindicated	Vaginoplasty	- Permanent hair removal on scrotum and penis	- Dilation multiple times a day at first, gradually moving to weekly dilation - Pelvic floor physical therapy for assistance with dilation as needed - Reintegration of sensation and exploration of sexuality is necessary before full sexual function is available
		Metoidioplasty and phalloplasty	- Understanding of multistage nature of surgery and possibility for revisions - Hair removal on phalloplasty donor site	- Extended catheterization may be necessary after surgery with urethral lengthening - Reintegration of sensation and exploration of sexuality is necessary before full sexual function is available

masculinizing facial surgeries, as well as surgeries for those with nonbinary gender goals.[17]

Hair Grafting and Hair Removal

Dermatological interventions are also powerful tools for those wishing to alter the secondary sex characteristics of the face.[17] The hairline, facial hair, and body hair are hormone-responsive secondary sex characteristics. Some reversal of alopecia and thinning of facial and body hair can occur when androgen levels are suppressed; however, many patients with gender incongruence related to these features seek more permanent and definitive dermatologic care.

Androgenic alopecia can be treated with hairline lowering or hair grafting. Hairline lowering leaves a scar; however, hair grafting may not be able to achieve the desired hair density. In patients taking testosterone, hair grafting can be used to address androgenic hair loss, or can be added to the beard and moustache in those who wish to increase androgenic hair patterns.

The removal of facial and body hair is an evolving industry with many technologies that may or may not be affordable or accessible in various locations. Insurers are beginning to cover permanent hair removal technologies for both the purposes of genital gender-affirming surgery (see page 7–11) and for any patient with gender incongruence regarding sexually dimorphic hair patterns.[15] **Electrolysis,** in which a cauterizing needle is inserted into the hair follicle, is the only permanent hair removal technology approved by the US Food and Drug Administration. **Laser hair removal** uses various wavelengths of light to destroy hair follicles. Patients with darker skin types have better results with longer wavelength Nd:YAG lasers than intense pulsed light (IPL) lasers.[17] Neither laser nor electrolysis can be expected to remove all hairs completely in a single session. Hair removal, regardless of the modality, takes several months to years.

Voice Surgery and Alteration of Thyroid Cartilage

Vocal fold surgery is done to raise or lower pitch, which is only one of many gendered aspects of voice and communication.[16] Risk of damage to the vocal cords exists but is rare when performed by those with appropriate training. Speech-language pathologists can assist patients in discerning if vocal fold surgery will adequately treat vocal gender incongruence. Participation in pre- and postoperative voice therapy is required for vocal surgery and is essential for surgical success. The thyroid cartilage can be reduced or augmented as a stand alone procedure or in combination with vocal surgery or other procedures to the lower third of the face.

Gender-Affirming Mastectomy

Gender-affirming mastectomy is one of the most frequently performed gender-affirming surgeries.[18] There are many described techniques, but the two most common techniques are periareolar and double incision with free nipple graft. The goals of gender-affirming mastectomy are to remove breast tissue, achieve a flat contour, and reshape the nipple-areola complex.[19]

In a **periareolar mastectomy**, the scar is confined to the nipple-areolar complex. The technique is best suited for patients with minimal glandular tissue and no skin laxity. The skin envelope is not significantly reduced, and the repositioning of the nipple-areola complex is limited. The rate of **revision surgery** using this technique is higher due to stretching of the areola; revision is also done to remove any remaining excess skin that may appear, particularly below the nipple-areolar complex.[20] It is important to wait 9 months to a year to allow for swelling to resolve and skin retraction to occur before undergoing revision surgery.

The **double-incision mastectomy** technique is the most common. Two incisions are made across the chest, and the nipple-areola complex is removed, resized, and placed back on the chest above the incision as a graft. Each of the incisions is ideally placed in the pectoral shadow, not the inframammary fold. Some surgeons offer a **pedicled graft** technique, in which the nipple is left attached to glandular tissue to preserve sensation. In this technique, glandular tissue is left behind to provide a blood supply, making it more difficult to create a flat chest contour.[19] Patients may select not to have the nipples placed back onto the body and undergo medical tattooing or eschew the appearance of nipples altogether.[21]

In both the periareolar and double-incision techniques, dissection is performed in the plane between the breast capsule and subcutaneous fat, removing all of the breast tissue.[20] Care is taken to obliterate the inframammary fold by dissecting beyond it and removing the fascial attachments. Complications include hematoma, which may require reoperation in approximately 7% of cases; seroma, or formation of a serous fluid pocket, which occurs in approximately 5% of cases; and partial or complete nipple loss, occurring in less than 3% of cases. Additionally, nipple hypopigmentation can occur, particularly among people of color. Poor scarring, excess tissue laterally ("dog ears"), or contour irregularities may lead to the need for revision surgery, which occurs in up to 22% of cases.[16]

Breast Augmentation

Insurance companies increasingly cover breast augmentation. Augmentation is most commonly achieved with implants, although there are descriptions of lipofilling alone.[16] Patients can select either saline or silicone, with silicone being the more common choice as the texture is more natural. It is preferred for patients to be on estrogen-based hormones for 1 year or longer before breast augmentation surgery.[7] This is both to provide a more certain idea of final size after breast tissue growth plateaus and aid in operative planning as natal tissue distribution is assessed. Trans feminine people may have a wider chest diameter, and an implant with a wider base diameter implant may be more appropriate. Additionally, widely set nipples cannot be easily corrected, and medial cleavage can be more difficult to achieve.

To help patients select the most appropriate implant size to meet their needs, sizers, or bags filled with grain measured to a specific volume, can be used as bra inserts to test sizing. Implants can be inserted through a variety of incisions, including a periareolar incision around the nipples, transaxillary incision in the armpit, or inframammary fold incision in the fold under the breast. The inframammary fold incision is the most common incision used. Implants can be placed in the subglandular plane below the breast tissue or submuscularly under the chest muscle. Submuscular placement is thought to provide a more gradual transition in the superior pole, but it can also result in animation deformity or lateral displacement of the implant with muscle activation. Patients should be aware of the risks, which include infection, implant malposition, implant rupture, capsular contracture, and breast implant-associated anaplastic large cell lymphoma (BIA-ALCL).[16]

Surgical Removal of Gonads and Internal Reproductive Organs

Gonadectomy can be performed due to gender incongruence related to these organs or to induce hormonal changes by removing the endogenous source of hormones supplied by these organs. Testicle removal or orchiectomy can be used to decrease the need for gender-affirming tucking, stowing the penis and testicles using tape or special garments. Orchiectomy is ideally done through a vertical midline incision into the scrotum. The spermatic cord is dissected and ligated at the level of the inguinal canal. The cord stumps are allowed to retract to the retroperitoneum, minimizing volume in the scrotal sac.

Hysterectomy is the surgical removal of the uterus only, although the term is often used colloquially to include removal of the ovaries. Careful discussion with patients during counseling regarding surgical choices or taking a surgical history is necessary to clarify remaining anatomy. In addition to treating gender incongruence, hysterectomy may be a strategy for managing new-onset pelvic pain after testosterone initiation without other etiology.[22] Subtotal hysterectomy leaves the cervix, which is a subunit of the uterus, and may be an option for patients who accept the ongoing need for cancer screening of this tissue and desire the retention of maximal vaginal length for receptive intercourse. Total hysterectomy resects the cervix along with the uterus, creating

a vaginal cuff at the previous cervix, which should not significantly impair receptive vaginal intercourse. Bilateral salpingectomy, removal of the fallopian tubes, is generally performed with hysterectomy. Oophorectomy, removal of the ovaries, is less standardized. Some clinicians advocate for retaining one or more ovaries in patients as an endogenous hormone source, particularly in patients with inconsistent access to hormone medication. Some surgeons advocate for prophylactic removal at the time of hysterectomy to prevent the need for future intervention, especially if there is a concern for increased cancer risk, cysts, or fibroids. If either orchiectomy or oophorectomy is performed, no further gamete production is possible, and fertility preservation referrals should be offered in advance (see Chapter 19, "Reproductive Health, Obstetrical Care, and Family Building").[7]

Vaginoplasty

Vaginoplasty refers to a set of techniques used to create the vulvar subunits, clitoris, urethral meatus, labia minora and labia majora, and the vaginal canal. Vulvoplasty, sometimes called zero- or limited-depth vaginoplasty, creates the vulvar subunits and introitus but not a canal or only a limited canal that does not extend beyond the level of the prostate. In all vaginoplasty techniques, the existing genital tissue is repurposed to create the vulva and line the canal. A portion of the glans is used to create the clitoris, preserving the deep dorsal artery, vein, and nerves. The urethra is shortened and opened at the new tip (meatus), and this new opening is inset above the entrance to the vagina. The excess urethral lining tissue lines the space between the urethral meatus and the clitoris. The corpora cavernosa is resected. Appropriate reduction of the corporal tissue and bulbospongiosus muscle is crucial to reduce swelling upon arousal, which may obstruct the vaginal canal. The penile skin is used to create clitoral prepuce and labia minora. A portion of the scrotal skin is used to create the labia majora and line a portion of the vaginal canal.

The vaginal canal is created between the rectum and the prostate. The canal can be lined with various autologous tissues, including penile and scrotal skin, peritoneum, or colon. The penile skin forms the proximal aspect of the vaginal canal. Most commonly, the scrotal skin is tubed and attached to the penile skin to line the remaining vaginal canal.[23]

There are instances in which there is limited natal tissue to line the vaginal canal. The peritoneal flap is a hairless, readily available donor site that can be used to deepen the canal.[24] A diagram of pre- and postoperative vaginoplasty anatomy using peritoneal flaps is shown in Figure 9-1. A bowel segment can also be used in primary and revision vaginoplasty, but there are additional risks of enteric surgery beyond the risks of vaginal canal dissection. Rectal injury occurs in 1–4% of vaginal canal dissections and may lead to rectovaginal fistula.[25] Use of robotic assistance in dissecting the vaginal canal

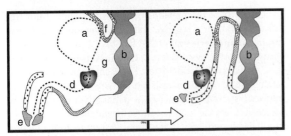

▲ **Figure 9–1.** Lateral view of pre- and postoperative anatomy in the robotic peritoneal flap vaginoplasty. The anatomy prior to and after vaginoplasty is shown. (a) Represents the bladder and urethra, (b) the rectum, (c) the prostate, (d) the urethra, and (e) the glans. The preoperative anatomy includes (f) the pouch of Douglas, the inferior aspect of the peritoneal cavity and (g) the position of Denovielliers' fascia, the space that is opened to create the vaginal canal. (Used with permission from Gaines Blasdel.)

improves visualization, avoiding rectal injury and facilitating greater and more consistent depth.

Clitoral sensation should be preserved and is usually partially available soon after surgery; however, it is not the only source of successful orgasm and sexual satisfaction (see the section "Sensation, Pleasure, and Orgasm"). Following vaginoplasty, future digital prostate exams should be performed through the vagina instead of the rectum, as the prostate now sits on the anterior vaginal wall. For any method that uses hair-bearing skin, hair removal should be completed prior to vaginoplasty (see the section "Hair Grafting and Hair Removal"). While follicle scraping intraoperatively can work to remove some hairs by electrocautery under direct visualization, this technique cannot be expected to completely remove hair.

Vaginal Dilation

In patients who choose to have a vaginal canal created, lifelong dilation should be expected to retain the ability to engage in receptive vaginal penetrative intercourse. After surgery, patients are initially instructed to dilate multiple times a day, with a gradual transition to once weekly after a year if the patient can maintain stable vaginal patency at that frequency. Rigid, medical dilators are recommended to provide sufficient resistance to the body's natural process of scarring and contracture. Dilation stretches the skin of the vaginal canal and also assists in retraining the pelvic floor musculature so that receptive penetration is pleasurable. Trauma-informed, proactive engagement with patients on possible barriers to dilation is an effective aspect of postoperative management. **Pelvic floor physical therapy** is a useful adjuvant in all patients, especially those who struggle

with dilation or have voiding or elimination disorders in the postoperative period.[26] **Case 1** explores this in further detail. In patients with a bowel segment lining the canal, discontinuation of dilation can lead to stenosis of the vaginal opening (introitus) while the bowel-lined segment of the canal remains patent, producing fluid, in some cases leading to mucocele formation requiring reoperation.[27] Some patients substitute receptive intercourse for dilation but may have less depth and width than could be maintained with long-term dilation.

Vaginal Depth Revision

Some patients seek depth revision surgery. This surgery is performed to open a stenotic canal that has closed due to difficulty with dilation, or it can be performed in patients whose canal dissection did not proceed past the level of the prostate in an initial surgery. In our practice, patients are assessed by a pelvic floor physical therapist to ascertain barriers to dilation adherence before undergoing depth revision, as unaddressed barriers will cause recurrent stenosis.

▶ Penile Reconstruction

Penile reconstruction involves a combination of several procedures that are customized to the patient under a modular framework.[10] Several goals of penile reconstruction have been described: standing to urinate, gender-congruent visual appearance of the new penis, and sexuality-related goals including erogenous sensation, sexual satisfaction, and intercourse as the penetrating partner.[28] Patients may not endorse every goal, and in these cases, surgical customization and risk minimization should be offered. Patients may also endorse a goal but be willing to compromise and forgo procedures for less potential morbidity or a shorter surgical process. It is rare for surgeries to be completed in a single stage, although the incorporation of fewer elements, particularly forgoing urethral lengthening and/or internal prosthesis, may allow for a single-stage procedure. Patients planning to undergo penile reconstruction should endeavor to verify the entirety of their treatment plan with surgeons they expect to be involved in their care before embarking on operations, as some methods foreclose future options.

Metoidioplasty

Metoidioplasty creates a penis using the **natal phallus,** comprised of external clitoral tissue that has undergone hormone-responsive hypertrophy in patients taking testosterone. Maximal hypertrophy can take 2–5 years to plateau, but the majority of growth occurs by 2 years. Penile length upward of 10 cm has been reported; however, most patients are in the 4–7 cm range.[29] During metoidioplasty, the ligamentous attachments of the natal phallus on the ventral side of the shaft are released, and the labia minora are used to

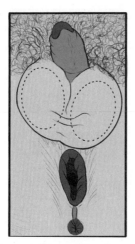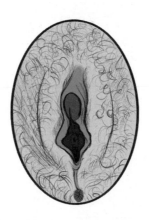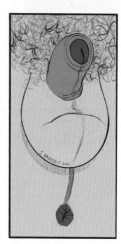

▲ **Figure 9–2.** Two possible combinations of metoidioplasty surgery. The presurgical anatomy (center) is shown. Metoidioplasty with urethral lengthening and vaginectomy (right) creates a smooth perineum and a urethral meatus at the tip of the penis. The labia minora are used to cover the penile shaft, and the labia majora become the new scrotum. Metoidioplasty without urethral lengthening or vaginectomy (left) shows the urethral meatus unmoved. The vaginal introitus is changed in appearance by the removal of the labia, but the ability to have receptive vaginal intercourse is usually not impacted. Testicular implants can be inserted in an additional stage, shown in the scrotum on the left as dashed lines. (Used with permission from Sami Brussels.)

tubularize the penile shaft. Although **urethral lengthening**, surgical extension of the urine channel, and **vaginectomy**, removal of the lining of the vagina and closure of the vaginal space, are often a part of metoidioplasty, this is not always the case (these procedures are explained below).[28] Figure 9-2 shows two possible options for metoidioplasty. Additional mobility of the penile shaft may be achieved by transecting the suspensory ligament along the dorsal aspect of the penile body. This maneuver risks the loss of erectile quality in both the perceived firmness and the directionality of the erection, since the phallus may point inferiorly after cutting the suspensory ligament. Metoidioplasty may be more challenging and fail to meet patient goals, such as standing to urinate or penetrative intercourse, in those with significant loose skin or subcutaneous adipose tissue in the region of the mons, as the resulting penis may be buried despite metoidioplasty.

Scrotoplasty and Testicular Prosthesis

Scrotoplasty is a procedure that uses the labia majora to create a scrotum in tandem with metoidioplasty or phalloplasty. Rotational labia flap techniques create a more forward, hanging scrotum; other techniques fuse existing labia, although this procedure may create functional issues with bicycle riding or other activities. While it is not a required aspect of penile reconstruction, the addition of the scrotum is desired by many. **Testicular prostheses**, also called testicular implants, are silicone or saline-filled implants of varying sizes used to fill the scrotum. Implantation is often done in a second stage to minimize the risk of infection or extrusion. Extrusion, infection, and malposition are possible complications of implants, which require surgical correction or implant removal.

Phalloplasty

Phalloplasty uses vascularized tissue from another part of the body to construct the penile shaft. The resulting penis is larger than can be expected from metoidioplasty and does not rely on clitoral hypertrophy from testosterone. Tissue from various donor sites, including the forearm, thigh, back, and abdomen, can be used, resulting in differing penile dimensions and secondary scarring. **Radial forearm phalloplasty** (RFF, forearm) is historically the most common donor site. Skin from the forearm, together with the radial artery, cephalic vein, and medial and lateral antebrachial cutaneous nerves, is harvested.[10] The tissue is tubularized once to form the urethra and again to form the penile skin envelope. The blood vessels and nerves are disconnected and reconnected in the groin or abdomen. A split-thickness skin graft, the outer layer of dermis from the thigh, is also needed to cover the donor site on the forearm. Figure 9-3 shows donor sites and resulting scarring in forearm phalloplasty.

In **anterolateral thigh phalloplasty** (ALT, thigh), skin and fat are harvested with the lateral femoral cutaneous nerve from the thigh. The blood supply is generally left connected

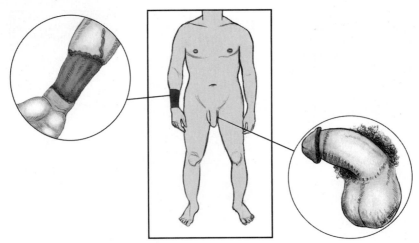

▲ **Figure 9–3.** Donor sites in radial forearm flap phalloplasty. Locations of donor sites utilized in radial forearm phalloplasty. The appearance of the forearm scar (left) is highly variable depending on individual scarring tendency and is expected to improve over several years if sun exposure is minimized. A several inch "leash" scar is utilized to create a neurovascular pedicle to attach to recipient vessels in the pelvis. A secondary split-thickness skin graft on the thigh (center) is expected to have less significant scarring and is utilized to cover the forearm donor site. Minor scarring at the base of the penis and along the ventral aspect represents suture lines (right). The glans and coronal sulcus are created using a secondary graft, which may flatten over time. (Used with permission from Sami Brussels.)

and pedicled into the groin. The donor site is often easier to conceal. The resulting penis has more girth and potentially more length but may be less sensitive. Depending on preoperative anatomy, the penis may be of a size that is difficult to fit into clothing and utilize during sexual intercourse.

The **musculocutaneous latissimus dorsi** phalloplasty (MLD, latissimus) uses skin and muscle from the back to create the penile shaft. This location has only a motor nerve, and while nerve coaptation can be performed, it is unlikely to provide equivalent sensation to a sensory nerve coaptation. Additionally, this donor site usually requires a split-thickness skin graft that can be conspicuous when shirtless. **Abdominal flap phalloplasty** (ABD, abdominal) is the oldest described donor site. This skin is elevated and rotated to the pubis without microsurgical techniques. For urethral lengthening, a second donor site is required, as a tube-in-tube approach is not possible. If a penile urethra is being created, donor sites should be evaluated for hair follicles, and hair removal should be undertaken in advance of surgery. Remnant hair follicles in the urethra can harbor detritus and contribute to lower urinary tract symptoms.[17]

External erectile devices or light compression wrapping may be sufficient for penetrative intercourse. Many individuals elect for placement of a **penile prosthesis**, which may be a malleable rod or an inflatable, closed saline system activated by a pump in the testicles. Insertion of the erectile device should occur in the last stage of surgery after any urethral or other revisions have been completed. Some patients

may not have enough subcutaneous fat on the forearm to allow for future placement of an erectile device.

Penile Sensation and Placement of Natal Phallus

The sensory nerves from the forearm or the lateral thigh are connected to the nerves supplying sensation to the natal phallus to provide erogenous, tactile, and thermal sensation along the length of the new penis. Regardless of the success or extent of erogenous and tactile sensation from nerve coaptation, if the natal phallus is incorporated into the design of the new penis, traction on the natal phallus from movement of the penis will provide some proprioceptive ability and erogenous sensation. The final position of the natal phallus in this strategy can be in the scrotum, the penoscrotal junction, or the base of the new penis, depending on surgical technique and patient anatomy. Patients can also elect to leave the natal tissue exposed, minimizing the risk of sensation loss from removing the outer skin of the natal phallus and adding layers of tissue (the skin of the penis) around it.

Vaginectomy and Urethral Lengthening

In patients who undergo phalloplasty but do not desire urethral lengthening, the urethra can be left in the perineum. **Urethral stricture**, or narrowing, can happen as part of an individual's predisposition to keloid formation or hypertrophic scarring, and can also result from insufficient vascular supply or other surgical shortcomings. Stricture can occur at the natal urethral meatus, at the neomeatus at the end of the penis, or along the urethral tract between them. **Urethral fistula**, or an opening in the urethra leading to urine leakage, can occur independently or concomitantly with stricture. The risk of urethrocutaneous fistula has been reported to be as high as 75% with forearm phalloplasty.[25] Some fistulae will resolve spontaneously, but others will require surgical intervention. A suprapubic and/or penile catheter is left in place for several weeks following surgery to allow the urethra to heal without urine exposure. Many surgeons perform urethral lengthening in multiple stages several months apart to reduce the risk of complications.

It is advisable to perform **vaginectomy**, or removal of the vaginal lining and closure of the vaginal space, when urethral lengthening is being done. There are many reasons for the pairing of these procedures. First, if the patient's goal is to have receptive vaginal penetration after surgery, this goal is difficult to guarantee. During urethral reconstruction, tissue from the anterior vaginal canal is used, creating a ring of scar tissue along the anterior rim of the vaginal introitus. Furthermore, the interposition of additional buttressing tissue, such as the gracilis muscle and/or bulbospongiosus muscle, is advised to ensure that a fistula does not occur at this location. Attempting to meet both goals (standing urination, receptive vaginal intercourse) may result in neither goal being met. Vaginectomy can be performed with complete excision of the mucosa, which we advocate, or fulguration (burning) the lining of the vaginal canal, which has an increased risk of late mucocele formation.[30] Vaginectomy can also be performed in those who select it due to gender incongruence but are not seeking urethral lengthening.

Urethral revision surgery is likely necessary for strictures or fistulae that do not resolve with conservative management. Symptoms of stricture include increased time to complete urination, urinary frequency, or the sensation of incomplete emptying. Downstream stricture can cause an upstream fistula, as well as a diverticulum or pouching of the urethra where urine pools. This diverticulum can also open into the former vaginal space, creating a pocket of urine. In these cases, dribbling or release of urine long after urination may indicate pooling urine. Although correcting a vaginal remnant or urethrocutaneous fistula is usually achieved in a single operation, strictures may require a two-stage operation. Patients can be offered **perineal urethrostomy** if they do not wish to undergo revision surgery, allowing for sitting urination from a perineal meatus. **Case 3** explores urethral revision in greater detail.

▶ Postoperative Care

Immediate management of postoperative concerns should be handled by the surgeon, or if not possible, through direct coordination of the surgeon and local medical providers. Many surgeries utilize surgical drains, which are removed in an outpatient setting once fluid output has decreased to the surgeon's specifications. Hematoma and seroma are best managed by the surgeon. Postoperative infection in the setting of implants is particularly concerning, as a biofilm of bacteria may develop and the implant may need to be removed. Imaging after gender-affirming surgery is best interpreted by a radiologist with knowledge of the patient's history of gender-affirming surgery.

Scars can be managed with silicone sheeting, scar massage, and sun protection. If hypertrophic or raised scars develop, steroid injections, laser treatment, and surgical revision can be considered.[17] Massage can aid in "softening" implants used in breast augmentation and testicular prosthesis, relaxing the scar capsule that surrounds the implant and allowing the implant to settle into a lower or relaxed position.

In genital surgery, patients may be catheterized in the immediate postoperative period. In vaginoplasty patients, the catheter usually remains in place for 5–7 days. In penile reconstruction involving urethral lengthening, a catheter is left in place for 2–4 weeks as the urethra heals. In the first several weeks following surgery, urinary frequency, urgency, and spraying during voiding can be expected. Although there are no validated screening tools for TGD patients, the American Urological Association Symptom Score or Urinary Distress Inventory can help identify and measure urological symptoms. Granulation tissue may be present in the vaginal canal following vaginoplasty. Patients with pain, bleeding, discharge, or odor should be evaluated with a speculum exam. Mechanical debridement with a curette, cauterization with silver nitrate, and application of steroid and antibiotic cream generally provide adequate treatment. Occasionally, significant granulation tissue requires surgery and even regrafting of the vaginal lining.

Sensation, Pleasure, and Orgasm

Many seek surgery partly as a sexual health intervention, because gender incongruence disrupted their sexual intimacy. Patients with sexual dysfunction before surgery may improve after surgery, but current literature rarely includes both pre- and postoperative measures of sexual health, and no sexual health measures have been robustly validated for populations seeking gender-affirming surgery.[6] Sensory issues following surgery include numbness or lack of sensation, hypersensitivity, pain, and referred sensation. After tissue rearrangement, nerves must reestablish both their biomechanical connections and their location within the cortical homunculus (brain-body map). It is expected for early sensation to include pain or discomfort, even past initial swelling and bruising.

Frequent, purposeful self-testing of sensation and other somatosensory therapy can encourage the reintegration of sensation into the bodily schema.[31] Although genital surgeries aim to convey maximal erogenous sensation, orgasm and sexual satisfaction are complex phenomena that are dependent on multiple factors beyond sensory input. The majority of patients report the ability to orgasm after surgery, but the literature is limited by short follow-up and cisnormative and heterosexist constructs in measures of sexuality.[6] Once cleared to return to sexual contact after genital surgery, patients should expect to spend several months exploring their new anatomy and establishing the brain-body connection before their full sexual function returns.

Penetrative Intercourse

While metoidioplasty has historically been considered insufficient for penetrative intercourse, this may not be the patient's experience after surgery, depending on definitions of penetration and the patient and partners' body habitus. Phalloplasty produces a penis of larger size; however, many phalloplasty patients need an erectile device to have satisfactory penetration, while arousal-response erections can occur after metoidioplasty. After vaginoplasty, emission by the glands of Littre or bulbourethral glands may produce fluid with arousal from the truncated urethra at the vaginal introitus. For most patients, this fluid is insufficient for sexual intercourse, and additional lubricant is useful for pleasurable receptive penetration. A vaginal canal containing a bowel segment secretes fluid that is thought to obviate the need for external lubricant. This fluid, however, is produced not just in response to arousal but continuously.

Revision Surgery

Patients who have had postoperative complications or for whom surgery has failed to treat their gender incongruence may seek revision surgery. This term can encompass a wide variety of interventions, ranging from a "complete redo" of the initial surgery to a minor refashioning of skin, which can be done in the surgeon's office. Functional deficits, such as with urination, and visual issues, such as asymmetry, can often be satisfactorily addressed in revision surgery.[30] Repeated revision surgery may reach a point of diminishing returns in reducing gender incongruence or in correcting the functional deficit. This issue is further explored in Case Study 3.

SUMMARY

- Surgery is not able to create a singular ideal of "female" or "male" bodies but is used to treat sources of gender incongruence unique to each patient.
- Gatekeeping should be avoided by centering patient autonomy while ensuring informed consent to the greatest extent possible.
- After vaginoplasty, ongoing dilation is necessary, and barriers to dilation adherence can contribute to loss of depth.

- After phalloplasty or metoidioplasty with urethral lengthening, complications such as stricture and fistula are common.
- While genital surgery preserves genital sensation, sexuality and orgasm are complex and require active reintegration of postoperative sensory inputs.

CASE STUDIES

Note: Answers are given to the case questions in this chapter to enhance learning and foster greater understanding of the complex issues inherent to gender-affirming surgical care.

CASE STUDY 1: CINDY

Cindy presents to a gender-affirming psychologist for a letter of support for vaginoplasty surgery after consulting with and selecting a surgeon. She is initially guarded but finds the psychologist to be welcoming and affirming. He states that as there is no valid "test" of transgender identity and that, given her clear capacity to consent to the intervention, he will provide her with the letter her surgeon requires before offering a surgical date. After it is clear that the letter will be provided, she discloses her fears regarding the hospitalization, stating that she was violently sexually assaulted several years ago after first starting estrogen and was consistently misgendered at the hospital afterward.

1. How should Cindy's fear be communicated to her surgeon, if at all?

     The psychologist offers Cindy ongoing care to discuss her trauma, which she declines at this time. The psychologist suggests briefly including this information in the letter to inform the surgeon of Cindy's need for trauma-informed care, but Cindy is hesitant to complicate her request for surgery before being offered a surgery date. They collaboratively decide that Cindy will disclose prior medical mistreatment after securing a surgical date and ask for support during hospitalization.

2. How might Cindy's prior trauma impact the postoperative course?

     After being given a date for surgery, Cindy discloses her hospital experience to her surgeon. The team is compassionate and proactive to ensure she will be comfortable. A nurse navigator offers Cindy a personalized tour of the hospital before her surgery day, walking her through registration, perioperative areas, and the floor on which she will recover, where she meets a charge nurse and other staff who will be involved in her inpatient care. After surgery, she expresses appreciation for the safety and respect she experienced throughout the hospital environment. As she begins to dilate at home, she has trouble meeting the dilation schedule and does not advance the dilator size as expected.

3. What type of supportive services could be offered to Cindy?

The surgeons continue to encourage Cindy and suggest that she attend pelvic floor physical therapy. The therapist identifies anxiety and muscular guarding as the source of dyspareunia. Returning for further follow-up with her surgeons, she becomes tearful and discloses that receptive penetration, both anal intercourse previously and now vaginal dilation, has been more painful and challenging since her previous sexual assault. Her surgeons provide support and empathy and connect Cindy to ongoing therapy to further explore her trauma. She returns to her previous assessing psychologist to begin to address the impact of trauma on her sexual function after surgery.

CASE STUDY 2: PASQUAL

Pasqual is a nonbinary patient who has long desired gender-affirming mastectomy and is beginning to plan for surgery, scheduling consultations with surgeons who take his Medicaid plan. He is unstably housed after leaving home due to conflict with his parents about his gender identity. During warmer months, he sleeps outside, on roofs or in parks, and in colder months, he stays with friends. He has an emotional support dog, a standard poodle named Tyler, and has struggled with entering the shelter system as he has been unable to find a placement with Tyler.

1. What needs to be in place for Pasqual to have a safe recovery from gender-affirming mastectomy?

While Pasqual is obtaining letters of support that he has been told he needs for surgical consultation, his primary care clinician cautions that the surgeons will screen for stable housing. Both his primary care clinician and his mental health clinician are forthright that they will mention current housing instability in their letters of support but offer Pasqual referrals to housing care coordination within the health center. Upon learning that the emotional support dog has previously been a barrier to emergency housing, they write accommodation letters to indicate the necessity for Tyler as an emotional support dog. The mental health clinician asks about who can help walk Tyler, and Pasqual has not yet considered that he may be unable to care for his support dog during the weeks after surgery.

2. Is Pasqual able to have a surgical consultation?

Pasqual and the referring clinicians strategize for the letter of support to include that Pasqual is being referred to a housing coordination program and can move forward with surgical planning while this coordination is underway. At the consult, in addition to operative planning, the surgeon asks about Pasqual's progress in securing housing. Pasqual is now on a waitlist for a supportive housing program. After case conferencing with the housing care coordinator, the surgeon agrees to schedule surgery for 2 months after Pasqual is anticipated to enter supportive housing. Pasqual understands that if he is unhoused at any point between his entering the program and his surgery, his surgery date will be postponed. To address the concern around care for Tyler, Pasqual sets up a care exchange with a friend who is having surgery with the same surgeon. Pasqual will provide his friend with support for hospital discharge and postoperative activities of daily living; in exchange, the friend will do the same for Pasqual, assisting at the hospital and walking Tyler.

CASE STUDY 3: THOMAS

Thomas has been on testosterone for 5 years and is now seeking a penile reconstruction procedure. He is clear that his priorities include having a large penis, at least 6.5 inches in length, and that standing to urinate is also a priority. For these reasons, he is researching surgeons who have experience with thigh donor flap phalloplasty and urethral reconstruction, attending informational conferences and support groups.

1. What surgical risks might Thomas need to be counseled on for his specific requests?

2. What strengths or resources might Thomas bring to the surgical planning process?

Thomas consults with a local academic medical center, where the surgical team members quickly see that Thomas has done extensive research and has a clear vision of the specific procedures which would produce his ideal outcome. They caution that given his body habitus, the thigh flap donor site could result in a girthy penis and may not meet his goals. Specifically, the healing of the larger penis and longer urethra might be compromised by insufficient blood supply and result in stricture or other complications. They advise that the forearm donor site would provide a more reliable option with fewer risks; however, the resulting penis would be thinner and less than 6.5 inches in length.

3. What compromises or risk reduction strategies might be offered to Thomas if he chooses to move forward with the thigh donor site?

The surgical team offers him the option to proceed with the thigh donor site but suggest either forgoing urethral lengthening entirely or placing the new urethral meatus at the ventral base of the phallus, which would still allow for standing urination but give a hypospadias-like appearance. Thomas elects to travel to a surgical team in another state who agrees to move forward with the thigh donor site and urethral lengthening to the tip of the penis. After an initially uneventful recovery, he finds that some urine dibbles from his penis, not only immediately after voiding but also for up to several hours after he finishes urinating.

4. What causes should be investigated given the urinary symptoms?

A voiding retrourethrogram shows that Thomas has a urethral stricture, and proximal to that, a diverticulum. The surgical team performs two revision urethroplasty surgeries in the year following the initial surgery. Thomas is supported by his mental health clinician, who is unclear about the likelihood of success of further surgical intervention as Thomas continues to have trouble urinating after the second procedure. Thomas has had a suprapubic catheter for 15 months and has recurrent bladder spasms.

5. What resources can the mental health clinician draw on?

Thomas's therapist reaches out to the surgical team to discuss further revisions. The surgical team explains that their first and second attempts at repair utilized the same technique and that a third attempt may not be successful. They recommend Thomas consult with the reconstructive urologist at the local medical center for alternative techniques. After reviewing records of the previous surgical interventions and examining Thomas's penis, which has extensive keloid scar tissue with minimal response to steroid injections, the local surgeons counsel that an additional revision urethroplasty using an alternative technique would require multiple procedures several months apart.

6. What choices are available if Thomas does not wish to proceed with an additional attempt at revision urethroplasty?

After Thomas elects not to try further urethroplasty, the local surgical team offers Thomas the choice of "starting over" with a new donor site or reversing his urethra to a perineal urethrostomy and sitting to urinate. Although Thomas ideally would like to stand to urinate with his penis, he has experienced so much relief from gender incongruence with his new penis, which is exactly the dimensions that he initially envisioned, that he no longer has as much distress about sitting to void. He elects to undergo a perineal urethrostomy.

7. When Thomas' catheter is removed, what side effects can he expect?

After his surgery at the local academic medical center, his surgeons refer Thomas to a pelvic floor physical therapist to help to regain bladder function after his lengthy catheterization. Thomas is able to regain complete bladder function in physical therapy and starts to carry an "STP" or stand-to-pee device so that he can stand to urinate when necessary.

REFERENCES

1. Bhinder J, Upadhyaya P. *Brief History of Gender Affirmation Medicine and Surgery*. Springer International Publishing; 2021:249–254.
2. Stone S. The empire strikes back: a posttranssexual manifesto. *Camera Obsc Femin Cult Media Studies*. 1992;10(2):150–176.
3. Bauer GR, Hammond R, Travers R, Kaay M, Hohenadel KM, Boyce M. "I don't think this is theoretical; this is our lives": how erasure impacts health care for transgender people. *J Assoc Nurses AIDS Care*. 2009;20(5):348–361.
4. Nolan IT, Kuhner CJ, Dy GW. Demographic and temporal trends in transgender identities and gender confirming surgery. *Transl Androl Urol*. 2019;8(3):184–190.
5. Passos TS, Teixeira MS, Almeida-Santos MA. Quality of life after gender affirmation surgery: a systematic review and network meta-analysis. *Sexual Res Social Policy*. 2020;17(2):252–262.
6. Dy GW, Nolan IT, Hotaling J, Myers JB. Patient reported outcome measures and quality of life assessment in genital gender confirming surgery. *Transl Androl Urol*. 2019;8(3):228–240.
7. Coleman E, Bockting W, Botzer M, et al. Standards of care for the health of transsexual, transgender, and gender-nonconforming people, version 7. *Int J Transgend*. 2012;13(4):165–232.
8. Rotondi NK, Bauer GR, Scanlon K, Kaay M, Travers R, Travers A. Nonprescribed hormone use and self-performed surgeries: "do-it-yourself" transitions in transgender communities in Ontario, Canada. *Am J Public Health*. 2013;103(10):1830–1836.
9. Ashley F. Surgical informed consent and recognizing a perioperative duty to disclose in transgender health care. *McGill J Law Health*. 2020;13(1):73–116.
10. Heston AL, Esmonde NO, Dugi DDIII, Berli JU. Phalloplasty: techniques and outcomes. *Transl Androl Urol*. 2019;8(3):254–265.
11. Gill-Peterson J. *Histories of the Transgender Child*. University of Minnesota Press; 2018.
12. Almazan AN, Keuroghlian AS. Association Between Gender-Affirming Surgeries and Mental Health Outcomes. *JAMA Surg*. Published online April 28, 2021. doi:10.1001/jamasurg.2021.0952
13. Poceta J, Cousins S, Wenzel C, et al. Effectiveness of a gender affirming surgery class for transgender and non-binary patients and their caregivers in an integrated healthcare setting. *Int J Transgend*. 2019;20(1):81–86.
14. Boskey ER, Taghinia AH, Ganor O. Association of surgical risk with exogenous hormone use in transgender patients: a systematic review. *JAMA Surgery*. 2019;154(2):159–169.
15. Ngaage LM, McGlone KL, Xue S, et al. Gender surgery beyond chest and genitals: current insurance landscape. *Aesthet Surg J*. 2020;40(4):NP202–NP210.
16. Van Boerum MS, Salibian AA, Bluebond-Langner R, Agarwal C. Chest and facial surgery for the transgender patient. *Transl Androl Urol*. 2019;8(3):219–227.
17. Marks DH, Awosika O, Rengifo-Pardo M, Ehrlich A. Dermatologic surgical care for transgender individuals. *Dermatol Surg*. 2019;45(3).
18. Nolan IT, Kuhner CJ, Dy GW. Demographic and temporal trends in transgender identities and gender confirming surgery. *Transl Androl Urol*. 2019.

19. Wolter A, Diedrichson J, Scholz T, Arens-Landwehr A, Liebau J. Sexual reassignment surgery in female-to-male transsexuals: an algorithm for subcutaneous mastectomy. *J Plast Reconstr Aesthet Surg.* 2015;68(2):184–191.

20. Bluebond-Langner R, Berli JU, Sabino J, Chopra K, Singh D, Fischer B. Top surgery in transgender men: how far can you push the envelope? *Plast Reconstr Surg.* 2017;139(4): 873e–882e.

21. Esmonde N, Heston A, Jedrzejewski B, et al. What is "nonbinary" and what do I need to know? A primer for surgeons providing chest surgery for transgender patients. *Aesthet Surg J.* 2019;39(5):NP106–NP112.

22. Grimstad FW, Boskey E, Grey M. New-onset abdominopelvic pain after initiation of testosterone therapy among trans-masculine persons: a community-based exploratory survey. *LGBT Health.* 2020;7(5):248–253.

23. Watanyusakul S. Vaginoplasty modifications to improve vulvar aesthetics. *Urol Clin North Am.* 2019;46(4):541–554.

24. Dy GW, Jun MS, Blasdel G, Bluebond-Langner R, Zhao LC. Outcomes of gender affirming peritoneal flap vaginoplasty using the Da Vinci Single Port versus Xi Robotic systems. *Eur Urol.* 2020.

25. Dy GW, Sun J, Granieri MA, Zhao LC. Reconstructive management pearls for the transgender patient. *Current Urology Reports.* 2018;19(6):36.

26. Jiang DD, Gallagher S, Burchill L, Berli J, Dugi DIII Implementation of a pelvic floor physical therapy program for transgender women undergoing gender-affirming vaginoplasty. *Obstet Gynecol.* 2019;133(5).

27. Brittain J, Dunford C, Miah S, Takhar M, Morley R, Rashid T. Enormous mucocele following colonic graft neovagina formation in a transwoman. *Urol Case Rep.* 2018;21:73–74.

28. Frey JD, Poudrier G, Chiodo MV, Hazen A. A systematic review of metoidioplasty and radial forearm flap phalloplasty in female-to-male transgender genital reconstruction: is the "ideal" neophallus an achievable goal? *Plast Reconstr Surg Glob Open.* 2016;4(12):e1131.

29. Djordjevic ML. Novel surgical techniques in female to male gender confirming surgery. *Transl Androl Urol.* 2018;7(4): 628–638.

30. Dy GW, Granieri MA, Fu BC, et al. Presenting complications to a reconstructive urologist after masculinizing genital reconstructive surgery. *Urology.* 2019;132:202–206.

31. Garcia MM. Strategies to optimize sexual function with feminizing and masculinizing genital gender-affirming surgery. In: Schechter LS, ed. *Gender Confirmation Surgery: Principles and Techniques for an Emerging Field.* Cham: Springer International Publishing; 2020:215–228.

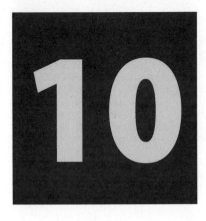

Case Studies in Gender Emergence and Affirmation

Jennifer Reske-Nielsen

INTRODUCTION

This chapter is unlike the other chapters in this book as it is comprised only of cases. The cases highlight and explore common scenarios encountered in the clinical care of **transgender and gender diverse (TGD)** populations. These cases can be used as self-study, in small groups for discussion, or in larger groups as prework to discussion. The goal of this chapter is to consider a variety of clinical scenarios of providing gender-affirming care and how a health care professional should respond to them.

CASE STUDY 1: Alex

Alex is 25 years old, new to the city, and presents to your clinic to establish care. Registration paperwork lists Alex's sex as female. Past medical history reveals mild asthma, and Alex's only medication is a rescue inhaler. Alex does not smoke, drink alcohol, or use any drugs. Alex has no family history of early coronary artery disease, blood clots, or cancer. You ask what Alex's pronouns are, and Alex tells you "they/them/their." You ask how they identify their gender, and they say "genderqueer." Alex explains that they are interested in starting testosterone to affirm their gender and want to know more about the changes it can lead to.

▶ Discussion Questions

1. You and your office staff assumed that Alex identifies as a woman because of the information in the electronic health record (EHR). If a mistake was made with pronouns as Alex checked in at the front desk, how could you address this within the visit? What changes could be made in the EHR to prevent another mistake when Alex returns to the clinic?

   It is awkward for both clinicians and patients when an incorrect assumption is made during a visit, especially when it concerns something as important as one's gender identity or pronouns. If a mistake is made, the best approach is for the clinician to recognize the error, apologize to the patient, and then move forward in a respectful manner. Documenting the patient's name and pronouns in the EHR prevents such mistakes. Doing so ensures that all patients are accorded respect and dignity throughout their contact with the health care system. Each EHR has different ways that this information can be collected.[1] If recording this information is not yet possible in the existing system, the health care team for the day should be notified about the patient's name and pronouns.

   Gender identity and pronouns should be collected as part of registration paperwork completed by patients new to the practice. This process, however, may miss existing patients. Since 2016, health centers have been required to collect sexual orientation/gender identity (SOGI) data.[1] If the SOGI information gathered is incorporated into the patient's EHR "banner" where it is readily visible each time the EHR is opened, all members of the health care team will be continually reminded to use the patient's correct identifiers.

   Additionally, clinicians can collect this information directly by asking two simple questions of all patients: "What is your gender identity?" and "What are your pronouns?" Some clinicians worry that asking these questions may offend some patients. Although patients who are unaware of various gender identities may sometimes be confused by the questions, they are unlikely to be offended when it is explained that asking about gender identity and pronouns is standard practice. Ways to show that this is an organizational standard of practice is to post signs about pronoun usage or to wear badges displaying one's pronouns.

2. What questions would you ask to gather a gender history?

   The key to taking a gender history is to be nonjudgmental and ask open-ended questions that do not require a patient to feel as though there is a right answer. The goal is to ascertain the patient's experiences and feelings about their gender so that the clinician can offer the appropriate options to help affirm the patient's gender. Possible prompting questions include:

- Can you tell me how you came to discover your gender identity?
- What was gender like for you as a child? As an adolescent? As a young adult?
- What is the earliest that you remember feeling that your gender identity differs from the sex you were assigned at birth?
- How do you feel about your body? (Follow-up questions could include asking about any gender dysphoria they may experience.)
- What are your goals for gender affirmation? In what ways are you thinking of achieving those goals?
- Are there specific changes that you are looking forward to? That you are hoping will not happen?
- There are many ways to affirm one's gender. Are there any that you have used to affirm your gender?
- Have you ever taken gender-affirming hormones?
- Have you had any procedures to affirm your gender previously?
- Have you disclosed your gender identity to anyone?

3. Alex is considering testosterone for gender affirmation but wants to know more about it. How would you counsel them on what physical changes to expect and the timing of these changes? What resources can you provide Alex to support them?

Establishing clear and realistic outcome-related expectations is a critical part of counseling for gender-affirming hormone therapy (GAHT). Otherwise, it can be discouraging if the patient feels that their anticipated changes are not happening fast enough or are not the changes they were hoping for. Expected masculinizing changes and the timing of their onset are discussed in Chapter 7, "Gender-Affirming Hormone Therapy in Adults."

CASE STUDY 2: Rebecca

Rebecca is a 55-year-old transgender woman who presents to establish care and start feminizing hormone therapy. Rebecca discloses that she has felt that she has identified as a girl and then a woman for "as long as I can remember" but only recently felt comfortable disclosing her gender identity to her wife and grown children. She uses the pronouns she/her/hers despite her insurance card listing her sex as male. She has been taking feminizing hormones purchased from online websites for over 10 years. Now that she is open about her gender identity, she would like to use medically prescribed hormones. She

has not had any gender-affirming surgeries or procedures. She has a past medical history of obesity, hypertension, and sleep apnea. She has no personal or family history of blood clots or early coronary artery disease. She takes lisinopril for her blood pressure, is trying to lose weight (her body mass index [BMI] is 48), and uses a continuous positive airway pressure (CPAP) machine for sleep apnea. She is up to date on colonoscopy screening. She asks what the next steps are so she can get a prescription for hormones.

▶ Discussion Questions

1. Is it safe to prescribe feminizing hormones (estrogen) to Rebecca given her age (55)? If so, what type? What dosage? Are there other considerations regarding her health history that raise concerns about the safety of estrogen, and if so, what are these? Are there other medications that could be prescribed to help affirm her gender identity?

Contraindications to estrogen therapy for gender affirmation are an active estrogen-sensitive cancer or an allergy to estrogen; Rebecca does not have any of these contraindications. The safety concerns of estrogen relate to her age (older than age 50 years) and her cardiovascular risk factors of obesity and hypertension. Data from the Women's Health Initiative indicated increased risks of cardiovascular and thrombogenic events when estrogen (in the form of conjugated equine estrogen) and medroxyprogesterone acetate were given to postmenopausal **cisgender** women aged 50–79 years.[2] It is unclear, however, if **trans feminine** people taking 17β-estradiol (the most commonly used oral formulation for gender affirmation) without progesterone have the same risks. Recent published reviews examining this question demonstrated mixed results.[3,4] There does appear to be an increased risk of blood clots; however, these studies examined patients taking conjugated equine estrogen, which is more thrombogenic compared with 17β-estradiol. For Rebecca, given her higher than average cardiovascular risks, the safest route would be to start her on transdermal estrogen, which is less thrombogenic, and work on controlling her modifiable cardiovascular risk factors of obesity and hypertension.

The feminizing effects of estrogen for gender affirmation cannot be accomplished by other medications. The decision to use estrogen therapy should be individualized by carefully considering the risks and benefits for each patient. It is also important to note that there are potential risks of psychological harm to individuals seeking gender affirmation who cannot attain it.

The baseline cardiovascular risk factors to consider when counseling patients about estrogen therapy include the following:

- **Smoking.** Smoking is a known independent risk factor for coronary artery disease and stroke. In individuals who smoke, the use of estrogen can also increase the risk of blood clots. This risk is higher with ethinyl estradiol (the type found in many combined oral contraceptive pills) than with 17β-estradiol (the oral formulation used for gender affirmation and in the estradiol patch). People wanting to start gender-affirming estrogen should be counseled to quit smoking tobacco, but this should not be a requirement to start on estrogen. A **harm reduction** approach is best used by using transdermal estrogen for individuals who are smoking tobacco.

- **Other cardiovascular risks (e.g., hypertension, diabetes, family history of cardiovascular or vascular disease).** The same recommendations for lifestyle modification and management of these conditions apply to TGD patients as they do to cisgender patients.

- **Personal history of blood clots.** Consensus guidelines recommend that TGD individuals with a personal history of blood clots seeking estrogen for gender affirmation use transdermal estradiol because it is associated with a lower thrombogenic risk.[5]

- **Type of estrogen.** Transdermal estradiol is less thrombogenic than oral or injectable estrogen formulations. Of the oral formulations, 17β-estradiol oral pills are less thrombogenic than ethinyl estradiol and conjugated equine estrogen.

- **Estrogen dosage.** Using lower doses of estrogen decreases the risk of thromboembolic events. One way to still maximize gender-affirming effects of estrogen with lower doses of estrogen is to block endogenous androgens with an antiandrogen such as spironolactone.

Although Rebecca is 55 years old, she does not have any absolute contraindications to estrogen use and is a nonsmoker. She has high blood pressure that is controlled with medication. She has no history of blood clots. Thus, starting her on low-dose transdermal estradiol would be appropriate as the safest method due to her age and comorbidities of hypertension and obesity.

Consideration should be given to adding an androgen blocker as an adjunct to estrogen therapy. The use of an androgen blocker lowers the levels of endogenous testosterone, allowing the administered estrogen to have greater gender-affirming effects at lower doses. Although increasing the estrogen dosage would decrease endogenous testosterone levels, it would also cause an increase in side effects. In the United States, the most common antiandrogen used for gender affirmation is spironolactone. Typical dosages of spironolactone are 50–200 mg/day. The use of spironolactone requires monitoring of potassium and kidney function through bloodwork (see Chapter 7). In Europe, a medication called cyproterone acetate is a commonly used antiandrogen, but it is not approved by the U.S. Food and Drug Administration for this indication.

2. What questions should you ask Rebecca about her previous hormone treatments?

Rebecca obtained estrogen from internet sources for more than 10 years. It is important to determine the type, dosage, and route of delivery of the estrogen she has been taking.

Oral: Rebecca may have been taking both conjugated equine estrogen and ethinyl estradiol (the form of estrogen in birth control pills), both of which are associated with increased cardiovascular risk. Neither of these formulations is detectable by blood tests for estradiol. Oral 17β-estradiol is detectable by blood testing. There is no consensus regarding the utility of measuring estradiol levels for gender affirmation. One of the arguments for testing is that it can determine whether the patient's estradiol levels are in the normal female range; if they are not, the dosage may be adjusted accordingly. However, the normal range of estradiol is not clear because levels vary in cisgender women. Arguments against testing are that it is inaccurate and that changes in dosage should be based on a patient's physical changes rather than laboratory values.

Estradiol patches: Patches are available in different dosages. It is important to ask which dosage Rebecca had been using, how many patches were used at a time, and how often they were changed. Transdermal estrogen is considered the safest form for gender-affirmation therapy.

Injection: Typical formulations are estradiol valerate and estradiol cypionate. It is important to determine when the patient's last injection was to decide when to initiate transdermal estrogen. Patients who have used injectable estrogen obtained through nonmedical sources should be tested for bloodborne pathogens such as hepatitis B and C and HIV.

3. What questions should you ask about Rebecca's gender affirmation history and goals?

You should ask the same questions that you would for anyone starting on hormones (see Case 1). You may also want to ask what made her decide to come out to her family and start medically monitored hormone therapy. It would also be helpful to ask if there were physical effects she has not experienced despite being on estrogen for 10 years that she would like to achieve (e.g., surgeries, voice therapy), or if there are other logistical affirmation goals that she needs help with, such as **gender marker** changes.

4. Will her blood pressure medication need to be adjusted while she is on feminizing hormones? What follow-up testing would you recommend? Would you make any changes if she undergoes an orchiectomy?

Rebecca's blood pressure medication may need to be adjusted after you add spironolactone for androgen suppression. Angiotensin-converting enzyme (ACE) inhibitors (such as lisinopril), angiotensin receptor blockers (ARBs), and spironolactone can increase serum potassium. If adding spironolactone to an ACE inhibitor or ARB, it is critical to closely track the potassium level for signs of hyperkalemia. For Rebecca, one option would be to stop the lisinopril and see how her blood pressure responds to the spironolactone alone. This option would decrease pill burden and reduce the risk of hyperkalemia. However, if she were taking multiple antihypertensive agents, you might consider replacing one of them with spironolactone and then following her closely to make sure her blood pressure remains well controlled. If she were to undergo **orchiectomy**, she would no longer require androgen suppression with spironolactone. She may then require reinitiation or an increased dosage of her antihypertensive medications.

5. What testing should you do before prescribing feminizing hormones for gender affirmation?

Basic metabolic panel. Checking potassium levels and kidney function is important before prescribing spironolactone, as it can result in elevated potassium. These labs should be checked at baseline and after starting or increasing the dose.

Cholesterol. Because estrogen can increase triglyceride levels, knowing the baseline levels can be helpful for older individuals to understand possible additional cardiovascular risks.

CASE STUDY 3: Blake

Blake is a 20-year-old transgender woman who presents to establish care. She has been socially affirmed as a woman for years but has never been on medications or used friends' medications. She had breast augmentation surgery last year outside the United States. When she disclosed her gender identity to her family 3 years ago, she was kicked out of the house. She was unable to finish school and has been exchanging sex for money to get by. Currently, she is staying with a friend but has no specific address of her own. She has good support from a few friends. She feels that she can blend in socially as a woman most of the time since her breast augmentation surgery. She would now like to start on feminizing hormones. Her goal is to get her GED and to be able to start working in the cosmetics industry.

▶ Discussion Questions

1. What social circumstances should be considered when initiating gender-affirming hormone therapy? Do Blake's social circumstances affect her choice of hormones?

A person's living situation should not prevent them from receiving gender-affirming care. However, in some situations, particularly when a patient lives with others (including family members) who may be unsupportive or even hostile to gender diversity, discovering the medications could place the patient in danger of physical violence or possible homelessness. One way to circumvent this potential problem is to provide injections for Blake in the clinic every 2 weeks. If undergoing physical changes from hormones might "out" her as being transgender and put her in danger or cause homelessness, an open discussion about the timing of onset of physical changes and options to defer hormones or initiate them at a lower dose may be warranted. The fact that Blake exchanges sex for money is not a factor in determining the safety of starting gender-affirming hormone therapy.

2. What questions should you ask as part of a sexual history for Blake? What type of counseling regarding the prevention of sexually transmitted infections (STIs) should be provided? Are there any medications that she should be offered?

The sexual history should be obtained in an open and nonjudgmental way. Instead of asking, "Do you have sex with men, women, or both?" it is more appropriate to ask, "Who are your sexual partners?" If a patient appears confused by this question, you can clarify by adding, "What are the genders of your sexual partners?" It is also important to ask about types of sexual behavior in an open-ended manner: "What types of sex do you have, and what body parts are involved?" Many clinicians providers may feel uncomfortable asking such sensitive questions, but they are important in assessing a patient's risk of acquiring STIs, including HIV, so that appropriate counseling, screening, and prevention can be offered. Other important parts of the sexual history include condom use, the ability to negotiate condom use with partners, and the use of alcohol or drugs in relation to sex.

Safer sex counseling should include increasing condom use with partners and decreasing alcohol or drug use involved in sex. Using drugs and alcohol during sex alters a person's decision-making ability about the use of condoms or the type of sexual behaviors engaged in. Safer sex counseling could also include a discussion of pre-exposure prophylaxis (PrEP) medication (tenofovir-emtricitabine). PrEP is a daily pill that can significantly decrease the risk of acquiring HIV, even if exposed. Because Blake has multiple sexual partners in the context of sex work and may also have limited ability to negotiate condom use with clients, she should be offered PrEP. Before initiating PrEP, patients should test negative for HIV and have normal renal function. They should also be tested for hepatitis B and other STIs, including chlamydia and gonorrhea testing from all anatomical sites, including the throat, rectum, and urethra (i.e., urine), and blood tests for syphilis and hepatitis C. Once on PrEP, Blake should be monitored every 3 months with repeat testing for HIV and other STIs (except for repeat hepatitis B testing if the patient is immune).

3. What other supports should be offered to Blake?

   Blake should be offered housing support. A referral for mental health counseling may also be appropriate given her history of family rejection.

4. After Blake is started on her gender-affirming medications, how often should she return for follow-up visits?

   Blake should initially return in one month to assess medication side effects and discuss any further support she may need. She should have a basic metabolic panel (BMP) to make sure her electrolytes and renal function remain normal on spironolactone. It is customary to start on 100 mg spironolactone daily at first, then increase the dose to 100 mg twice a day at the follow-up visit. Her next visit can be in 3 months, at which time the testosterone level and BMP can be checked again. This 3-month visit is also an appropriate time to perform STI testing if she is now taking PrEP. Even if she is not on PrEP, she should receive STI testing every 3 months if she engages in high-risk sex.

CASE STUDY 4: Jake

Jake is a 40-year-old transgender man whom you have seen for a few appointments to discuss his readiness to start masculinizing hormones. His pronouns when speaking with you are he/him/his, and his pronouns in other settings are she/her/hers. He has disclosed that his chest is very upsetting to him. He menstruates regularly, which also causes him distress. He has a friend who started testosterone and then had top surgery the next year; he would like to receive this same gender-affirming medical and surgical care. He is not interested in having facial hair and reports he would do electrolysis if he developed facial hair. He is worried about his voice deepening because he feels that this would "out" him in his work as a hairstylist. He is only out to his partner and presents in feminine-styled clothing with baggy shirts to cover his chest. When he cannot wear a baggy shirt, he often wears a binder. He has had dysphoria about his body since he was younger and is very worried about his family, friends, and coworkers' reaction if he presents as masculine. He reports that his family took some time to get used to him being "gay," and he has heard them make biased comments about gender diversity. There is no family history of breast cancer. He has social anxiety and depression and takes sertraline, which he reports has been effective. He has been told he needs a behavioral health letter before he can start on masculinizing hormones.

▶ Discussion Questions

1. Given the gender history that Jake discloses to you, do you think he is prepared for the physical changes of masculinizing hormones?

   Because Jake is worried about irreversible changes associated with testosterone (e.g., facial hair, voice deepening), the effects of testosterone do not seem to align with his gender affirmation goals at this time. This does not mean that we cannot help him affirm his gender. Jake appears to be most dysphoric around his chest and his monthly bleeding. (Jake refers to his periods or menstruation as "monthly bleeding" as the other two terms seem too gender typing. It is important to find out what terms individuals use for their body.) Both issues that Jake mentions can be managed without masculinizing hormones, as discussed below.

2. What methods of gender affirmation may help Jake affirm his gender even if he is not ready to be fully open about his gender in all realms of life?

   For his chest, Jake could have chest masculinization surgery ("top surgery"). There is a common misconception that top surgery is only done for people on testosterone therapy: this is not the case. Letters documenting the medical necessity of top surgery should indicate that masculinizing hormones are not indicated for him at this time. Because top surgery requires time for postoperative recovery, you may want to explore how he plans to explain his recovery to the people he lives with and coworkers before the surgery. As for Jake's monthly bleeding, options include the use of a combined oral contraceptive taken continuously (no placebo) or progestin-only (e.g., progestin-only pill, implant, or hormonal intrauterine device [IUD]).

3. What counseling would you offer regarding possible health issues associated with chest binding?

   Binding is a form of compression of the chest tissue with a tight garment to create a flatter top. Binders come in many styles. Patients should be counseled to minimize the amount of time they are worn and avoid wearing them continuously. Particularly in hot climates, sweating can cause skin irritation, fungal infections, and skin breakdown if worn for an extended time.

4. What additional supports would you recommend to Jake?

   Jake would likely benefit from attending a peer support group with other **trans masculine** people who have also navigated gender affirmation and disclosure. Groups can be found either online or in different communities.

5. How would you help Jake further explore his gender affirmation goals at his next visit?

   At the next visit, you could explore how he views himself and what things he could do to live in accordance with his self-perception even though he is not out to everyone. It may also be helpful to explore his ultimate goals in gender affirmation and to highlight the fact that he is engaged in a change process. These discussions may help him feel that he is progressing in his gender affirmation despite not taking masculinizing hormones.

6. What do the World Professional Association for Transgender Health (WPATH) guidelines say about

"requirements" for starting on masculinizing hormones? What do the WPATH guidelines say about clearance for gender-affirming top surgery?

WPATH's criteria for hormone therapy in adults are:

- Persistent, well-documented gender dysphoria.

- Capacity to make a fully informed decision and to give consent to treatment.

- Age of majority in their country.

- If significant medical or mental health concerns are present, they must be reasonably well controlled.

A letter from a mental health professional is not needed to start hormone therapy in adults.[6]

7. Consider the impact of intersectional identities on gender affirmation. Would you change your approach to counseling Jake depending on his race/ethnicity? His religious or spiritual beliefs?

It is important to understand a patient's multiple intersecting identities when providing gender affirmation counseling. The way a patient's communities view people who are TGD may influence their internal view of themselves, what gender diversity means to them, and, ultimately, their gender-affirmation goals. Concepts of gender diversity may differ across cultural contexts. For example, some Native American tribes recognize two-spirit people, and some Asian cultures acknowledge a third gender. These cultural norms may make it easier for someone to express their gender diversity. Other cultures may be less likely to accept gender diversity, which can lead to internalized transphobia. As health care professionals, it is important to understand that an individual may hold a multiplicity of identities and to help each person recognize the ramifications that a visible gender change may have in all aspects of their lives.

REFERENCES

1. Grasso C, McDowell MJ, Goldhammer H, Keuroghlian AS. Planning and implementing sexual orientation and gender identity data collection in electronic health records. *J Am Med Inform Assoc.* 2019;26(1):66-70.
2. Manson JE, Chlebowski RT, Stefanick ML, et al. Menopausal hormone therapy and health outcomes during the intervention and extended poststopping phases of the Women's Health Initiative randomized trials. *JAMA.* 2013;310(13):1353-1368.
3. Connelly PJ, Marie Freel E, Perry C, et al. Gender-affirming hormone therapy, vascular health and cardiovascular disease in transgender adults. *Hypertension.* 2019;74(6):1266-1274.
4. Seal LJ. Cardiovascular disease in transgendered people: a review of the literature and discussion of risk. *JRSM Cardiovasc Dis.* 2019;8:2048004019880745.
5. UCSF Transgender Care, Department of Family and Community Medicine, University of California San Francisco. *Guidelines for the Primary and Gender-Affirming Care of Transgender and Gender Nonbinary People.* 2nd ed. Deutsch MB, ed. June 2016. transcare.ucsf.edu/guidelines.
6. Coleman E, Bockting W, Botzer M, et al. Standards of care for the health of transsexual, transgender, and gender-nonconforming people. Version 7. *Int J Transgend.* 2012;13(4):165-232.

Primary, Preventive, and Specialty Care

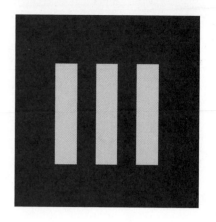

Primary Preventive,
and Specialty Care

Basic Principles of Trauma-Informed and Gender-Affirming Care

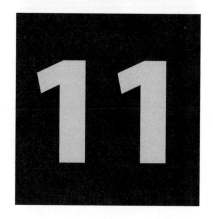

Samara Grossman
Sarah Berman
Jennifer Potter

INTRODUCTION

I believe that telling our stories, first to ourselves and then to one another and the world, is a revolutionary act. It is an act that can be met with hostility, exclusion, and violence. It can also lead to love, understanding, transcendence, and community. I hope that my being real with you will help empower you to step into who you are and encourage you to share yourself with those around you.

Janet Mock, Redefining Realness: My Path to Womanhood, Identity, Love & So Much More[1]

This chapter begins reviewing the high prevalence of trauma and adversity among transgender and gender diverse (TGD) people and explaining the potential effects of trauma on their overall health and well-being. The chapter then describes how clinicians can support the healing and recovery of their TGD patients by incorporating principles of trauma-informed care during health care encounters and by advocating for trauma-informed changes at both institutional and systems levels.

TRAUMA AND ITS EFFECTS

The concept of **trauma** has evolved over time; currently, it describes events that overwhelm ordinary human stress responses and "involve threats to life or bodily integrity, or a close personal encounter with violence or death."[2] For example, the Substance Abuse and Mental Health Services Administration (SAMHSA) defines trauma as resulting from "an event, series of events, or set of circumstances that is experienced by an individual as physical or emotionally harmful or life-threatening and that has lasting adverse effects on the individual's functioning and mental, physical, social, emotional, or spiritual well-being."[3] Traumatic events include violence (e.g., sexual, physical, and emotional abuse and other violent crimes), political acts (e.g., war, genocide, and torture), natural disasters and accidents (e.g., car crashes, house fires), and experiences with illness and disease (e.g., intensive care stays, birth trauma). Discrimination and **structural violence,** defined as social structures that stop individuals, groups, and societies from reaching their full potential, can also be experienced as traumatic.[4] Studies estimate that approximately 90% of American adults will experience at least one traumatic event in their lifetime according to the *Diagnostic and Statistical Manual of Mental Disorders*, 5th edition criteria.[5] More than one-half of Americans have reported a traumatic experience related to interpersonal violence (child abuse, physical assault, and sexual violence).[5]

Adverse childhood experiences (ACEs), as defined by the landmark ACE study conducted by researchers at Kaiser Permanente, are specific types of trauma that occur before age 18. These include abuse (physical, emotional, or sexual), neglect (physical or emotional), and household dysfunction (exposure to divorce; a member of the household with mental illness, a substance use disorder, or who is incarcerated; or witnessing violence in the home).[6] ACEs are common: over one-half of participants in the original Kaiser study reported at least one ACE. Moreover, ACEs were associated with increased health risk behaviors; mental illness; substance use disorders; heart, lung, and liver disease; and cancer. The number of ACEs was positively correlated with the risk for developing adverse health effects; the higher the number of ACEs reported, the greater the risk for later health effects.[7] The original ACEs study enrolled a predominantly white population; subsequent studies have proposed expanded ACEs to be more accurate across socio-demographic groups. Expanded ACEs include community-level indicators such as experiencing racism, bullying, or foster care; witnessing violence; and living in an unsafe neighborhood.[8] The prevalence of expanded ACEs is also high; for example, in a community study performed in Southeast Pennsylvania, 63.4% of participants reported at least one expanded ACE.[8]

All forms of trauma may be associated with adverse effects on physical, psychological, and social health.[9] A major consequence of trauma is the development of **posttraumatic stress disorder (PTSD)**, a disorder characterized by intrusive symptoms, avoidance behaviors, mood and cognitive alterations, and alterations in arousal and reactivity after experiencing a traumatic event or acute stressor.[10] A survey of almost 3,000 U.S. adults found an 8.3% lifetime prevalence of PTSD overall, with a prevalence of 11% and 5.4% among presumed **cisgender** women and men, respectively.[5] It is generally thought that traumatic experiences involving rape, genocide, and combat are more likely to lead to the development of PTSD.[10] Beyond the negative health outcomes, clinicians must also be aware that health care itself can be difficult for people with trauma histories. Patients with trauma histories may be negatively affected by health care encounters; adverse experiences may in turn lead to decreased engagement in future health care or outright health care avoidance.[11,12] Experiences in health care, such as critical illness and birth, can also be traumatizing to people and may lead to symptoms of PTSD.[13,14]

Several biological systems are impacted by trauma (Figure 11-1). Dysregulation of the autonomic nervous system and the hypothalamic-pituitary-adrenal (HPA) axis, which mediate stress responses, has been observed.[15] Neural circuits may also be altered after traumatic exposure, and emerging theories have implicated fear learning, threat detection, and emotion regulation systems in the pathogenesis of PTSD.[15,16] Additionally, studies have suggested "a genetic component" to the development of PTSD after experiencing trauma and have identified several gene variants of interest, many of them involved in neurotransmitter and HPA axis signaling.[17] However, because structural and social contexts influence exposure to trauma and experiences of trauma can cluster in families and environments, it is difficult to determine the degree of genetic inheritability. Early life stressors, including stress in the prenatal period, have been linked to epigenetic changes in DNA methylation patterns that may make an individual more susceptible to trauma-related health effects later in life.[17]

Despite the harmful effects of trauma, healing and recovery are possible. Psychotherapy is the mainstay of treatment: both prolonged exposure therapy and cognitive processing therapy have been found to be effective modalities.[16,18] Additionally, a growing emphasis is being placed on the identification, development, and utilization of **resilience** to mitigate the effects of trauma and promote healing.[19] Resilience can be thought of as the ability of survivors to access their strengths in order to facilitate recovery.[19] Strengths or protective factors that foster resilience include individual characteristics (e.g., emotional regulation skills, self-esteem, self-efficacy), social supports (e.g., family support, feeling

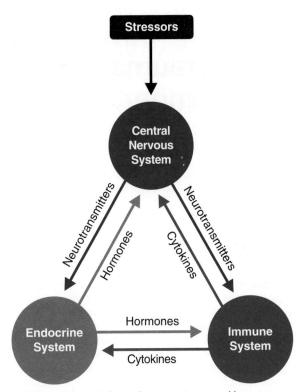

▲ **Figure 11-1.** Biological systems impacted by trauma.

loved by caregivers, support from friends), and community circumstances (e.g., social cohesion of the community, resourced school environments).[20] Finally, studies have increasingly shown that survivors of trauma may experience posttraumatic growth, which is the development of positive psychological change after a traumatic event that may surpass a person's pretrauma baseline. Some, but not all, survivors may, through the process of coping with and healing from trauma, find that they have a greater appreciation for their lives, a changed understanding of what is important, an increased sense of personal strength, and improved experience relating to others.[21]

HEALING AND RECOVERY IN TGD POPULATIONS

Healing and recovery from trauma are especially relevant for TGD people, who experience disproportionately higher rates of trauma and adversity across the life course compared to their cisgender peers. For example, TGD youth report higher ACE scores than cisgender sexual minority youth and are disproportionately affected by interpersonally mediated ACEs (i.e., emotional abuse, physical neglect, and emotional neglect) in particular.[22] Transgender youth also report greater severity of ACE exposure (i.e., childhood polyvictimization) compared with nontransgender youth.[23] Nonwhite TGD youth report the highest average ACE scores.[24]

In addition to ACEs, other forms of childhood adversity—including school-based bullying and harassment,[25,26] weight-based victimization,[27] and dating violence[28,29]—are disproportionately prevalent in TGD youth and young adults. High levels of structural stigma and interpersonal violence persist throughout adulthood across a wide range of societal contexts, including education, employment, housing, public accommodations (e.g., restaurants, transportation, public bathrooms), law enforcement, military service, and health care.[30] Consequently, TGD people, and especially TGD people with multiple intersecting stigmatized identities, such as transgender women of color,[31] are vulnerable to risk factors independently associated with violence, such as poverty, homelessness, survival sex, and incarceration.

Hendricks and Testa adapted Meyer's Gender Minority Stress and Resilience (GMSR) model[32] to explain how exposure to **gender minority stress** might account for disparities in mental and physical health (e.g., depression, PTSD, suicide attempts, substance use disorders, high-risk sexual activity, HIV) observed among TGD populations (see Chapter 3, "Health Disparities," for more information about this model).[33] This adapted model is supported by empirical data.[34–38] As described succinctly in a recent review,[39] gender minority stress: (1) is unique to the experience of TGD people; (2) is a chronic process stemming from lifetime experiences of stigma, discrimination, and violence; and (3) has a social basis formed by structural, institutional, and policy-level conditions. The processes that contribute to gender minority stress exist on a continuum extending from distal stressors that originate in the environment to proximal stressors that arise within the individual. From distal to proximal, these processes include objective discriminatory events that can be acute or chronic; the expectation of discrimination or victimization; concealment of minority identity status (e.g., gender identity); and internalization of discriminatory social views. Gender minority stress exists in a larger environment of social advantages and disadvantages that interact with a person's gender minority status. These additional sources of stress, which include both general stressors and those of other marginalized statuses (e.g., race, ethnicity, sexual orientation, etc.), combine with gender minority stress to determine an individual's cumulative stress burden and coping resources. Inclusion of resilience factors in the GMSR model helps to explain how, despite exposure to adversity across the lifespan, TGD people are able to achieve positive health outcomes.

INJUSTICE WITHIN THE HEALTH CARE SYSTEM

Historically, the health care industry has done a poor job of meeting the health care needs of TGD people. Even as recently as 2015, a U.S. survey of >27,000 transgender people revealed that 33% of respondents did not seek care in the past year when they needed to because they could not afford

it. The 33% of respondents who did seek care reported being verbally harassed or refused treatment or needing to educate their clinicians about transgender health.[31] Lack of clinician respect for a TGD patient's gender identity and body, clinician actions that reduce a TGD patient's agency and control during the encounter (e.g., gatekeeping bargains such as "I'll only prescribe hormones after you've had your Pap test"), and systemic barriers such as disaffirming care environments and lack of insurance coverage for gender-affirming procedures collectively have an adverse impact on care.[40] As clinicians, we have a professional duty to do a better job, both during our interactions with TGD patients and by advocating for their needs more broadly. Fortunately, there is now guidance on how we can do so.

As shown in Figure 11-2, the formation of a productive therapeutic alliance and patient engagement in care may depend on how successfully the clinician and patient navigate gender and power dynamics during the encounter. This figure was derived from results of qualitative interviews with trans masculine participants in regard to undergoing cervical cancer screening.[41] Attention to power enactment and gender construction can be woven into an overall trauma-informed approach to patient care in order to establish productive clinician–patient relationships that provide a foundation for healing and recovery.

TRAUMA-INFORMED CARE AS A FOUNDATION FOR HEALING AND RECOVERY

Building off of previous work in the study and treatment of trauma, SAMHSA developed **trauma-informed care (TIC)** as a framework for health care professionals and systems to address trauma in patients and communities. In 1994, SAMHSA convened the Dare to Vision Conference, where trauma survivors shared their experiences with being retraumatized and triggered by standard hospital practices.[3] Later, in 1998, SAMHSA initiated the Women, Co-occurring Disorders, and Violence Study (WCDVS), a 5-year study that enrolled 2,729 women who had experienced trauma or violence and who had co-occurring substance use and mental health disorders. They found that patients in comprehensive trauma-informed treatment programs had improved substance use, trauma, and mental health symptoms at 6- and 12-month follow-up as compared to patients undergoing standard treatment. This improvement in care occurred with no added cost.[42] This study promoted a trauma-informed approach to delivery of services to treat addiction, and brought heightened attention to the need for trauma-informed health care services overall.[43] Subsequently, in 2014, SAMHSA outlined a framework for TIC and advocated for the implementation of TIC into health care services and systems.[3]

TIC aims to understand, address, and alleviate the trauma burden faced by patients. A trauma-informed approach is based on a set of assumptions known as the four "R's": *realizing*

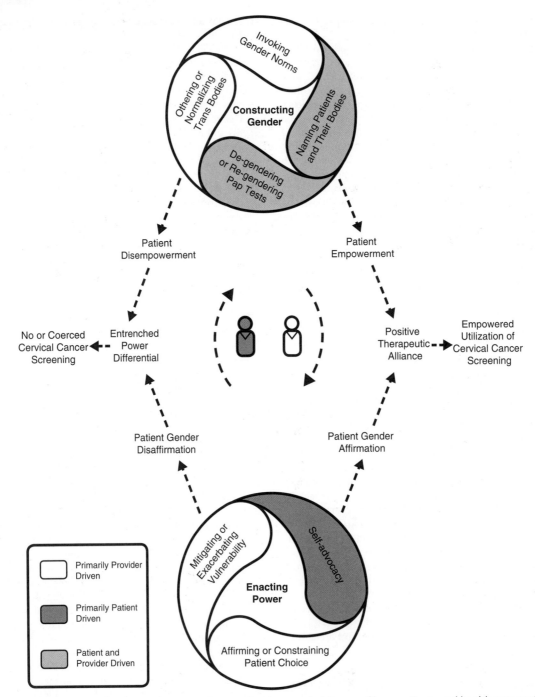

▲ **Figure 11-2.** Enacting power and constructing gender. A grounded theory of how patients and health care professionals interact in a cervical cancer screening encounter to produce patient (dis)empowerment and gender (dis)affirmation, and accordingly, a therapeutic alliance that does not support the patient decision to undergo cervical cancer screening. (Reproduced with permission from Peitzmeier SM, Bernstein IM, McDowell MJ, et al: Enacting power and constructing gender in cervical cancer screening encounters between transmasculine patients and health care providers. *Cult Health Sex* 2020;22(12):1315-1332.)

the impact of trauma; *recognizing* the signs and symptoms of trauma; *responding* through policies, procedures, and practices; and actively *resisting* retraumatization.[3] Essentially, clinicians and systems should consider that any patient's health may be impacted by trauma, their experience of health care may be affected by trauma, and that "difficult" behaviors might represent survival adaptations in the face of trauma. This requires a shift in focus for clinicians from thinking, "What is wrong with you?" to considering, "What has happened to you and how has that affected you?" when working with patients.

TIC should be adopted as a "universal precaution"—used for every person in every situation, whether or not there is a known trauma history. TIC can be distinguished from trauma-specific care, which focuses on clinical interventions for individuals with trauma histories. Trauma-informed approaches are guided by six principles outlined by SAMHSA that will be highlighted throughout this chapter:

1. Safety
2. Trustworthiness and Transparency
3. Peer Support
4. Collaboration and Mutuality
5. Empowerment, Voice, and Choice
6. Cultural, Historical, and Gender Issues

In addition to promoting sensitive and patient-centered practices, TIC also emphasizes self-care as an important tool for clinicians. Health care workers are commonly affected by vicarious or secondary traumatization, which occur when an individual is negatively affected by hearing about or being exposed to aversive details of a traumatic event (e.g., a social worker may experience secondary traumatization when hearing about a client's experience with child abuse).[44] **Vicarious traumatization** presents with changes in beliefs about the world that resemble those held by patients with trauma histories (e.g., "The world is not a safe place"). **Secondary traumatization** presents with PTSD-like signs and symptoms, including intrusive symptoms like nightmares and distressing thoughts, avoidance behaviors, changes to mood and cognition, and changes in arousal (e.g., a person may startle easily or have angry outbursts). Compassion fatigue and burnout may also occur when treating patients with histories of trauma. Clinician self-care has been shown to reduce levels of burnout and to increase compassion.[45]

Given the high prevalence of trauma in TGD patients and the history of health care discrimination, TIC is a vital approach for all clinicians working with TGD patients.[46,47] Throughout this chapter, TIC principles and approaches, particularly around communicating with patients, will be illustrated via case examples. For more detailed information about trauma-informed physical exam techniques for TGD patients, see Chapter 13, "Performing a Trauma-Informed Physical Examination."

UNIVERSAL APPLICATION OF TIC PRINCIPLES

Universal application of TIC principles is accomplished by applying SAMHSA's six principles of TIC to each and every interpersonal, institutional, and community/societal-level interaction a patient has across the health care and health care policy continuum (Table 11-1). While TIC principles apply to all patients, the table highlights areas where TGD-specific education and training of the workforce, intentional inclusion of TGD voices in systems redesign, and TGD-focused advocacy efforts are needed to transform the health care sector so that it can fully respond to the health care needs of TGD patients. Resources that may be helpful during systems transformation efforts include the National LGBTQIA+ Health Education Center[48] and the Health Equity Index Scoring Criteria.[49]

TIC principles can also be applied at numerous junctures within a clinician-patient encounter to optimize patient safety and well-being. The remainder of this chapter provides specific case-based examples.

▶ Avoiding Assumptions

Case (*Part 1*)

Excited to incorporate what you are learning into the care of your patients, you make a commitment to remember SAMHSA's four "R's" during everyday practice.[3] Back in clinic, as you look over the paperwork for your next patient, you see that they are 22-year-old, have a "male" insurance sex, and a nonbinary name. According to your medical assistant (MA)'s notation, the reason for the patient's visit is "difficulty sleeping" and "feels tired all the time." After knocking on the door and entering the room, you encounter an individual who does not make eye contact with you as you introduce yourself.

▶ Discussion Questions

1. What is the likelihood that this individual has experienced trauma or adversity at some point during their lifetime?
2. What is the likelihood that this individual has experienced trauma or adversity *within the health care system* in the past?

We cannot make assumptions about whether or not any patient has a history of trauma or adversity either within or outside the health care system; we know from population statistics, however, that the overall likelihood is high. Therefore, it makes sense to incorporate SAMHSA's six principles of TIC into every health care encounter as universal precautions. A basic first step is to *attend to gender dynamics* by avoiding assumptions about a patient's gender identity based on their insurance sex, name, gender presentation, or any other factors. In this case, you as the clinician do not yet have information about the

Table 11-1. Universal Application of TIC Principles across the Health Care Continuum to Optimize Care for TGD Patients

Trauma-Informed Care Principle	Level of Application		
	Interpersonal	Institutional	Community and Societal
SAFETY: Ensure physical and emotional safety.	Demonstrate respect and accord dignity (e.g., ask for and affirm gender identity by using the correct patient name, pronouns, and anatomical terms). Stay within the patient's line of vision and ask permission to touch the patient throughout the examination, i.e., when moving from one part of the body to the other. Maintain awareness of potential triggers and help patients de-escalate at the first sign of distress. Make sure patients have clear access to the door in exam rooms and can easily exit if desired. Tailor follow-up visit content and frequency to patient preference and tolerance.	Create an environment that allows TGD individuals to feel safe, secure, validated, and affirmed during every contact with the health care institution. Apply a trauma- and TGD-informed lens to all institutional policies and procedures. Explicitly describe TIC principles in the Patient Bill of Rights. Include gender identity in institutional diversity, inclusion, and equity statements. Adopt a zero-tolerance policy toward instances of identity-based stigma and discrimination. Create a physical environment that is safe, inclusive comfortable, and warm and that offers privacy for TGD individuals. Train the institution's entire workforce to deliver services that are effective, efficient, timely, respectful, and TGD-centered, taking into account that health care professionals also have histories of trauma.	Advocate for coverage of gender-affirming treatments and procedures. Provide education and training on trauma-informed practices to community organizations, insurance companies, and policymakers to enhance their ability to provide safe and effective services and protections for TGD people. Advocate for legal protections for TGD individuals people (e.g., to ban harmful practices such as conversion therapy efforts and enact nondiscrimination legislation in health care and other sectors).
TRUSTWORTHINESS AND TRANSPARENCY: Create clear and consistent expectations and boundaries.	Clarify patient and clinician roles and responsibilities. Establish and maintain consistent professional boundaries. Provide anticipatory guidance regarding sensitive questions, exams, tests, and procedures. Invite patients to bring a trusted companion to appointments. Explicitly discuss documentation and confidentiality concerns.	Continually seek feedback about patients' care experiences via TGD-inclusive patient satisfaction surveys. Address patients' concerns about their care experiences via TGD-inclusive patient relations processes.	
PEER SUPPORT: Provide ready access to peer support.	Refer TGD patients to TGD-sensitive trauma recovery services.	Embed TGD-sensitive trauma healing and recovery services (e.g., "safe bed," violence recovery, and prevention program) within the institution to ensure a "warm handoff." Offer meeting space for TGD-sensitive, peer-led recovery groups at the institution.	Partner with community organizations to ensure availability of TGD-sensitive trauma healing and recovery services in the greater TGD community.

(Continued)

Table 11-1. Universal Application of TIC Principles across the Health Care Continuum to Optimize Care for TGD Patients (*Continued*)

Trauma-Informed Care Principle	Level of Application		
	Interpersonal	Institutional	Community and Societal
COLLABORATION AND MUTUALITY: Maximize collaboration among patients, families, and health care staff in organizational and treatment planning.	Work with the patient to decide what is documented and what language is used in the documentation, with increased sensitivity to terms used for sexual and reproductive anatomy. Recognize that "challenging" symptoms and behaviors may be a person's way of coping with trauma (shift from blaming the patient ["What is wrong with you?"] to productively effectively engaging the patient ["How has what has happened affected you?"]. Participate in shared decision-making with TGD patients and their families regarding all aspects of their care.	Involve TGD recipients of services in numerous roles at the institution (e.g., as paid employees, volunteers, Patient Advisory Committee members, peer recovery specialists, etc.)	Engage in external community outreach and relationship-building to identify and address the health care needs of the greater TGD community.
EMPOWERMENT, VOICE, AND CHOICE: Inform patients of treatment options so they can choose the options they prefer. Attend to power dynamics to ensure that patients retain locus of control at all times.	Sit at eye level to avoid adopting a "power over" stance Ask permission before proceeding with sensitive questions, exams, tests, and procedures. When screening for trauma, always include an opt-out option. Offer choices in care and respect patients' preferences.	Incorporate feedback from TGD stakeholders into continuous quality improvement.	Support TGD stakeholders in advocating for their own needs with community organizations, insurance companies, and policymakers.
AWARENESS OF CULTURAL, HISTORICAL, AND GENDER ACKNOWLEDGEMENT: Recognize the impact that culture, history, and gender have on a patient's experiences. Explore one's biases to ensure that they do not interfere with a patient's care.	Acknowledge the harms caused by historically TGD-phobic health care practices. Recognize that patients carry intersectional identities that are also subject to bias and prejudice. Regularly reflect on one's implicit biases and work to mitigate them.	Provide institution-wide implicit bias training that includes gender identity bias. Provide institution-wide TIC training to enable staff to respond to patients' "challenging" behaviors in a trauma-informed manner. Provide institution-wide bystander training to enable staff members who observe coworkers making TGD-phobic microaggressions and/or non-trauma-informed missteps to respond in an effective productive manner. Ensure that trainings explicitly address the ways in which Black, Indigenous, and TGD patients of color have increased trauma histories due to both individual and societal/structural traumas, including experiences of racism; increase awareness about the ways these traumas overlap.	Disseminate best practices to other institutions and sectors.

patient's current gender identity or sex assigned at birth. *All* patients should be asked for their gender identity, sex assigned at birth, pronouns, and how they wish to be addressed at the outset of the health care encounter.[50] This information can be obtained verbally or on forms during the registration process, on intake/medical history forms at the office, or when a clinician greets the patient in person (see Chapter 4, "Harnessing Information Technology to Improve Clinical Care," for detailed information about how to collect and record gender identity information in health care practices). In the spirit of transparency and mutuality, it can be helpful for the clinician to greet the patient by sharing their full name, how they wish to be called, and what their pronouns are, before asking the patient to share these details. In addition to attending to gender dynamics, it is also crucial to *attend to power dynamics* throughout the encounter. A good way to start is to avoid "power-over" stances, by sitting at eye level whenever possible, facing the patient directly, making eye contact, and using open body gestures that communicate a welcoming attitude (i.e., relaxed body posture rather than arms crossed over chest).

▶ Obtaining a Relevant History

Case (*Part 2*)

Proceeding further with the interview, you ask for the patient's sex assigned at birth (assigned female at birth; AFAB), gender identity (genderqueer), and pronouns (they/them/theirs). Now that you know their gender identity, you find yourself wondering if they are using any gender-affirming hormones or have had any gender-affirming surgeries.

▶ Discussion Questions

1. Is it relevant to ask TGD patients about hormones and surgeries?
2. If so, how and when would you obtain this information?

   It is important to refrain from asking TGD patients about gender affirmation practices unless it is clinically relevant, to avoid being perceived as intrusive or voyeuristic. In this case example, it *is* relevant to obtain information about gender affirmation, because one of the patient's symptoms ("tired all the time") could be related to diagnoses (e.g., excess menstrual blood loss, pregnancy) that require knowledge of the patient's sexual and reproductive anatomy, sexual practices, and medications (including hormones). When it is relevant to ask about sexual and reproductive issues, a TGD-sensitive organ inventory can be obtained via medical history forms or asking questions during the encounter. Following TIC principles, it is helpful to start with a ubiquity statement ("I'd like to take an organ inventory to know what body parts we need to consider when evaluating your current symptoms. I ask all of my patients for this information"), and obtain permission

("Is that OK with you?"), before proceeding to ask specific questions (e.g., "Please take a look at this list and check off the body parts you have present"). To demonstrate respect for the patient's gender and to accord their body dignity, it is also important to ask what terms they use to refer to their sexual and reproductive anatomy ("What words do you use to refer to these body parts?") and to remember to use these terms throughout the encounter and in your medical documentation. Please refer to Chapter 12, "Obtaining a Gender-Affirming Sexual History," and Chapter 5, "Gender Identity Emergence and Affirmation in Adults," for additional helpful details on taking a TGD-sensitive sexual history and instituting electronic health record fields for documentation of sex assigned at birth, pronouns, and organ inventory.

▶ Using Trauma-Informed Principles to Repair Gender and Power Missteps

Case (*Part 3*)

The patient volunteers that they started taking testosterone a year ago and stopped bleeding shortly thereafter. They haven't had any gender-affirming surgeries yet but hope to do so in the future. They use the nongendered anatomical terms "chest" rather than "breasts" and "front hole" rather than "vagina." As you begin to explore the patient's presenting symptoms in more depth, one of the medical assistants knocks on the door and brings the patient a jacket they left in the waiting room. In thanking the medical assistant, you use the wrong pronouns by mistake ("Thanks so much for noticing that she left her jacket out there").

▶ Discussion Questions

1. How would you feel after misgendering the patient?
2. How might you utilize TIC principles to handle this situation?
3. If it had instead been the medical assistant who misgendered the patient, how could you have used TIC principles to supportively educate the medical assistant and the rest of the office staff?

   After misgendering a patient, many clinicians may feel embarrassed, possibly even humiliated or ashamed. In addressing this issue, it is important to remember that a trauma-informed environment supports the learning needs of both patients and staff. It is normal to be confused at first. It may actually be helpful to use a mistake like this to level power dynamics between clinician and patient ("I'm sorry I made that mistake. I will be [conscious][diligent] going forward to be correct in my use of your pronouns. I am open to talking about how that felt to you just now, if you would like."). Similarly, TIC principles can be used in all interactions to respectfully educate other members of the care team without causing shame, by using a warm and nonjudgmental tone, and making clarifications ("I noticed you said 'she' to that patient. I wanted to let you know that their pronouns are 'they/them/theirs'. I am happy to discuss pronouns further with you anytime if you have questions"). The National LGBTQIA+ Health Education Center provides resources to support staff education and training.[48]

▶ Recognizing and Responding Effectively When a Patient Becomes Distressed

Case (*Part 4*)

After you offer a straightforward apology, the patient responds by saying "I'm used to it," continues to avoid making eye contact, and slumps back into their chair.

▶ Discussion Questions

1. How do you interpret the patient's reactions?

2. How might you respond?

TGD patients who have experienced repeated exposure to discriminatory experiences are at increased risk for developing PTSD compared to the general population.[36] PTSD is characterized by intrusive memories that lead to re-experiencing the trauma, avoidance of potential triggers, changes in thoughts and feelings, and alterations in arousal and reactivity (Box 11-1).[10]

Hypervigilance leads trauma survivors to make ongoing assessments of their safety level in every new environment, and they are more likely than people without a trauma history to perceive the presence of danger. Once threat is perceived, a person's body may respond automatically. The resulting physical responses can be grouped into three different categories according to underlying physiological mechanism and behavioral manifestations.

Fight or flight reactions result from sympathetic nervous system activity (hyperarousal, "stuck on high"), while freeze reactions result from parasympathetic nervous system activity (hypoarousal, "stuck on low"). All three of these responses are "normal reactions to the abnormal circumstances of trauma"—coping behaviors that may once, quite literally, have enabled the individual to survive.[9] Under other circumstances, however, these reactions may no longer be adaptive and are often referred to as "dysregulated." Because these reactions can be unexpected or extreme, clinicians sometimes interpret them in judgmental and unhelpful ways. Ineffective clinician responses can be averted by remembering that a patient's fight, flight, or freeze reaction is occurring because they do not feel safe; their reactions were adaptive and necessary in the past; and their behavior represents an unconscious, physiologic reaction to current perceived threat (Table 11-2). For the patient in this case example, the avoidance of eye contact and the shutdown behavior could be viewed as a freeze

| BOX 11-1 | Characteristics of Posttraumatic Stress Disorder |

Intrusion (Re-experiencing the Trauma)
Involuntary memories
Traumatic nightmares
Flashbacks
Intense or prolonged distress after exposure to reminders (triggers)

Avoidance of Potential Triggers
Avoiding trauma-related:
- Thoughts and feelings
- Conversations and activities
- People and places

Changes in Thoughts and Feelings
Inability to remember key features of events
Distorted beliefs about self or others ("I am bad," "No-one can be trusted")
Ongoing fear, horror, anger, guilt, or shame
Lack of interest in activities previously enjoyed
Sense of alienation and detachment from others

Arousal and Reactivity Changes
Irritable behavior and angry outbursts
Reckless or self-destructive behavior
Hyperarousal and hypervigilance
Exaggerated startle response
Sleep and concentration problems

reaction, occurring as a consequence of being reminded of previous trauma during the health care encounter.

When a patient starts to become dysregulated, there are a number of simple statements and behavioral interventions the clinician can utilize to help the patient reestablish a sense of power and control, with improvement in acute distress (see Figure 11-2).

When a patient manifests a fight response, first offer them understanding and validation. Next, facilitate their empowerment and control to support them in a trauma-informed manner as they move back into their "window of tolerance" where it is easier to engage with other people effectively. **Window of tolerance** is a term coined by Daniel Siegel to describe the zone of arousal in which an individual is able to effectively manage the range of emotion without becoming either physiologically hyperaroused (e.g., high energy, anxious, angry, overwhelmed, hypervigilant, or in fight-or-flight mode) or hypoaroused (e.g., shut down, numb, depressed, passive, withdrawn, ashamed, or in freeze mode).[51]

Sample statements to demonstrate understanding and validation:

Table 11-2. Trauma-Informed Interpretation of Fight, Flight, and Freeze Reactions

Reaction	Behavioral Manifestations	Unhelpful Clinician Interpretations	Trauma-Informed Interpretations
Fight	Animated Impatient Irritable, angry Loud voice	"Aggressive" "Combative" "Resistant" "Provocative" "Sullen"	Hyperaroused "Stuck on high" Attempting to regain or hold on to personal power
Flight	Anxious Confused Forgetful Restless Fidgeting Easily startled Eyes darting	"Nonadherent" "Noncompliant"	Hyperaroused "Stuck on high" Attempting to avoid or escape from those in power
Freeze	Acquiescent Withdrawn Distracted, not paying attention Distant look to eyes Quiet/faint voice	"Passive" "Disengaged"	Hypoaroused "Stuck on low" Shutting down in response to power

– "You have every right to feel upset. I would like to understand what you need."

Sample statement to demonstrate that the patient maintains power and control:

– "You can decide if you want to proceed with me or not, it is OK either way."

When a patient has escalated, and you are not sure if it is safe for you or the patient to remain engaged, you can say:

– "I think we should stop for today."

When a patient manifests a flight response, offer reassurance, followed by empowerment and control to help them decrease their acute distress.

Sample statement to demonstrate reassurance:

– "I appreciate how difficult coming to this appointment may have been, and how being here now may still be difficult. Would you like to take a pause?"

Sample statement to demonstrate that the patient maintains power and control:

– "You do not have to stay if you do not want to, it is OK for us to end whenever you want."

When a patient manifests a freeze response, offer guidance, followed by empowerment and control to help the patient recenter in the present.

Sample statements to demonstrate guidance through grounding skills include the following:

– "Could you remind me of your address, birthdate, and phone number?"

– "Can you tell me the day, month, year, and time it is right now?"

– "Could you describe the poster on my wall?"

Next, once the patient has engaged verbally and responded in an accurate manner, you can continue, using empowerment and control to help the patient return to their "window of tolerance":

– "Let's take a break and check in. Is there anything you would like me to adjust right now?"

▶ Recognizing Symptoms and Exam Findings that Suggest a History of Trauma

Case (Part 5)

In recognition of the patient's strength in coming to the appointment and to restore their sense of power and control in the moment, you say, " I appreciate how difficult coming to this appointment may have been, and how being here now may still be difficult." "Let's take a break and check in. Is there anything you would like me to adjust right now?" Your question seems to ease the uncomfortable feeling in the room, and the patient agrees to tell you more about their presenting complaints. You learn that they have fatigue, periods of forgetfulness, chronic undiagnosed stomach pain, and difficulty sleeping.

▶ Discussion Questions

1. Describe common presenting symptoms that may suggest a history of trauma among TGD patients.

2. Describe physical exam findings that may suggest a history of trauma among TGD patients.

3. Describe how a clinician can utilize TIC principles to avoid responding reactively when a patient presents with multiple somatic complaints or describes dissatisfaction with their previous health care professionals.

In addition to mental health complaints, such as anxiety, depression, and manifestations of PTSD, common physical symptoms that may suggest a history of trauma in any patient include fatigue, headaches, jaw pain related to teeth grinding, palpitations, gastrointestinal symptoms, pelvic floor dysfunction, sleep disturbance, and chronic pain. Few studies have examined PTSD-related symptoms among TGD people specifically; gender minority stress, however, has been linked to sleep disturbance among TGD people.[52] Some of these complaints (e.g., pelvic floor symptoms and sexual dysfunction) may be linked to physical injuries that occurred during a traumatic event (e.g., sexual assault), whereas others are related mechanistically to activation of more distal (e.g., neurological, endocrine, immune) trauma pathways. Many patients have undergone extensive previous medical work-ups for their symptoms and have been told that "nothing is wrong" or "it's all in your head." Lack of diagnosis can lead patients to feel deeply disillusioned and dissatisfied with health care; a clinician's compassion and belief that an underlying explanation (i.e., exposure to trauma) can be identified and addressed can go a long way toward establishing a therapeutic connection.

A number of physical exam findings may also suggest a history of acute or chronic trauma. For example, among cisgender women, head, neck, and facial injuries are suggestive of intimate partner violence,[53] and the abdomen is often targeted during pregnancy. Few published data exist describing interpersonal injuries experienced specifically by TGD people; anecdotal reports, however, suggest that the face is a commonly targeted site of injury for transgender women, while the chest and genitalia are commonly targeted among transgender men. Non-suicidal self-injury (NSSI), such as cutting or burning, is more common among TGD people than cisgender people[54-56] and has been linked to a history of both perceived and enacted stigma and discrimination[57]; the chest and genitals are also commonly targeted sites. It has been suggested that NSSI plays a functional role in coping with trauma symptoms by diverting one's attention from intrusive thoughts and aversive emotional states, and reducing dissociation and numbness by generating feelings.[58] Among TGD people,

NSSI may also be a manifestation of gender dysphoria. Thus, when working with a TGD patient who engages in NSSI, it is important to gain an appreciation of the underlying psychological function of the behavior.

For TGD patients who discuss suicidal ideation, plans, and intent, it is important to use TIC tenets to help them access higher levels of care (e.g., emergency department [ED] for further evaluation). Clinicians should be as transparent and collaborative as possible, as there are times the patient may be unwilling to go to the ED, yet due to safety reasons the clinician makes a decision to involuntarily evaluate or hospitalize the patient. Sample statements during this time include, "Based on what you are saying I am going to need to call the ambulance to bring you to the ED. Do you have any questions about the process? Normally… [then describe each step that you reasonably think the patient can expect to experience]. Would you like to take a moment to call anyone to meet you at the hospital/alert them that you are going? I will call ahead to the clinicians at the ED and explain to them why I sent you. Is there anything else you would like me to tell them?"

When a patient presents with longstanding symptoms that have gone undiagnosed or describes prior experiences of feeling misunderstood or misdiagnosed by health care professionals, it can be daunting, and at times frustrating. The following trauma-informed reflections and techniques can be used to illuminate potential paths forward:

- **Safety**: In what ways have this patient's life experiences contributed to their current symptoms/behaviors?

- **Trustworthiness and transparency**: How can I build trust with this patient so that they feel comfortable disclosing their experiences to me?

- **Peer support**: Who in the patient's life might be able to [provide support to the patient during their evaluation][provide additional information to help me understand their presentation]?

- **Collaboration and mutuality**: How can I work with the patient to find the source of their symptoms, instead of leaning toward an "expert" or "top-down" model of care?

- **Empowerment, voice, and choice**: State to the patient: "You are the expert of your body's sensations and signs—what would you like me to know?"

- **Cultural, historic, and gender acknowledgment**: How do my patient's identities (e.g., race, ethnicity, ability status, class, gender identity, and sexual orientation identity) impact their experiences? What assumptions am I making about the patient based on their identities? What are my biases based on these assumptions? What can I do to make sure my biases do not interfere with their care?

Obtaining a Trauma History in a Trauma-Informed Manner

Case (*Part 6*)

Based on the symptoms the patient is reporting, you begin to suspect a trauma history. You believe that it is important to obtain a more thorough, trauma-oriented history, but you are unsure how or if you should proceed.

Discussion Questions

1. What are the potential benefits of trauma inquiry in this situation? What are the potential complexities?

2. If you decided to obtain a trauma history, how would you proceed?

3. How would you respond to positive disclosure?

4. How would you respond if the patient became acutely distressed?

5. What is the evidence to support routine screening for trauma (in any patient)?

Potential benefits of obtaining a trauma history include identification of the events that set the patient's trauma cascade in motion, and the opportunity to normalize trauma responses, describe pathways to healing and recovery, and offer linkage to trauma recovery services.[59,60] Trauma inquiry, however, can be complicated. It is important to address clinician barriers (fear that disclosure might harm the patient, that the patient might become distressed during the interaction, that there will not be enough time to respond to trauma disclosure, and that lack of knowledge, skill, and resources will hamper the clinician's ability to provide appropriate assistance) before proceeding.[61] It is also important to provide appropriate framing before asking questions about trauma exposure, as the patient may not otherwise understand why their past experiences are relevant to their current symptoms. In addition, many patients with trauma histories have blamed themselves, been pathologized, or received inadequate attention for their trauma-based symptoms.[61] It is therefore crucial to apply trauma-informed principles when offering responses (e.g., "It makes sense that your body is reacting this way," "It's not your fault," "You can get better") throughout the process of trauma inquiry.

One of the most important things to consider when deciding whether or not to pursue a trauma history is the patient's current state: if they are exhibiting signs of distress, or beginning to show these signs, it is important to slow down, check in, or stop the history-taking. If the patient is already distressed, as in the case of the misgendering episode discussed above, it is highly likely that trauma inquiry will move their physiologic response into a fight, flight, or freeze reaction. In order to avoid this, the clinician should follow TIC principles to learn if the patient is willing and physiologically able to tolerate questions about prior trauma.

There are several ways to pursue trauma inquiry. One way is to ask open-ended questions so that the patient can lead the discussion at the pace and to the level that they feel comfortable.[59,60,62] The inquiry should be based on trauma symptoms as they relate to the patient's health, rather than focusing on a chronological recounting of traumatic events ("I would like to learn more about when these symptoms started. Is there any context to what was going on in your life then that relates to what you are feeling now?"). The patient's strengths and resilience should be emphasized by validating their skills in navigating their trauma history (e.g., "Just coming to an appointment is often an act of courage. I want to acknowledge the effort you took in coming here. To me, this marks your commitment to yourself and your health." Or, if a trauma history is disclosed, "I want to acknowledge all that you have been through, and your dedication to your own healing, as evidenced by your coming in today"). The patient's choice to come for the current appointment can also be highlighted as an inherent strength. During the process of inquiry, the patient can be educated about different types of trauma and their effects, and interventions can be offered as needed, with the patient guiding the selection of specific services.[59,60,62] The following trauma-informed questions and responses to disclosure may be useful in guiding such discussions:

- **Safety**: If during our talk today you feel uncomfortable at any time, please say "pause" and we will take a break. You get to lead this discussion.

- **Trustworthiness and transparency**: I would like to find out more about what has happened to you so I can more fully understand your symptoms; I will ask you some questions and you can answer in the ways that feel most comfortable for you. If you feel overwhelmed or I notice you are overwhelmed, I may suggest we take a break.

- **Peer support**: Would you like anyone with you while we talk about your history? If I ask anything that you would rather not answer, please feel free to say "pass."

- **Collaboration and mutuality**: We can work together today to find a pace that works for you in telling me about your past as it relates to your current symptoms. You decide what is important for me to know.

- **Empowerment, voice, and choice**: You get to decide what you share, even if I ask something directly. [After disclosures]: I am so glad you had the courage to share ___ with me, thank you.

- **Cultural, historic, and gender acknowledgment**: All of your identities are important to me. Please feel free to share with me any identities that you would like, such as your race, ethnicity, gender identity, and sexual orientation, as well as any other identities that you think I should know. [After disclosures]: The traumas you've experienced are part of a larger system of issues in society, often called structural violence. The traumas you've experienced are not your fault.

Another way to approach trauma inquiry is to use a validated screening tool. A potential advantage of this practice is that screening can be performed electronically (i.e., via iPad or computer interface), which allows clinicians to pursue more in-depth discussions with those patients who screen positive. When conducting screening in this manner, it is crucial to attend to the patient's safety (i.e., explain the purpose of the screening, what will be done with the information, provide an opt-out option, and conduct the screening when the patient is alone, as a companion could be an abuser of the patient). Similarly, it is important to provide prompt in-person follow-up with a clinician so that additional information can be obtained and trauma-informed education and resources can be provided. It is crucial when screening TGD adults to make sure that the screening tool used is culturally relevant. Screening tools that have been validated in clinical TGD populations include the IPV-4, a four-question, gender-inclusive screener for intimate partner violence that has been validated among mixed-gender people living with HIV,[63] and the PC-PTSD-5, a five-item screener for PTSD which has been validated among veterans [64] and used with transgender adults in the primary care setting.[36] Some clinicians are beginning to screen adults for ACEs using the original ACE questionnaire[7]; there are, however, no data yet to validate the use of the ACE questionnaire as a screening tool among TGD adults in a clinical setting.

Issues related to legally mandated reporting requirements can arise during disclosure (e.g., abuse or neglect of children, elders, or persons with intellectual disabilities; interpersonal violence when children are present; expression of suicidal or homicidal intent) and should always be addressed appropriately. To maintain transparency, it is imperative for clinicians to discuss documentation of sensitive information with patients and the possibility of mandatory reporting when abuse or neglect is disclosed or suspected. In addition, it is important for clinicians to have a list of TGD-affirming trauma recovery services available so that patients can be seamlessly referred to appropriate services.

No matter which screening method is selected, for some patients, being asked about traumatic exposure can be a relief, and they may begin to share detailed histories in response. It can be important to gently help patients establish boundaries around the nature and extent of the information they reveal, to prevent inadvertent triggering of a fight, flight, or freeze reaction, and to remain cognizant of clinical time constraints. Sample statements to help patients contain information include:

- "This information is really important and I wonder if telling it right now might be overwhelming to you or your body? Let's take a moment to breathe and then tell me what you think. Does it feel right to keep talking about this now, or would you like to address this at another appointment?"

- "This is/was a really important event in your life; right now I unfortunately cannot give it the attention it deserves due to (be transparent). In order to best respect your history, can we both make a commitment to return to this on (date you can)?"

- "I am really glad you are able to share this important information with me. I wonder if you might also want to talk to a social worker I know, one who has specialized training that I do not have in addressing histories like the one you are sharing with me. Would you like me to help you connect with this person?"

If a patient manifests acute distress during the process of trauma inquiry, one can use simple grounding exercises to reestablish equilibrium. Examples include helping the patient to focus on their breathing ("Take 3 mindful breaths [4 in, hold 3, 5 out]"), or asking the patient to take an inventory of their immediate environment to connect back to the present ("List 5 things you see, 4 things you hear, 3 things you can touch, 2 things you can smell, 1 thing you can taste"). Alternatively, one can ask the patient to describe one object in great detail, as if you can't see it or have never encountered it before.

It is important to help patients who have disclosed trauma or have exhibited signs of being outside their window of tolerance during the medical encounter to create a self-care plan for after the encounter. Useful strategies include: validating that the encounter might have been difficult for the patient, encouraging the patient to take time after their appointment to take a slow walk, talk to a friend, eat or drink something soothing, and take a moment to themselves before moving on to the regular activities of their day. This is especially important if the patient seems disoriented, slowed, or activated.

▶ Facilitating Connection to Trauma-Informed Support Services

Case (*Part 7*)

After you ask an open-ended question, the patient discloses a history of penile-frontal sexual assault 6 months prior. Luckily, a friend took them to the emergency room immediately afterward, where they received appropriate care, including medications, to prevent sexually transmitted infections and pregnancy. The walk-in clinic also gave the patient a list of recovery programs, but they did not follow up, stating that: "None of the programs out there are going to want to see a person like me."

Discussion Questions

1. What barriers might a TGD patient encounter when trying to access trauma recovery services?

2. How would you locate TGD-affirming trauma recovery services?

3. What could you do to facilitate your patient's connection to care?

TGD people face substantial barriers when trying to access support after experiencing violence. Stigma and discrimination in the criminal justice system and criminalization of sex work impede assistance when TGD people are victims of a crime. TGD people may also have difficulty accessing intimate partner violence services, since women's shelters often deny entry to anyone who is not a cisgender woman. Fortunately, organizations such as FORGE[65] and The Network/La Red[66] provide violence prevention and recovery services that are tailored to the needs of TGD people; their websites are a good place to begin when making a referral. In cases in which a patient has experienced discrimination in accessing needed care, consultation to an organization that provides legal assistance to TGD people, such as the National Center for Transgender Equality[67] and Transcend Legal,[68] may be helpful.

When seeking to make a referral to trauma recovery services, be sure to use trauma-informed principles. Use transparency to state, "I was thinking that a next step that might be useful is to give you some referral options to individual experts/agencies that specialize in trauma recovery for [issue the patient presented with]." Follow this up with collaboration: "Do you feel this would be helpful to you right now?" Then end with empowerment: "Are there resources you know of that you would like my help in accessing? The next steps in referral are entirely up to you."

Incorporating Trauma-Informed Principles into the Physical Exam

Case (Part 8)

After responding appropriately to the patient's disclosure and offering a referral, they thank you for the suggestion but say they want to think about it more before taking action. The patient then reiterates their presenting concerns: "First, I want to make sure we do something about what I came in here for today."

Discussion Question

1. How would you approach the performance of a physical exam to evaluate the patient's symptoms?

A trauma-informed approach to the physical exam includes: providing anticipatory guidance (reasons for performing the exam, what the exam will entail); reviewing options to optimize patient comfort during the exam, including the presence of a trusted companion if the patient so desires; obtaining permission before proceeding; according respect to the patient's body by using their self-designated anatomical terms; maintaining safety during the exam by avoiding potentially triggering language (e.g., words with sexual or violent connotations), staying within the patient's line of sight at all times, and maintaining an appropriate physical distance; checking in periodically to ask how the patient is doing; and stopping immediately if the patient requests it or manifests distress (refer to Chapter 13, "Performing a Trauma-Informed Physical Examination," for additional details). Similar techniques can be applied when performing diagnostic tests and procedures.

Trauma-Informed Evaluation and Treatment Planning

Case (Part 9)

The patient agrees to a physical exam, except for examination of their chest and genitalia, which you agree are not relevant to perform at this visit. Examination of their head, neck, lymph nodes, lungs, heart, abdomen, extremities, skin, and neurological system is normal. Following completion of the exam, you leave the room so the patient can dress: "I'll return in a few minutes so we can talk about next steps." After waiting a suitable period, you knock on the door to see if the patient is ready, and they give you permission to enter.

Discussion Questions

1. How would you incorporate TIC principles into the discussion of possible explanations for the patient's presenting symptoms and decision-making regarding the next steps in their evaluation/treatment?

2. What follow-up plans would you make?

Decision-making regarding next steps in the patient's evaluation and care should always be a collaborative process in which potential diagnostic considerations and evaluation options are carefully discussed and the patient chooses the path that makes sense to them (empowerment, voice, and choice). In this case, it is appropriate to discuss the differential diagnosis of the patient's presenting symptoms (fatigue, periods of forgetfulness, chronic undiagnosed stomach pain, and difficulty sleeping) and to offer testing for common causes of these symptoms (e.g., anemia, thyroid illness). In addition, it may be reasonable to talk about evidence-based interventions (e.g., cognitive behavioral strategies to enhance sleep), if the patient is interested in learning about and trying these modalities.

When patients present with symptoms that could be based on somatic reactions to trauma/chronic stress (otherwise known as "normal reactions to abnormal situations"), it is always important to explain this possibility alongside other diagnostic considerations. This provides an opportunity to educate the patient about the impact of trauma on health and explain the emergence of symptoms as manifestations of chronic stress, including explaining the adverse health effects of chronic stress and chronic PTSD-type symptoms). When concluding the encounter, it is crucial to develop a longitudinal follow-up plan that will enable mutual respect, safety, and ongoing engagement. Examples of trauma-informed language to use when discussing diagnostic, evaluation, and treatment possibilities, and next steps in follow-up are listed below:

- **Safety**: May I share some information with you about how experiences from the past might be manifesting as symptoms in your body today?

- **Trustworthiness and transparency**: May I share information now about how past experiences, especially difficult or traumatic ones, impact physical health, and may be contributing to your symptoms today? Please let me know if at any point you have questions, disagree, want me to slow down, or repeat or change the subject.

- **Peer support**: Is there anyone you would like here with you while we discuss your symptoms and next steps to take? Or anyone you would like me to contact after our visit today?

- **Collaboration and mutuality**: I consider everything we decide to do to address your current symptoms to be a plan we create together. I may make suggestions, including lab work or specialists to visit, and I understand you may disagree with these suggestions—please let me know if you do. I am completely open to this.

- **Empowerment, voice, and choice**: I consider you to be in the "driver's seat" of your care. I want to hear your ideas about how to approach your current symptoms so that I can figure out how to best support you.

- **Cultural, historic, and gender acknowledgment**: The symptoms you are having now may stem from prior experiences, but they are not your fault. They reflect a society that permits discrimination, oppression, and

targeting of people on the basis of their identities and social circumstances to happen.

Case (*Part 10*)

Following discussion, the patient chooses to have a panel of lab tests checked (all of which return normal) and to try cognitive behavioral techniques to improve their sleep (with subsequent improved quality of sleep). They decide to return for monthly follow-up visits, during which they continue taking testosterone, gradually accomplish all of their recommended health screenings, begin seeing an individual therapist for cognitive processing therapy, and join a recovery group at a local TGD-affirming violence recovery program. Six months later, they are feeling much better and making plans for top surgery.

▶ Discussion Question

1. What else might you do to support the patient's ongoing recovery and resilience?

   It is important to support the patient's ongoing engagement in health care and self-care between in-person encounters. The clinician can inquire if the patient would like to check in by phone or secure email between visits and codevelop a safety plan to help them cope with distress when they become triggered. Clinicians should explain and normalize the fact that trauma-related symptoms are likely to wax and wane over time so that the patient does not retreat from care out of shame and understands that recovery will be a lifelong process. In addition, clinicians can emphasize that resilience is related to community, social, environmental, and political factors, and that not all elements of health and well-being are tied to the individual's coping skills or efforts at recovery. For example, if new government policies arise that negatively impact the human rights of TGD communities, it is common for TGD patients to experience increased distress, worsening anxiety and depression, or other adverse health consequences. It is important to check in with TGD patients at such times, both to encourage an office visit and promote connection to TGD community and activist groups.

   Overall, a strength- and empowerment-based approach that incorporates understanding of the nonlinear aspects of healing and recovery will help foster a trauma-informed, collaborative approach to the patient's health and healing. Clinicians should educate the patient on resilience factors, name and celebrate aspects of resilience they observe in the patient, and help the patient build on their strengths by engaging in positive coping skills of the patient's choice (e.g., connecting with peers, building community, and engaging in activities that promote health and bring pleasure and joy).

Incorporating Trauma-Informed Principles Into Self-Care

Case (*Part 11*)

Because of the work you have been doing to enhance care for TGD patients with trauma histories, you find that you are receiving progressively more and more referrals of patients with trauma-related experiences and symptoms to your practice. Over time, you notice that you are starting to dread your long clinic days.

Discussion Questions

1. What are the signs and symptoms of vicarious and secondary traumatization?
2. How can you utilize TIC principles to optimize your own health and well-being?

Trauma and its health effects are not experiences limited to the patients we see. Raja et al specifically highlight the need for all clinicians to examine and understand their own trauma histories, so that discomfort with taking a trauma history in patients and fear of self-triggering is reduced.[69] Mindfulness of our own trauma histories permits us to attend to our own healing and recovery and take precautions so that we do not suffer from vicarious or secondary traumatization associated with repeated exposure to patients' trauma histories. While research has not yet examined this question, it is possible that TGD clinicians may be at increased risk of experiencing distress when witnessing the trauma narratives of their TGD patients; thus, attention to self-care may be especially important for this group. There are a number of ways in which clinicians can utilize TIC principles to prevent vicarious and secondary traumatization and to optimize their own health and well-being:

- **Safety**: Find a calm area to self-regulate and rest between interactions with patients. Allow yourself time to re-regulate when you move out of your window of tolerance.
- **Trustworthiness and transparency**: Acknowledge when you are experiencing symptoms of vicarious trauma.
- **Peer support**: Find like-minded and empathetic professional peers with whom you can talk candidly about your feelings and experiences working with patients who report trauma. Access reflective supervision, mentoring, or coaching relationships that emphasize TIC principles.
- **Collaboration and mutuality**: Find ways to connect with peers who are doing similar work, as validation and normalization of your reactions to the traumatic narratives you are encountering are crucial.

- **Empowerment, voice, and choice**: If you are feeling overwhelmed, know that you can ask for support and help as needed. You do not have to experience distress alone.
- **Cultural, historic, and gender acknowledgment**: Understand that your intersectional identities affect how you could be triggered by the traumatic narratives you are witnessing with your patients.

Through attention and self-awareness, clinicians can develop emotional regulation skills and other self-care techniques. Most importantly, clinicians need to be aware of their own stress levels and limits when feeling overwhelmed. While training and medical environments may create a culture or norm of pushing past one's own limits, downplaying emotional reactions or emotional toll, or showing emotion or reactivity to clinical work, these responses are not trauma-informed. TIC asks that we as clinicians acknowledge our typical reactions to stressful circumstances (i.e., fight/fight/freeze) and allow ourselves time to re-regulate as needed. Recognizing and allowing for reaction allows balance and fosters the ability to stay within one's window of tolerance so that therapeutic connections with patients and our own self-care remain healthy, vital, and healing.

Both patients and clinicians can grow and find meaning in their traumatic experiences. For patients, this can be measured by the Posttraumatic Growth Inventory,[70] which seeks to itemize for patients the ways their traumatic experiences have helped them change and grow in ways that they could not have experienced before their traumatic experiences. Hernandez et al[71] describe a related concept among clinicians called vicarious resilience, which describes the positive impact of exposure to patient resilience. This effect can be measured by the Vicarious Resilience Scale.[72]

At the same time, it is important to acknowledge that existing health professional training programs and health care practice settings often focus solely on care of the patient and forget to attend to the needs of the health care workforce. We are all affected by the same systemic stressors, and while we are often trained to ignore our own emotions and even physical needs in order to serve our patients, we are subject to the same responses to difficult clinical procedures, unjust policies, unhealthy hierarchies, and difficult work dynamics as our patients.

Incorporating Trauma-Informed Principles into Advocacy and Systemic Change

Case (*Part 12*)

Your institution asks you to serve on a task force that will apply a trauma-informed lens (i.e., SAMHSA's six principles) to recommend systems changes to support the safety, security, validation, and affirmation of TGD people during every contact they have with your institution. In preparation for the first meeting, each task force member has been asked to perform a homework assignment.

▶ Discussion Question

1. Trace the journey of a hypothetical TGD patient through your [institution][practice]. What aspects of the care environment may not be trauma-informed? What improvements can you suggest? Table 4-1 can be used as a guide.

When addressing systemic issues that impact TGD people, it is important to factor in historical trauma and structural violence.[73] Understanding the impact of systematic oppression and violence as part of the context in which TGD patients' trauma has occurred is crucial and also helps to begin to undo the shaming and blaming of victims that often creeps into conversations about trauma.

SUMMARY

- Trauma exposure is highly prevalent in transgender and gender diverse (TGD) communities.
- TGD patients with identities subject to additional oppressions (race, class, immigration status, etc.) are at increased risk for trauma exposure.
- Exposure to trauma and gender minority stress may be associated with both adverse health effects and development of resilience.
- Trauma-informed care (TIC) provides a model for responding to trauma appropriately, reducing retraumatization and setting the stage for healing and recovery.
- TIC is guided by six principles: safety; trustworthiness and transparency; peer support; collaboration and mutuality; empowerment, voice, and choice; and cultural, historical, and gender issues.
- Universal application of TIC principles is essential when caring for TGD patients and includes:
  - Affirming the patient's gender identity throughout the encounter
  - Attending to power dynamics throughout the encounter
  - Obtaining the history in a patient-led manner
  - Asking about trauma in a manner that resists retraumatization
  - Responding appropriately to trauma disclosure
  - Performing the physical examination in a collaborative manner that resists retraumatization
  - Recognizing symptoms and exam findings that may suggest a history of trauma
  - Recognizing and responding effectively when the patient becomes distressed

- Codeveloping care plans that are patient empowering and enable mutual respect, safety, and ongoing engagement
- Facilitating connection to TGD-affirming trauma recovery services
- Recognizing, celebrating, and building on the patient's strengths over time
- Continuously attending to the self-care of the clinician

- TIC principles apply to both TGD patients' clinical encounters and institutional, community, and societal responses to TGD populations.
- Clinicians can play a key role in advocating for TIC at the systems level, to ensure that the health care sector is fully responsive to the needs of TGD patients.

REFERENCES

1. Mock J. *Redefining Realness: My Path to Womanhood, Identity, Love & So Much More.* Simon & Schuster, Inc.; 2014.
2. Herman J. *Trauma and Recovery.* Basic Books; 1992.
3. *SAMHSA's Concept of Trauma and Guidance for a Trauma-Informed Approach.* Published online 2014.
4. DiPlacido J. Minority stress among lesbians, gay men, and bisexuals: a consequence of heterosexism, homophobia, and stigmatization. In: *Stigma and Sexual Orientation: Understanding Prejudice against Lesbians, Gay Men, and Bisexuals.* Sage Publications, Inc.; 1998:138-159. *Psychological Perspectives on Lesbian and Gay Issues*; Vol. 4.
5. Kilpatrick DG, Resnick HS, Milanak ME, Miller MW, Keyes KM, Friedman MJ. National estimates of exposure to traumatic events and PTSD prevalence using DSM-IV and DSM-5 criteria. *J Trauma Stress.* 2013;26(5):537-547.
6. Dube SR, Felitti VJ, Dong M, Chapman DP, Giles WH, Anda RF. Childhood abuse, neglect, and household dysfunction and the risk of illicit drug use: the adverse childhood experiences study. *Pediatrics.* 2003;111(3):564-572.
7. Felitti VJ, Anda RF, Nordenberg D, et al. Relationship of childhood abuse and household dysfunction to many of the leading causes of death in adults. The Adverse Childhood Experiences (ACE) Study. *Am J Prev Med.* 1998;14(4):245-258.
8. Cronholm PF, Forke CM, Wade R, et al. Adverse childhood experiences: expanding the concept of adversity. *Am J Prev Med.* 2015;49(3):354-361.
9. Substance Abuse and Mental Health Services Administration. Understanding the Impact of Trauma. In: *Trauma-Informed Care in Behavioral Health Services.* Treatment Improvement Protocol (TIP) Series 57. Substane Abuse and Mental Health Services Administration; 2014:59-89.
10. Trauma- and Stressor-Related Disorders. In: *Diagnostic and Statistical Manual of Mental Disorders.* DSM Library. American Psychiatric Association; 2013.
11. Schnur JB, Dillon MJ, Goldsmith RE, Montgomery GH. Cancer treatment experiences among survivors of childhood sexual abuse: a qualitative investigation of triggers and reactions to cumulative trauma. *Palliat Support Care.* 2018;16(6):767-776.
12. Stalker CA, Russell BDC, Teram E, Schachter CL. Providing dental care to survivors of childhood sexual abuse:

treatment considerations for the practitioner. *J Am Dent Assoc.* 2005;136(9):1277-1281.

13. Righy C, Rosa RG, da Silva RTA, et al. Prevalence of post-traumatic stress disorder symptoms in adult critical care survivors: a systematic review and meta-analysis. *Crit Care.* 2019;23(1):213.

14. Nakić Radoš S, Matijaš M, Kuhar L, Anđelinović M, Ayers S. Measuring and conceptualizing PTSD following childbirth: validation of the City Birth Trauma Scale. *Psychol Trauma.* 2020;12(2):147-155.

15. Liberzon I, Abelson JL. Context processing and the neurobiology of post-traumatic stress disorder. *Neuron.* 2016;92(1):14-30.

16. Shalev A, Liberzon I, Marmar C. Post-traumatic stress disorder. *N Engl J Med.* 2017;376(25):2459-2469.

17. Ryan J, Chaudieu I, Ancelin M-L, Saffery R. Biological underpinnings of trauma and post-traumatic stress disorder: focusing on genetics and epigenetics. *Epigenomics.* 2016;8(11):1553-1569.

18. Bisson JI, Roberts NP, Andrew M, Cooper R, Lewis C. Psychological therapies for chronic post-traumatic stress disorder (PTSD) in adults. *Cochrane Database Syst Rev.* 2013;2013(12).

19. Harvey MR. Towards an ecological understanding of resilience in trauma survivors. *J Aggress Maltreatment Trauma.* 2007;14(1-2):9-32.

20. Gartland D, Riggs E, Muyeen S, et al. What factors are associated with resilient outcomes in children exposed to social adversity? A systematic review. *BMJ Open.* 2019;9(4).

21. Elderton A, Berry A, Chan C. A systematic review of posttraumatic growth in survivors of interpersonal violence in adulthood. *Trauma Violence Abuse.* 2017;18(2):223-236.

22. Schnarrs PW, Stone AL, Salcido R, Baldwin A, Georgiou C, Nemeroff CB. Differences in adverse childhood experiences (ACEs) and quality of physical and mental health between transgender and cisgender sexual minorities. *J Psychiatr Res.* 2019;119:1-6.

23. Baams L. Disparities for LGBTQ and gender nonconforming adolescents. *Pediatrics.* 2018;141(5).

24. Stone A, Schnarrs PW, Salcido R. Assessing differences in adverse childhood event scores between transgender/nonbinary individuals and cisgender sexual minorities. In: Population Association of America; 2019.

25. Earnshaw VA, Bogart LM, Poteat VP, Reisner SL, Schuster MA. Bullying among lesbian, gay, bisexual, and transgender youth. *Pediatr Clin North Am.* 2016;63(6):999-1010.

26. Kosciw J, Greytak E, Zongrone A, Clark C, Truong N. The 2017 National School Climate survey: the experiences of lesbian, gay, bisexual, transgender, and queer youth in our nation's schools. Published online 2018.

27. Puhl RM, Himmelstein MS, Watson RJ. Weight-based victimization among sexual and gender minority adolescents: findings from a diverse national sample. *Pediatr Obes.* 2019;14(7):e12514.

28. Valentine SE, Peitzmeier SM, King DS, et al. Disparities in exposure to intimate partner violence among transgender/gender nonconforming and sexual minority primary care patients. *LGBT Health.* 2017;4(4):260-267.

29. Scheer JR, Baams L. Help-seeking patterns among LGBTQ young adults exposed to intimate partner violence victimization. *J Interpers Violence.* Published online May 14, 2019:886260519848785.

30. Grant J, Mottet L, Harrison J, Herman J, Keisling M. Injustice at every turn: a report of the National Transgender Discrimination Survey. Published online 2011.

31. James S, Herman J, Rankin S, Keisling M, Mottet L, Anafi M. The report of the 2015 U.S. Transgender Survey. Published online 2016.

32. Meyer IH. Prejudice, social stress, and mental health in lesbian, gay, and bisexual populations: conceptual issues and research evidence. *Psychol Bull.* 2003;129(5):674-697.

33. Hendricks ML, Testa RJ. A conceptual framework for clinical work with transgender and gender nonconforming clients: an adaptation of the Minority Stress Model. *Professional Psychology: Research and Practice.* 2012;43(5):460-467.

34. Nuttbrock L, Bockting W, Rosenblum A, et al. Gender abuse, depressive symptoms, and HIV and other sexually transmitted infections among male-to-female transgender persons: a three-year prospective study. *Am J Public Health.* 2013;103(2):300-307.

35. Klein A, Golub SA. Family rejection as a predictor of suicide attempts and substance misuse among transgender and gender nonconforming adults. *LGBT Health.* 2016;3(3):193-199.

36. Reisner SL, White Hughto JM, Gamarel KE, Keuroghlian AS, Mizock L, Pachankis JE. Discriminatory experiences associated with posttraumatic stress disorder symptoms among transgender adults. *J Couns Psychol.* 2016;63(5):509-519.

37. Bockting WO, Miner MH, Swinburne Romine RE, Hamilton A, Coleman E. Stigma, mental health, and resilience in an online sample of the US transgender population. *Am J Public Health.* 2013;103(5):943-951.

38. White Hughto JM, Pachankis JE, Willie TC, Reisner SL. Victimization and depressive symptomology in transgender adults: the mediating role of avoidant coping. *J Couns Psychol.* 2017;64(1):41-51.

39. Fuchs M, Potter J. Societal experiences of LGBT people. In: *The Plasticity of Sex: The Molecular Biology and Clinical Features of Genomic Sex, Gender Identity and Sexual Behavior.* Academic Press; 2020.

40. Agénor M, Peitzmeier SM, Bernstein IM, et al. Perceptions of cervical cancer risk and screening among transmasculine individuals: patient and provider perspectives. *Cult Health Sex.* 2016;18(10):1192-1206.

41. Peitzmeier SM, Bernstein IM, McDowell MJ, et al. Enacting power and constructing gender in cervical cancer screening encounters between transmasculine patients and health care providers. *Cult Health Sex.* 2020;22(12):1315-1332.

42. Noether CD, Finkelstein N, VanDeMark NR, Savage A, Reed BG, Moses DJ. Design strengths and issues of SAMHSA's Women, Co-occurring Disorders, and Violence Study. *Psychiatr Serv.* 2005;56(10):1233-1236.

43. Clark HW, Power AK. Women, co-occurring disorders, and violence study: a case for trauma-informed care. *J Subst Abuse Treat.* 2005;28(2):145-146.

44. Beck CT. Secondary traumatic stress in nurses: a systematic review. *Arch Psychiatr Nurs.* 2011;25(1):1-10.

45. Salloum A, Kondrat DC, Johnco C, Olson KR. The role of self-care on compassion satisfaction, burnout and secondary trauma among child welfare workers. *Child Youth Serv Rev.* 2015;49:54-61.

46. Scheer JR, Poteat VP. Trauma-informed care and health among LGBTQ intimate partner violence survivors. *J Interpers Violence.* Published online December 29, 2018:886260518820688.

47. Brezing C, Ferrara M, Freudenreich O. The syndemic illness of HIV and trauma: implications for a trauma-informed model of care. *Psychosomatics.* 2015;56(2):107-118.

48. LGBT Health Education Center. https://www.lgbthealtheducation.org/. Accessed February 14, 2020.

49. Human Rights Campaign. HEI scoring criteria. https://www.hrc.org/hei/hei-scoring-criteria/. Accessed February 14, 2020.

50. Goldhammer H, Malina S, Keuroghlian AS. Communicating with patients who have nonbinary gender identities. *Ann Fam Med.* 2018;16(6):559-562.

51. Siegel D. *The Developing Mind: How Relationships and the Brain Interact to Shape Who We Are.* Guilford Press; 1999.

52. Kolp H, Wilder S, Andersen C, et al. Gender minority stress, sleep disturbance, and sexual victimization in transgender and gender nonconforming adults. *J Clin Psychol.* 2020;76(4):688-698.

53. Wu V, Huff H, Bhandari M. Pattern of physical injury associated with intimate partner violence in women presenting to the emergency department: a systematic review and meta-analysis. *Trauma Violence Abuse.* 2010;11(2):71-82.

54. Claes L, Bouman WP, Witcomb G, Thurston M, Fernandez-Aranda F, Arcelus J. Non-suicidal self-injury in trans people: associations with psychological symptoms, victimization, interpersonal functioning, and perceived social support. *J Sex Med.* 2015;12(1):168-179.

55. Davey A, Arcelus J, Meyer C, Bouman WP. Self-injury among trans individuals and matched controls: prevalence and associated factors. *Health Soc Care Community.* 2016;24(4):485-494.

56. McDowell MJ, Hughto JMW, Reisner SL. Risk and protective factors for mental health morbidity in a community sample of female-to-male trans-masculine adults. *BMC Psychiatry.* 2019;19(1):16.

57. Jackman KB, Dolezal C, Levin B, Honig JC, Bockting WO. Stigma, gender dysphoria, and nonsuicidal self-injury in a community sample of transgender individuals. *Psychiatry Res.* 2018;269:602-609.

58. Smith NB, Kouros CD, Meuret AE. The role of trauma symptoms in nonsuicidal self-injury. *Trauma Violence Abuse.* 2014;15(1):41-56.

59. Machtinger EL, Cuca YP, Khanna N, Rose CD, Kimberg LS. From treatment to healing: the promise of trauma-informed primary care. *Womens Health Issues.* 2015;25(3):193-197.

60. Machtinger EL, Davis KB, Kimberg LS, et al. From treatment to healing: inquiry and response to recent and past trauma in adult health care. *Womens Health Issues.* 2019;29(2):97-102.

61. Clark C, Classen CC, Fourt A, Shetty M. *Treating the Trauma Survivor: An Essential Guide to Trauma-Informed Care.* Routledge/Taylor & Francis Group; 2015.

62. Lewis-O'Connor A, Warren A, Lee JV, et al. The state of the science on trauma inquiry. *Womens Health (Lond).* 2019;15:1745506519861234.

63. Fitzsimmons E, Loo S, Dougherty S, et al. Development and content validation of the IPV-4, a brief patient-reported measure of intimate partner violence for use in HIV care. *AIDS Care.* 2019;31(sup1):1-9.

64. Prins A, Bovin MJ, Smolenski DJ, et al. The Primary Care PTSD Screen for DSM-5 (PC-PTSD-5): development and evaluation within a veteran primary care sample. *J Gen Intern Med.* 2016;31(10):1206-1211.

65. Anti-Violence. FORGE. https://forge-forward.org/anti-violence/. Accessed February 14, 2020.

66. The Network. http://tnlr.org/en/. Accessed February 14, 2020.

67. Know Your Rights | Health Care. National Center for Transgender Equality. https://transequality.org/know-your-rights/health-care. Accessed February 14, 2020.

68. Resources | Transcend Legal. https://transcendlegal.org. Accessed February 14, 2020.

69. Raja S, Hasnain M, Hoersch M, Gove-Yin S, Rajagopalan C. Trauma informed care in medicine: current knowledge and future research directions. *Fam Community Health.* 2015;38(3):216-226.

70. Tedeschi RG, Calhoun LG. The posttraumatic growth inventory: measuring the positive legacy of trauma. *J Traumatic Stress.* 1996;9(3):455-472.

71. Hernández P, Gangsei D, Engstrom D. Vicarious resilience: a new concept in work with those who survive trauma. *Fam Process.* 2007;46(2):229-241.

72. Edelkott N, Engstrom DW, Hernandez-Wolfe P, Gangsei D. Vicarious resilience: complexities and variations. *Am J Orthopsychiatry.* 2016;86(6):713-724.

73. Farmer PE, Nizeye B, Stulac S, Keshavjee S. Structural violence and clinical medicine. *PLoS Med.* 2006;3(10):e449.

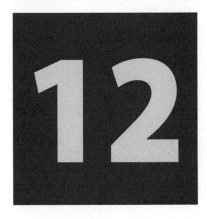

12

Obtaining a Gender-Affirming Sexual History

Danielle O'Banion

Sebastian Mitchell Barr

INTRODUCTION

Transgender and gender diverse (TGD) individuals deserve high-quality health care in which they feel safe and empowered. Critical to achieving this aim is creating a clinical space where a comprehensive health history can be discussed, free of judgment or shame. No such history is complete without a respectful understanding of patients' sexual experiences and behaviors; therefore, it is recommended that a **sexual history** be obtained from all patients. Because all patients need an open-minded and nonjudgmental approach to feel comfortable discussing their sensitive personal experiences, use of a gender- and sexuality-inclusive framework is of paramount importance. Studies suggest that many TGD people do not disclose their gender identity to a health care professional; as many as 60% of TGD patients do not disclose they are transgender or gender diverse to some of their health care professionals, and 30% do not disclose to any of them.[1] Other patients may not yet be aware of being TGD when they first begin care with a health care professional. Therefore, it is not uncommon for many health care professionals to have TGD patients whom they inaccurately believe to be **cisgender**. Due to the spectrum of possibilities in clinical practice, it is important to maintain an open and neutral approach with all patients that fosters opportunities for disclosure instead of creating barriers. This chapter has been written particularly with primary health care professionals in mind; those in other specialties and disciplines, however, may also benefit from incorporating aspects of obtaining a gender-affirming sexual history into their practice.

IMPORTANCE OF GENDER AFFIRMATION IN HEALTH CARE ENCOUNTERS

Currently, few clinical training programs offer instruction on how to provide health care that is affirming for TGD people.[2,3] Most education and practice models have been developed with cisgender people in mind and do not consider the different identities, experiences, bodies, and needs of TGD individuals. Given that at least 1 out of 200 people identify as TGD,[4] such neglect means that a large population of people receives suboptimal health care, leading to delayed or missed diagnoses and worse health outcomes than their cisgender peers.

Additionally, although familiarity with gender diversity is increasing, the majority of Americans report that they do not personally know an openly transgender person.[5,6] Clinicians likely mirror this statistic, though most see TGD patients throughout their careers whether they know it or not. Without personal familiarity or dedicated training, it is likely that even those health care professionals who have some working knowledge of trans health still do not have an understanding of the adverse impacts of gender non-affirmation, particularly when it occurs in a health care setting.

In this chapter, gender non-affirmation comprises behaviors and actions—either intentional or unintentional—that signal to a person that they are not being viewed as the gender that they identify as or know themselves to be. Such behaviors include using the incorrect name or pronouns, interacting with a person's body in ways that center the sex they were assigned at birth (e.g., referring to a **trans masculine** person as "biologically female" or assuming the presence of certain anatomy), or using gender-coded language misaligned with a person's identity (e.g., "buddy" or "dear").[7] For many TGD people, instances of non-affirmation, especially as they accumulate, are experienced as painful invalidations of one's sense of self. In the 2015 U.S. Transgender Survey,[1] a transgender respondent is quoted describing their experience of a hospital stay: "I was consistently misnamed and **misgendered** throughout ... I passed a kidney stone during that visit. On the standard 1–10 pain scale, that's somewhere around a 9. But not having my identity respected, that hurt far more." This profound hurt is not a passing emotion. Perceived disrespect and mistreatment by health care professionals is associated with depression and suicidal thoughts among TGD people,[8] while the cumulative effect of non-affirmation (within and outside of health care contexts) is predictive of symptoms of **posttraumatic stress disorder (PTSD)**.[9,10] Unfortunately, such non-affirming health care experiences are common among TGD communities, even more so among those with additional intersecting marginalized identities and experiences: specifically for trans women who are Black, Indigenous, and people of color (BIPOC); those with **nonbinary** gender identities; and sex workers and others who exchange sex for money and resources.[1,11]

In addition to the negative impact on psychological well-being, receiving non-affirming health care functions as a barrier to the patient–clinician relationship and impairs health outcomes in TGD communities. Many TGD people report avoiding or delaying needed health care to protect themselves from mistreatment or disrespect. Again, avoiding or delaying health care is even more likely among BIPOC and sex workers.[1] Studies have found that between 20% and 50% of TGD people decided not to seek care within the past year because they feared **discrimination** and non-affirmation. The risk of avoidance is understandably higher in individuals who have already directly experienced mistreatment in a health care setting or who know of other transgender adults who have.[12] Conversely, TGD people who report being treated with respect by health care professionals and feeling understood are more likely to be engaged with continuous health care, be up-to-date on preventive screening, and report better health outcomes.[13-15]

This research suggests that using a gender-affirming approach to interacting with patients not only allows health care professionals to offer the most appropriate and holistic care but also reduces harm. Interactions that are respectful and validating empower patients to participate more effectively in medical decision-making. Building a trusting and respectful relationship with patients creates an accepting environment in which sensitive topics, particularly those related to sex and sexuality, can be discussed with patients.

INTERSECTION OF MEDICINE AND SEXUAL HEALTH

Medical professionals, educated in a culture steeped in scientific inquiry and academic assessment, have met with challenges in addressing the more sensitive aspects of the human lives they serve. Possibly the most frequently omitted part of a patient's clinical history is that of their sexual practices and behaviors. Clinicians tend to struggle with this element of discussion due in part to academic medical education: instruction in obtaining a sexual history is usually linked to identifying pathology, such as sexually transmitted infections (STIs), or providing contraception to reduce the risk of unintended pregnancy. Little to no instruction is given on how to holistically and meaningfully engage with a patient on the topic of sexuality, including discussions of pleasure

and pain. Most health care professionals cite a lack of training and awareness about sexual issues while also minimizing their importance.[16]

In addition, many sociological and cultural factors complicate the task of discussing sex with patients. Western medicine invariably centers cisgender heteronormativity with few exceptions, which puts any patient who does not adhere to these norms at a significant disadvantage in clinical spaces. Clinicians' discomfort or lack of knowledge about the sexual practices of **LGBQIA+** and TGD patients often leads to patient dissatisfaction with how their medical care is handled.[15] A survey of health care professionals at U.S. Veterans Affairs hospitals found that 40% avoided asking about sexuality because they believed a patient's sexual orientation was not relevant to their health care.[17] Clinicians are also less likely to obtain sexual histories in patients who are older, BIPOC, and/or have disabilities.[16] Anecdotal experience suggests this avoidance is likely true for larger-bodied patients, as well. Additionally, in the United States (and many other societies), there is a prevalent culture of shame around sex that serves as a challenging backdrop to having these conversations, regardless of the gender identities and sexual orientations of those involved.

Despite these challenges, obtaining a comprehensive sexual history is crucial to understanding the overall health and well-being of a patient.[18] A necessary first step for health care professionals is to identify and address potential sources of personal discomfort or avoidance of this topic. Next, it is important to expand the working definition of sexual health. Most medical models of sexual behavior identify the absence of disease as evidence of "sexual health," but this description is only a fraction of what should be a multidisciplinary paradigm. In contrast, the World Health Organization defines sexual health as:

> … a state of physical, emotional, mental and social well-being in relation to sexuality; it is not merely the absence of disease, dysfunction or infirmity. Sexual health requires a positive and respectful approach to sexuality and sexual relationships, as well as the possibility of having pleasurable and safe sexual experiences, free of coercion, discrimination and violence. For sexual health to be attained and maintained, the sexual rights of all persons must be respected, protected and fulfilled.[19]

This approach creates a holistic view of a patient's sexual health that can offer key insights into other aspects of their general well-being. A person's experience of sexuality—attraction, desire, arousal, intimacy, pleasure—is heavily informed by their overall health.[20-22] A disruption of any of these components can be secondary to mental health changes, medication side effects, progressive medical conditions, or surgical sequelae. For example, painful receptive vaginal or anal intercourse can be a signal of infection or high-tone pelvic floor disorder. A loss of libido can be secondary to relational issues, mental health concerns, or medication side effects. Impaired clitoral/penile erections or vaginal lubrication can be due to physiologic or age-related changes; these can also be secondary to hormonal contraception, gender-affirming hormones, or postoperative alterations to natal anatomy. Similarly, pleasurable sexual experiences can both demonstrate and contribute to positive aspects of a patient's health. Sexual satisfaction is associated with healthier stress responses and well-being,[23] and there is a large body of literature on the health benefits of sex and pleasure in multiple aspects of patients' sex lives.[24] For discussions of these topics to happen effectively, health care professionals must make space for them. When patients can discuss this sensitive topic freely and without shame in the clinical encounter, they will come to a deeper understanding of the relationship between their sexual lives and general health. Comprehensive sexual histories reduce the possibility of missed diagnoses and improve opportunities for patients to participate in their sex lives with autonomy.

Patients *want* their health care professionals to make more space for these conversations. In a study of Swiss patients, more than 90% of surveyed patients reported wanting to talk to health care professionals about their sex lives, but only 41% of those patients had ever had such discussions.[25] U.S. surveys show that between 25% and 63% of health care professionals routinely obtain or document sexual history, and often these inquiries do not include exploration of patients' satisfaction, sexual orientation, or even sexual dysfunction.[26] Because most patients feel uncomfortable bringing up sexual health concerns, the task ultimately falls on the health care professional to incorporate it as part of the general approach to health care. In addition to asking about sleep, nutrition, and mental health at an annual physical, a simple question, such as, "Do you have any concerns about sex or intimacy?" can also be asked. Respectful, affirming questions about sex can be incorporated into any clinical encounter, provided that all experiences of gender and sexuality are considered, including those on the asexuality spectrum.

TRUST AND TALKING ABOUT SEX

Discussions about sex, sexuality, and sexual health are sensitive in nature. Furthermore, they may involve or be adjacent to topics that elicit shame or trigger emotional reactions from patients. Assessing sexual health and history cannot be done effectively without specific attention to building trust. Patients deserve to know why such information is relevant to clinical decision-making, and they should be allowed space to decline to share if they feel uncomfortable. Building trust may be particularly important when working with TGD patients, who report being asked invasive, unnecessary, and voyeuristic questions in health care settings.[27] Some patients need several sessions with a health care professional to build

enough trust to discuss this topic. Because each patient has different requirements for feeling safe enough to have these conversations, health care professionals must be flexible in their approach and center the patient's needs at all times.

Possibly the most important aspect of building trust is in equalizing the traditional power dynamic inherent in clinician–patient relationships. The classic model of obtaining a history centers the clinician as entitled to the information the patient has to give. The reality is that patients possess the power to share or withhold information based on the level of comfort and trust that they have in the clinical space.[28] Although clinicians have the expertise necessary to guide patients toward healthy decision-making, it is important to remember that the patient is the expert on their own body, behaviors, and needs. Starting the patient interview with a statement such as, "I know it can be hard to talk about sensitive topics with a clinician, but please know that I am here to serve as a facilitator for your needs, not to judge you" can help to equalize the dynamic and put the patient at ease.

Further complicating clinician-patient power dynamics are the insidious impacts of oppression. Distrust of health care professionals and medical institutions is particularly high in marginalized communities.[29] The medical community has historically failed to meet the needs of patients who hold intersecting marginalized identities, especially with regard to race and **gender identity**. Patients, particularly those who are Black, Indigenous, and Latinx, have experienced extensive **trauma** at the hands of the American medical community. These traumas include being subjected to nonconsensual medical experimentation, involuntary sterilization, and having pain dismissed by clinicians, resulting in delayed or missed diagnoses of serious illnesses.[30] Experiences of **bias**, including microaggressions, can lead to a poor clinician–patient relationship and low levels of trust. In addition to BIPOC patients, other marginalized groups such as people with disabilities, people with larger bodies, sex workers, and TGD individuals report distrust that results from discrimination and disrespect in clinical visits.[31,32]

Western medical and mental health professionals have long pathologized noncisgender identities and gender diverse presentations; health care professionals and institutions have thus been complicit in labeling TGD people's identities as abnormal, wrong, or bad. Currently, despite a growing movement (and some victories) to depathologize TGD identities, many TGD individuals still report having health care professionals who are not culturally responsive or clinically skilled in caring for them.[27] Although awareness of TGD patients' needs is growing among the general medical community, a large majority of health care professionals still report insufficient knowledge to deliver high-quality transgender health care.[3,12] Understandably, TGD patients may enter health care encounters with a protective skepticism that can make more sensitive and vulnerable discussions (like a sexual history) challenging.

Similarly, individuals who have experienced sexual or physical violence may struggle with conversations about sex due to a guardedness that stems from trauma. Hypervigilance is a common symptom of PTSD that can manifest in the clinical encounter as suspicion or a reluctance to engage. Reminders of trauma can trigger an emotional response in patients that leads to avoidance and fear, thereby shutting down the clinical encounter. TGD people are more likely than the general population to have experienced trauma, so awareness of the potential for these responses is particularly relevant when providing care for TGD populations.[33]

In general, TGD patients are more likely to feel trusting and comfortable when they are affirmed in their identities and experiences. For this reason, it is imperative to make the clinical space affirming of all gender identities and sexual orientations from the moment a patient engages. The entire patient experience should be affirming, including an inquiry of correct name and pronouns at each level of access, from the front desk staff to medical assistants to clinicians (see Chapter 11, "Basic Principles of Trauma-Informed and Gender-Affirming Care"). If a patient feels affirmed throughout their engagement with a clinical setting, they are more likely to trust the health care professional with their personal information and feel empowered to choose what information is relevant to disclose.

Given the likelihood that TGD patients, particularly those with intersecting marginalized identities, have had negative health care experiences, health care professionals must work to create an environment that alleviates or calms distrust. It is important to let patients set the rate of disclosure of sensitive information; they should never be pushed to say more than they are ready to. Recognition of potential trauma-related responses can help defuse stressful encounters with patients who may be defensive or shutting down. Importantly, creating a holistically gender-affirming patient experience offers the strongest chance of building trust with a patient. Use of gender- and sexuality-inclusive language during the sexual history is especially important.

▶ Case Study 1: KB

27-year-old KB, a white-presenting person, sits in Nurse Practitioner Johnson's office with eyes downcast, arms folded. NP Johnson asks KB why they are in clinic today. "I just don't feel right," KB replies. KB is listed as "female" in the electronic health record and has a close-shaved haircut, traditionally masculine clothing, and does not wear makeup. They also smell strongly of cigarettes. NP Johnson reviews the chart and notes the patient has a history of irregular menstrual periods but otherwise no major issues. She asks the patient some follow-up questions about physical symptoms, but KB shrugs repeatedly and does not offer much of an answer to anything. NP Johnson sees the patient identified as "lesbian" in the chart and asks, "How is your personal life? Are you dating any new women? Having relationship troubles?" KB looks up angrily and replies, "What?" then looks back down at the floor and shrugs further into their coat. NP Johnson, realizing she has made a mistake, backtracks. "KB, I'm sorry. I really want to help you today, but I'm definitely asking the wrong questions. I realize that must be stressful for you. Did I miss something?" KB looks up at NP Johnson and says, "Well for starters, you can ask me if I've had sex with any dudes lately, and that might be something." NP Johnson then says gently, "Ok, then. Have you had sex lately with any people who have penises?" KB then quietly tells her that they had sex with a guy at a party and are worried because they have chest tenderness and their menstrual period is late. "I have periods that are all over the place, but this is different." NP Johnson asks, "Was the sex consensual?" KB replies that they had a lot to drink at the party, so they're not entirely sure. "It was a friend of mine. I'm not sure what happened exactly. I'm pretty messed up about it." NP Johnson then obtains a urine pregnancy test, checks for STIs, and refers KB to her clinic's social worker for counseling. KB's test results confirm pregnancy. KB opts not to continue the pregnancy, and NP Johnson refers them to an abortion provider within a manageable distance. KB starts counseling with a queer-affirming violence recovery program.

▶ Discussion Questions

- NP Johnson, informed by the patient's chart and perhaps by their presentation, assumed that KB was not having sex with people with penises and, therefore, might have missed their pregnancy risk. What initial assumptions might you make about KB in a similar situation, and how might they lead to misdiagnosis or inadequate treatment?

- If you were seeing this patient, how might you assess KB's chief complaint of "not feeling right" to avoid some of the initial missteps NP Johnson made?

- A turning point occurs in the encounter when NP Johnson says, "KB, I'm sorry. I really want to help you today, but I'm definitely asking the wrong questions. I realize that must be stressful for you. Did I miss something?" What about this approach might have opened up the interaction between KB and NP Johnson? What language and tone do you use when you need to course-correct during a challenging dynamic with a patient?

- How might KB's whiteness affect this encounter and subsequent follow-up? Consider what might be different in this case if they were Black, Indigenous, or Latinx? What communities access your clinical space and how might your perceptions influence your care of non-White populations?

- Multiple aspects of the follow-up plan in this case are dependent on access to resources: (1) a social worker with immediate availability who is able to work with KB in a way that feels affirming; (2) available and affordable abortion care; (3) a violence recovery or survivors network/program that is queer-affirming. What factors limit access to or availability of these resources for patients where you practice? Are you familiar with similar resources in your community, particularly those that focus on BIPOC communities? How would you adapt this case if any or all of these resources were not options for KB?

OBTAINING A GENDER- AND SEXUALITY-INCLUSIVE HISTORY

Perhaps the most important principle in obtaining an affirming sexual history is to do so in a gender- and sexuality-inclusive way. As reviewed in the chapter introduction, TGD people experience trauma from micro- and macroaggressions in the clinical space. Much of this trauma occurs when they are misgendered or assumptions are made about their lives and bodies, which happens because the standard health care space operates from a norm of cisgender heterosexuality. Most health care professionals assume that the patient in front of them has a binary gender identity, anatomy traditionally associated with their outward gender expression, and a sex life that involves penile-vaginal intercourse. Conversely, clinicians may assume that patients who present in a more gender-expansive way (e.g., a more masculine-presenting woman or a more feminine-presenting man) are lesbian- or gay-identified with cisgender partners, and potentially miss pregnancy or STI risk. Such false assumptions may in turn lead to frustration and distrust among patients. At worst, mistaking a patient's gender identity or sexual behaviors can rupture a clinician–patient relationship, but more commonly it leads to patients withholding information from clinicians, thereby impairing the level of care they ultimately receive.

Of paramount importance to the gender-affirming paradigm is the detachment of clinical vocabulary from gendered language.[7] First, it is necessary to recognize and then unlearn the gendered ways in which clinicians engage with patients. Words like "sir" or "ma'am" have the potential to cause harm to a patient for whom those words are non-affirming of their gender. Using gendered terms of endearment (e.g., "buddy" or "dear") are equally problematic. It is critically important to have systems in place so that all office staff use the correct names and pronouns for all patients, but the subtle ways in which health care professionals engage with gender are just as important to evaluate as they can cause significant harm. Similar to this, using terms like "female-bodied" and "male-bodied" to describe people's anatomy is another common pitfall.[34] For example, a clinician might describe a transgender man or nonbinary person as "female-bodied" in discussing the patient with a colleague, or document a transgender woman or nonbinary person as "male-bodied" to indicate these individuals have their natal organs. Health care professionals often use the terms "biologically male" and "biologically female" in similar ways. For most surveyed

TGD people, this terminology is problematic and harmful as these terms are incongruent with the patient's gender identity. They center patients' sex assigned at birth and potentially dysphoria-inducing parts of their bodies, while invalidating their affirmed gender.[34,35] Such practices also contribute to the erasure of people with differences of sex development, whose biologic milieu can transcend binary male/female designations. See Table 12-1 for suggestions on ways to adapt sexual health and history terminology to be gender-inclusive and affirming.

In assessing sexual behaviors, open-ended, anatomy-driven questions should be asked to allow space for a patient to disclose the breadth of experiences they might have. It is important to start from an inclusive framing that considers diverse potential experiences of asexuality, physical or emotional intimacy, and romance, as well as nonmonogamy,

Table 12–1. Adapting Sexual Health and History Terminology

Use Gender-Neutral or Less-Gendered Language	In Lieu of...
People with vaginas People who menstruate People with ovaries People with penises/testes People with prostates People who produce sperm	Women, men, females, males
Assigned male sex at birth	Biologically male, male-bodied
Assigned female sex at birth	Biologically female, female-bodied
Pregnant person/people	Pregnant woman/women
Parent, birth/gestational parent Parent, nonbirth/gestational parent	Mother, father
External genitals/genitalia, external pelvic area[4]	Vulva, clitoris
Genital opening, frontal opening, internal canal, front hole	Vagina
Outer folds	Labia, lips
Uterus, ovaries, internal reproductive organs	Female reproductive organs
External genitals/genitalia	Penis, testes
Chest	Breasts
Chest-feeding	Breastfeeding
Menstruation, bleeding	Period
Internal condom	Female condom

kink, and sex work. (These terms and concepts are defined in a later section.) Health care professionals should be aware that relationships and behaviors can be complex and traditional labels are restrictive. Before embarking on this part of the discussion, consent should be obtained from the patient to discuss their sexual history as part of establishing trust with the patient and equalizing the power dynamic in the encounter.

Once consent is obtained to ask about sex, the health care professional should begin by asking the patient what terms should be used when discussing the patient's sexual practices. TGD patients can have complex relationships with the gendered parts of their bodies, so it is important for them to dictate how their bodies are discussed. The foundation of this approach is to have a clear idea of what information is relevant and necessary for medical decision-making. When obtaining a sexual history, it is important to be flexible and allow the patient to determine the rate of disclosure. Sexual and romantic relationships exist in countless permutations. The health care professional's task is to assess the risks and positive aspects of a patient's sexual behaviors and offer recommendations that facilitate harm reduction and improve well-being. The following section illustrates how to structure a comprehensive sexual history using a gender- and sexuality-inclusive framework.

▶ Case Study 2: JW

Dr. Brown washes her hands, turns toward her new patient, JW, and says, "Hi there! I'm Dr. Brown. My pronouns are she and hers. Do you mind sharing your name and pronouns with me?" JW replies uncertainly, "I go by Jessica and my pronouns are she and hers, too." Dr. Brown sits, opens the patient's electronic health record chart, and asks about JW's medical, surgical, and family histories, which are all unremarkable. She looks kindly at JW and says, "For the next bit, I'd like to ask you some sensitive questions about your personal life, including sex, if you have any. Is that ok? You need only tell me the things you think are relevant to your health." JW assents. Dr. Brown asks, "What words should I use to refer to body parts, whether they are yours or someone else's?" JW asks her to use formal anatomic terms for body parts, like "penis" and "vagina." "Thank you, I certainly will. Are you currently emotionally or sexually intimate with anyone?" JW replies that she does not really date much, as she has been out and socially affirmed as a woman for a few years, and it has made dating a bit tough. "Do you typically prefer folks with penises or vaginas, or do you not have an anatomy preference?" JW is a bit confused at that question, but replies that in general she prefers women, as far as she knows, "women with vaginas, but I'm open to seeing all women... I just don't know yet because I'm new at this." Dr. Brown reassures her that sexual exploration is a normal part of life, particularly with new lived experiences, and offers her

counseling on pleasure and STI prevention when the time comes. JW thanks her and schedules a follow-up in 6 months.

▶ Discussion Questions

- Imagine yourself as Dr. Brown. How different is this encounter from the ways in which you currently practice? Which parts of this encounter feel uncomfortable for you? Explore potential sources of your discomfort and whether there are situations or language with which you need more practice.

- How does Dr. Brown work to build trust in this initial visit? Is Dr. Brown effective? How do you know?

- Although you read that JW is trans, the case did not provide any information about her various intersecting identities or cultural background. Who did you picture when you read this case, and what might that signify about your internalized norms? In what ways might this case look different depending on a patient's race, class, geographic location, age, body size, disability? Are there other factors that might impact the interaction between clinician and patient?

THE EIGHT P'S OF A GENDER-AFFIRMING SEXUAL HISTORY

The sexual history can consist of one question or several. The approach can be modified depending on the context of the visit, how much time is allotted, and the relationship with the patient. For example, sexuality can be addressed as part of a general physical exam with a simple, "Do you have any concerns about sex or intimacy?" If, however, someone has presented specifically with a physical symptom such as dysuria or rectal pain, the specifics of sexual practices and past history of STIs have more relevance. Health care professionals should always be prepared to incorporate aspects of obtaining a sexual history into an encounter, because symptoms that patients themselves have not linked to sexual function may very well be related (e.g., painful stooling due to herpes proctitis, or a cough from undiagnosed HIV).

The Centers for Disease Control has outlined five "P's" of obtaining a sexual history to assess behaviors and risk: Partners, Practices, Protection from STIs, Past History of STIs, and Prevention of Pregnancy (Table 12-2).[36] In this chapter we present an adapted version, with a few changes made to promote an affirming and holistic clinical space. The last item has been changed to "Pregnancy considerations," rather than "prevention," and three items have been added that offer important insight into sexual well-being: Preferences, Pleasure, and Power dynamics. Their meaning and importance are outlined below. All of the items noted do not need to be addressed in each clinical encounter. In most settings, there is insufficient time and bandwidth to do so. Additionally, the suggested questions should not be considered a rigid "script" that must be followed

Table 12–2. Eight "P's" of Obtaining a Sexual History

Preferences	Patients' needs for a safe and empowering discussion about sex (e.g., preferred terminology for anatomy and behaviors)
Partners	Number and type of intimate partners a patient has, thinking beyond traditional labels for sexual orientation
Practices	The sexual behaviors in which a patient engages, inclusive of various anatomy permutations and nontraditional relationships
Pleasure and Pain	Degree to which patients enjoy or do not enjoy sexual activity, including the presence or absence of arousal and orgasm
Protection from STIs, HIV	Respectful identification of barriers to STI prevention methods, including PrEP and PEP
Past History of STIs	Prior STIs—especially syphilis, herpes, and rectal gonorrhea/chlamydia—can predict future HIV and STI risk
Pregnancy Considerations	Facilitation of healthy pregnancies when childbearing is desired; protection against pregnancy when it is not desired
Power Dynamics and Partner Violence	Universal, gender-inclusive screening of patients for IPV to increase uptake of resources and improve outcomes

Data from Centers for Disease Control and Prevention. A Guide to Taking a Sexual History https://www.cdc.gov/std/treatment/sexual-history.pdf.

without modifications. Rather, this list presents a menu of options that can be adapted to fit a health care professional's own style and context, bearing in mind the core framework of gender- and sexuality-inclusive language.

Preferences

The first task is to obtain consent from the patient to discuss their sexual history and clarify what words should be used to discuss sensitive topics like anatomy. A patient may prefer the term "breasts" instead of "chest" (or vice versa) or "front hole" instead of vagina, for example. If certain terms are off-limits (e.g., breast, vagina, or penis), the clinician should ask open-ended, inclusive questions to allow the patient to disclose information on their own terms. Eliciting preferences offers patients autonomy in this exchange and is key to minimizing experiences of dysphoria.

- "Is it ok for me to ask about your sexual history today?"
- "Do you have sex? Are you physically intimate with anyone?"
- "In asking about your sex life, I need to know specific information about what you do during sex. How would you like for me to discuss this with you?" "What words should I use to refer to your anatomy or specific things you do sexually? Are there words I should try to avoid?"

Partners

Sexual dynamics and relationship structures can be complex and require more specific inquiry than the label a patient uses for their sexual orientation identity. Traditional labels like "lesbian," "gay," "bisexual," and "straight" may insufficiently capture the practices of a particular person; simultaneously, more recent sexual orientation identity terminology (e.g., "pansexual," "queer") does not communicate necessary details about partners and practices. While these labels may be critical for identity development and sense of self, clinicians need specific information for a thorough sexual history. It is now common practice for health care professionals to ask, "Do you have sex with men, women, or both?" Unfortunately, this question is inadequate because it does not sufficiently capture the breadth of intimate experiences that two or more bodies can have with each other. First, it erases people who do not identify as men or women. Second, it suggests that the clinician assumes the sexual anatomy of "women" and "men." And third, this question also misses those who do not have sex, who identify as asexual, or both.

An additional challenge is that nontraditional sexual orientations and relationship structures, such as asexuality and nonmonogamy, have historically been omitted from clinical consideration. These are common, however, and require space and affirmation to be discussed. Asexuality includes a diversity of sexual orientations for which sexual activity is not centered as paramount in a person's life. Many people on the asexuality spectrum are intimate or romantic with people with whom they do not have traditional sexual intercourse. Ethical nonmonogamy involves a system of multiple simultaneous relationships in which there are clear consensual boundaries around how people engage with each other in romantic and sexual ways, which can be different for each set of relationships. Nonmonogamy may also be relevant in **kink** and bondage/discipline, dominance/submission, sadism/masochism (**BDSM**) communities, which include a wide range of consensual activities that center particular fetishes or power dynamics. For example, a person may exist in a monogamous sexual relationship with one partner and engage in activities like spanking or bondage, which do not necessarily involve sexual intercourse, with outside partners (these activities are discussed in more detail in a subsequent section). People engaged in sexual activity outside of the agreed-upon boundaries of their relationship(s) (e.g., people having extramarital affairs or any intimate interactions outside their established relationship rules) also need to be able to discuss those aspects of their sex lives with health care professionals. It is important to always ask about outside intimate partners, even if patients describe themselves as married or monogamous.

The language used in determining a patient's sexual partners is crucial to understanding their range of practices and experiences. Do not assume that a patient has sex, and if they do, do not assume that a patient has sex with only one partner. Avoid restrictive labels and instead ask anatomy-based questions. Finally, assess a patient's level of comfort with their partners as this can help to uncover potential challenges they may be having with intimacy or relationship dynamics.

- "Are you currently intimate or sexual with anyone? Have you been in the past?"

- "Do you typically have one partner or multiple partners? What about currently?"

- "Can you tell me what anatomy your sexual partners have? Is it likely you will have future partners with different anatomy?" (Or, "can you tell me what body parts your sexual partners have?" if "anatomy" feels too cumbersome.)

- "Are you comfortable discussing your sexual needs with your partners?"

Practices

Once the clinician has ascertained the anatomy involved in the patient's sexual behaviors, the next task is to discuss the behaviors themselves. The clinician's job in the sexual history is to assess a patient's sexual well-being and risk. It is important not to become mired in labels for sexual orientation. Use of a consensual, anatomy-based approach to obtaining a history allows the health care professional to understand which body parts are involved in sex, and how.

It is important to be mindful of sexual or sex-related practices that are commonly stigmatized by health care professionals. Patients may use recreational drugs, like methamphetamine, MDMA ("ecstasy"), or amyl nitrite ("poppers"), to augment their experience of penetration and orgasm. It is important to create a judgment-free clinical space to determine whether drugs are used as part of sex. Patients often withhold details of their substance use from health care professionals because of fear of stigma and inadequate medical care. Sex work is similarly often stigmatized by the medical profession, with consequently high rates of patient nondisclosure.[32] Sex work is different from sex trafficking, which is nonconsensual. Transgender people enter survival sex work at a higher rate than the general population because anti-trans discrimination can make it difficult to find adequate employment elsewhere. Sex work is not protected by federal employment agencies and is illegal and unregulated in most of the world.[37] It is important that, in an affirmative clinical model, drug use and sex work are regarded respectfully by health care professionals. These practices are relevant to patients' sexual and general health, and patients must be able to feel safe when discussing them with their health care professionals.

Another highly stigmatized area of sexual practices is BDSM and kink. BDSM is an umbrella term for an array of erotic behaviors that center interpersonal power dynamics. Sometimes these behaviors involve bodily striking (e.g., impact play) that can leave injuries. BDSM is a consensual practice. Patients can present with consensual bruising and abrasions that may be incorrectly interpreted as abuse. Kink is an even wider catch-all term for non-normative sexual behavior, including everything from fetish to fantasy, some of which can make nonpractitioners uncomfortable. Health care professionals must strive to depathologize their understanding of consensual nontraditional sex practices. Creating an affirming clinical space in which these practices are normalized will help patients trust and engage more effectively with their health care. All patients should be asked about nonmainstream practices and informed that such questions are a routine part of obtaining a history so they do not think they are being singled out due to stereotypes about TGD people.

- "What parts of your body touch your partners when you are having sex? What parts of your partners' body/bodies touch you?"

- "Do you prepare for sex in any way? Do you use lubricants or use an anal douche? Do you use medications or drugs to help sex feel better?"

- "Do you ever have sex in exchange for money or housing?"

- "Are drugs or substances part of your sex life?"

- Are you part of any BDSM or kink communities that would impact your medical health?"

- "Is there anything about your sex life that you feel might be relevant to your health?"

Pleasure and Pain

The experience of sexual pleasure and pain is a significant part of a patient's overall well-being. The World Health Organization deems sexual pleasure to be a human right, but many clinicians do not have the vocabulary or knowledge to engage with this topic effectively.[16] Furthermore, due to shame and stigma, many patients who experience pain or impaired pleasure do not mention it to their health care professionals. Pleasure and pain may be particularly relevant to TGD individuals' health care needs, because a patient's experience of their body can deeply impact their sexual experiences. Trauma can lead to dissociative episodes that impair a patient's ability to experience pleasure or pain. Trauma responses may also lead to physical hypervigilance, causing increased musculoskeletal tension throughout the spine and pelvic floor; this tension can reduce the experience of pleasure and increase risk of injury. **Gender dysphoria** can similarly lead to dissociation and physical tension, thereby heightening negative sensations during sex. Additionally, painful sex can be a signal of treatable medical conditions, such as STIs, other infections, pelvic floor dysfunction, neuropathy, postoperative healing changes, and medication side effects. A wide range of medical interventions can impact a person's ability to feel pleasure during sex, the most common being antidepressant medications. All gender-affirming medical and surgical interventions can significantly affect sex in both negative and positive ways. There are some specific considerations to bear in mind for those experiencing changes in physical sensations or pain during sex and intimacy. Note that the effects listed below are risks and not at all universal outcomes of these interventions.

- Estrogen, androgen blockers: altered or reduced libido, fewer or less firm erections, thinned or nonexistent ejaculate, testicular aching

- Testosterone: altered or increased libido, clitoral swelling and sensitivity, increased incidence of vaginitis and urinary tract infections (UTIs) or dysuria

- Assigned Male at Birth genital reconstruction: change in orgasm sensation, different stimulation to orgasm, increased incidence of pelvic floor dysfunction, pain with penetration of neovagina due to granulation or scar tissue, changes in urinary stream and control, increased incidence of UTIs and dysuria

- Assigned Female at Birth genital reconstruction: change in orgasm sensation, different stimulation to orgasm, increased incidence of pelvic floor dysfunction and pelvic pain, changes in urinary stream and control, increased incidence of UTIs and dysuria

- Gonadectomy: fatigue, change in libido, hot flashes (both), erectile changes (orchiectomy) and vaginal dryness, vaginitis, UTIs (oopherectomy);

- Hysterectomy: possible increase in vaginitis, postoperative pain

It is important to remember that the majority of TGD people who engage in sexual activity report satisfaction with sexual functioning and are able to achieve orgasm, regardless of whether they have had genital surgery.[38] Accordingly, impaired orgasm and sexual pain or dysfunction should not be assumed to be solely related to gender-affirming medical or surgical interventions. Such concerns should be fully evaluated. It is important to note, however, that sexual satisfaction is not always centered on achieving orgasm and should be defined by the patient. Although an assessment of sexual function may seem like a time-consuming endeavor, it is nonetheless an important component of a patient's overall health and well-being and worth the health care professional's attention. Straightforward questions can open the topic with ease. Because pleasure and pain are such large topics to discuss, it may be wise to dedicate an entire patient encounter to this subject.

- "Are you able to enjoy your sex life?"
- "Do you experience any pain during sex or intimacy?"
- "Is orgasm important to your sex life? Are you able to experience orgasm, either alone or during partnered sex?"

Protection from STIs and HIV

Safer sex behaviors rely heavily on access to health care and education, as well as multiple social and economic factors like family support and financial stability. Marginalization at systemic, institutional, and interpersonal levels leads to increased experiences of trauma due to violence, as well as substance use disorder, both of which can increase risky sex practices such as unprotected receptive anal intercourse.[39,40] Furthermore, a marginalized sex industry means that sex workers may engage in condomless sex to satisfy the requirements of maintaining survival income. An additional barrier to protection from STIs is that most HIV prevention strategies have been formulated with cisgender men who have sex with other cisgender men in mind. These strategies have been shown to be insufficient to meet the needs of the TGD community, particularly Black trans feminine people, who are 50 times more likely to contract HIV than the general population.[41] For these reasons, it is important to have community members who are affected by HIV at the table when preventive strategies are being formulated. In the individual clinical encounter, it is important to check in with patients about what safer sex practices they are currently using and if not, identify barriers and troubleshoot with them about possible changes. Offering protection like condoms, lubricant, and dental dams for free in the office is very important. All health care professionals should feel comfortable discussing and prescribing **preexposure prophylaxis (PrEP)** against HIV. Nonoccupational postexposure prophylaxis against HIV, or nPEP, should be offered as well, with workflows to allow patients to access this therapy as soon as possible after an exposure. If a clinic consults with affected community members about best practices to reach the intended target population, they should be paid for this work. Community outreach programs should be helmed by these same community members to improve the chance of success.

Starting the conversation about safer sex practices is best done using a straightforward, affirmative approach:

- "Are you interested in discussing ways to protect yourself against STIs?"
- "What percentage of the time do you use condoms [or dental dams, other barriers] during sex? 50%? 25%? Do you understand how these things work to protect you

from STIs?" "What prevents you from using condoms during sex?"

- "Do you know about the pill that protects against getting HIV?"

Past History of STIs

The most significant predictor of a patient's future STI risk is having had an STI in the past. For all of the reasons stated above, TGD people have a higher rate of STIs than the general population.[42,43] A history of syphilis, rectal gonorrhea, or genital herpes puts patients at a higher risk of contracting HIV in the future. Unprotected receptive anal intercourse confers a 14-fold higher risk for acquiring HIV than insertive anal and receptive vaginal intercourse taken together. Unprotected insertive vaginal intercourse carries twice the risk for HIV acquisition than receptive vaginal intercourse.[44] Therefore, the anatomy involved in sex is the primary concern for risk assessment. Open-ended and anatomy-driven questions about sexual practices and partners, as outlined above, are critical. The following questions about STI history are direct and affirmative:

- "Have you ever been treated for an STI?"
- " Do you know if any of your contacts have an STI?"

Pregnancy Considerations

Although research about pregnancy intention and reproductive planning in the TGD community is sparse, surveyed patients have reported wanting to know more from their medical professionals. TGD people often want to have children and deserve access to information on assisted reproduction, adoption, and foster parenting.[45] Although gender-affirming hormones can impair fertility, many TGD people have successfully used their gametes to achieve pregnancy, both with and without assisted reproduction. It is also important to educate TGD people on potential risks of pregnancy and methods of pregnancy prevention if they do not wish to have a child. In the United States, 45% of pregnancies are unintended, which increases the risk of the carrying parent's mortality as well as infant health outcomes.[46] People who are on gender-affirming hormones can either impregnate or become pregnant if they are engaging in penile-vaginal intercourse. For sperm-producing people, any ejaculate deposited into a partner's vagina can carry sperm that may fertilize an egg, regardless of whether their ejaculate has diminished in amount or changed in color or consistency. For people with ovaries, ovulation can occur even if they are amenorrheic or have therapeutic levels of testosterone. Should a pregnancy occur while a patient is on testosterone, the testosterone can have a teratogenic effect on the fetus and should be immediately stopped if the pregnancy is desired. Options counseling and referrals should be used in the event of pregnancy. It is important to assess for pregnancy intention at regular intervals with all patients, as intention can change with time and circumstances.

- "Do you plan on having children in the next year?"
- "Do you have any kinds of sex that can lead to pregnancy, bearing in mind that hormones are not sufficient birth control?"
- "Are you interested in discussing pregnancy planning or prevention today?"

See Chapter 19, "Reproductive Health, Obstetric Care, and Family Building," for more information about contraception, pregnancy, and other aspects of reproductive health and family building.

Power Dynamics and Partner Violence

TGD people experience violence, including **intimate partner violence (IPV)**, at much higher rates than their cisgender peers due to antitrans bias and systemic risk factors.[47] Furthermore, IPV is particularly damaging to TGD communities because legal assistance, criminal justice pathways, and social services are often inadequate and even harmful when TGD victims seek support—especially if they are members of marginalized and stigmatized racial or ethnic groups.[48,49] Screening for IPV reduces the incidence of physical and emotional violence through increased uptake of helpful interventions. It is important to be aware of TGD-specific resources in your community, as mainstream organizations may be insufficiently trained to meet the needs of the TGD community. Universal IPV screening of all patients is recommended, but it is critical to ensure that this measure sufficiently reaches your TGD patients with gender- and sexuality-inclusive language:

- "In the past year, did a current or former partner…"
- "…make you feel cut off from others, trapped, or controlled in a way that you did not like?"
- "…make you feel afraid that they might try to hurt you in some way?"
- "…pressure or force you to do something sexual that you didn't want to do?"
- "…hit, kick, punch, slap, shove, or otherwise physically hurt you?"

HOW TO REPAIR A MISSTEP

For many, shifting from existing practices to an affirming framework can be difficult. Cis-heteronormativity has been deeply centered in most aspects of culture and society. It may take time for health care professionals to adapt their terminology to be gender- and sexuality-inclusive. Mistakes and missteps happen, so health care professionals must plan for recovery to alleviate patient distress and maintain the relationship. In the event of a negative event, the health care professional should apologize swiftly and simply and proceed with the encounter. Doing anything more centers the health care professional and may increase the level of non-affirmation the patient may be experiencing. Efforts should be made not to repeat the mistake, which may lead to further distress for the patient. It is important for all health care professionals to undergo basic training in transgender health care and terminology to minimize the risk of patient non-affirmation.

SUMMARY

- A thorough understanding of patients' sexual histories and sex lives is a fundamental component of comprehensive, high-quality health care.

- Patients from marginalized groups, including TGD people, may enter clinical encounters with suspicion and guardedness due to traumatic prior experiences; it is the clinician's responsibility to help patients feel safe and empowered in the clinical space, which is crucial to effectively obtaining an sexual history.

- Health care professionals should avoid assumptions about the gender, reproductive anatomy, and sexual behaviors of their patients, and must approach obtaining a sexual history in an anatomy-based, gender- and sexuality-inclusive way.

- Holistic evaluation of patients' sexual health and history includes the eight P's: Preferences, Partners, Practices, Pleasure/Pain, Protection from STIs, Past History of STIs, Pregnancy Considerations, and Power Dynamics and Partner Violence.

► Case Study 3: LB

LB, a Black, 30-year-old, masculine-presenting person wearing a suit, had been struggling with a cough for 3 weeks. He was very reluctant to seek medical care due to countless bad experiences with health care professionals in the past. Nonetheless, he felt sick enough to schedule an appointment at a nearby free clinic. As part of the intake paperwork, LB was asked which pronouns he wanted to be used for him, and he wrote "he/him/his." Soon, a physicians' assistant named Jerry came to interview him. Jerry asked LB the usual questions about his health, then moved on to the personal questions. "Do you mind sharing some personal information with me?" Jerry asked. LB had never been asked if he minded before, but it felt nice to be consulted first. He said he did not mind. Jerry then asked, "Before I ask you any questions, what terms should I use to talk about your bottom parts?" LB replied, "Well, I'd prefer you call my front part my 'front hole' and my back part my 'back hole,' but everything else is ok I guess." Jerry asked him if he had one partner or more than one partner. LB thought for a second, "I have a

boyfriend, but sometimes we have sex with other people, like if we're at a party or something." Jerry: "What bottom parts does your boyfriend have?" LB chuckled nervously and replied, "He has a penis. All of my partners have penises." Jerry then asked, "Do penises go in your front or back hole, or both?" LB replied, "I only use my back hole for sex. Not the front." Jerry then asked, "Do you ever use drugs to help sex feel better? Like poppers or anything?" LB had never been asked this before, but nervously replied, "Uh, yeah, poppers, a little cocaine if it's around, sometimes crystal but I try not to mess with that stuff too much." Jerry nodded, then asked if LB would be willing to get an HIV test that day given he's been feeling run down and has had receptive anal intercourse with new partners lately. LB's test was negative, so Jerry took that time to discuss pre-exposure prophylaxis for HIV (PrEP) with him after he treated his cough.

► Discussion Questions

- Given what you've learned about LB, what factors might have contributed to his previous negative experiences with health care professionals? Why else might he be nervous and avoidant of care? Can you name his separate and intersecting identities that put him at risk for suboptimal medical care?

- How likely is it that you would explore a sexual history with a patient who presents with a benign-seeming cough? What are the benefits of Jerry obtaining a sexual history in this case? What could have been the consequences of Jerry *not* obtaining a sexual history?

- What steps did Jerry take to begin to build trust with LB? Did they work? How do you know?

- What do you imagine would be different about this case vignette if you were in Jerry's place? LB is a Black masculine-presenting person. If you were seeing LB in a clinic, how might your own race, gender, and appearance affect the clinician–patient relationship and aspects of this encounter?

- Jerry never explicitly asks about words LB uses to describe his gender or sexuality. Are these relevant? Do you find yourself making assumptions about these identities or being curious? What would be some potential benefits and consequences of explicitly inquiring about labels for sexual orientation and gender identity?

- LB reported recreational use of poppers and occasional use of cocaine. What follow-up assessment would be beneficial here? What are the risks and benefits of engaging LB in a motivational interviewing intervention around his substance use?

► Case Study 4: DJ

DJ thought it was time to go to the clinic to get her HIV levels checked, so she called to set up an appointment. She saw a new health care professional, Dr. G, who seemed ok. DJ wasn't going to tell them anything unless they asked, though. She was tired of doctors acting like she owed them her personal information. Dr. G asked her about her antiretroviral medication adherence, and DJ rolled her eyes and told them that yes, she takes her medications every day, and has done so consistently for 10 years. (DJ believes everyone suspects she doesn't take her meds the way she's supposed to and finds this frustrating.) Dr. G asked DJ if it was ok to talk about her sex life. DJ raised an eyebrow and said, "Why do you want to know?" Dr. G replied, "You don't need to tell me anything you don't want to. Sex is a really important part of people's health, and sometimes it's helpful to talk about it." DJ thought it over for a moment and said it would be ok to discuss sex, as long as it is relevant to the appointment. Dr. G then said, "Thank you for understanding. To start with, do you have sex with one partner or more than one partner?" DJ replied, "Depends on how you mean." Dr. G replied, "Well, what does sex look like for you?" DJ mulled it over and then said, "Well, it depends. I have a life partner who's a man. We have sex the old-fashioned way, like he goes into me. But I'm also an escort." Dr. G: "What do you mean when you say, 'he goes into you?' Can you be more specific about body parts?" DJ: "His penis or whatever. My vagina. I had the surgery a few years ago, so since then nothing goes into my back part." Dr. G: "Ah ok, thank you. I get it. When you are escorting, do you have sex the same way?" DJ: "Oh no, I'm a dominatrix who just bosses people around for money. I don't have any other sex partners." Dr. G: "Ok then. Do you have any concerns about STIs? Are you worried about transmitting HIV?" DJ replied that she had no concerns, that she has been virally suppressed for years, and neither she nor her partner are worried about that. "I don't have sex with anybody but my husband, and I know I'm his only partner." Dr. G replied, "That sounds great. I trust you to know what is best for your health. Remember that STIs usually don't have symptoms and that sometimes it's good to get checked even when you are confident in your partner. If you ever change your mind, I'm happy to help, no questions asked." DJ thanked Dr. G for their advice and exited the exam room, meeting her smiling husband in the waiting area.

▶ Discussion Questions

- What do you think of Dr. G's response to DJ's "Why do you want to know?" How might you have responded? What would you say to provide DJ with a rationale for obtaining a sexual history?

- How did Dr. G attempt to build trust with DJ? Did it work? How do you know?

- You learn halfway through this case vignette that DJ has "had the surgery" and has a vagina. How does learning this information affect your thinking about this case and her health needs? How, if at all, is her surgical history

relevant to her needs in this encounter? How, if at all, is it relevant to her sexual health overall?

- Dr. G decided to follow DJ's lead with regard to STI testing. What factors do you think contributed to that decision? What benefits and consequences are there to Dr. G's approach? Would you handle this differently? And if so, what are the potential benefits and consequences to your chosen approach?

REFERENCES

1. James S, Herman J, Rankin S, Keisling M, Mottet L, Anafi M. *The Report of the U.S. Transgender Survey.* National Center for Transgender Equality; 2016.
2. Johnston CD, Shearer LS. Internal medicine resident attitudes, prior education, comfort, and knowledge regarding delivering comprehensive primary care to transgender patients. *Transgender Health.* 2017;2(1):91-95.
3. Safer J, Chan K. Review of medical, socioeconomic, and systemic barriers to transgender care. In: Porestsky L, Hembree W, eds. *Transgender Medicine: A Multidisciplinary Approach.* Totowa, NJ: Humana Press; 2019:25-38.
4. Flores AR. How many adults identify as transgender in the United States? 2016. https://williamsinstitute.law.ucla.edu/publications/trans-adults-united-states/. Accessed November 15, 2020.
5. Adam S, Goodman M. Number of Americans who report knowing a transgender person doubles in seven years, according to new GLAAD survey. 2015. https://www.glaad.org/releases/number-americans-who-report-knowing-transgender-person-doubles-seven-years-according-new. Accessed November 15, 2020.
6. Vast majority of Americans know someone who is gay, fewer know someone who is transgender. 2016. https://www.pewforum.org/2016/09/28/5-vast-majority-of-americans-know-someone-who-is-gay-fewer-know-someone-who-is-transgender/. Accessed November 15, 2020.
7. Hagen DB, Galupo MP. Trans* individuals' experiences of gendered language with health care providers: recommendations for practitioners. *Int J Transgender.* 2014;15(1):16-34.
8. Kattari SK, Bakko M, Hecht HK, Kattari L. Correlations between healthcare provider interactions and mental health among transgender and nonbinary adults. *SSM Popul Health.* 2020;10:100525.
9. Barr SM, Snyder KE, Adelson JL, Budge SL. Post-traumatic stress in the trans community: The roles of anti-transgender bias, nonaffirmation, and internalized transphobia. *Psychology Sex Orientat Send Divers.* 2021 Advance online publication; doi: https://doi.org/10.1037/sgd0000500.
10. Richmond KA, Burnes T, Carroll K. Lost in translation: interpreting systems of trauma for transgender clients. *Traumatology (Tallahass Fla).* 2012;18(1):45-57.
11. Cicero EC, Reisner SL, Silva SG, Merwin EI, Humphreys JC. Healthcare experiences of transgender adults: an integrated mixed research literature review. *ANS Adv Nurs Sci.* 2019;42(2):123.
12. Lerner JE, Robles G. Perceived barriers and facilitators to health care utilization in the United States for transgender people: a review of recent literature. *J Health Care Poor Underserved.* 2017;28(1):127-152.

13. Heng A, Heal C, Banks J, Preston R. Transgender peoples' experiences and perspectives about general healthcare: a systematic review. *Int J Transgend.* 2018;19(4):359-378.

14. Sevelius JM, Keatley J, Calma N, Arnold E. "I am not a man": trans-specific barriers and facilitators to PrEP acceptability among transgender women. *Glob Public Health.* 2016;11(7-8):1060-1075.

15. Hines DD, Laury ER, Habermann B. They just don't get me: a qualitative analysis of transgender women's health care experiences and clinician interactions. *J Assoc Nurses AIDS Care.* 2019;30(5):e82-e95.

16. Dyer K, das Nair R. Why don't healthcare professionals talk about sex? A systematic review of recent qualitative studies conducted in the United kingdom. *J Sex Med.* 2013; 10(11):2658-2670.

17. Sherman MD, Kauth MR, Shipherd JC, Street RLJr. Provider beliefs and practices about assessing sexual orientation in two veterans health affairs hospitals. *LGBT Health.* 2014;1(3):185-191.

18. Nusbaum MR, Hamilton CD. The proactive sexual health history. *Am Fam Physician.* 2002;66(9):1705-1712.

19. World Health Organization. Defining sexual health: Report of a technical consultation on sexual health. 2006. https://www.who.int/reproductivehealth/publications/sexual_health/defining_sh/en/. Accessed November 15, 2020.

20. Avis NE, Zhao X, Johannes CB, Ory M, Brockwell S, Greendale GA. Correlates of sexual function among multi-ethnic middle-aged women: results from the Study of Women's Health Across the Nation (SWAN). *Menopause.* 2018;25(11):1244-1255.

21. *Male Sexual Dysfunction: Pathophysiology and Treatment.* CRC Press; 2007.

22. *Textbook of Female Sexual Function and Dysfunction: Diagnosis and Treatment.* John Wiley & Sons Ltd; 2018.

23. Rosen RC, Bachmann GA. Sexual well-being, happiness, and satisfaction, in women: the case for a new conceptual paradigm. *J Sex Marital Ther.* 2008;34(4):291-297; discussion 8-307.

24. Brody S. The relative health benefits of different sexual activities. *J Sex Med.* 2010;7(4 Pt 1):1336-1361.

25. Meystre-Agustoni G, Jeannin A, de Heller K, Pécoud A, Bodenmann P, Dubois-Arber F. Talking about sexuality with the physician: are patients receiving what they wish? *Swiss Med Wkly.* 2011;141:w13178.

26. Sobecki JN, Curlin FA, Rasinski KA, Lindau ST. What we don't talk about when we don't talk about sex: results of a national survey of U.S. obstetrician/gynecologists. *J Sex Med.* 2012;9(5):1285-1294.

27. Baldwin A, Dodge B, Schick VR, et al. Transgender and genderqueer individuals' experiences with health care providers: what's working, what's not, and where do we go from here? *J Health Care Poor Underserved.* 2018;29(4):1300-1318.

28. Murray B, McCrone S. An integrative review of promoting trust in the patient-primary care provider relationship. *J Adv Nurs.* 2015;71(1):3-23.

29. Halbert CH, Armstrong K, Gandy OHJr, Shaker L. Racial differences in trust in health care providers. *Arch Intern Med.* 2006;166(8):896-901.

30. How the bad blood started. In: Hannah-Jones N, editor. *The New York Times*; 2019.

31. Gudzune KA, Bennett WL, Cooper LA, Bleich SN. Patients who feel judged about their weight have lower trust in their primary care providers. *Patient Educ Couns.* 2014;97(1):128-131.

32. Roche K, Keith C. How stigma affects healthcare access for transgender sex workers. *Br J Nurs.* 2014;23(21):1147-1152.

33. Mizock L, Lewis TK. Trauma in transgender populations: risk, resilience, and clinical care. *J Emotional Abuse.* 2008;8(3):335-354.

34. Spade D. Some very basic tips for making higher education more accessible to trans students and rethinking how we talk about gendered bodies. *Radical Teacher.* 2011;92:57-62.

35. Peitzmeier SM, Bernstein IM, McDowell MJ, et al. Enacting power and constructing gender in cervical cancer screening encounters between transmasculine patients and health care providers. *Cult Health Sex.* 2020;22(12):1315-1332.

36. Centers for Disease Control and Prevention. A Guide to Taking a Sexual History. https://www.cdc.gov/std/treatment/sexualhistory.pdf. Accessed November 15, 2020.

37. Nadal KL, Davidoff KC, Fujii-Doe W. Transgender women and the sex work industry: roots in systemic, institutional, and interpersonal discrimination. *J Trauma Dissociation.* 2014;15(2):169-183.

38. Holmberg M, Arver S, Dhejne C. Supporting sexuality and improving sexual function in transgender persons. *Nat Rev Urol.* 2019;16(2):121-139.

39. Crepaz N, Marks G. Towards an understanding of sexual risk behavior in people living with HIV: a review of social, psychological, and medical findings. *AIDS.* 2002;16(2):135-149.

40. Ekstrand ML, Coates TJ. Maintenance of safer sexual behaviors and predictors of risky sex: the San Francisco Men's Health Study. *Am J Public Health.* 1990;80(8):973-977.

41. Baral SD, Poteat T, Strömdahl S, Wirtz AL, Guadamuz TE, Beyrer C. Worldwide burden of HIV in transgender women: a systematic review and meta-analysis. *Lancet Infect Dis.* 2013;13(3):214-222.

42. Nuttbrock L, Hwahng S, Bockting W, et al. Lifetime risk factors for HIV/sexually transmitted infections among male-to-female transgender persons. *J Acquir Immune Defic Syndr.* 2009;52(3):417-421.

43. Toibaro JJ, Ebensrtejin JE, Parlante A, et al. [Sexually transmitted infections among transgender individuals and other sexual identities]. *Medicina (B Aires).* 2009;69(3):327-330.

44. Patel P, Borkowf CB, Brooks JT, Lasry A, Lansky A, Mermin J. Estimating per-act HIV transmission risk: a systematic review. *AIDS.* 2014;28(10):1509-1519.

45. von Doussa H, Power J, Riggs D. Imagining parenthood: the possibilities and experiences of parenthood among transgender people. *Cult Health Sex.* 2015;17(9):1119-1131.

46. Finer LB, Zolna MR. Declines in unintended pregnancy in the United States, 2008-2011. *N Engl J Med.* 2016 Mar 3; 374(9):843-852.

47. Garthe RC, Hidalgo MA, Hereth J, et al. Prevalence and risk correlates of intimate partner violence among a multisite cohort of young transgender women. *LGBT Health.* 2018;5(6):333-340.

48. Kattari SK, Walls NE, Whitfield DL, Langenderfer-Magruder L. Racial and ethnic differences in experiences of discrimination in accessing health services among transgender people in the United States. *Int J Transgend.* 2015;16:68-79.

49. Seelman KL. Unequal treatment of transgender individuals in domestic violence and rape crisis programs. *SW Publications.* 2015;59.

Performing a Trauma-Informed Physical Examination

Sadie Elisseou
Jennifer Potter

INTRODUCTION

The physical examination is a core component of most medical encounters. For centuries, physicians have used the physical examination to determine the cause of a patient's symptoms and develop a treatment plan. Despite its critical role in patient care, the physical examination may potentially cause patients harm. Consider a patient sitting on a table, naked under a thin gown, answering personal questions, being touched by a stranger, and wondering what bad news they may discover about their health. This routine scenario makes patients physically and emotionally vulnerable and may provoke feelings of embarrassment, shame, or fear. The risk of discomfort is amplified when patients have experienced previous psychological, physical, or sexual **trauma**, including prior traumatic encounters in the health care system itself.

Some medical procedures are inherently uncomfortable for most patients. For example, in one study, 73% of presumed cisgender patients undergoing digital rectal examination for prostate cancer screening reported experiencing moderate or higher discomfort during the exam.[1] Such "sensitive" examinations can be more complicated for people with trauma histories: in another study, nearly one-half of presumed cisgender adult survivors of childhood sexual abuse reported experiencing triggered memories of abuse during pelvic examinations.[2] For **transgender and gender diverse (TGD)** people, physical examination may be particularly fraught due to high rates of exposure to previous trauma and physical and emotional vulnerability related to being asked to reveal body parts that are not concordant with gender identity.[3]

Sexual and gender minority (SGM) individuals are disproportionately burdened by trauma, stress, and violence, and are at increased risk of exposure to adversity on intrapersonal, interpersonal, and institutional levels.[4,5] In one survey, 98% of transgender participants ($N = 97$) experienced at least one potentially traumatic event, and 17.8% of those individuals reported clinically significant symptoms of **post-traumatic stress disorder (PTSD)**.[6] Higher rates of violence and **intimate partner violence (IPV)** represent important forms of trauma affecting SGM communities, though the narrative of adversity is more complex and embedded in social systems.[7] Community-focused **stigma** and **discrimination** are increasingly identified as causes of health disparities in marginalized populations.[8] They have been proposed as modifiable risk factors for the higher rates of poor physical health, disability, depressive symptoms, and perceived stress that are seen among transgender older adults.[9] On an individual level, internalized homophobia and transphobia and identity concealment contribute to gender minority stress and negative health outcomes.[10,11] Historically, the medical system has been a perpetrator of trauma among SGM people in many different ways, which include misgendering patients, labeling them as pathological, and outright refusing to provide them care. In a national survey on transgender discrimination, 24% of transgender respondents reported unequal treatment in health care settings, 33% did not seek preventive health services, and 19% reported being denied medical care altogether.[12]

SGM people comprise 4.5% of the general U.S. population; however, medical professionals to date have lacked adequate training in SGM patient care.[13] Clinicians are largely unaware of pertinent, potential findings on physical examination for TGD patients. This relative unfamiliarity may lead to surprise, fumbling, speaking or behaving inappropriately, or being unsure how to inquire about the physical characteristic without causing the patient offense. In addition to lacking proficiency with SGM health, clinicians generally find it challenging to deliver care for trauma survivors. Barriers may include lack of time, lack of perceived proficiency or comfort, and difficulty building trusting relationships.[14] Acknowledging gaps in knowledge and attempting to uncover underlying biases are key steps in moving forward in a patient-centered alliance.

Given the prevalence of trauma and its impact on health, what can be done to address it? **Trauma-informed care (TIC),** discussed in detail in Chapter 11, Basic Principles of Trauma-Informed and Gender-Affirming Care, is an organizational and treatment framework for providing quality care to survivors of trauma that fosters healing through safe and collaborative relationships. The concept emerged in the 1980s to address substance disorders among homeless cisgender women, using a systems-based approach to trauma and recovery.[15] TIC has since evolved into a rapidly growing social movement that encompasses the breadth of trauma-related experience for patients and communities in the healthcare system and beyond. It emphasizes physical and psychological safety for both health care professionals and survivors. The Substance Abuse and Mental Health Services Administration (SAMHSA) defines a trauma-informed system as one that realizes the widespread impact of trauma, recognizes the signs and symptoms of trauma, responds by fully integrating knowledge about trauma into practice, and resists retraumatization.[16] Resisting retraumatization is especially relevant during the physical examination, where inherent features of the clinical environment and maneuvers performed have increased potential to trigger memories of abuse and even cause new traumatization. SAMHSA's six guiding principles to a trauma-informed approach to patient care are: (1) Safety, (2) Trustworthiness and Transparency, (3) Peer Support, (4) Collaboration and Mutuality, (5) Empowerment, Voice, and Choice, and (6) Cultural, Historical, and Gender Issues.

Health care professionals have the opportunity to provide TIC in each of these categories, in a variety of ways, from the individual to the societal level. At its core, TIC requires us to shift from the traditional, pathologizing paradigm of "What's wrong with you?" to the compassionate inquiry, "What happened to you?"[17] Creating welcoming and affirming clinical environments, training staff in culturally sensitive terminology and use of chosen names and pronouns, and assessing personal biases are measures that can facilitate patient-centered care for all patients, including TGD patients.[18] Clinicians can also incorporate trauma-informed principles into the physical examination by creating a safe and trusting environment, using language and maneuvers that enhance patient autonomy and affirm choice, and avoiding triggering memories of previous maltreatment.

INCORPORATING A TRAUMA-INFORMED APPROACH INTO THE PHYSICAL EXAMINATION

A trauma-informed approach to the physical examination does not necessarily confer a radical shift in thinking or practice from the traditional method. At its core, TIC is a form of patient-centered care that is focused on empathy and communication. When a physical examination is trauma-informed, it is considerate—considerate of patient

preference, patient comfort, patient safety, and overall patient experience. TIC aims to deconstruct the preexisting power differential between patient and health care professional to align with the principle of "empowerment, voice, and choice." Clinicians who are newly learning about TIC may argue that they have been practicing TIC all along—and they may not be wrong. Consider routine practices such as handwashing, helping a patient out of a chair, providing a pillow for a patient's back, and adjusting the exam table to a comfortable position; these practices help build trust and reinforce a sentiment of care. The nearly universal use of drapes and curtains in exam rooms communicates respect for patient privacy. Even the clean, padded exam table sets a reassuring boundary between touch during the examination and conversing in chairs during the medical interview. Beyond these practices, however, there is still room for improvement of examination style, particularly for patients who are trauma survivors.

COMPONENTS OF A TRAUMA-INFORMED APPROACH TO PHYSICAL EXAMINATION

A trauma-informed approach necessitates an understanding of the importance of trauma screening, appropriate referrals, and avoidance of retraumatization. Certain aspects of trauma-informed physical examination are not intuitive; rather, they are learned skills. Ultimately, trauma-informed physical examination is about excellent communication between the examiner and the patient. In simple terms, be polite, explain what you are doing and why, ask permission before proceeding, be mindful of draping and positioning, and use gender-affirming language. Table 13-1 identifies specific strategies that can be employed before, during, and after a trauma-informed physical examination that are aligned with SAMHSA's six core principles of TIC. The following sections describe these strategies in more detail.

▶ Before the Examination

Screening for traumatic exposure before the physical examination is a valuable consideration for patients in any medical setting. At present, there are no standard recommendations for routine screening for trauma in all adults. The ultimate goal is for TIC to become a "universal precaution," a patient-centered protocol to be followed as standard care for all-comers.[19] Several tools have been developed to screen for signs and symptoms of PTSD, which may be used if adequate mental health resources are available for follow-up in a given clinical setting.[20] Clinicians can also consider asking patients a broader question, as demonstrated in Table 13-1. It is not necessary—and may not be appropriate—for the medical team to identify the details of a person's trauma history; however, knowing a patient's status can help to facilitate a trauma-informed physical examination and appropriate referrals for treatment, if needed.

Table 13–1. Trauma-Informed Strategies for the Physical Examination Aligned With SAMHSA's Six Guiding Principles[10,45,50]

SAMHSA's Six Guiding Principles to a Trauma-Informed Approach	Before the Examination	During the Examination	After the Examination
Safety	Consider screening for trauma. "Sometimes, people have experienced something difficult in childhood or as an adult that has had a lasting impact on physical or mental wellbeing. Do you think that is relevant for you?" Ensure effective non-verbal skills—speak clearly and slowly, appear engaged, maintain appropriate eye contact, sit/stand at eye level with the patient, avoid sudden movements, keep hands out of pockets, avoid blocking exit doors. Be aware of patient cues (e.g., tensing muscles, trembling, fidgeting, breathing heavily, appearing distracted or disinterested, crying), and respond appropriately. "I notice that you're tensing up. Is something making you uncomfortable?"	Be mindful of time spent during examination maneuvers that may be triggering, checking in with the patient as needed. "I'll be checking the teeth and gums now to make sure there are no signs of infection. This can take a minute. Please let me know at any point if you'd like a break." Respect personal space. "You can have a seat on the exam table. I'm going to stand here at your side to listen to the heart." Ensure patient privacy when the patient is undressing/dressing, and knock prior to re-entering the room. "I'm going to close this curtain and exit the room to allow you to change. I'll come back in a few minutes. I'll knock before I come in." Stay within the patient's eyesight. "Let's elevate the head of the exam table so that you can see better for this exam. We can also offer you a mirror if that would be helpful."	Establish a self-care plan if patient distress occurs, and arrange follow-up as appropriate. "Let's think of what you can do this afternoon to start feeling a little better, and I'll call you tomorrow to check in."
Trustworthiness and Transparency	Set an agenda for the exam, with the patient still clothed and seated in a chair. "I'd like to transition to the physical exam, where we'll be checking the heart and lungs. This will involve listening to the chest with a stethoscope, while you're sitting up and then lying down. In total, this should take about 5 minutes." Make it clear that this is standard procedure for all patients and is not being done for this patient alone. "This is a standard exam that we do for all patients who come in with symptoms of a sexually-transmitted infection, or STI."	Introduce each exam component, and explain why it is being done. "Next, I'll stand here at your side while we check the thyroid gland. You'll feel some firm pressure on the front of the neck. When you can, please swallow." Prepare the patient for sensations they may experience. "This tuning fork will feel like a vibration."	Discuss results, once the patient is seated in a chair in their regular clothes. "I did hear some wheezing when I listened to the lungs with my stethoscope. I think we should get a chest x-ray to make sure you don't have pneumonia."
Peer Support	Offer the presence of a chaperone, friend, or loved one. "Would you like anyone else to be present for this exam, such as a friend or loved one?"	Ensure that any chaperone and/or loved one is positioned to the patient's comfort. (To partner): "I'm going to ask you to have a seat over here, if that's alright." (To patient): "Does that feel ok for you?"	Offer relevant referrals as appropriate, based on positive screening tools and/or other disclosures of trauma exposure. "Sometimes speaking with others about difficult experiences can help in the road to recovery. How would you feel about speaking with a mental health specialist or a peer advocate?"

(Continued)

Table 13–1. Trauma-Informed Strategies for the Physical Examination Aligned With SAMHSA's Six Guiding Principles[10,45,50] (*Continued*)

SAMHSA's Six Guiding Principles to a Trauma-Informed Approach	Before the Examination	During the Examination	After the Examination
Collaboration and Mutuality	Identify any patient concerns, offering space for disclosure of trauma or prior negative experiences with the examination. "Are there concerns regarding the exam that you'd like to share with me before we move forward? Have you had any difficulties with this type of exam in the past?"	Check in periodically and as needed. "How are you doing?" Ask the patient to move clothing/draping on their own, when possible. "Could you please raise the pant leg to just above the knee so that we can see the rash? When we're finished, you can roll it back down."	Express thanks to the patient for their active participation. "Thanks very much for coming to this appointment and for helping me perform a thorough exam."
Empowerment, Voice, and Choice	Ask if anything can be done to enhance patient comfort. "Is there anything I can do to make you more comfortable?" Reassure the patient that they are in control of the pace and can stop at any time. "Let me know at any point if you feel uncomfortable, and we will stop—you are in control."	Consider alterations to physical exam technique to enhance patient autonomy and comfort. "Some people prefer to insert the swab privately, on their own—would that be helpful for you?" Ask permission before touching the patient. "I'm going to press on various parts of the ankle to make sure everything is intact. Is that alright?" Give the patient choices and freedom to adjust their physical environment. "You can have a seat wherever you're comfortable. I'm going to step out for a minute to bring you a handout about our patient portal. Would you like the door open or closed?"	Use open-ended inquiry to identify any patient questions. "What questions do you have?"
Cultural, Historical, and Gender Issues	Choose only to perform exam components that are medically necessary. "I've confirmed in your medical record that the cervix was removed during your recent bottom surgery. It is no longer necessary for you to be screened for cervical cancer." Acknowledge and validate any identified concerns expressed by the patient regarding the physical examination, and proceed only with patient permission. "I'm aware that this type of exam can be difficult for many people. Our goal is to keep you healthy, while also keeping you as comfortable as possible. What do you think we should do?"	Speak with gender-affirming and normalizing language. Use patient-identified pronouns and patient-determined terms for anatomy and gender-related paraphernalia. Extend sensitive language to written documentation of physical examination findings. "I want to make sure I'm using terms that feel right for you. How do you refer to your body parts?"	Offer after-care instructions and a follow-up plan that is clear and understandable to the patient. "I'm going to print out a summary of what we've discussed, and we'll review it together so that we're on the same page."

In the age of electronic health records, quality measures, and billing using medical documentation, clinicians often perform a head-to-toe physical examination for all medical follow-up visits. A trauma-informed approach would be to perform only those components of the physical examination that are deemed medically necessary, and to proceed with patient consent. What is considered "standard medical practice" is constantly evolving; examination components that were once considered medically necessary may no longer be viewed as such. For example, there is growing evidence that digital rectal exams may not provide helpful information during the secondary survey of Advanced Trauma Life Support (ATLS) protocols.[21,22] While pelvic exams were once performed routinely for asymptomatic, **cisgender** women, the American College of Obstetricians and Gynecologists (ACOG) now recommends using shared decision-making to perform a pelvic examination when indicated by medical history or symptoms.[23]

Deciding which components of the physical examination to perform should take into account sex assigned at birth, gender identity, body parts present, and the use of gender-affirming hormone therapies or surgeries. Clinicians should proceed with the examination after weighing potential harms (e.g., exposure, shame, discomfort) and benefits (e.g., aid in diagnosis, evidence-based or expert consensus-based screening) with the patient. At present, there is insufficient evidence to determine whether TGD persons are at an increased or decreased risk for certain cancers. Preventive health measures should include organ-specific cancer screening (e.g., age- and risk-appropriate cervical cancer screening for patients with a cervix). Patients should be screened for illness according to standard screening guidelines for each current body part, regardless of exposure to hormone therapy.[24] Programs such as the University of California-San Francisco Center of Excellence for Transgender Health provide resources to help clinicians determine which screening elements to perform.

Before examining a patient, the clinician should know about the presence or absence of sexual organs. This knowledge ensures that recommended preventive health measures are performed (e.g., cancer screening) and directs screening for and diagnosis of sexually transmitted infections (STIs). Clinicians can ask about sexual organs once for every patient, after first establishing rapport, which can be done as early as the initial visit. These questions can be repeated in the future if deemed necessary or appropriate. Framing this question may be challenging, as the conversation is generally considered sensitive and may be emotionally charged. Consider a broad transition statement to begin: "I ask all my patients about sexual health because it's an important part of our health overall. Is it all right for us to discuss that today?" To ensure the usage of the patient's correct pronouns, consider setting the example: "My name is ___, and my pronouns are ___. What are your pronouns?" To obtain an **anatomical inventory**, consider starting with a broad question: "What terms should I use or avoid when referring to your body?" Alternatively, consider: "I want to make sure that I'm providing healthcare that is specific to your own body's needs. Can you confirm which sexual organs you have, such as a penis, vagina, testes, cervix, etc.? This is a standard question we ask all our patients." As a general rule, it is best to use the terminology for body parts that a patient provides (Table 13-2). However, further assessment may be appropriate if these terms are self-critical or derogatory.[25]

A physical examination of sexual anatomy has the potential to either invoke or relieve **gender dysphoria** in TGD persons. For example, a trans masculine patient may experience emotional or psychological distress during an examination of retained anatomical structures that are not in alignment with their current gender identity. This experience may be vastly different from that of a trans feminine patient who has undergone gender-affirming vaginoplasty and has a postprocedure pelvic

Table 13–2. Suggested Trauma-Informed Alternatives to Common Language Used During the Physical Examination[17,37]

Sample Language	Suggested Trauma-Informed Phrasing
"For me" (e.g., "Lift up your shirt for me")	(Nothing) (e.g., "Could you raise the shirt to just below the bra, so that we can examine the abdomen?")
"Your" (e.g., "Your penis")	"The" (e.g., "The penis")
"Butt," "Boobs"	"Buttocks," "Breast," and/or patient-determined terms, as appropriate
"Vagina," "penis," "labia"	Patient-determined term or gender-inclusive term (e.g., "canal," "inside," "front," "back," "outer folds")
"Bed," "Sheet"	"Exam table," "Drape"
"Provocative tests"	"Additional tests"
"Gynecologic exam"	"Pelvic exam"
"Normal"	"Healthy"
"Stirrups"	"Footrests"
"Blades" of speculum, "probe"	"Speculum"
"That looks good."	"That looks healthy."
"I want to…"	"I am going to…," "Would it be ok if…"
"Look at"	"Check," "Inspect"
"Feel," "Touch," "Palpate"	"Examine," "Check"
"Don't let me…"	"Resist this motion."
"Push me away."	"Push forward."
"Push my finger out."	"Bear down and push, like you're having a bowel movement."
"Put up your arms like you're going to fight."	"Bend the elbows."
"Open your legs."	"Allow the knees to fall to the side."
"Now I'm going to come into you."	"I'm going to place the speculum now; you may feel some pressure."
"Pretend you're at the beach."	"Some find it helpful to take a deep, relaxing breath."
"Relax. Relax. Relax!"	"Allow the knees to relax."

examination. Some trans feminine patients may even request a pelvic examination because it has historically correlated with a "well-woman exam." In this circumstance, the clinician should explore the patient's wishes through compassionate inquiry and counsel them regarding medical procedures that are relevant for their individual needs. While TIC cannot be provided to TGD patients without gender-affirmative language and behaviors, physical examination components should not be performed for the sole purpose of gender affirmation without underlying medical necessity.

If a support person, chaperone, caregiver, or translator is present for the physical examination, they should be positioned in the room according to the patient's wishes (e.g., behind a curtain, if desired).[26] Confirm that this person is also comfortable in their positioning, keeping in mind that witnessing certain maneuvers (e.g. rectal exam) may be uncomfortable for some and may trigger painful memories. When examining a patient after an assault, recognize that persons accompanying the patient may actually be perpetrators of violence. The patient has the right to include or deny their presence during the examination, and any personal health information, including gender status, should not be discussed without the patient's explicit permission to do so.

Traditionally, a nonclinician member of the health care team (e.g., medical assistant) is present during a pelvic examination as a "chaperone" serving multiple roles. Chaperones can assist the clinician in the mechanics of the exam (e.g., setting up equipment, handing the clinician swabs during the speculum exam, labeling specimens); help reduce patient anxiety with friendly conversation or encouragement; and ensure that the interaction is ethical and safe as a third party. In their role in ensuring ethical practice, chaperones may be called on to provide legal testimony in the event of a future malpractice lawsuit. Clinicians should discuss the presence of a chaperone with patients before the examination: "I usually ask our medical assistant to join us and hand me the tools I need. Would it be all right if that person were here in the room today?" If a patient refuses to have a chaperone present, clinicians must respond using their best judgment while operating within the guidelines of their institution. For a variety of historical and legal reasons, certain clinical facilities have mandated the presence of a medical professional as chaperone for a breast, pelvic, or rectal examination for patients who identify as women. These types of policies should be reassessed to account for the prevalence of sexual violence and other forms of trauma among patients and clinicians of all genders.[3] A trauma-informed approach to any clinical encounter reinforces patient agency and choice and aims to foster physical, psychological, and emotional safety.

▶ During the Examination

The following sections explain techniques, approaches, and language that can be used during a trauma-informed physical examination.

Physical Examination Technique

It is important to be mindful of time spent during a particular examination component, so that the examiner is neither rushing nor lingering too long.[27] For example, if a patient reports a lump on the scrotum, it may be more efficient to ask the patient to identify its location for the examiner, rather than the clinician attempting to do so. Setting up the room ahead of time for a speculum exam can help expedite the examination, omitting the need to obtain or adjust equipment mid-procedure. While it is important to move steadily through each step of a pelvic exam, the examiner should take care to remove the speculum slowly to avoid surprise or pain. If a blood pressure measurement needs to be repeated, the patient's permission should be sought, and the examiner should try to minimize delays in inflating and deflating the cuff, which can resemble a restraint.[28] Forced oral sex is an under-recognized barrier to patients seeking routine dental care; therefore, requiring the patient to keep the mouth in an open, fixed position for an extended time should be avoided. Explaining what you are doing, offering breaks, and efficiently gathering data can communicate care and help minimize any patient distress.[29,54]

Small adjustments in the examiner's body positioning can help establish a feeling of safety in the room during a physical examination. For example, clinicians often stand hidden behind the patient when examining the thyroid gland or auscultating the posterior lung fields. The same information can be gathered while standing at the patient's side, within their field of vision. Rather than standing directly in front of a patient to auscultate the heart, the examiner can stand at the patient's side to allow them more personal space. Many health care professionals measure heart rate (i.e., pulse) while the patient's hand is resting in their lap. Consider having the patient rest their hand on their knee or next to them on the exam table, to avoid positioning the examiner's hand too close to the patient's groin.

Clear communication is vital in establishing a sense of safety and inclusiveness in the medical environment. It is appropriate to prepare the patient for sensations they might experience at each stage of the examination, such as vibration from a tuning fork or a tight squeeze from a blood pressure cuff. It is generally best to explain each component of the physical examination before it is performed to the patient. However, some trauma survivors may prefer not to know this information and request that the examination is completed as quickly as possible. Ultimately, a trauma-informed physical examination is collaborative when the patient and health care professional communicate about the process and make adjustments to meet the patient's individual needs.

Clinicians should consider alterations to standard physical examination procedures that might increase patient comfort and reduce emotional or physical distress that do not compromise the gathering of data. For example, a study of transgender men's preferences regarding cervical cancer screening identified the following potential modifications: (1) self-insertion of the speculum, (2) use of a pediatric speculum, (3) having a trusted support person as a chaperone,

(4) alternative positioning, and (5) use of antianxiety medications.[30] Self-collected frontal (vaginal) swabs for STI testing are preferred by some patients and may even provide enhanced sensitivity and specificity compared to physician-collected samples.[31] If a pelvic exam is deemed medically necessary for trans feminine patients with a neovagina, an anoscope or pediatric speculum may be more comfortable, as the neovagina has a blind cuff, lacking fornices and a cervix.[32] If a "transvaginal ultrasound" is performed as part of the medical evaluation, the patient should be offered the option of inserting the ultrasound probe themselves, rather than having the technician do so. Being open to such options, and having appropriate medical equipment available, can reduce the preexisting power differential between patient and health care professional and communicate a commitment to mutual respect and collaboration.

A clinician's touch during a medical visit can be interpreted anywhere along a spectrum from therapeutic to harmful. A touch of the forearm during a patient's poignant expression of sorrow can be a powerful demonstration of empathy when appropriate, while touch can also be the cause of litigation against clinicians in accusations of assault. A trauma-informed approach to the physical examination aims for touch to be healing and recognizes that, for many trauma survivors, no touch is considered routine. When touch is too gentle, it may be read as sexually suggestive, while a touch that is too firm may be interpreted as aggressive.[33] When standing directly at the patient's side to auscultate the posterior chest, consider placing fingers of an outstretched hand on the patient's shoulder, to reduce the surprise of touch by the stethoscope on their back.[34] Consider the same firm touch on the shoulder if moving a step behind the patient to reach for something, such as an otoscope or other tool, so that the patient still knows where you are in the room. Prior to inserting a finger, swab, or speculum in a genital or rectal orifice, start by placing the side of your hand or a few fingers several inches away, while telling the patient what they will feel next: "First you will feel my hand on the buttock" or "You will first feel my hand on the inner thigh." This procedure can help to reduce the surprise of touch in sensitive areas. When a physical examination requires that a seeing patient closes their eyes, be sure to explain the examination adequately beforehand, showing them any tools you will use while their eyes are still open. For example, when performing a monofilament test of the feet: "Next we are going to test sensation of the feet, using this plastic device (examiner uses it on their hand in front of the patient). With the eyes closed, please point to the foot I am touching."

Using Trauma-Informed Language During the Physical Examination

Language is a powerful tool that clinicians can utilize during the physical examination to enhance trauma-informed principles of safety, empowerment, and trustworthiness. Trauma-informed language should be easy to understand; avoid medical jargon, triggering imagery, and sexual connotation; minimize the power differential between patient and health care professional; accommodate patients who speak other languages; and aim to be professional rather than personal.[35] It is particularly important to ensure that the examiner speaks using the patient's self-determined terms. Clinicians should also refrain from comments that seem too personal, bring unnecessary attention to the patient's body, or seem to suggest that the clinician is taking pleasure in the examination. For example, instead of "now I want to look at your breasts," consider, "Next, I will examine the chest to make sure everything is healthy." Creating a trauma-informed space in the examination room requires language that is neutral and free of judgment. As TGD patients face both external and internalized scrutiny, normalizing all bodies can help to establish a therapeutic alliance, promote body positivity, and ultimately offer healing.

Physical Characteristics on Examination

Medical professionals have been traditionally trained to identify "normal" versus "abnormal" findings on physical examination using standard female and male prototypes. This approach poses a challenge to providing quality care for SGM patients, as findings that deviate from the norm may still be healthy. Many patients adjust their gender presentation using simple, mechanical means, with or without the addition of hormones or gender-affirming surgery (see Chapter 8, "Nonmedical, Nonsurgical Gender Affirmation"). Examples include tucking the testicles and penis using an undergarment called a "gaff," taping the penis back between the buttocks, and binding the breasts (for trans feminine people), and for trans masculine people, adding packing to the genitals, wearing padded bras, and using chest binders. These practices can carry certain health risks that may be assessed on physical examination. For example, prolonged use of a chest binder may lead to skin breakdown, and tucking the testicles has been associated with hernias and scrotal pain.[36,37] TGD people seeking an immediate, body-contouring effect may also inject silicone or other filler materials into the body, often without supervision from licensed professionals. The physical examination may reveal evidence of the risks of these practices, including infection, allergy, scarring, or disfigurement.[38] Alterations of speech may be noted during the physical examination, as some patients work with speech-language pathologists to achieve gender-affirming speech and communication. As nonsuicidal self-harming behaviors are more common among TGD people, particularly trans men, clinicians should be attuned to evidence of self-cutting, burning, and hitting.[39]

In partnership with primary care providers or specialists, adult patients can elect to pursue **gender-affirming** hormone therapy (GAHT) that alter anatomic function or appearance. These therapies may cause changes in baseline physical characteristics on examination and can be monitored and discussed with patients over time with primary care providers or specialists. TGD patients receiving feminizing hormone therapy with estrogen and an antiandrogen may observe breast development, feminine fat redistribution, and the reduction of muscle mass, body hair, libido, and testicular size.[40] TGD patients receiving masculinizing hormone therapy with testosterone may develop masculine fat redistribution, clitoromegaly, androgenic alopecia, acne, and an increase in muscle mass and body hair.[41] Note that testosterone therapy may also lead to vaginal atrophy and dryness, and adequate lubrication using a water-soluble, non–carbomer-based product can help to minimize local discomfort when performing a pelvic exam for trans masculine patients.

Finally, gender-affirming surgery is a growing practice and area of research. For some people, gender-affirming surgical procedures can be pivotal in relieving gender dysphoria. A range of surgical options may be considered, including mastectomy, breast augmentation, facial and laryngeal surgery, and genital surgery. Genital construction surgeries may include the following[16,42–44]:

- Vaginoplasty (creation of a neovagina) with or without labiaplasty (creation of neolabia) and/or clitoroplasty (creation of a neoclitoris)
- Orchiectomy (removal of the testes)
- Phalloplasty (creation of a neophallus)
- Hysterectomy (removal of the uterus) with or without salpingectomy (removal of the fallopian tubes) and/or oophorectomy (removal of the ovaries)
- Glansplasty (creation of a neoglans penis)
- Vaginectomy (vaginal mucosal ablation)
- Scrotoplasty (creation of a neoscrotum)
- Metoidioplasty (using local tissue to create a smaller phallus)

Chapter 9, "Surgical Gender Affirmation," provides a complete overview of the types of gender-affirming surgeries that are available, including surgical techniques and potential complications.

Managing Reactions During the Physical Examination

Both patients and clinicians may experience challenging thoughts or feelings during the physical examination. As TIC emphasizes safety for everyone in a health care organization, it is worthwhile to describe strategies for managing these reactions. If a patient demonstrates or verbalizes discomfort at any point, pause the examination and address the patient's individual need (see Table 13-1). Patients often prefer to proceed with the examination if the discomfort

---

BOX 13–1   Grounding Techniques to Use During a Physical Examination

Grounding Techniques

Speak in a calm voice and avoid sudden movements.

Ask (or remind) the patient where they are and what you are doing.

Use self-talk to emphasize safety (e.g., "I am safe right now").

Ask the patient to state what they observe in the room using their senses (e.g., objects, sounds, colors, smells, temperature).

Use counting or other tools for distraction.

Use somatosensory techniques (e.g., toe-wiggling, gripping a table, clenching fists, planting feet on the ground).

Use breathing techniques.

Offer the patient a drink of water, and extra gown, or a wet washcloth for their face.

Change the environment by bringing the patient into a different room.

---

is mild, particularly if it is physical in nature (e.g., shoulder pain during an examination to evaluate a rotator cuff injury). If a patient demonstrates severe discomfort, emotional distress, or evidence of dissociation (e.g., spacing out, appearing detached, starting to cry), stop the examination.[45] Grounding techniques can be used to help an emotionally overwhelmed person become aware of the present time and space (Box 13-1).[46–48] Additional information about assisting patients with grounding after the examination and before the end of the visit is provided in the section "After the Physical Examination."

Regardless of their expertise and experience, clinicians may still encounter unfamiliar findings on physical examination at times. Managing reactions to what is found on physical examination is, in part, an exercise in addressing one's implicit biases. TIC emphasizes the importance of respect, dignity, and collaboration in all patient-clinician interactions.[49] It involves resisting and not contributing to abuse, victimization, and structural stigma. When encountering a physical examination finding that is unexpected or unknown, consider enlisting the patient's help: "I notice that you're wearing a tight garment on your chest. I'm still learning—would you be comfortable telling me what it is and how you use it?" This type of question is likely to be received better than a perplexed look and asking, "What's this thing?" Taking a moment to respond thoughtfully, rather than reacting impulsively, is a skill that clinicians can exercise to aid in rapport-building and effective communication. Note that comments about patients' bodies that are intended to be complimentary may be inappropriate and interpreted as offensive (e.g., "Your boobs look great! You must be so glad you had that surgery!"). In general, sharing personal opinions about patient's bodies should be avoided to avoid stigmatizing the patient or being perceived as a voyeur. Take care not to overemphasize sexual organs during the physical examination, especially when not medically pertinent. Asking to see or lingering when examining patient bodies due to curiosity about anatomical findings or hormonal or surgical results is unprofessional and a form of harassment.[50]

For some clinicians, performing a physical examination with TGD patients may generate strong emotions toward the patient. For example, a physician with religious opposition to LGBTQIA+ rights may be at risk for providing suboptimal LGBTQIA+ care. Continual self-reflection is encouraged as a routine part of professional development in medicine. It takes skill to recognize when one's thoughts or feelings are due to personal matters, rather than those related to the patient. Working with trauma as a professional may lead to retraumatization, burnout, or vicarious trauma. Creating a social support network, engaging in self-care activities, and having a positive outlook can be helpful strategies for clinicians.[51] Sometimes, a single experience of examining a trauma survivor can generate strong feelings of empathy, sadness, or even hopelessness. Know that we do not speak about trauma without also speaking about resiliency. Exploring the patient's strengths, self-help strategies, and protective factors may be healing for both patient and health care professional. Healing can occur in healthy relationships, including those that take place in the health care setting. Offering verbal expressions of empathy, holding space for a patient's emotions, thanking them for sharing their experience, coordinating a relevant referral, and partnering with them for next steps can be life-changing. Sometimes, simply being present is enough.

▶ After the Examination

If a patient verbalizes or otherwise demonstrates emotional distress during the physical examination, take time afterward to help them reconstitute. Allow time for debriefing about their experience. This debriefing should be done once the patient has put on their regular clothes, is seated in a comfortable chair, and expresses readiness to talk. Reassure the patient that it is common for people who have experienced something difficult in the past to have a hard time with the physical examination; it should not be considered a sign of weakness or failure.[52] Develop a plan for self-care that they can use after leaving the office. Some options include speaking with a counselor, reciting a prayer, engaging in a soothing activity (e.g., aromatherapy, listening to music), or repeating a positive affirmation (e.g., "I am resilient," "I can do this"). If using guided imagery, ask the patient to identify what a safe space looks like for them. Avoid offering imagery to patients (e.g., "Just pretend you're at the beach"), because we cannot assume what images are or are not connected to a particular patient's trauma narrative.[53] Ensure that the patient is conscious of their current environment and that they have a plan for maintaining personal safety.[16] Consider scheduling a follow-up appointment in the near future explicitly to check in, without performing an additional physical examination. Future physical examinations should be done with advanced planning, informed consent, and adherence to basic trauma-informed principles. Finally, reaffirm to the patient your commitment to working together as a team to ensure that they receive the best possible care.[41]

PHYSICAL EXAMINATION FOLLOWING A SEXUAL ASSAULT

Sexual violence is a common and complex cause of trauma, with significant short- and long-term effects on patient health. Sexual assault is a broad term that includes unwanted genital touching, forced viewing of or involvement in pornography, and rape, the latter being a legal term referring to nonconsensual penetration of any bodily orifice with force or threat of force.[43] According to the 2015 National Intimate Partner and Sexual Violence Survey (NISVS), 43.6% of presumed cisgender women and 24.8% of presumed cisgender men in the United States experienced some form of contact sexual violence in their lifetime.[43] TGD people are at even higher risk—an astonishing 44% of trans men and women and 55% of individuals identifying as nonbinary are sexually assaulted at some point in their lifetime.[55] Immediately following a sexual assault, patients can present to an emergency department, urgent care setting, or primary care setting. Health care practitioners have a responsibility to follow a standard, established protocol for postassault care while keeping in mind additional best practices for TGD patients.

Various organizations have published detailed guidelines for the care of patients following a sexual assault.[46,47] A multifaceted approach involves participation by health care institutions, law enforcement agencies, courts, and other relevant organizations. Some health care facilities have access to professionals who are highly trained and experienced in responding to sexual assault, including sexual assault nurse examiners (SANE), rape crisis counselors, or sexual assault response teams (SART). Providing TIC following a sexual assault includes consideration of patient choice (e.g., accommodating preferences for gender of the health care professional, when possible, and allowing a loved one to be present, if desired), confidentiality, informed consent, establishing physical and psychological safety, providing explanation throughout the physical examination and respectfully allowing the patient to opt out, demonstrating cultural sensitivity, and responding empathically to a broad range of patient emotions.

Informed consent is first obtained, and the clinician interviews the patient about their general medical history and details of the assault, using a calm tone of voice and a nonjudgmental, empathic communication style.[16] The clinician then performs a head-to-toe physical examination to assess for acute traumatic injury, documenting all findings comprehensively and precisely, with the use of body diagrams or photographs (for which informed consent has been obtained). Medical records may serve as critical evidence in criminal proceedings. A trained team member may collect forensic evidence using a meticulous, multistep process. All patients with confirmed or presumed anogenital contact should be offered prophylaxis for STIs. Patients with a vaginal canal and uterus who have experienced penetration should be offered emergency contraception. Finally, the team arranges mental health and primary care follow-up as appropriate, with the understanding that one-third of sexual assault survivors may go on to experience PTSD (30%), depression (30%), and/or suicidal ideation (33%), as well as chronic physical ailments.[48,49]

All survivors of sexual assault should be asked about reproductive anatomy for the specific purpose of providing focused medical treatment, emergency contraception, and illness risk reduction. While determining risk for pregnancy is an important component of a postassault assessment, TGD adults may not visibly present as patients who require a "gynecologic history." Consider phrasing such as the following: "When people experience an assault, it's important for us to assess each person's unique needs. For example, a sexual assault may put us at risk for certain injuries, sexually transmitted infections, or even pregnancy. What reproductive body parts do you have, such as a penis, vagina, uterus, etc.? We ask this question because it will help us take care of you."

When assessing for injuries during a postassault physical examination, it is important to note that most rape-related injuries are found on areas of the body other than the genitalia. In one study, less than 30% of premenopausal women had genital injuries visible to the naked eye after nonconsensual penetration.[56] Therefore, the absence of anogenital lesions does not negate the occurrence of a sexual assault. Staff who work in a setting where assaults are frequently reported may witness health care professionals conveying skepticism as to whether a sexual assault truly occurred. This unfortunate consequence likely arises from a variety of complex factors. Ultimately, the determination of whether a sexual assault has taken place is not within the scope of the medical team. In a trauma-informed approach to postassault care, health care professionals should welcome all patients who disclose in an empathic, nonjudgmental manner and universally offer these patients the best practices in care.

Examination of the back, chest, breasts, external and internal genitalia, buttocks, and rectum can be particularly sensitive following an assault. In these circumstances, the health care professional should rely on the core principles of TIC and a framework for examining patients using a trauma-informed approach (see the section "Incorporating a Trauma-Informed Approach into the Physical Examination"). Ensure privacy for the visit by closing a curtain or door and by allowing the patient to change in and out of clothes privately. Be mindful of appropriate draping technique to preserve patient dignity, such as exposing only the minimum body surface area required at any time and replacing the drape before moving to other areas. Ask the patient to move their clothing, gown, or drape to facilitate the examination, rather than reaching to do so. If it would be more comfortable for the patient to have assistance (e.g., untying a gown with an arm injury), offer and await permission to help. Providing fabric gowns, whenever possible, may provide better coverage and comfort than paper gowns. In the setting of acute physical injury, it can be helpful to prepare the patient for uncomfortable sensations, such as pain with palpation of affected body parts. If a cervical swab is recommended for STI screening, consider self-collection of a blind swab if preferred by the patient. For examination components that require lubrication, provide tissues for the patient to use as needed.

A trauma-informed physical examination of sexual assault survivors must be accurate and thorough while also being patient-centered and gender-affirming. Health care professionals should recognize that some people may be wearing gender-affirming clothing or accessories, such as wigs or binders. These items may contain forensic evidence and need to be removed carefully to preserve evidence; they may also need to be removed to check the patient for injuries. Asking patients to remove these items must be done in a sensitive way. For example, removing a wig may exacerbate feelings of shame, vulnerability, and gender dysphoria. Clinicians can reassure the patient by explaining the underlying medical need and can strive to preserve patient dignity by providing privacy and using empathic, validating language: "Do you happen to be wearing a wig today? We ask this question so that we can check the scalp for any injuries. We understand that this might be difficult. Thank you for being patient with the process. We respect you, and our goal is to take care of you as best we can." If the patient insists on keeping the wig or other gender-related accessories, consider taking a sample or collecting a swab to contribute as forensic evidence. Some facilities offer clean clothes and underwear following a SAFE exam. Providing additional items, such as makeup, a wig, or a voucher for financial compensation of such items, may serve as a compassionate gesture and help preserve patient dignity.[49]

SUMMARY

- TGD patients experience increased rates and unique forms of stress, adversity, and trauma compared with cisgender patients. These experiences can have significant, lasting impacts on physical and mental health.

- Health care professionals have a responsibility to approach all patients with dignity and respect. Trauma-informed care (TIC) is a framework that helps clinicians partner with patients to enhance their sense of safety and empowerment in the health care setting.

- The physical examination has the potential to retraumatize trauma survivors. TGD patients may face additional difficulty due to negative prior experiences with the health care system, ongoing gender dysphoria, and higher rates of sexual assault and IPV.

- Clinicians can learn and use sensitive and effective language (e.g., patient's choice of anatomical terms; free of jargon, triggering imagery, and sexual connotation) and behavioral strategies (e.g., informed consent; patient-centered adaptations; grounding techniques) during the physical examination to mitigate vulnerability, communicate cultural sensitivity, and create a healing space.

CASE STUDY 1: Sidney Murphy

▶ Part 1

A 29-year-old U.S. military Veteran named Sidney Murphy is scheduled to see a primary care provider at a local U.S. Department of Veterans Affairs (VA) ambulatory clinic to establish care. Sidney is new to the VA system and is interested in obtaining treatment for service-related disabilities. An initial primary care visit, including a history and physical examination, is required to become vested and eligible for a range of VA services.

▶ Discussion Questions

1. What do you know about Sidney's identities and experiences? What do you not know?

2. How should you greet and personally address Sidney when you meet in the exam room?

3. What is your approach to soliciting Sidney's goals and expectations for the visit, as well as setting your own agenda for a history and physical examination?

▶ Part 2

During the medical interview, you learn that Sidney has been deployed twice and served in combat. Sidney states that "things have been really difficult" postdeployment due to severe headaches and mood swings. You reaffirm your commitment to evaluating and treating these health concerns. A brief review of the electronic health record reveals that Sidney was recently rated by the VA Compensation and Pension Department for service-connected disabilities, including PTSD and **military sexual trauma (MST)** [trauma caused by sexual assault or harassment experienced during military service]. As you transition to the physical examination, you wonder about the best approach.

▶ Discussion Questions

1. How relevant is the patient's history of PTSD and MST to your performing a head-to-toe physical examination?

2. How might you phrase your transition to the physical examination? Consider which body parts might be medically relevant to examine today and how to set this agenda with Sidney.

3. What can you ask to better understand the patient's prior experiences with physical examinations in order to inform the experience today?

▶ Part 3

Sidney has short hair and a tall stature, and is dressed in a baggy sweatshirt, baseball hat, and sweatpants. You recognize this as a typical appearance of other young, male Veterans you see in clinic. You ask Sidney to remove the sweatshirt and have a seat on the examination table. Sidney pauses, seeming suddenly uneasy. Slowly moving toward the table, Sidney does as you ask, and you are surprised to find that Sidney is wearing an athletic chest binder.

▶ Discussion Questions

1. What underlying biases are at play in the initial assumption that Sidney is a cisgender man?

2. How can you manage your own mental and physical reactions to discovering that Sidney has chest tissue?

3. How would you inquire about pronouns, gender identity, and presence of body parts prior to starting the physical examination?

4. How can the physical examination serve as a potentially healing experience for individuals who are grappling with body positivity?

5. Is it possible to predict which components of the physical examination might be triggering for Sidney? What universal precautions can you take to ensure that the overall experience feels safe for everyone in the room?

CASE STUDY 2: The Patient in Room 18

You are working a shift in the emergency room when a team member approaches you with a smirk to report, "Room 18 is another claim of sexual assault. Wait until you see this one!" You glance over to the exam room to find a patient crying in a chair and saying, "I knew I never should have come." The patient is a muscular person wearing a red dress, fishnet stockings, stiletto boots, and a pink wig.

▶ Discussion Questions

1. Should you address your colleague's remarks? If so, what might you say that would help this and other patients

receive trauma-informed care, while still fostering a positive working relationship?

2. Review the interpersonal, intrapersonal, and institutional factors that may have contributed to trauma in this patient and in TGD communities at large.

3. What are the core components of a standard examination immediately following a sexual assault?

4. Describe your overall approach to examining body parts and gender-related prostheses that may be sensitive in this patient.

REFERENCES

1. Romero FR, Romero AW, Brenny Filho T, Bark NM, Yamazaki DS, de Oliveira FCJ. Patients' perceptions of pain and discomfort during digital rectal exam for prostate cancer screening. *Arch Esp Urol.* 2008;61(7):850-854.

2. Robohm JS, Buttenheim M. The gynecological care experience of adult survivors of childhood sexual abuse: a preliminary investigation. *Women Health.* 1996;24(3):59-75.

3. Potter J, Peitzmeier SM, Bernstein I, et al. Cervical cancer screening for patients on the female-to-male spectrum: a narrative review and guide for clinicians. *J Gen Intern Med.* 2015;30(12):1857-1864.

4. McKinnish T, Burgess C, Sloan C. Trauma-informed care of sexual and gender minority patients. In: Gerber M, ed. *Trauma-Informed Healthcare Approaches.* Switzerland, UK: Springer; 2019:93.

5. Poteat T, Singh A. Conceptualizing trauma in clinical settings: iatrogenic harm and bias. In: *Trauma, Resilience, and Health Promotion in LGBT Patients: What Every Healthcare Provider Should Know.* Cham: Springer International Publishing; 2017:26.

6. Shipherd JC, Maguen S, Skidmore WC, Abramovitz SM. Potentially traumatic events in a transgender sample: frequency and associated symptoms. *Traumatology.* 2011;17(2):56-67.

7. Alessi E, Martin J. Intersection of trauma and identity. In: Eckstrand K, Potter J, eds. *Trauma, Resilience, and Health Promotion in LGBT Patients: What Every Healthcare Provider Should Know.* Cham: Springer International Publishing; 2017:9.

8. Meyer IH. Prejudice, social stress, and mental health in lesbian, gay, and bisexual populations: conceptual issues and research evidence. *Psychol Bull.* 2003;129(5):674-697.

9. Fredriksen-Goldsen KI, Cook-Daniels L, Kim H-J, et al. Physical and mental health of transgender older adults: an at-risk and underserved population. *Gerontologist.* 2014;54(3):488-500.

10. Meyer IH. Prejudice, social stress, and mental health in lesbian, gay, and bisexual populations: conceptual issues and research evidence. *Psychol Bull.* 2003;129(5):674-697.

11. Hendricks ML, Testa RJ. A conceptual framework for clinical work with transgender and gender nonconforming clients: an adaptation of the Minority Stress Model. *Prof Psychol Res Practice.* 2012;43(5):460-467.

12. Grant J, Mottet L, Tanis J, Harrison J, Herman J, Kiesling M. Injustice at every turn: a report of the National Transgender Discrimination Survey. http://www.thetaskforce.org/static_html/downloads/reports/ reports/ntds_full.pdf.

13. LGBT Data & Demographics—The Williams Institute. https://williamsinstitute.law.ucla.edu/visualization/lgbt-stats/?topic=LGBT#density.

14. Bergman AA, Hamilton AB, Chrystal JG, Bean-Mayberry BA, Yano EM. Primary care providers' perspectives on providing care to women veterans with histories of sexual trauma. *Womens Health Issues.* 2019;29(4):325-332.

15. Fallot RD, Harris M. The Trauma Recovery and Empowerment Model (TREM): conceptual and practical issues in a group intervention for women. *Community Ment Health J.* 2002;38(6):475-485.

16. SAMHSA's Concept of Trauma and Guidance for a Trauma-Informed Approach. 27.

17. Bloom S. The sanctuary model: developing generic inpatient programs for the treatment of psychological trauma. In: Williams M, Sommer J, eds. *Handbook of Post-Traumatic Therapy, a Practical Guide to Intervention, Treatment, and Research.* Connecticut, US: Greenwood Publishing; 1994:474-449.

18. Klein DA, Paradise SL, Goodwin ET. Caring for transgender and gender-diverse persons: what clinicians should know. *AFP.* 2018;98(11):645-653.

19. Gerber M, Gerber E. An introduction to trauma and health. In: Gerber M, ed. *Trauma-Informed Healthcare Approaches.* Switzerland, UK: Springer; 2019:3.

20. Prins A, Bovin MJ, Smolenski DJ, et al. The Primary Care PTSD Screen for DSM-5 (PC-PTSD-5): development and evaluation within a veteran primary care sample. *J Gen Intern Med.* 2016;31(10):1206-1211.

21. Esposito TJ, Ingraham A, Luchette FA, et al. Reasons to omit digital rectal exam in trauma patients: no fingers, no rectum, no useful additional information. *J Trauma.* 2005;59(6):1314-1319.

22. Docimo S, Diggs L, Crankshaw L, Lee Y, Vinces F. No evidence supporting the routine use of digital rectal examinations in trauma patients. *Indian J Surg.* 2015;77(4):265-269.

23. The utility of and indications for routine pelvic examination. https://www.acog.org/en/Clinical/Clinical Guidance/Committee Opinion/Articles/2018/10/The Utility of and Indications for Routine Pelvic Examination.

24. General approach to cancer screening in transgender people | Transgender Care. https://transcare.ucsf.edu/guidelines/cancer-screening.

25. Bates CK, Carroll N, Potter J. The challenging pelvic examination. *J Gen Intern Med.* 2011;26(6):651-657.

26. Schachter C, Stalker C, Danilkewich A, Teram E, Lasiuk G. *Handbook on Sensitive Practice for Health Care Practitioners: Lessons from Adult Survivors of Childhood Sexual Abuse—Principles of Sensitive Practice*; 2008. https://www.canada.ca/en/public-health/services/health-promotion/stop-family-violence/prevention-resource-centre/children/handbook/handbook-sensitive-practice-health-care-practitioners-lessons-adult-survivors-childhood-sexual-abuse-13.html.

27. Schachter J, Chernesky MA, Willis DE, et al. Vaginal swabs are the specimens of choice when screening for Chlamydia trachomatis and Neisseria gonorrhoeae: results from a multicenter evaluation of the APTIMA assays for both infections. *Sex Transm Dis.* 2005;32(12):725-728.

28. Reisner SL, Deutsch MB, Peitzmeier SM, et al. Test performance and acceptability of self- versus provider-collected swabs for high-risk HPV DNA testing in female-to-male trans masculine patients. *PLoS One.* 2018;13(3):e0190172.

29. Peitzmeier S, Gardner I, Weinand J, Corbet A, Acevedo K. Health impact of chest binding among transgender adults: a community-engaged, cross-sectional study. *Cult Health Sex.* 2017;19(1):64-75.

30. Wesp L. Transgender patients and the physical examination. In: Deutsch MB, ed. *UCSF Transgender Care*. 2nd ed.; 2016:21-22.

31. Aguayo-Romero RA, Reisen CA, Zea MC, Bianchi FT, Poppen PJ. Gender affirmation and body modification among transgender persons in Bogotá, Colombia. *Int J Transgend*. 2015;16(2):103-115.

32. Marshall E, Claes L, Bouman WP, Witcomb GL, Arcelus J. Nonsuicidal self-injury and suicidality in trans people: a systematic review of the literature. *Int Rev Psychiatry*. 2016;28(1):58-69.

33. Vaginoplasty procedures, complications and aftercare | Transgender care. https://transcare.ucsf.edu/guidelines/vaginoplasty.

34. Phalloplasty and metoidioplasty: overview and postoperative considerations | Transgender care. https://transcare.ucsf.edu/guidelines/phalloplasty.

35. Hysterectomy | Transgender care. https://transcare.ucsf.edu/guidelines/hysterectomy.

36. Transgender Health Care Nexus. Understanding the transgender and gender-diverse physical exam. Published online 2018. TransgenderHealth.com.

37. Peitzmeier SM, Potter J. Patients and their bodies: the physical exam. In: Eckstrand K, Potter J, eds. *Trauma, Resilience, and Health Promotion in LGBT Patients: What Every Healthcare Provider Should Know*. Cham: Springer International Publishing; 2017:195-196.

38. Sexual Trauma: Information for Women's Medical Providers—PTSD. National Center for PTSD. https://www.ptsd.va.gov/professional/treat/type/sexual_trauma_women.asp.

39. Melnick SM, Bassuk EL. Identifying and responding to domestic violence among poor and homeless women. 22.

40. Sciolla A. An overview of trauma-informed care. In: Eckstrand K, Potter J, eds. *Trauma, Resilience, and Health Promotion in LGBT Patients: What Every Healthcare Provider Should Know*. Cham: Springer International Publishing; 2017:177.

41. Peitzmeier SM, Potter J. Patients and their bodies: the physical exam. In: Eckstrand K, Potter J, eds. *Trauma, Resilience, and Health Promotion in LGBT Patients: What Every Healthcare Provider Should Know*. Cham: Springer International Publishing; 2017:192.

42. Katsounari I. The road less traveled and beyond: working with severe trauma and preventing burnout. *Burnout Research*. 2015;2(4):115-117.

43. Linden JA. Care of the adult patient after sexual assault. *N Engl J Med*. 2011;365(9):834-841.

44. The National Intimate Partner and Sexual Violence Survey: 2015 Data Brief—Updated Release. 32.

45. James SE, Herman JL, Rankin S, Keisling M, Mottet L, Anafi M. The Report of the 2015 U.S. Transgender Survey. National Center for Transgender Equality. Published online 2016.

46. A National Protocol for Sexual Assault Medical Forensic Examinations, Adults/Adolescents. Washington, DC: Department of Justice. Published online 2004.

47. WHO | Guidelines for medico-legal care for victims of sexual violence. WHO. https://www.who.int/violence_injury_prevention/publications/violence/med_leg_guidelines/en/. Accessed October 23, 2020.

48. National Victim Center. *Rape in America: A Report to the Nation*. National Victim Center; 1992.

49. Paras ML, Murad MH, Chen LP, et al. Sexual abuse and lifetime diagnosis of somatic disorders: a systematic review and meta-analysis. *JAMA*. 2009;302(5):550-561.

50. Bowyer L, Dalton ME. Female victims of rape and their genital injuries. *BJOG: Int J Obstet Gynaecol*. 1997;104(5):617-620.

51. Peitzmeier SM, Potter J. Patients and their bodies: the physical exam. In: Eckstrand K, Potter J, eds. *Trauma, Resilience, and Health Promotion in LGBT Patients: What Every Healthcare Provider Should Know*. Cham: Springer International Publishing; 2017:200.

52. Sadie E, Sravanthi P, Meghna N. A novel, trauma-informed physical examination curriculum for first-year medical students. *MedEdPORTAL*. 2019;15. https://www.mededportal.org/doi/10.15766/mep_2374-8265.10799.

53. Ravi A, Little V. Providing trauma-informed care. *AFP*. 2017;95(10):655-657.

54. Stalker CA, Carruthers-Russell BD, Teram E, Schachter CL. Providing dental care to survivors of childhood sexual abuse. Treatment considerations for the practitioner. *J Am Dent. Assoc*. 2005;136:1277-1281.

55. James SE, Herman JL, Rankin S, Keisling M, Mottet L, Anafi M. (2016). The Report of the 2015 U.S. Transgender Survey. Washington, DC: National Center for Transgender Equality.

56. Bowyer L, Dalton ME. Female victims of rape and their genital injuries. *Br J Obstet Gynaecol*. 1997;104:617-620.

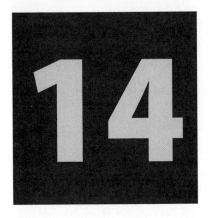

Recognizing and Addressing Intimate Partner Violence

Xavier Quinn

INTRODUCTION

Although there is a dearth of research on **transgender and gender diverse (TGD)** people and **intimate partner violence (IPV)**, current research suggests rates much higher than those of straight, **cisgender** women, with 30%–50% of TGD people experiencing IPV compared to 28%–33% in the general population.[1] IPV is also known as domestic violence, dating violence, or partner abuse. The Network/La Red, an organization at the forefront of work with **LGBTQIA+** survivors, defines partner abuse as "a systematic pattern of behaviors where one person tries to control the thoughts, beliefs, and/or actions of their partner.[2]" Included in their definition is the recognition that aside from partners, the abusive person can be "someone they are dating or someone they had an intimate relationship with.[3]" The Network/La Red suggests using the term "survivor" for a person who is experiencing or has experienced abuse from their partner explaining, "for many who have experienced abuse, "survivor" can be much more empowering than "victim.[2]" Additionally, the words "victim" and "perpetrator" are inaccurate and sometimes dangerous to use as they are legal terms that refer to "single incidences of criminal behavior" rather than a pattern of power and control.[2]

While this definition of IPV may be accurate if there is an act of physical violence, many of the tactics of abuse explored in this chapter are not criminal in nature.[2] Additionally, a survivor may use violence to resist abuse, which may legally make them the perpetrator of a crime.[2] For these reasons, they suggest using the terms "abuser" or "abusive partner" to identify the person in the relationship choosing to use "nonconsensual power over their partner."[2]

Attention to IPV by nonprofits, medical organizations, and police has been relatively recent, only unfolding in the past 40 years through the work of feminists bringing the issue to public consciousness.[3] Even as awareness has grown, the majority of the narratives told about IPV focus on straight cisgender women as the survivors, victimized by straight cisgender heterosexual men.[3] Through the work of LGBTQIA+-specific programs such as The Network/La Red, The Northwest Network, and the National Coalition of Anti-Violence Programs, there is a growing awareness that LGBTQIA+ individuals can also be survivors of IPV. Much of the research on LGBTQIA+ survivors of IPV, however, has focused on cisgender gay men and lesbian women. Studies focused specifically on the experiences of TGD people have only emerged recently. Because of this, existing knowledge on the specific experiences of TGD people must be drawn from a combination of the limited existing research, the organizations that specialize in supporting TGD survivors of IPV, and the stories of survivors themselves.

Given the general lack of awareness of the experiences of TGD survivors, it is not surprising that one study shows that 27% of trans survivors did not identify their experience as IPV.[4] Therefore, raising awareness of this issue is a key element in getting survivors the services they need. Medical and mental health care professionals are in a unique role to identify and support TGD survivors of IPV, yet are often unequipped to do so. One trans survivor speaks to this phenomenon: "[Health care professionals could use] **lots** more education and understanding about transgender issues, the variety of experience, and the unique way it may impact the way we feel or cope as survivors."[5] This chapter aims to familiarize health care professionals with the dynamics of IPV, the tactics perpetrators use to target TGD individuals, methods clinicians can use to screen for IPV in medical or mental health settings, and how to respond to disclosure in helpful and supportive ways.

THE CYCLE OF VIOLENCE

Understanding IPV starts with understanding the **cycle of violence** (Figure 14-1). Domestic violence survivors first conceptualized the cycle of violence in the 1970s, and since

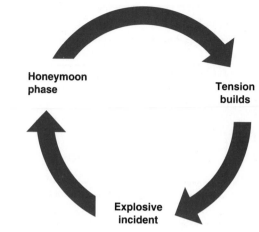

▲ **Figure 14-1.** Cycle of violence.

then, it has become a useful model to help IPV survivors understand their experiences.[6] Although this model may not fit all survivors, many report finding their experience echoed in the cycle. The first phase in the cycle is often called the "honeymoon stage" or "hearts and flowers," reflecting the early part of the relationship. During this time, the abusive partner is on their best behavior, showing attention and affection.[2] At some point, tension starts to build, moving the cycle into the second phase. The survivor will often notice a feeling of "walking on eggshells" or trying to avoid upsetting their partner.[2] This tension continues to build until phase three, the "explosive incident," when the abusive partner uses one or more tactics of abuse.[2] These tactics can include emotional, financial, sexual, physical, and identity-based abuse. For example, the explosive incident could be the abusive partner screaming at the survivor in public, stealing their money, threatening them, sexually assaulting them, or physically attacking them. It is at this point in the cycle that a survivor is most likely to identify the abuse or consider leaving the relationship. Because of this shift in awareness, the abusive partner quickly returns to phase one, the "honeymoon" stage, offering apologies or promises to change, returning to affectionate behavior, or lulling the survivor into a sense that the recent incidents were just a temporary loss of control.[2] However, the tension begins to build again, leading to another set of abusive incidents.[2] Rotation through the cycle of abuse can happen in as quickly as a few minutes or as slowly as a year or more.[2] However, many survivors report that the abusive incidents become more frequent and extreme over time.[2] Throughout the cycle of abuse, a TGD survivor might vacillate between feelings of love for their partner, fear of another episode of abuse, and hope that the partner will change and be the person they met in the initial honeymoon stage.[2]

This cycle can be illustrated through an abusive partner who may criticize or attack the survivor's gender minority identity during an explosive episode and then show remorse and display signs of acceptance of the survivor's gender minority identity in the honeymoon stage.[3] One trans man explains this part of the cycle as follows: "Several times she told me I was triggering her because she hated men... But at the same time, she also told me...to do whatever steps in transition I needed to do, without worrying about what she or anyone else thought".[7]

COMMON TACTICS OF ABUSE IN IPV

Is it important to recognize that IPV is not a single incident, but a pattern of behaviors where the abusive partner employs a variety of tactics, including emotional, financial, sexual, physical, and identity-based abuse.[3] Physical violence in IPV, including hitting, kicking, disrupting sleep, strangulation, or even threatening physical violence, is perhaps the most identifiable tactic of abuse. However, physical violence is only one of many tactics that an abusive partner might employ to exert power and control,[3] and it may or may not be present (Figure 14-2). Emotional abuse is nearly always present. Common tactics of emotional abuse include an abusive partner isolating the survivor, controlling what they do, and damaging their self-esteem with name-calling, accusations, and blame. Often an abuser uses *gaslighting*, or lying to cause the survivor to question their own reality. One common example of gaslighting is denying that the abusive episode occurred or turning the situation around to blame the survivor for the abuse. Isolation is often a key aspect of emotional abuse and how an abusive partner maintains control, by disrupting friendships, monitoring calls, and not allowing a survivor to have contact with others.

Other tactics of IPV include financial abuse, such as controlling money, disrupting work or school, or not paying bills. Sexual abuse can include sexual coercion, assault, or nonconsensually sharing nude photos or videos with sexual content. One genderqueer survivor shared her experience of sexual abuse and coercion: "I didn't want to engage in penetrative sex. Zie would say that I wasn't really meant to be in a relationship. Like that all relationships had to be about sex and that I wouldn't really attract anyone unless I was willing to do things that people expect of me, sexually that is."[8,9]

Additionally, identity-based tactics target the survivor's marginalized identities. For example, an abusive partner may target the survivor's race with stereotypes and slurs, threaten to deport them or expose their immigration status if they are undocumented, or target their disability by taking away a crutch, wheelchair, or hearing aid. One young **trans masculine** survivor explains their experience of their abusive partner, who used a combination

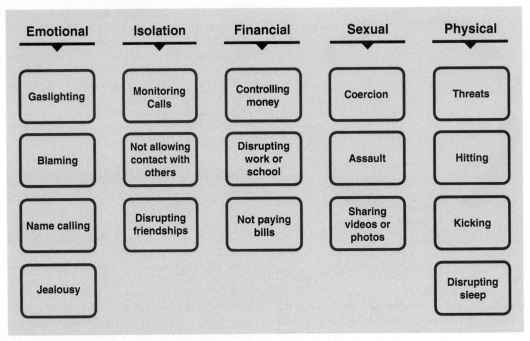

Emotional	Isolation	Financial	Sexual	Physical
Gaslighting	Monitoring Calls	Controlling money	Coercion	Threats
Blaming	Not allowing contact with others	Disrupting work or school	Assault	Hitting
Name calling	Disrupting friendships	Not paying bills	Sharing videos or photos	Kicking
Jealousy				Disrupting sleep

▲ **Figure 14-2.** Examples of common tactics of abuse.

of identity tactics, sexual tactics, and emotional tactics of abuse:

> It is difficult to describe because it was a pattern of behaviors, but some examples are: she pressured me/guilted me into sex ("if you loved me, you would do it"); she would continue touching my chest after I told her it made me uncomfortable; she would get mad at me for being depressed (I have clinical depression) and make me feel like everything was my fault, and my feelings were not valid, and imply that she must know better because she was older. She also made me afraid to leave the relationship by using emotional manipulations such as threatening suicide if I left.[5]

As illustrated in this example, abusers use a combination of tactics to control their partner. This example includes threatening suicide, which is a common tactic of abuse. In this case and in the case of self-harm, the abusive partner directs the physical violence toward themselves but blames their actions on the survivor.

To better identify abuse, health care professionals need to recognize the variety of tactics an abusive partner might employ against TGD individuals. While many of the above tactics apply regardless of the identity of the survivor, often the abusive partner weaponizes transphobia to control the survivor. These tactics of identity abuse specific to a survivor's

gender identity can be categorized as denial of transgender identity, control of gender expression, insinuated transphobia, and blatant antitrans attacks (Figures 14-3 and 14-4).

▶ Denial of Trans, Gender Diverse, or Nonbinary Identity

One way that an abuser partner can weaponize transphobia to exert power over the survivor is to deny their **gender identity**.[3] This type of abuse may be carried out explicitly by insisting that the survivor's gender identity is not real[8,9]; 25% of transgender survivors in one study had experienced this form of abuse.[4] Similarly, 33% of survivors experienced their partner refusing to use their correct name and pronouns.[4] Intentional use of the wrong name and pronouns, particularly by someone as close as a partner, can have a profoundly detrimental effect on the survivor, increasing feelings of dysphoria and isolation.[3] In the intimate context of sexual situations, an abusive partner may also deeply injure the survivor through denial of their gender identity. Examples include intentional usage of the wrong gender-based terminology during sex, wrongly naming the survivor's body parts, or demanding sex acts that go against the TGD person's understanding of themselves.[10,11]

Denial of the survivor's gender identity can include attempts to block their gender affirmation. When an abusive partner disapproves of the survivor's need for **gender**

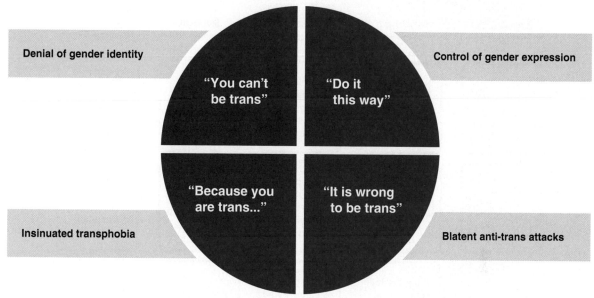

Denial of gender identity

"You can't be trans"

Control of gender expression

"Do it this way"

"Because you are trans..."

"It is wrong to be trans"

Insinuated transphobia

Blatent anti-trans attacks

▲ **Figure 14-3.** Types of trans-specific identity abuse.

affirmation, they may respond with a variety of tactics in order to keep them from being affirmed in their gender. They might demand that the survivor remain closeted, a tactic that 30% of transgender people reported experiencing.[4] They may refuse to allow the survivor to seek gender-affirming medical treatment such as hormones or surgeries.[8,10,12] One transgender survivor spoke about his partner's methods of keeping him from **gender-affirming hormone therapy**: "He prevented me from getting on testosterone until the relationship ended with numerous threats of suicide and other things."[8,10] Along with threats of suicide, abusive partners often threaten to leverage transphobia either by outing the survivor at work or to their family or by using the legal system against them.[13] One transgender survivor shares her experience of this tactic of abuse as follows: "My ex had me convinced she could turn everyone against me and take my kids and eventually grandkids away from me."[14]

Denial of gender can also manifest in preventing the partner from expressing their gender through their appearance. Nearly one-third of transgender people reported this experience in an intimate relationship.[4] One trans woman survivor explained how her partner would use the guise of saving money to persuade her not acquire gender-affirming items: "If I wanted to buy, or bought, anything feminine for me (such as a lipstick), all hell would break loose as I'd be wasting money that should be spent on the family."[7] Another trans masculine survivor, explained, "Sometimes she would hide my chest binder all day, knowing I couldn't

go out without it.[8] Other abusive partners move beyond manipulation and guilt into the realm of physical destruction, by disposing of or destroying clothing, makeup, wigs, or prosthetics.[7,10,12]

Other forms of gender identity denial include openly mocking or questioning a survivor's gender identity. One trans masculine survivor shared the following account: "My ex-girlfriend who was emotionally, sexually, and physically abusive used to use my gender-questioning as ammunition. She would embarrass me by telling people about it in front of me. She made fun of my attempts to present as a boy."[4] In this case, the survivor's partner was trans as well, demonstrating that denial of a partner's gender and other forms of trans-specific tactics can be perpetrated by either cisgender or transgender abusive partners. The survivor shared, "She is transsexual, and she always said I was just making things up for attention."[5]

▶ Control of Gender Expression

Identity abuse that leverages transphobia also includes an abusive partner attempting to control the **gender expression** of the survivor. Control of gender expression can take a variety of forms, including controlling who knows about the survivor's gender identity, enforcing stereotypes of gendered clothing or behavior, and limiting access to spaces where the survivor can get support from other TGD people. An abusive partner may take control of who knows the survivor is transgender or gender diverse, by outing the survivor to others.[15]

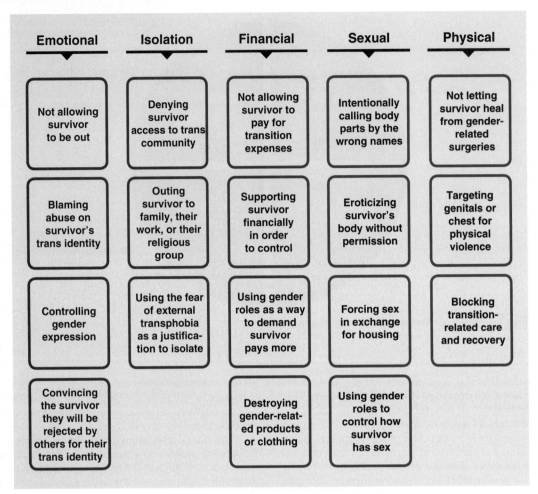

Emotional	Isolation	Financial	Sexual	Physical
Not allowing survivor to be out	Denying survivor access to trans community	Not allowing survivor to pay for transition expenses	Intentionally calling body parts by the wrong names	Not letting survivor heal from gender-related surgeries
Blaming abuse on survivor's trans identity	Outing survivor to family, their work, or their religious group	Supporting survivor financially in order to control	Eroticizing survivor's body without permission	Targeting genitals or chest for physical violence
Controlling gender expression	Using the fear of external transphobia as a justification to isolate	Using gender roles as a way to demand survivor pays more	Forcing sex in exchange for housing	Blocking transition-related care and recovery
Convincing the survivor they will be rejected by others for their trans identity		Destroying gender-related products or clothing	Using gender roles to control how survivor has sex	

▲ **Figure 14-4.** Examples of trans-specific tactics of abuse by type of tactic of abuse.

The impact of outing can be the survivor losing work, community, family, or a sense of safety and privacy.[3]

To attempt to control a TGD survivor, an abusive partner may use gender stereotypes to influence how a TGD survivor dresses.[12] At times, this tactic may take the form of explicit criticism or instructions, but it can also include manipulation. In the same way that the honeymoon stage in the cycle of abuse plays a part in maintaining control, an abusive partner's flattery and gifts can persuade the survivor to present their gender in a particular way.[3] One transgender woman, describes this dynamic in her relationship:

I started doing [wearing] some of the things he got, like, the better bras and silicone; I even did more on my face, like the lips and cheeks [referring to surgeries], that were just easy one day things. He would praise me for that… I started to just lose myself; I was just now this thing. This, like experiment or something, of his to use and "Doll Up." It only made me more depressed, which made him more angry, and then that's when he got colder, more distant, more angry and kind of like violent.[12]

The control of gender expression can extend to gendered behaviors as well as appearance. Abusive partners may use gender roles as a means of manipulating the survivor to perform labor, demanding a trans woman to do housework to be womanly, or insisting that a trans man "be a man" by financially supporting his partner.[3]

These dynamics can occur in sexual situations as well. The abusive partner may insist that the survivor has sex in a particular way to affirm their gender or use gender stereotypes to coerce the partner sexually. For example, they might insist that a transgender man must prove his masculinity by always being willing to have sex.[15] This coercion can occur regardless of whether the abusive partner is cisgender or transgender. For example, an abusive trans man may insist that their partner act in feminine ways or take on feminine roles for the purpose of affirming *his* gender.[16] One survivor explained: "His abusers had been female, and as a nontrans person and nonsurvivor I 'owed' him sexually. It was my duty to provide for his pleasure, any needs and boundaries of my own were supposedly abusive."[17] In this example, the abusive partner used both his vulnerabilities as a trans man and his vulnerabilities as a survivor to manipulate and control the survivor's gender expression and behavior.

Attempts to control a TGD survivor's gender expression can also translate to controlling the process of gender affirmation.[8] One survivor shared,

> He would use [gender affirmation] as a constant scare tactic. When I had finally gotten the means to pay for top surgery, for example, he would talk about how he and I would go to the surgeon place together and take care of me, but that wasn't my plan at all. I had someone else in mind, and when I told him that, he would do dramatics like "why am I not good enough for you?" or regarding the hormones, it would be like "why do you have to do this? We could go talk to a therapist together." It was what I felt personal, my personal thing to do, he would turn it about him or both of us together, and he would just sort of use it. He would try to keep something that was personal and for me to deal with, he would turn it into like, an issue to talk about with me, he would just use it a guilt trip thing regularly.[8]

In this example, the abusive partner tried a variety of tactics to control the survivor's gender affirmation first by offering to take control of his top surgery and recovery process and then by pathologizing his desire to start hormones and using guilt to keep him from starting gender-affirming hormone therapy.

Subtle Transphobia

IPV often includes manipulation and gaslighting, convincing a survivor to question their own reality. This manipulation and gaslighting manifests through **transphobia** as well. Rather than direct assaults on TGD identities, abusers may insinuate that the survivor is unlovable or vacillate between acceptance and rejection of their partner's gender.[11] One trans survivor's partner would tell them "it was very difficult to date a trans person" making them "feel like it was a burden," and that this subtle transphobia "affected [their] self-image negatively and impacts [them] to this day."[8] Another

survivor, a transgender woman, shared that her partner "was careful to tell me how beautiful I was to *her*. She was occasionally subtle and often not so subtle about using my trans status to tell me how no one could really love or accept me like her."[11] In a similar way, an abusive partner may eroticize the trans, **nonbinary**, or gender diverse person's body nonconsensually or focus on parts of the body that the survivor does not feel comfortable with.[11]

Another tactic of IPV directed toward TGD survivors is to use the existence of transphobia to persuade or isolate their partner.[11] Under the guise of protectiveness or concern for their partner, the abusive partner may evoke transphobia as a reason to keep them from events or social situations.[3] They might warn their partner that LGBTQIA+ communities do not include trans, nonbinary, or gender diverse people to dissuade them from connecting to others.[18] An extreme example of this could be trying to convince the survivor to remain closeted, and even to lead them to dispose of any clothing, books, or other articles related to their gender identity, ostensibly for the safety of the survivor.[4] When both partners are trans, nonbinary, or gender diverse, this form of abuse can also manifest as the abusive partner acting as a "gatekeeper" to TGD communities, controlling access or implying that they know the "right way" to be transgender or gender diverse.[16]

Blatant Transphobia

Blatant transphobia can come in many forms and can include the open use of antitransgender slurs, criticism, or attacks on the survivor's gender identity, and even extreme acts of violence.[10,11] In one survey, 52% of trans people reported a partner had made them feel that their trans identity was shameful or wrong, and 45% reported a partner using repeated verbal abuse to make them feel worthless.[4] Some abusive partners blame the abuse on the survivor's gender identity. One client shared the abuse they experience from their partners echoed the broader pattern of transphobia in their lives: "I, all my life, was told that I brought on such assaults because of who and what I was."[5]

Blatant transphobia can lead to acts of violence, including attacks to the chest and genitals with the intent of causing increased psychological distress.[19] This type of violence can take place while a survivor is healing from a gender-affirming surgery. Forcing a survivor to work or not allowing a survivor to rest after surgery can have a detrimental impact on the survivor. Some abusive partners go to a more violent extreme. For example, one trans man shared: "He slapped me and pushed on my chest and pushed on my surgical scars and made them bleed."[12] While all violence is impactful to survivors, violence that includes targeting vulnerabilities after surgery or gendered areas of the body can be particularly emotionally distressing.

BARRIERS TO SUPPORT

Trans survivors face a range of barriers to accessing support, the majority of which are a result of real or perceived transphobia in needed services. TGD people are subject to discrimination in a variety of settings. Many have firsthand experiences of bias from police, hospitals, and employers or have faced familial rejection.[20] Because of the experiences, TGD survivors may be hesitant to seek help from domestic violence programs, police, or medical professionals.[8] One survivor explained, "I would never have called the police. I mean, like, what are they going to do? I am a transsexual[1] woman, and I'm an immigrant, and also, I mean, I was doing illegal things like hormone sharing, and I don't think they would've believed that my ex was forcing me to have sex for money."[8] When working with TGD survivors, it is important to acknowledge any fears or concerns about transphobia or discrimination, to advocate for fair services on behalf of the survivor when possible, and to accept the fact that the survivor may choose not to access certain systems.

Another unique barrier is the impact of small communities. LGBTQIA+ communities are small, but TGD people make up an even smaller portion of those communities. One survivor recounts how their partner weaponized this fact: "My trans ex and I are part of a very small trans community, and as a result of our breakup, I have become largely alienated from our community. He is a respected leader in the trans community. He spreads rumors about me."[5] In this example, the survivor's partner acted to permanently cut them off from the local trans community.

Being part of a small community can also negatively affect a survivor's ability to reach out to trans-specific programs and services. Another survivor recounts, "I called the local LGBTQIA+ domestic violence project after I was being stalked by my abusive [trans] ex. The person I talked to there, a trans woman, said 'is your ex a member of the trans community?' I said he was, and she said, 'I can't help you; that's a conflict of interest.'"[5] While LGBTQIA+-specific services are often desirable for TGD survivors, it is important to recognize that accessing these services may not be the safest option. In cases such as this, a service provider can reach out to the LGBTQIA+-specific program to get referrals for mainstream IPV programs that are trans-inclusive that may offer more confidentiality and anonymity from other LGBTQIA+ community members.

---

[1] While it is not recommended that clinicians use the term transsexual as a general rule, it is important to reflect the language used by each individual patient. The term "transsexual" is more likely to be used by patients who speak languages other than English such as Spanish and Portuguese.

BEST PRACTICES FOR WORKING WITH TGD SURVIVORS

When working with TGD survivors, it is important to use principles of trauma-informed care ([TIC], discussed in Chapter 11, "Basic Principles of Trauma-Informed and Gender-Affirming Care") This approach acknowledges the impact that past trauma may have on the patient and uses patient-centered policies, procedures, and practices in response that actively resist retraumatization. TIC includes asking for and using the name and pronouns aligned with the survivor's gender identity. It also includes basic knowledge of terms related to TGD communities. Health care professionals must not ask questions about gender affirmation or body parts needlessly and should be aware of the systemic issues facing TGD people. Knowledge of local and national resources for TGD individuals is also an important factor.

▶ Screening for IPV

Identifying TGD survivors of IPV is the first step to supporting them. The United States Preventive Services Task Force (USPSTF) recommends screening for IPV in health care settings for women of reproductive age.[21] While this recommendation includes transgender women of that age group, there is less evidence suggesting that health care professionals should screen all adults for IPV.[21] The USPSTF, however, also acknowledges that there is little or no risk in screening all adults.[21] Additionally, the American Medical Association recognizes that all patients may be at risk for IPV and recommends that physicians screen patients regularly.[22] Considering the high rates of IPV experienced by TGD individuals, screening this population is an emerging best practice.

Screening for IPV can identify survivors and enable them to connect to the counseling and supportive services they need and can improve clinical outcomes for survivors.[23] Fenway Health created a four-question screener with gender-inclusive language, adapted from the Abuse Assessment Screen (AAS), to address the needs of IPV survivors of all genders[24] (Figure 14-5). This universal screener has been distributed to all patients aged 18 and older at Fenway Health since 2014.[22] During this time, it has also been validated for use with TGD patients.[25] The Fenway Health's IPV screener has the following questions:

In the past year, did a current or former partner...

Q1:...make you feel cut off from others, trapped, or controlled in a way that you did not like?"

Q2:...make you feel afraid that they might try to hurt you in some way?"

Q3:... pressure or force you to do something sexual that you didn't want to do?"

Q4: ...hit, kick, punch, slap, shove, or otherwise physically hurt you?"

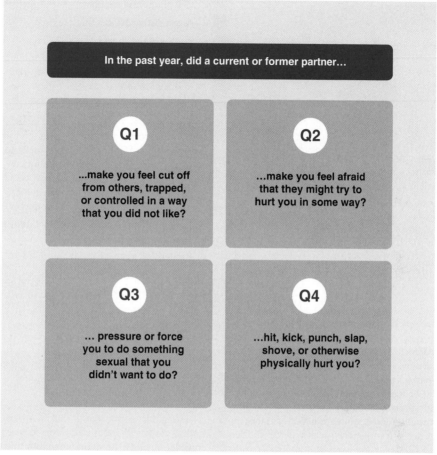

In the past year, did a current or former partner...

Q1

...make you feel cut off from others, trapped, or controlled in a way that you did not like?

Q2

...make you feel afraid that they might try to hurt you in some way?

Q3

... pressure or force you to do something sexual that you didn't want to do?

Q4

...hit, kick, punch, slap, shove, or otherwise physically hurt you?

▲ **Figure 14-5.** Fenway health IPV screening questions.

Throughout the implementation of this IPV screener, feedback from health care professionals at Fenway Health has been positive.[24] They report that the screener introduces the topic of IPV, making it easier for patients to talk about it.[24] Negative screening results do not lengthen the visit, and most patients react neutrally or positively to the screener.[24]

As overwhelming as it can be to hear a disclosure of IPV, it is probably more frightening for the survivor to share this information. They may fear your judgment, be concerned that you do not believe them, or fear that you will report the IPV to police or others without their permission. The best way to respond is to listen and provide brief supportive statements such as, "I'm sorry this is happening" and "How can I help?" Depending on your role and the amount of time you have with the TGD survivor, you can also provide safety planning and referrals to appropriate resources. Some examples of supportive responses to survivors are shown in Figure 14-6.

▶ Safety Planning

Safety planning is not based on a checklist but rather a series of conversations that address the specific needs of the TGD survivor in front of you.[5] Safety planning focuses on multiple components. First, safety planning helps the survivor prepare for a violent or abusive incident by helping them plan for how they can respond in the moment.[5] For example, part of safety planning can be advising the survivor to stay away from areas with weapons or knives, like the kitchen, or enclosed areas, like a closet or bathroom.[5] In addition, survivors are encouraged to move any confrontations into areas with multiple exits, and to stay close to the door when possible.[5] Other areas of focus in a safety plan entail enlisting the support of neighbors and friends to help should they receive a signal or code word.[5] A neighbor who sees violence or hears yelling may know to call the police.[5] A friend may get a particular text or call with a preset phrase

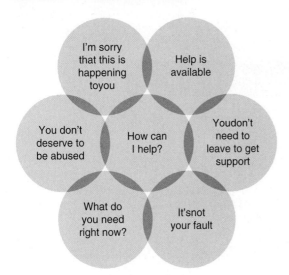

▲ **Figure 14-6.** Responding to disclosures.

that signals them to pick up the survivor or bring others to help.[5]

Another area of focus in safety planning involves preparing to leave an abusive partner. This part of the plan may entail storing important paperwork, medications, or belongings with a friend or family member or creating an emergency bag that the survivor can store in the car or at work. FORGE, an organization focused on the needs of transgender survivors, created a transgender-specific guide entitled *Safety Planning: A Guide for Transgender and Gender Non-Conforming Individuals Who are Experiencing Intimate Partner Violence* (http://forge-forward.org/wp-content/docs/safety-planning-tool.pdf).[5] This guide includes ideas for what any survivor might wish to include in their emergency bag such as "driver's license/state identification card, car registration, and proof of insurance, work ID/work permit, health care insurance or Medicaid/Medicare ID cards, social security card, birth certificate, passport, Green card, visa, or other immigration papers."[5] The guide also includes specific considerations for TGD survivors, such as letters from a surgeon, a "carry letter" from a doctor, and paperwork from the court for a name or gender change.[5] FORGE's emergency bag description includes essential resources:

- Keys to car, house, work, safety deposit/post office boxes
- List of possible service organizations (see Laying the Groundwork)
- Friends' and therapist's addresses and phone numbers
- Spare glasses or contact lenses
- Medications, prescriptions, contact information for doctor(s) and pharmacy

- Cell phone and charger
- Any assistive devices that are used
- Photos of the abuser
- Record or journal of the abuse, if you do not already store it elsewhere, and/or photos of injuries your partner has inflicted on you
- Public transportation schedule[5]

The FORGE safety plan also includes a list gender-affirmation items, both nonmedical and medical (i.e., hormones), that a TGD survivor may need to include in their emergency bag (for more information on nonmedical and medical gender affirmation, please see Chapter 8, "Nonmedical, Nonsurgical Gender Affirmation," and Chapter 7, "Gender-Affirming Hormone Therapy for Adults"):

- Hormones, prescriptions, contact information for doctor and pharmacy
- Binders
- Stand-to-pee devices
- Packers or penile prosthetics
- Wigs
- Gaffing materials
- Shaving and plucking tools
- Breast/hip forms or other feminizing prosthetics
- Makeup
- Clothing

The guide also suggests that if a person has difficulty finding clothes or shoes in the correct size then they should consider buying extra items when they find them and asking friends or colleagues to store them. A list of favorite clothing sources can be added to the emergency list of addresses and phone numbers.[5]

It can be helpful to have a copy of FORGE's safety plan available to consult when working with a TGD survivor as it addresses many of their specific needs and considerations. It is also one of the more thorough safety plans available and includes tips on technology safety, emotional safety, and getting emotional support.[5]

▶ Continuum of Care

When working with a TGD survivor of IPV, it is important to assess where their needs are on the continuum of care. Figure 14-7 shows four stages in the IPV continuum and the needs of survivors for each stage.

Survivors Who Are in a Relationship

When the survivor is currently in a relationship with an abusive partner, they may not have identified their partner's behavior as abusive.[26] If they have not, it can be helpful

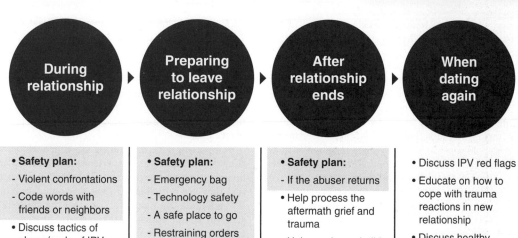

During relationship ▶ **Preparing to leave relationship** ▶ **After relationship ends** ▶ **When dating again**

- **Safety plan:**
  - Violent confrontations
  - Code words with friends or neighbors
- Discuss tactics of abuse/cycle of IPV
- Refer to IPV hotlines, support groups, advocacy

- **Safety plan:**
  - Emergency bag
  - Technology safety
  - A safe place to go
  - Restraining orders
  - Risk assessment
- Refer to IPV hotlines, support groups, and advocacy

- **Safety plan:**
  - If the abuser returns
- Help process the aftermath grief and trauma
- Help survivor rebuild self-esteem
- Refer to IPV support groups, counseling, advocacy

- Discuss IPV red flags
- Educate on how to cope with trauma reactions in new relationship
- Discuss healthy relationship skills
- Explore the survivor's needs and wants in new relationship

▲ **Figure 14-7.** Continuum of care for IPV survivors.

for the health care professional to reflect on the partner's behaviors that could be abusive and check in with the survivor about how they feel in the relationship. Mirroring the client's language can be helpful, for example, "I notice that you said your partner doesn't use 'she' for you and criticizes your 'feminine look.'"[26] These statements can be paired with information about abuse and follow-up questions, such as, "From my training, I know that this can be a warning sign of abuse. Do you have any concerns about your relationship?" If the survivor does not wish to engage in this conversation, the clinician can let them know that they can bring the topic up in the future, for example by saying: "If you ever want to talk about your relationship, I am open to it and can offer resources that might be helpful."

If the survivor has already identified their partner's behavior as abusive, the clinician can reflect their concerns and provide additional information. For example, "You mentioned you are afraid because she threatened to take your kids away if you move forward with medical gender affirmation. Abuse is often a pattern. Are there other times in your relationship when you were afraid of your partner?" It can be difficult not to move into immediate action about how the survivor can leave the relationship or get a restraining order. It is important, however, to ensure what the survivor wants first. Are they ready to leave the relationship right now? Survivors in this stage may not want to leave; more often, a survivor is ambivalent. They may be just beginning to feel concerned. They may want more information on what IPV is, or they may not have the resources to leave. Let the survivor take the lead by asking them what they need.

If they want more information, you can explain the cycle of abuse. Clinicians may wish to use motivational interviewing techniques to reflect the survivor's concerns and assess the survivor's motivation to act. If they are ambivalent but want information, they can be directed to a hotline or program for LGBTQIA+ survivors of IPV (see the "Resources" section later in the chapter for more information).[26] If a survivor asks for referrals for couples counseling, it is important to inform them that couples counseling is not recommended in cases of IPV.[26] Couples counseling can put the survivor at greater risk of retaliation from their partner if they share their true feelings in what they believe to be a safe environment.[26]

Preparing to Leave the Relationship

A highly dangerous time for survivors of IPV is when they are leaving their abusive partner.[5] When an abusive partner believes they are losing the survivor, they may respond with increased violence or even attempts to kill the survivor.[5] Safety planning during this time should focus on strategies for leaving, where the survivor can go, and how to reduce the chances of further abuse or injury.[5]

At this point, it is also helpful to guide the survivor through a risk assessment, such as *The Danger Assessment* (DLA), a tool created by nurses to assess for the risk of intimate partner homicide.[27] This assessment can help the survivor better grasp the level of danger they face and can alert them to their risk for homicide. Indicators of risk for lethality include the abuser threatening suicide or homicide; past incidents of strangulation, sexual assault, drug use, or jealousy; and owning weapons.[28] One limitation of the DLA is that it is gender specific. The original guide is written for a straight, female audience and includes questions like, "Does he own a gun?" However, a new version is available in which the abusive partner is a woman (e.g., "Does she own a gun?").[28] While these two assessments may be helpful to use with TGD survivors whose partners use binary pronouns of "he" or "she," there are currently no risk assessments with nonbinary pronouns. Nevertheless, these assessments could be adapted with use of a nonbinary pronoun such as "they" to meet the needs of all survivors. Further research is needed to determine if there are additional warning signs of risk that are specific to trans, gender diverse, or nonbinary survivors and to create a tool designed specifically for this population.

After the Relationship Ends

After the relationship ends, safety planning should continue and focus on what the survivor can do if the abuser attempts to contact them or is continuing the abuse.[5] In the aftermath of abuse, many TGD survivors need resources to recover financially.[26] Financial recovery can be particularly pertinent for survivors who have faced familial rejection and cannot use their family as a source of support. Survivors may require assistance with basic needs such as housing, food, and health insurance as well as help with finding employment, enrolling in school, or repairing credit.[26] Many programs that support IPV survivors can assist with connection to resources and support for these basic needs.[26]

In addition to safety and basic needs, survivors need emotional support in the aftermath of abuse.[5] After the focus of day-to-day survival in the relationship is gone, the survivor is often overwhelmed with emotions that were previously contained, including grief, anger, and fear. Many survivors experience grief for the loss of companionship, the dreams they had with their partner, and the aspects of their partner that they loved. There may also be grief over what they may have lost because of the abuse, whether it be possessions, their home, physical mobility, freedom from injury, and a sense of safety and trust. Sometimes it can mean the loss of a job, important friendships, or custody of children. Paired with this grief is often anger that the abuser treated them this way, or that they got away with the abuse. Often, the survivor misdirects anger toward themselves. They may ask, "Did I choose this person because they are abusive?" "Did this happen because I am trans?" "Should I have known they were abusive?" or "Will anyone healthy want to be with me?"

Many survivors develop **posttraumatic stress disorder (PTSD)**. PTSD includes symptoms such as intrusive thoughts and memories about the abuse, as well as nightmares and flashbacks; avoiding people, places, and things associated with the abuse; feeling detached or numb; and hypervigilance, negative emotional states, and a distorted sense of self-blame[29] (see Chapter 11, "Basic Principles of Trauma-Informed and Gender-Affirming Care," for more information). These symptoms can last for years after the relationship ends and often spike during anniversaries, such as the day the survivor met their abusive ex-partner or the day the relationship ended. They can also worsen if the abuser reappears in the survivor's life in any way, particularly if there are continued interactions, such as ongoing court cases.

Supporting survivors during this time includes normalizing their reactions and experiences and letting them know how they can access support.[26] The survivor needs to know that they are not alone. During this time, speaking to an IPV advocate can help[26] validate that the abuse is not the survivor's fault and help the survivor process what they experienced, with tools such as the *cycle of abuse* and the *power and control wheel*.[26] A gender-affirming counselor can also be an important asset during this time. Psychoeducation on trauma, cognitive processing therapy, eye movement desensitization and reprocessing (EMDR), dialectical behavior therapy, and cognitive behavior therapy for trauma are evidence-based interventions to aid survivors in stabilizing symptoms and processing traumatic experiences.[30]

Reconnecting with supportive people in one's life is also an important step for survivors of IPV to rebuild trust.[5] TGD survivors may have been isolated due to the abuse and may need help connecting with others.[5] Social supports can include trans support groups, IPV support groups, addiction recovery groups (when appropriate), and linking to regional social events that are inclusive of and center TGD people.[14] Communities of faith may be another area of support for TGD survivors, and it can be helpful to know of welcoming religious communities in the area.[5] When the survivor is in a region with no services designed specifically for TGD people, online chat rooms, phone meetings, and hotlines, such as Trans Lifeline, can be a place for the survivor to get support.[14]

When Dating Again

Many survivors seek counseling services for recovery from IPV when they start a new relationship. Often, the new relationship brings up fears and memories of the abuse. One trans survivor shared that their past abuse "now plays a part in physical aspects of [their] relationship with [their] current partner. There are many things that trigger panic attacks, and there is always caution to avoid these triggers."[14] When dating again, survivors may fear that their new partner is abusive or wonder about how to disclose their experience of IPV to their new partner. During this time, it can help survivors to review red flags, talk about boundaries, reflect on healthy relationships and communication skills, and process the past abuse with a skilled professional counselor.

RESOURCES

The following resources are divided into two broad groups: LQBTQIA+-specific hotlines and programs, and resources that provide information about IPV for survivors.

▶ LGBTQIA+-Specific IPV Programs

When concerns about small communities arise, it can be helpful to offer national LGBTQIA+ IPV hotline information that is not specific to a particular region. Due to the shortage of LGBTQIA+-specific services, most national LGBTQIA+-specific antiviolence programs are accustomed to supporting people from all areas.

The Network/La Red: 24-hour hotline: 617-742-4911, www.tnlr.org

National Coalition of Anti-Violence Programs: 212-714-1141, www.avp.org

Fenway's Violence Recovery Program: 617-927-6250, fenwayhealth.org/care/behavioral-health/violence-recovery

The Northwest Network: 206-568-7777, nwnetwork.org

FORGE trans-specific antiviolence resources: forge-forward.org

Trans lifeline (a trans-specific peer support and crisis hotline): 877-565-8860

Trans-specific resources for survivors:

Transgender Sexual Violence Survivors: A Self Help Guide to Healing and Understanding, FORGE. https://forge-forward.org/2015/09/24/trans-sa-survivors-self-help-guide/

Let's talk about it! A Transgender Survivor's Guide to Accessing Therapy, FORGE.

http://forge-forward.org/wp content/docs/Lets-Talk-Therapist-Guide.pdf

VAWA special collections: Serving trans and nonbinary survivors of domestic violence. https://vawnet.org/sc/serving-trans-and-non-binary-survivors-domestic-and-sexual-violence/resources-survivors

SUMMARY

- TGD people experience IPV at higher rates than other populations. Because health care professionals are in a unique role to identify and support TGD survivors of IPV, they must educate themselves about how to identify TGD survivors of IPV and provide evidence-based support to these patients in the context of gender-affirming and trauma-informed care.

- Abusive partners often use identity abuse tactics, such as denying or denigrating the survivor's gender identity.

- Screening for IPV with gender-inclusive questions is an effective way to identify when TGD patients have experienced abuse. Fenway Health's screening tool for IPV has four questions written in gender-inclusive language and has been validated for use with TGD clients.

- Health care professionals can support TGD survivors of IPV with gender-affirming and trauma-informed care, safety planning, consistent support, and appropriate referrals.

CASE STUDY 1: Loretta

Loretta is a 65-year-old White transgender woman who is meeting with her primary care health professional Dr. Song to pursue gender-affirmative hormone therapy (GAHT). Loretta tells Dr. Song that "there is nothing I want more than to start transition" but that "my wife is against it." She tells Dr. Song that her wife responds with hostility and rage and tells her she is "not really a woman." Loretta says "she destroys any make-up, wigs, or dresses that she finds and threatens to take our kids if I transition." Dr. Song listens and thinks about how she would feel if her husband transitioned. She says to Loretta, "I can understand why your wife is upset. This is a huge change." Loretta responds, "I know, but this isn't new information for her. I have been talking about this for years." Dr. Song says, "Maybe you just need to give her time" and suggests she tell her wife to go to PFLAG, a group for friends and family of LGBTQIA+ people. Loretta becomes withdrawn and upset and says, "I've waited long enough. I shouldn't have to put this on hold any longer" and starts to move toward the door. Dr. Song realizes that she has said something to upset the patient and calls Loretta back. Dr. Song says, "Loretta, wait. I am sorry I have upset you. Clearly, I don't understand what you are going through and how this is impacting you." Loretta stops and sits back down. Dr. Song says, "You are right that you should not have to wait for your wife to be ready for you to take steps to transition" and begins to talk with Loretta about her options for GAHT. When Loretta is calmer, she asks her, "Do you have any other concerns about your wife's reaction to this?" Loretta says, "I'm afraid she is going to use this against me to try and get me fired." Dr. Song recognizes that there may be abuse present and says, "It sounds like there are some significant challenges in your marriage, and that your wife may be treating you in ways that are not okay. Let me give you a number you can call to talk more about this situation and get support" and offers the number for an LGBTQIA+ hotline for survivors of IPV.

▶ Discussion Questions

- Dr. Song identified with Loretta's wife in this situation instead of aligning herself with Loretta, who is her patient, and therefore missed the red flags that Loretta's wife may be abusive. Whom might you empathize with in this scenario, and how might this lead to inadequate treatment?

- If you were seeing this patient, what question might you ask about her wife's behavior to avoid the initial missteps Dr. Song made?

- A turning point occurs in the encounter when Dr. Song says, "Loretta, wait. I am sorry I have upset you. Clearly, I don't understand what you are going through and how this is impacting you." What about this approach might have opened up the interaction between Loretta and Dr. Song? What language and tone do you use when you need to course-correct during a challenging dynamic with a patient?

- How might Loretta's whiteness affect this encounter and subsequent follow-up? Consider what might be different in this case if Loretta were Black, Indigenous, or Latinx? What communities access your clinical space, and how might your perceptions influence your care of Black, Indigenous, and People of Color (BIPOC)?

CASE STUDY 2: Ray

Susie is the case manager for Ray, a 38-year-old undocumented Haitian transgender man. Toward the end of the appointment, Ray tells Susie that his boyfriend keeps pressuring him to get married so he can sponsor him for U.S. citizenship. Ray says, "My boyfriend keeps telling me that I will get deported if I don't marry him." Susie asks Ray, "How do you feel about this?" Ray responds, "I am not sure I want to. He is already very controlling. I think if we lived together, it would get even worse." Susie responds, "How is he controlling?" and Ray answers, "He always wants to know where I am and what I am doing. He wants me to do everything his way." Susie asks, "Do you worry that he might be abusive?" Ray sighs and answers, "I don't know. He tells me no one else will want to be with me because I am trans and undocumented and he wants to marry me. Maybe I should just count my blessings and do it." Susie nods and says, "It sounds pretty confusing. On the one hand, he says he is offering you security from immigration, but on the other hand, he is controlling and puts you down. Are you open to talking to a counselor about this?" Ray looks hesitant and says, "I'm not crazy. I don't need a counselor." Susie explains, "Here in the United States, people see counselors for a lot of different reasons. Sometimes it is for mental health issues, but other times it is just to get help with difficult situations, like this one. I can give you information for a program that works with trans survivors of abuse and offers counseling if you are interested." Ray shakes his head and says "no counselors." Susie replies, "Okay, but if you change your mind, let me know… and you can always talk about this with me."

▶ Discussion Questions

- Imagine yourself as Susie. How different is Susie's approach from how you currently practice? Which parts of this encounter feel new to you? Explore potential sources of your discomfort and whether there are situations or language with which you need more practice.

- How does Susie start to explore the issue of IPV with Ray? What skills does she use? Is Susie effective? How do you know?

- In what ways did Susie demonstrate cultural sensitivity in this scenario?

- The follow-up plan in this case is dependent on knowledge of a violence recovery program or survivors network that is LGBTQIA+-affirming. What factors limit access to or availability of these resources for patients where you practice? Are you familiar with similar resources in your own community? How might you adapt this plan if not?

REFERENCES

1. Brown T, Herman J. Intimate Partner Violence and Sexual Abuse among LGBT People. 2015. Williams Institute. https://williamsinstitute.law.ucla.edu/research/violence-crime/intimate-partner-violence-and-sexual-abuse-among-lgbt-people/. Accessed November 7, 2020.

2. Santiago S. Power With Power For. 2016. Boston: The Network/La Red. https://www.tnlr.org/en/publications/. Accessed November 7, 2020.

3. Quinn X. Tactics and Justifications for Abuse. In Messinger A, Guadalupe-Diaz XL, eds. *Transgender Intimate Partner Violence: A Comprehensive Introduction*. New York: New York University Press; 2020.

4. Roch A, Morton J, Ritchie G. Out of Sight, Out of Mind? Transgender People's Experiences of Domestic Abuse. 2010. LGBT Youth Scotland and The Scottish Transgender Alliance. Accessed November 7, 2020. https://www.scottishtrans.org/wp-content/uploads/2013/03/trans_domestic_abuse.pdf.

5. Munsun M, Cook-Daniels L. Transgender Sexual Violence Survivors: A Self Help Guide to Healing and Understanding. September 2015. Accessed November 7, 2020. https://forge-forward.org/2015/09/24/trans-sa-survivors-self-help-guide/.

6. Walker LE. *The Battered Woman*. New York: Harper Perennial; 1979.

7. Rogers M. Challenging cisgenderism through trans people's narratives of domestic violence and abuse. *Sexualities*. 2019;22(5–6):803–820.

8. Guadalupe-Diaz XL. *Transgressed: Intimate Partner Violence in Transgender Lives*. New York: New York University Press; 2019.

9. Goodmark L. Transgender people, intimate partner abuse, and the legal system. 48 Harvard Civil Rights-Civil Liberties Law Review 51, 2013.

10. Cook-Daniels L. Intimate partner violence in transgender couples: "power and control" in a specific cultural context. *Partner Abuse*. 2015;6(1):126–139.

11. Greenburg K. Still hidden in closet: transgender women and domestic violence. *Berkley J Gender Law Justice*. 2012;27(2):198–251.

12. Guadalupe-Diaz XL, Koontz Anthony A. Discrediting identity work: understandings of intimate partner violence by transgender survivors. *Deviant Behavior.* 2017;8(1):1–16.

13. Cooper L. *Protecting the Rights of Transgender Parents and Their Children: A Guide for Parents and Lawyers.* New York City: American Civil Liberties Union and National Center for Transgender Equality; 2013.

14. Munson M, Cook-Daniels L. Let's talk about it! A transgender survivor's guide to accessing therapy. 2015. forge-forward.org/wp-content/docs/Lets-Talk-Therapist-Guide.pdf. Accessed November 7, 2020.

15. Quinn X. *Open Minds Open Doors: Transforming Domestic Violence Programs to Include LGBTQ Survivors.* Boston: The Network/La Red; 2010.

16. Brown N. Holding tensions of victimization and perpetration: partner abuse in trans communities. *Intimate Partner Violence in LGBTQ Lives.* In: Ristock JL, ed. New York: Routledge; 2011.

17. FORGE. A Guide for Partners and Loved Ones of Transgender Sexual Violence Survivors. 2016. http://forge-forward.org/wp-content/docs/partners-guide.pdf. Accessed November 7, 2020.

18. Bornstein DR, Fawcett J, Sullivan M, Senturia KD, Shiu-Thornton S. Understanding the experiences of lesbian, bisexual and trans survivors of domestic violence: a qualitative study. *J Homosex.* 2006;51(1):159–181.

19. Yerke AF, DeFeo J. Redefining intimate partner violence beyond the binary to include transgender people. *J Family Violence.* 2016;31:975–979.

20. Grant JM, Mottet JA, Tanis J, et al. *Injustice at Every Turn: A Report of the National Transgender Discrimination Survey.* Washington, DC: National Center for Transgender Equality and National Gay and Lesbian Task Force; 2011.

21. Screening for Intimate Partner Violence and Abuse of Elderly and Vulnerable Adults: U.S. Preventive Services Task Force Recommendation Statement. *Ann Intern Med.* 2013;158:478–486.

22. National Advisory Council on Violence and Abuse. Policy Compendium. American Medical Association; 2008.

23. McCloskey LA, Lichter E, Williams C, Gerber M, Wittenberg E, Ganz M. Assessing intimate partner violence in health care settings leads to women's receipt of interventions and improved health. *Public Health Rep.* 2006;121(4):435–444.

24. Basham C, Presley C, Potter J. Implementing routine intimate partner violence screening in a primary care setting. Fenway Health. https://www.lgbthealtheducation.org/wp-content/uploads/Screening-for-IPV-in-Primary-Care-Webinar.pdf. Accessed November 8, 2020.

25. Fitzsimmons E, Loo S, Dougherty S, et al. Development and content validation of the IPV-4, a brief patient-reported measure of intimate partner violence for use in HIV care. ISOQOL 26th Annual Conference, October 20-23, 2019; San Diego, CA.

26. Messinger A. *LGBTQ Intimate Partner Violence.* Oakland, CA: University of California Press; 2017.

27. Northcott M. *Intimate Partner Violence Risk Assessment Tools: A Review.* Ottawa, Canada: Department of Justice; 2012.

28. Campbell JC. Danger assessment. 2004. www.dangerassessment.com. Accessed November 7, 2020.

29. American Psychiatric Association. *Diagnostic and Statistical Manual of Mental Disorders.* 5th ed. Arlington, VA: APA; 2013.

30. Richmond KS, Burnes T, Carroll K. Lost in translation: interpreting systems of trauma for transgender clients traumatology. *Traumatology.* 2012;18(1):45–57.

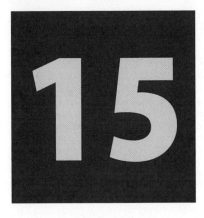

Eating Disorders, Body Image, and Body Positivity

Heidi J. Dalzell

Kayti Protos

Stacy K. Hunt

INTRODUCTION

Traditional treatment paradigms and research regarding patients with **disordered eating** (a range of irregular eating behaviors that do not meet *Diagnostic and Statistical Manual of Mental Disorders, 5th edition [DSM-5]* criteria for a specific eating disorder) and **eating disorders** (clinical presentations that meet DSM-5 clinical criteria for specific eating disorders) focus primarily on white, **cisgender**, and straight girls and women. Although knowledge about eating disorders among lesbian, gay, bisexual, and queer patients[1] cisgender straight men,[2,3] and Black, Indigenous, and People of Color[4,5] is increasing, information about eating disorders among **transgender and gender diverse (TGD)** patients remains scarce.

Published studies often combine gender minority and sexual minority groups in their samples. As a result, the sample of TGD patients included is frequently too small to produce statistically significant or generalizable information.[2,6,7] There is nevertheless a need to develop culturally responsive best practices on clinical care, given the number of TGD individuals with clinical and subclinical disordered eating.

In 2014, a large-scale study surveyed approximately 300,000 college students at risk for **anorexia nervosa** and **bulimia nervosa**,[8] revealing that transgender students had a risk of developing these disorders that was four times greater than their cisgender peers. This study suggests that mental health professionals are likely to encounter TGD patients who experience concerns with disordered eating and eating disorders.

Another area of risk for TGD patients involves **gender minority stress**[9] and the marginalizing nature of social environments for TGD people. Such discriminatory or marginalizing experiences have been linked to various mental health concerns, including depression,[10] substance use disorders,[11] and **posttraumatic stress disorder (PTSD)**. Depression and substance use disorders often co-occur with eating disorders.

Some people with eating disorders may also exhibit symptoms of PTSD.[12]

This chapter examines the connections between **gender identity**, gender minority stress, **body image**—particularly the experience of a body that does not align with gender identity—and the development and treatment of eating disorders. The chapter reviews themes available from the current literature and includes clinical observations and case studies that highlight eating disorders among TGD patients.

BODY IMAGE

Body image concerns are key factors for TGD persons presenting for mental health treatment.[13] Concerns range from body dissatisfaction—which can be considered a normative experience when the body and gender identity do not align—to body hatred, a more complex clinical presentation in which there is extreme body aversion. Body image is considered to be a primary but not the only factor leading to eating disorders in TGD communities.[13]

It is helpful to understand the concept of body image when considering the intersection of eating disorders and gender identity. Thomas Cash, an expert in the field of body image, defines it as "the multifaceted psychological experience of embodiment, especially but not exclusively related to one's physical appearance."[14] Cash describes body image as a phenomenon that encompasses one's body-related self-perceptions and self-attitudes, including thoughts, beliefs, feelings, and behaviors, all of which are unique to identity. Racial and cultural values also impact these beliefs, adding to the complexity and nuance of the concept. Body image, therefore, is an experience of physical self that affects self-concept, self-esteem, and one's sense of autonomy in the world.

In cisgender populations, negative body image is a key factor in the development and maintenance of clinical and subclinical eating disorders,[15] as well as low self-esteem and general mental health problems.[16] Negative body image is also a key factor for these effects in TGD populations. Body image exists on a continuum, ranging from more positive experiences of body ownership or acceptance to more negative experiences of body preoccupation, hatred, distortion, or dissociation.[17] Body image develops throughout the life cycle, with notable changes in late childhood and adolescence, a time of rapid physical change. Body image difficulties can affect people of all ages and have also been associated with physical and hormonal changes[18] as well as life changes and transition.[19] Body image concerns can arise in childhood, adolescence, young adulthood, and midlife[20] as well as in older adults.

Studies of body image have been conducted mainly with presumed cisgender samples, and while care should be taken in extrapolating to TGD populations, many causal factors appear to be similar. People receive information about bodies from many sources: family, peers, media, and culture[14,21–23] and develop a sense of acceptability based on these messages. These venues expose people to information about gender and gender norms, as well as societal body ideals. In the mainstream media, bodies are generally depicted as cisgender; in the United States, body image is based on White and Western ideals, while other areas of the world have different body image ideals. The White and Western cisgender male body ideal is tall and shaped as a reversed pyramid, with broad shoulders and a narrow waist. The White and Western cisgender female body ideal is petite and hourglass-shaped, with a small waist-to-hip ratio.[24]

These gendered ideals of body image are powerful, and for some, provide a standard that is impossible to attain or can be attained only through disordered eating. These ideals can be especially damaging to people whose gender identities are nonbinary, or whose inner sense of self differs from society's expectations based on their sex assigned at birth. Many TGD men, for example, have reached a peak height that is considerably shorter than their average cisgender counterparts. Some TGD women may be taller than cisgender women. Similarly, there may also be differences in body shape whereby people assigned female sex at birth who have undergone endogenous puberty sometimes having a "curvier" body shape than people assigned male sex at birth, who may have a narrower, more mesomorphic (muscular) frame. While these differences vary from person to person, they may immediately "out" TGD patients to peers.[13] Research has found that TGD people who tend to blend in visually based on a more traditional binary gender expression may be more accepted by others.[25]

Gendered ideas about the body are particularly complex when working with TGD patients. Some patients may have difficulty cultivating body acceptance when their bodies and gender identities are not congruent. For these patients, the focus is to work toward caring for their bodies and treating their current bodies in a respectful way. Patients may ultimately decide to pursue medical or surgical affirmation.

Body image development begins in infancy with self/other differentiation[26] and continues throughout the lifespan. Children as young as 19 months of age are aware of gender differences and use gender labels.[26,27] They may engage in play involving gender expression and roles. Many social cues projecting "boy" and "girl" are based on gendered physical differences, such as stereotypical hairstyles or clothing. Body size norms also develop early: children as young as age 5 who identify as girls express preferences for a small/thin body size and shape, another culturally mediated factor.[26] TGD children may begin to label themselves as the nonassigned sex or may express TGD behaviors as early as age 6, with a mean age of 10.4 years.[28] Retrospectively, adolescents may describe childhood as a time when they began to experience body discomfort and discontent. Examples are the desire to wear clothing more aligned with their gender identity, which helps them to feel more comfortable. Many **trans masculine** people express envy about the ways that cisgender peers are permitted to run, jump, or roughhouse.[13] Adolescence is a time of particular developmental significance for body image. A confluence of events occurs in the teen years. Adolescents are acutely aware of societal body ideals and can feel pressured by peers to look a certain way.[29] Awareness of these societal expectations may be heightened in the context of puberty when physical and hormonal changes peak.

Adolescents who are assigned female sex at birth gain weight as body fat increases and hips widen, develop secondary sex characteristics such as breasts, and begin menstruating as a result of increased body fat and maturation of gonadal function. These changes may be perceived negatively and as incongruent with the culturally prescribed "thin ideal."[30] Menstruation can be challenging. Trans masculine adolescents may experience menstruation as a frustrating reminder of sex assigned at birth. Similarly, trans feminine adolescents may experience the lack of menstruation as an indicator that their body does not match their gender identity.[13] Adolescents who are assigned male sex at birth may also experience body changes such as increased height, body and facial hair, changes in vocal register, and increased muscle mass. While cisgender adolescent boys may desire these changes, and late-maturing cisgender boys who have not achieved male body ideals report greater body dissatisfaction than their counterparts,[31] trans masculine and trans feminine adolescents often express body dissonance due to short and tall stature, respectively. TGD patients also describe dissatisfaction with vocal pitch and speaking patterns, which may remain a gender cue even after initiating masculinizing and feminizing hormones.[13]

Adolescence is also a time of increased awareness of social and self-identity, in which there is an intensive focus on asking the question, "Who am I?" Gender plays a role in answering this question, and socially constructed gender roles may feel incongruous to TGD teens.[13] Additionally, adolescents often begin to recognize, explore, and consolidate their gender identities at this time. Gender identity is a person's core sense of being "male," "female," another gender, or no gender. Some TGD adolescents are aware of their gender identities for some time. Others gain awareness at puberty and in response to hormonal changes and the development of secondary sex characteristics. **Gender dysphoria** refers to the distress that some TGD people may experience as a result of incongruence between their gender identity, physical bodies, and sex assigned at birth. Adolescents may engage in food restriction or compensatory eating behaviors as a means to prevent puberty onset or progression.[32]

EATING DISORDERS

Eating disorders are serious and often fatal mental illnesses. They are associated with severe disturbances in thoughts (e.g., "I am fat" even when severely underweight, emotions (i.e., irritability or emotional withdrawal), and eating behaviors (e.g., restricting food intake, binge eating, etc.). Common accompanying symptoms include preoccupation with food, body weight, and shape, as well as measures to control weight or compensate for food consumption. In cisgender adolescent samples, the lifetime prevalence of eating disorders is estimated to be 2.7%, and eating disorders are more than twice as prevalent among adolescents assigned female sex at birth (3.8%) than adolescents assigned male sex at birth (1.5%).[33]

This section briefly defines common eating disorders, using the American Psychiatric Association (2013) DSM-5 descriptors where available. It also introduces common patterns of eating disorder symptomatology among TGD people. Eating disorders include binge-eating disorder, bulimia, anorexia, and other specified feeding and eating disorders (a diagnosis that encompasses unhealthy dieting practices and subclinical disordered eating). According to the National Institute for Mental Health, binge-eating disorder is the most common eating disorder, with a prevalence of 1.2%, followed by bulimia at 0.3% and anorexia at 0.6%.[34]

▶ Binge-Eating Disorder

Binge-eating disorder is characterized by eating large quantities of food (often quickly and to the point of physical discomfort); feeling a loss of control during the binge; experiencing shame, distress, or guilt afterward; and not regularly using compensatory measures to counter the binging. Behaviorally, people with binge-eating disorder may demonstrate concern with body weight and shape, although they may be of average weight. Binge-eating may be a way to comfort or numb, distract from painful feelings, or intentionally make the body larger or less gendered.

▶ Bulimia Nervosa

Bulimia nervosa is characterized by a cycle of binging and compensatory behaviors such as self-induced vomiting,

laxative or diuretic use, or compulsive exercise that are designed to undo or compensate for the effects of binge eating. People with bulimia generally have excessive concern about body shape and weight.[26] Binge/purge behaviors may be used to discharge anger; to numb; to attempt to cleanse or purify the self (especially when there is also trauma); to release tension; or to communicate frustration.

▶ Anorexia Nervosa

Anorexia is characterized by restrictive eating patterns; weight loss (or lack of appropriate weight gain in children); difficulties maintaining a suitable body weight for height, age, and stature; and often a distorted body image. Restrictive eating often leads to the cessation of menses among people assigned female sex at birth.[26] One change from the DSM-IV criteria to the DSM-5 criteria is that menstruation is no longer a required criterion for anorexia, making the definition more gender-inclusive. Anorexia may provide increased control, identity, and self-esteem, distract from painful feelings, make the body smaller, or reduce the appearance of certain body parts.

Avoidant/Restrictive Food-Intake Disorder

Predominately seen in younger people (although not limited to this age range), **avoidant/restrictive food-intake disorder** (ARFID) involves highly selective ("picky") eating. This selectivity can be due to food textures or taste. People with ARFID often have difficulty consuming adequate calories. In children, these behaviors may affect growth and development.[26] Those with ARFID often do not express body image concerns. ARFID may progress to another eating disorder.

Orthorexia

Although not a formal DSM diagnosis, **orthorexia** (a term coined in 1998 by Steven Bratman, MD) is an obsession with "healthful" eating and an inability to eat foods that do not meet the person's definition of healthful. People with orthorexia would be diagnosed with Other Specified Food and Eating Disorder (OSFED), as described below. Weight may or may not be compromised, and people with orthorexia often do not have body image concerns. These factors may help distinguish between anorexia and orthorexia.[26]

Other Specified Food and Eating Disorder (OSFED) and Unspecified Feeding and Eating Disorder (UFED)

Other specified food and eating disorder (OSFED) and **unspecified feeding and eating disorder** (UFED) are diagnostic categories added to the DSM-5 to capture a range of subclinical diagnoses that cause significant clinical distress or negatively impact social or occupational functioning. This may include disordered eating of lower frequency than one would need to meet full clinical criteria and/or limited duration. The diagnosis of OSFED is generally followed by a description of the disordered eating behavior (e.g., OSFED: bulimia nervosa of low frequency). OSFED can include a range of disorders, including muscle dysmorphia, in which a person "bulks up" and focuses on muscularity. OSFED includes "atypical anorexia," in which people eat restrictively but are not weight-compromised, and "atypical bulimia," in which people may purge but not binge, as well as night eating syndrome, in which there are recurrent episodes of excessive food consumption occurring after awakening. In contrast, UFED is a catch-all that is typically used for brief contacts when a clinician is uncertain about the clinical presentation, such as in an emergency room setting, or when there is not sufficient information to make a specific diagnosis. In the only study of cisgender women published to date, the lifetime prevalence of OSFED/UFED was 1.5%.[35]

Anecdotally, patients have mentioned engaging in dieting practices aimed at redistributing body fat. One example is *fat cycling*. This practice involves alternating periods of consuming very low-fat foods or eating restrictively, resulting in weight loss, followed by consuming high-fat or high-calorie foods to redistribute body fat. TGD people may believe that fat cycling promotes a body that conforms more closely to gendered ideals. To date, no scientific studies of fat cycling have been done in TGD populations. As with other dieting practices, preoccupation/obsession, flexibility, and overall physical health are ways to distinguish healthy versus unhealthy practices.

PSYCHOLOGY OF EATING DISORDERS AND BODY DISSATISFACTION

Much of the literature about eating disorder development and body dissatisfaction among TGD people stems from three meta-analyses of available research,[3,7,36] ten quantitative studies, and a handful of case studies. Seven studies included TGD adolescents, and twelve included TGD adults. Additionally, four qualitative studies expanded on the experience of TGD patients with eating disorders, with one study reporting responses from an online questionnaire[37] and three studies analyzing interviews with TGD people.[38-40]

Based on this preliminary research, four themes have emerged to describe psychological motivations linked to eating disorders among TGD patients: (1) using eating disorder behaviors to manage body dissatisfaction related to gender dysphoria; (2) striving for the thin-ideal of femininity (trans feminine patients); (3) seeking to decrease feminine physical characteristics and increase the toned, muscular ideal of masculinity (trans masculine patients); and (4) utilizing eating disorder behaviors to cope with stigmatizing experiences related to being transgender or gender diverse. These studies provide the basis and foundation for the synthesis that follows.

▶ The Role of Gender Minority Stress and Trauma in the Development of Eating Disorders

The Gender Minority Stress and Resilience (GMSR) model was developed to describe the impact of **stigma** on the mental health of members of TGD communities.[9,41] The GMSR model is based on Ilan Meyer's Minority Stress Model,[42] which explored three domains of stress impacting the lesbian, gay, and bisexual community: external and environmental factors, anticipation of upsetting events, and internalized homophobic prejudices. The goal of this model was to explain sexual minority health disparities, including mental health concerns, as a function of outside determinants rather than individual-level factors. Stressors such as discrimination and stigma, and the mechanisms developed to cope with these stressors, are seen to underlie psychological disorders. Expanding this approach to TGD populations, the GMSR model identifies external (distal) and internal (proximal) stressors associated with stigma and mental health concerns and outcomes, as well as resiliency factors that protect transgender and TGD people from harm.[9,41,43] The GMSR model is discussed in more detail in Chapter 3, "Health Disparities."

Although the gender minority stress model was developed to help support TGD patients with depression, suicidal ideation, and general mental health concerns,[41] it is directly applicable to TGD patients with eating disorders.[13] While previous research highlights the heightened risk for using unhealthy coping skills to navigate stigma, such as substance use disorders or self-harm behaviors,[44] only a handful of articles exist that identify the connection between eating disorders as a coping response to stigma and trauma.[38]

The link between eating disorder symptoms and trauma has been well documented. **Trauma** is defined as an event experienced by a person as emotionally overwhelming and has deleterious adverse effects on the person's functioning (see Chapter 11, "Basic Principles of Trauma-Informed and Gender-Affirming Care"). Exposure to traumatic events can lead to clinical symptoms of PTSD, a clinical disorder that includes symptoms such as flashbacks, nightmares, or severe anxiety.[26] Research has shown that a history of trauma, in childhood or adulthood, is more frequent among people with eating disorders than healthy controls.[45] Traumatic experiences are connected to more severe eating disorder presentations and poorer long-term outcomes.[46] The most commonly researched type of trauma delineated in the literature is sexual abuse[47,48]; other types of trauma linked to eating disorders include physical abuse,[49] bullying,[50] and emotional abuse.[51] Such experiences may lead to heightened or blunted arousal states, even in the case of subclinical posttraumatic stress. Eating disorder symptoms, such as food restriction, binge eating, and purging, may be used as a way to numb trauma-related memories, thus decreasing trauma-related hyperarousal.[45]

Examples of trauma experienced by TGD populations include being misgendered by family members or colleagues, being forced to hide TGD identities, or receiving threatening, transphobic comments on social media.[13] Such traumas often occur chronically and over a long period of time. TGD people experience trauma at elevated rates.[52] Many such traumas, such as physical abuse, sexual abuse, or bullying, are directed to or about the body. Traumas may result in increased body hatred or dissociation from the physical body and also intensify feelings of gender or body dysphoria. People often use eating disorder behaviors to cope with the impact of traumatic events or to anchor themselves back into their bodies, shifting the focus away from the trauma. These behaviors may also be used to decrease the gender dysphoria aggravated by the traumatic experience.[53]

Conceptualization Model of Eating Disorders

TGD patients are at increased risk of developing eating disorders due to the myriad factors outlined previously. In gender-expansive patients with eating disorders, the body may be described as a potential source of confusion and distress. The conceptualization model depicted in Figure 15-1 characterizes the trajectory of eating disorder development that may occur with this population.

A thorough assessment of TGD patients with eating disorders must include exploration of the impact of gender dysphoria as well as identity-based traumas. Among people who have this exposure to gender minority stressors and body dissatisfaction, some will have baseline predisposing factors that place them at higher risk for eating disorders. Frequently, TGD patients describe a combination of these factors as central to the development of their eating disorders. By appreciating the complexity of each of these phenomena, independently and concurrently, it is possible to design a treatment approach that meets the unique needs of the TGD with an eating disorder.

Building a Dialectic Model

The treatment model described here for treating TGD patients with disordered eating has evolved over many years. The framework integrates traditional eating disorder treatment models, like Health At Every Size,[54] with core concepts of Marsha Linehan's Dialectical Behavioral Therapy (DBT).[55] While Health at Every Size is applicable to all body types, it can be especially helpful given the complexity that weight stigma brings to the burden of shame a gender-expansive person with other minority stresses may experience if their body is larger than societally accepted.

Health at Every Size promotes size acceptance, seeks to end weight discrimination, and challenges cultural expectations connected to thinness and diet culture. It is a body-positive approach that celebrates body diversity. Some of the core tenets of the Health at Every Size approach are self-acceptance and appreciation of bodies at all sizes; trust of internal body cues, emphasizing mind/body/spirit fulfillment to reduce the emphasis on food; tuning in to body cues; and eating foods that bring pleasure.[54] These principles are applicable to all genders.

Dialectical behavioral therapy (DBT) has also been influential in the creation of this treatment model. The basic tenet of DBT is that an individual can hold two opposing beliefs or truths at the same time. The fundamental principle of DBT is to create a dynamic that promotes two seemingly opposed goals for patients: change and acceptance.[55] Patients are encouraged to integrate these two important positions. Linehan's approach has been applied to many situations and populations, including work with substance use and personality disorders.

Society has different expectations for what body characteristics should be associated with a given gender identity. In working with patients with eating disorders, two theoretical poles are often evident: (1) a sense of body dissatisfaction (focus is on *acceptance*) and (2) the current body is worthy of care and nurturance (focus on *change* from disordered eating). DBT allows gender-expansive patients to explore the connections between gender identity and body image. This

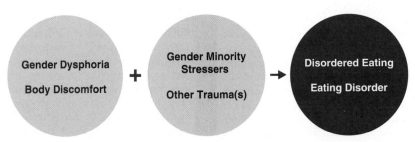

▲ **Figure 15-1.** Conceptualization for patients with eating disorder and gender-identity concerns.

approach neither assumes nor negates a patient's desire to change the body and instead focuses on developing healthier eating and self-care patterns as the initial steps to change.

When working with a patient who feels that their current body does not meet societal expectations based on sex assigned at birth, the therapist must acknowledge that a desire to change is appropriate and reasonable. While this acknowledgment of change is important, equally key is the importance of nurturing the current body. This may require the client to work on radically accepting the current body. Radical acceptance is another term borrowed from Linehan (2014).[55] Radical acceptance is the idea of accepting situations when there is little change that can be effected by the individual. Thus, patients are encouraged to radically accept both the drive to change the body to better support **gender affirmation** and to respect and nurture the bodies they are in at this moment.

▶ Treatment Strategies

At its core, treatment involves supporting patients in practicing safe and healthy ways to effect desired change(s) without unhealthy eating behaviors. Techniques and strategies that are used to work with patients are explained in this section and summarized in Table 15-1. Figure 15-2 is a diagram depicting overlapping paths in the treatment journey.

Acknowledge Links Between Body Image, Gender Identity, and Trauma

Initial eating disorder treatment with TGD patients focuses on the development of a rapport and alliance between the patient and the therapist or clinician.[56] Although clinicians working with individuals with eating disorders are generally familiar with rapport-building, special care and focus are needed in working with TGD patients. Clinicians need to spend time on their own or in groups exploring their own biases and developing cultural responsiveness with TGD populations.[13] Use of identity-affirming language and terminology and a strengths-based, egalitarian, and mutually empowering dynamic[57] is key in working with many populations but is particularly relevant with TGD patients, whose prior treatment experiences may have been invalidating. Other ways of providing a safe space include intake forms that allow patients to use their own terms for gender identity and provide their self-determined names and pronouns. These factors create what Winnicott termed the "holding environment," a space of safety, understanding, and alignment. This sense of emotional safety allows for collaborative exploration and acknowledgment of the body-gender incongruence.[58]

After establishing rapport, the clinician and patient begin the work of radical acceptance around the feeling of body-gender incongruence. Radical acceptance, as mentioned earlier in the chapter, plays an important role in reducing body dysphoria. While the eating disorder may be an effort to change the body, it is an unhealthy one that can have deleterious effects over time. Health care professionals work with patients to reduce and ultimately to suspend these harmful efforts to change the body. An example is exploration of social gender affirmation (such as changes in clothing). The process of radically accepting the current body allows the patient to reduce conflict and distress.

Another helpful facet of clinical work in this stage involves assisting patients in exploring how disordered eating is potentially helpful or unhelpful in their lives, rather than simply right or wrong. Using a nonjudgmental approach,

Table 15-1. Summary of Components of Treatment

Acknowledge Links: Body Image, Gender Identity, and Trauma
Initial discussions of gender identity
Identify specific areas of identity/body incongruence (e.g., menstruation, body shape)
Explore functions of eating disorder (e.g., desire for body changes, self-harm; need to ground and distract)
Discuss and validate experiences of past and present trauma, including misgendering, internalized transphobia, identity nondisclosure, discrimination
Nurture Body in Current State
Radical acceptance of current body
Psychoeducation about eating disorders
Active work on eating disorder symptom reduction, such as weight restoration, reduction/elimination of binge episodes, and/or purging
Increase interoceptive awareness and connection to body cues (hunger, satiety, fatigue, etc.)
Provide alternate coping skills and encourage use; support healthy ways to self-soothe
Promote body pleasure through enjoyable activities
Safe Ways to Affect Change (Short and Long Term)
Discussion of initial body change that may positively create change (e.g., binding to reduce chest and create less reliance on eating disorder)
Discussing transition and importance or overall health; what will best promote congruence
Social affirmation: binding, haircuts, name change, clothing
Medical affirmation: HRT, surgeries
Moderate and pleasurable exercise

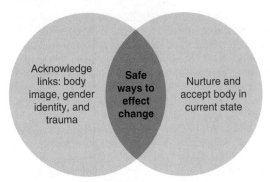

▲ **Figure 15-2.** Model for treating eating disorders in TGD populations. The left and right sides of the diagram are simultaneous tasks, while supporting body change is a later therapeutic task.

the clinician asks questions like: How does this style of eating help with the distress? How does this behavior serve you? As a result of this inquiry, patients may discover that their behaviors serve to reshape their body, increase their self-esteem, or distract from their experience of trauma(s).[53] These insights can often reduce eating disorder symptoms.

At this time, clinicians can also provide psychoeducation about eating disorders. Education can include the idea that eating disorder behaviors provide only temporary relief from psychological distress and that restrictive eating, binging, and purging can result in potential harm to the body.[59] Clinicians can acknowledge how difficult it is for the patient to think about reducing or eliminating such behaviors, particularly if the behaviors support a person's emotional regulation or shape-changing goals, whether specific to gender or size in general. Thus, when letting go of disordered eating behaviors, the person may experience distress due to removal of the short-term coping function, albeit maladaptive, that their disordered eating behaviors had previously performed.

Acknowledge and Treat Trauma-Based Symptoms

As therapy proceeds, the patient is likely to expose areas of hurt, harm, discomfort, and potential traumas that have contributed to the development of their eating disorder. Clinicians working with TGD and/or eating disorder patients must therefore have skills in providing trauma-informed care. Trauma-informed care, described in more detail in Chapter 11, is a treatment framework that emphasizes physical and emotional safety and focuses on supporting a sense of empowerment for trauma survivors, decreasing the potential for harm or retraumatization. Six key principles of trauma-informed care include safety; clinician trustworthiness and transparency; peer support (such as through group therapy), collaboration and mutuality; empowerment, voice,

and choice; and a focus on cultural, historical, and gender choices.[60]

Patients often report past negative experiences with therapy. The reasons for past negative experiences are varied, but one key theme that emerges is that treatment settings that are not trauma-informed can be harmful. For example, TGD patients often report past experiences where trust has been violated, such as being outed or misgendered in binary gender-specific programs, being prompted to share trauma narratives prematurely without attention to therapeutic pacing, or being criticized for choices such as choosing not to pursue romantic relationships. These incidents can contribute to or intensify trauma symptoms. Thus knowledge of trauma principles, such as the importance of pacing and attention to the patient's window of tolerance, is key.[61]

Clinicians can utilize many modalities when working with trauma in this population. While a comprehensive discussion of trauma-informed care is provided elsewhere in this book, some key areas of focus when working with TGD patients with eating disorders include developing safe ways to modulate emotion, grounding and being in the body, discussing traumatic experiences related to their identities, and addressing symptoms of posttraumatic stress related to misgendering and discrimination. There may also be traumas connected to a body that functions in a manner that does not align with their gender identity. For example, a trans masculine patient may be traumatized and deeply affected by the experience of being in a body that menstruates, and a trans feminine patient may experience the trauma of being in a body that does not.

Nurture the Body in Its Current State

The techniques and strategies that clinicians can cultivate for nurturing and nourishing the body are derived from work with eating disorders. Important in this effort is helping the gender-expansive patient reduce symptoms of the eating disorder, creating a healthier body. Other key areas in this stage of treatment involve fostering body positivity and acceptance, exploring gendered influences, encouraging healthy ways for the patient to self-soothe, and connecting the patient to their body through awareness of physical cues, including those that signal hunger and satiety. Because of the risk for medical complications, it is important to seek collaboration with a dietitian and medical professionals[7] who are also trained in working with TGD populations. Several questions may need to be considered. For example, consultation may be necessary to determine the appropriate goal weight for a TGD patient (based on sex assigned at birth or on gender identity). In all cases, patients are assisted in eating balanced meals that are appropriate for their caloric goals,[62] are nutritionally balanced, and taste good.[54]

A goal at this stage is to increase interoceptive awareness. Tribole and Resch define interoceptive awareness as a "process through which the brain receives physical sensations within the body ... and also includes physical sensations triggered by emotions."[63] Patients can increase interoceptive awareness through a focus on cues, such as those of hunger, satiety, fatigue, and other internal sensations.[64,65] Metrics such as hunger and fullness scales can help quantify such physical experiences. Another tool is a food diary, in which patients log emotions before and after eating. These tools teach patients to rely on their body's needs, eat balanced meals and snacks, and decrease food judgments.

Connection to the current body also includes supporting body and self-affirmative activities such as self-care and nurturance.[13] Clinicians can support patients by working on self-compassion and helping them decrease judgments of self and body. The work of Kristin Neff and Christopher Germer provides many excellent resources on self-compassion.[66] These goals relate directly to gender-expansive patients, who may struggle with self-esteem, interpersonal functioning, and social support.[67] Supporting pleasurable, body-based activities can also be helpful. To this end, patients are encouraged to generate lists of enjoyable activities (e.g., mindful walks, yoga, baths) and to engage in them. When patients do things that are good for their bodies (even without feeling that they want to), they affirm the fact that they deserve self-care,[68] thereby increasing body and self-positivity.

Effect Change Safely

Finally, the center of the diagram contains the overlap and middle path: safe ways to effect change. Work that is done in this area is patient-specific and requires an ongoing dialogue between clinician and patient, as well as with other professionals on the treatment team. For adolescent patients, parents, when supportive, should also be part of this discussion.[69] For consenting adolescent patients, parents may be invited to a family meeting or therapy session. In most cases, the conversation begins with an exploration of gender and an understanding of what gender-body congruence might look and feel like. Some patients may experience a sense of body-gender congruence by taking hormones, while others seek gender-affirming surgical care. The idea of safe body changes is explored, and patients are educated about the fact that extreme or risky behaviors do not constitute safe ways to change the body. For example, if the eating disorder is a way to decrease the gendered appearance of the chest, binding or ultimately chest construction surgery may be discussed as safer ways to affirm gender.

Social gender affirmation can also be very helpful as a safe way to change the body. Social affirmation is the process of making others aware of one's gender by expressing gender in a way that is congruent with gender identity,[13] such as name and pronoun changes or changing the body's outward expression. Cutting or growing hair, wearing more

gender-congruent clothing, and chest binding are examples of changes that help with gender expression. Clinicians should be mindful, however, of the fact that even these social affirmation interventions can be used in unhealthy ways. One example is overbinding, in which trans masculine patients may bind too tightly or for longer periods than are healthy. In these cases, it can be helpful to provide education about safe binding practices (e.g., limiting binding to 8–12 hours, not sleeping with binders) and about the adverse consequences of overbinding (e.g., pain, dermatological conditions, numbness or impaired circulation, or shortness of breath).[70] For more information on gender-affirmation practices such as binding, see Chapter 8, "Nonmedical, Nonsurgical Gender Affirmation."

Social and nonmedical/nonsurgical gender affirmation often supports a healthier body image but may not be sufficient in and of itself. Medical gender affirmation may also be desired and has been found to improve life satisfaction, increase gender-body congruence, and support a more positive body image.[38,71] Patients may be referred to a medical team to discuss hormone therapy and possible surgeries, including risks and possible outcomes. Again, coordination with medical professionals is key, and several gender-affirming surgical procedures continue to require a letter of support.[71]

Finally, there are other safe ways to affect changes in the body and relationship with the body. These may include healthy, moderate exercise that focuses on joy and body confidence rather than a drive to burn calories,[72] as well as activities that allow people to be in the body nonjudgmentally, such as yoga or meditation practices.[68]

SUMMARY

- Body image is a key factor for TGD patients. While dissatisfaction is a normative experience when body and gender identity do not match, it may be a factor leading to eating disorders.

- Eating disorders may be clinical or subclinical and have various functions, including decreasing body dissatisfaction, numbing emotions, distraction, and control.

- Eating disorder symptoms may be related to efforts to cope with identity-based traumas associated with the patient's gender minority status. Recovery efforts need to concurrently address the patient's struggle with posttraumatic stress, gender dysphoria, and eating disorders.

- Treatment of eating disorders with TGD patients requires a dialectical approach that includes acknowledging body-gender incongruence and trauma and nurturing the body in its current state to effect change safely. Eating disorder symptom reduction is important. Social, nonmedical/nonsurgical, or medical gender affirmation can help increase congruence in safe ways.

CASE STUDY 1: ALANA

Alana, a 40-year-old White-presenting married patient, assigned female sex at birth, presents to therapy for support. On the intake form, Alana indicated that their pronouns are they/them, and that they identify as nonbinary and pansexual. Alana appears to establish positive rapport quickly, mentioning that while some of their prior therapy experiences have been difficult, the intake form, magazine selection, and safe space indicators in the waiting area helped them to feel more at ease.

During the intake, Alana appears open and forthcoming. Alana's primary reason for therapy is support connected to some difficult family situations. Alana is estranged from their family of origin and extended family, has recently moved to the area, and is having some marital issues. Alana is also the primary caregiver for a preteen who can be emotionally volatile. Alana has limited supports.

Alana has a history of an eating disorder in their teens but did not initially disclose that the eating disorder was active. As a teen, Alana lost a significant amount of weight and had been in counseling. The counselor was a practitioner who "sided with my parents." Alana grew up in a conservative, "almost cult-like" family, where strict gender norms were harshly enforced. Norms for women included pleasantness and passivity, long skirts and blouses, and education around the expected roles of wife and mother. Nonadherence to these norms in their community resulted in a collective shunning and public berating of the offending party. Teenaged Alana, a feminist, did not connect with these gendered norms and reacted strongly both internally and externally. "I hated seeing myself dressed in those horrific outfits. My skin would crawl," they said. "At first I thought it was just rebelling against my parents' values. Then I realized that it was that I was not meant to wear skirts." Alana did not feel female nor male, yet they did not have words for this feeling.

At age 20, Alana married a man they met at a church retreat. Alana's husband Kurt "seemed really different at first, like I could breathe." Alana cut ties with their family, which Kurt encouraged. Quickly, however, Alana began to feel like the escape from their parents led to a similar, if not worse, prison. After the marriage, Kurt demanded that Alana not use birth control and begin the process of starting a family. After several pregnancy losses, Alana had a child, and they found parenting to be difficult from the start. Alana's unhappiness led to overeating and eventually to purging. Alana was able to connect with a "mom's group" and credits this support to stopping the overeating and purging, although the respite was temporary.

As Alana began to branch out socially, Kurt became more needy and demanding. He began to limit Alana's access to money. Alana learned that they could change Kurt's treatment by once again taking on the persona of the passive wife and mother. "I started to hate myself," Alana said. Alana projected this hatred onto their body, sticking pins into their breasts and hips. Alana also began to eat more restrictively, losing a noticeable amount of weight. Kurt did not comment on the self-injury but did berate Alana about the weight loss, telling them they looked like a boy. "Eventually I realized it was less the things I did, and more so my very identity that did not feel 'female.'" Alana grew increasingly depressed but credits these insights as pivotal to identifying as a nonbinary person.

▶ Discussion Questions

1. Alana provided significant detail in the initial session for the clinician to identify some factors that may be significant factors in their eating disorder. What factors are you considering? What are some past/current traumas evident in this case?

2. What are your diagnoses in this case? Your treatment plan?

3. Consideration of cultural factors is important in providing care. What cultural factors need to be considered here? How will you manage the role of church/religion? Despite the difficulties of Alana's upbringing, could spirituality still be a resource or source of support?

4. Alana is a married parent who is also a nonbinary person. Based on Alana's upbringing they may see these identities as conflicting with one another. Should that be the case, how can the clinician support Alana in better understanding this?

5. Alana has discussed restrictive eating and binging and purging symptoms as well as self-harm. These have occurred at various junctures in Alana's life. How do you understand Alana's multiple relapses? Differing eating disorder presentations? Connection to self-harm? What further questions may you need to ask?

6. Treatment involves nurturing the body and healthy body changes. What suggestions do you have to support Alana in greater body/self-care? This is a case where medical affirmation may not be desired, but there are healthy changes that could be helpful. What changes may support healthier body image? How will you discuss them with Alana?

CASE STUDY 2: JAYSON

Nora (she/her) is a licensed clinical social worker in private practice who specializes in helping patients who struggle with eating disorders and trauma and has a special interest in working with LGBTQIA+ patients. Her office is located within a building that houses a local LGBTQIA+ center as well as numerous other health care professionals. After returning a few calls from medical doctors and dietitians that she collaborates with regarding her patients, Nora greets her next patient in the lobby. "Welcome back, it's nice to see you again," she says to the 22-year-old Latinx client wearing an oversized blue sweatshirt and matching athletic pants who stands as she opens the door. Once they are in her office, Nora asks "How are you today, Jayson?"

Jayson started seeing Nora several months ago due to struggling with restrictive eating, excessive exercise, and gender dysphoria. While he identifies as male, has he/him/his pronouns, and presents with a masculine gender expression, Jayson's family, which espouses more "traditional" and binary ideals, does not support Jayson's desire to change his physical body. Jayson cannot move forward with gender affirmation. As a young adult and college student, Jayson is financially dependent on his relatively affluent parents. His parents are working with another therapist in the practice to process their feelings about Jayson being transgender and wanting to physically affirm his gender identity. He shares that his parents are making progress with using his name and pronouns more consistently, although they continue to refuse to support medical affirmation at this time. Jayson describes struggling with eating as his gender dysphoria is intensifying, naming multiple experiences of bullying and being misgendered during high school and continuing within the college environment. He reports feeling hopeless about his ability to navigate the next few years without beginning medical gender affirmation and knows he cannot risk the financial support of his parents.

In previous sessions, Jayson shared that he began restricting his food intake to create a more androgynous appearance, resulting in a welcomed reduction in chest tissue and the disappearance of his body curves. Last month, he was thrilled to experience amenorrhea. He lamented the loss of physical strength that came with restrictive eating and was concerned for his health after injuring himself in the gym while working out. Jayson did not endorse the fear of fat or weight gain typical in patients with symptoms of anorexia, nor did he experience body image disturbance outside of his gender dysphoria. He hoped to gain muscle that would help him appear masculine and did not care about the number on the scale. Instead, Jayson articulated a fear of appearing feminine and being misgendered due to his physical appearance. Now that his monthly bleeding had stopped, he did not want it back.

As Nora was concerned about the increasing severity of his anorexia symptoms and potential for medical consequences, she began discussing with Jayson options for higher levels of care. Jayson fidgeted nervously with the drawstrings of his sweatshirt for several moments before saying, "But I can't go to treatment for this, only women go to eating disorder treatment." Nora acknowledged Jayson's fears and provided information about the gender-inclusive treatment options in the area, including several that accepted his insurance.

Jayson shared anxiety about being misgendered in a treatment program by staff or peers. Nora offered to assist him with calling programs to ascertain their ability to provide a safe space for Jayson to address his eating disorder without being misgendered. Jayson agreed to discuss the possibility of going to treatment with his parents as long as Nora would only recommend places to them that worked with patients of all genders. With this in mind, Nora brought Jayson's parents into the session. Their conversation centered on the overlap of gender dysphoria, eating disorder behaviors, and Jayson's fears of being misgendered. Several local programs that treated patients with eating disorders of all genders were mentioned as treatment options. Jayson's mother acknowledged the difficulty of the situation and related her observations of Jayson increasing his food restrictions whenever anyone misgendered him, such as his grandparents who live at home with them. Jayson's father agreed as well, speaking to the impact of the bullying on the rigidity of Jayson's food intake and hyperfocus on his body. Nora noticed that Jayson had tears in his eyes and offered him space to share his thoughts. "I didn't know you guys noticed that stuff. I… I just… I thought you didn't care." Nora affirmed the importance of the family discussing this further and suggested a family session to continue this conversation while figuring out details around treatment.

While Jayson's journey would continue over the next many months as he completed a local partial hospitalization program for his eating disorder and entered into early recovery, this marked a turning point for Jayson and his family. Although his parents continued to have concerns about medical gender affirmation during young adulthood, they were willing to purchase Jayson a binder to help soothe this aspect of his gender dysphoria. They agreed to set up an appointment with a primary care physician specializing in gender identity and to learn more information about gender affirmation before finalizing their decision. In therapy, Jayson continued to process the impact of being misgendered and bullied at college, as well as how to manage his gender dysphoria without engaging in eating disordered behaviors.

▶ Discussion Questions

1. How does your own professional and clinical background relate or differ from Nora's experience? Does your professional training alter your approach to working with Jayson in any way? How so? Where is your practice located? How might the setting of the clinical provider impact the relationship with the patient? Are there other factors, such as your own identities, that may impact this relationship? How so?

2. In what way(s) would you alter treatment to support Jayson/his family's Latinx heritage? Are there other family members you would like to include in treatment? Outside supports?

3. Nora works to create options for Jayson that assuage his fears about seeking a higher level of care for his eating disorder. What are the options for eating disorder treatment in your area, and do the programs available take patients of all genders?

4. What was the role of the family? How might Jayson's situation be different if his parents were less supportive of his transgender identity? How would it differ if they were more supportive of his request to begin medical gender affirmation?

5. Other aspects of identity are relevant in this case discussion. What barriers might exist if Jayson came from a family that did not have insurance or were economically disadvantaged? What opportunities might arise if Jayson was able to achieve financial independence from his parents?

REFERENCES

1. Bell K, Rieger E, Hirsch JK. Eating disorder symptoms and proneness in gay men, lesbian women, and transgender and gender nonconforming adults: Comparative levels and a proposed mediational model. *Front Psychol*. 2019;9:1–13.
2. Conner M, Johnson C, Grogan S. Gender, sexuality, body image and eating behaviors. *J Health Psychol*. 2004;9(4):505–515.
3. Thapliyal P, Hay P, Conti J. Role of gender in the treatment experiences of people with an eating disorder: a metasynthesis. *J Eating Disord*. 2018;6(18):1–16.
4. Mitchell KS, Mazzeo SE. Evaluation of a structural model of objectification theory and eating disorder symptomatology among European American and African American undergraduate women. *Psychol Women Quarter*. 2009;33(4):384–395.
5. Rodriguez R, Marchand E, Ng J, Stice E. Effects of a cognitive dissonance-based eating disorder prevention program are similar for Asian American, Hispanic, and White participants. *Int J Eating Disord*. 2008;41(7):618–625.
6. Guss CE, William DN, Reisner SL, Bryn Austin S, Katz-Wise SL. Disordered weight management behavior, nonprescription steroid use, and weight perception in transgender youth. *J Adolesc Health*. 2017;60:17–22.
7. McClain Z, Peebles R. Body image and eating disorders among lesbian, gay, bisexual, and transgender youth. *Pediatr Clin North Am*. 2016;63(6):1079–1090.
8. Diemer EW, White Hughto JM, Gordon AR, Guss C, Austin SB, Reisner SL. Beyond the binary: differences in eating disorder prevalence by gender identity in a transgender sample. *Transgender Health*. 2018;3(1):17–23.
9. Testa RJ, Rider GN, Haug NA, Balsam KF. Gender confirming medical interventions and eating disorder symptoms among transgender individuals. *Health Psychol*. 2017;36(10):927–936.
10. Reisner SL, Katz-Wise SL, Gordon AR, Corliss HL, Austin SB. Social epidemiology of depression and anxiety by gender identity. *J Adolesc Health*. 2016;59(2):203–208.
11. Parent MC, Arriaga AS, Gobble T, Wille L. Stress and substance use among sexual and gender minority individuals across the lifespan. *Neurobiol Stress*. 2018;10:100146.
12. Killeen TK, Greenfield SF, Bride BE, Cohen L, Gordon SM, Roman PM. Assessment and treatment of co-occurring eating disorders in privately funded addiction treatment programs. *Am J Addict*. 2011;20(3):205–211.
13. Dalzell H, Protos K. *A Clinician's Guide to Gender Identity and Body Image: Practical Support for Working with Transgender and Gender-Expansive Clients*. Philadelphia, PA: Jessica. Kingsley Publishers; 2020.
14. Cash TF. Cognitive behavioral perspectives on body image. In: Cash TF, Smolak L, eds. *Body Image: A Handbook of Science and Prevention*. New York: The Guilford Press. 2011: 39–47.
15. Stice E, Shaw HE. Role of body dissatisfaction in the onset and maintenance of eating pathology: a synthesis of research findings. *J Psychosom Res*. 2002;53(5):985–993.
16. Paxton SJ, Damiano SR. The development of body image and weight bias in childhood. *Adv Child Develop Behav*. 2017;52:269–298.
17. Arizona Board of Regents (1997). Eating issues and body image continuum. https://health.arizona.edu/sites/default/files/continuum2.pdf
18. Hughes EK, Mundy LK, Romaniuk H, et al. Body image dissatisfaction and the adrenarchal transition. *J Adolesc Health*. 2018;63(5):621–627.
19. Howard LM, Romano KA, Heron KE. Prospective changes in disordered eating and body dissatisfaction across women's first year of college: the relative contributions of sociocultural and college adjustment risk factors. *Eat Behav*. 2020;36:101357.
20. McLean SA, Paxton SJ, Wertheim EH. Factors associated with body dissatisfaction and disordered eating in women in midlife. *Int J Eat Disord*. 2010;43(6):527–536.
21. Meier EP, Gray J. Facebook photo activity associated with body image disturbance in adolescent girls. *Cyberpsychol Behav Soc Netw*. 2014;17(4):199–206.
22. Vitelli R. (2013). Media Exposure and the "Perfect" Body. https://www.psychologytoday.com/us/blog/media-spotlight/201311/media-exposure-and-the-perfect-body.
23. Voges MM, Giabbiconi CM, Schöne B, Waldorf M, Hartmann AS, Vocks S. Gender differences in body evaluation: do men show more self-serving double standards than women?. *Front Psychol*. 2019;10:544.
24. Bockting WO, Miner MH, Swinburne Romine RE, Hamilton A, Coleman E. Stigma, mental health, and resilience in an online sample of the US transgender population. *Am J Public Health*. 2013;103(5):943–951.
25. Smolak L. Body image development in childhood. In: Cash TF, Smolak L, eds. *Body Image: A Handbook of Science and Prevention*. New York: The Guilford Press; 2011; 67–75.
26. Keo-Meier C, Ehrensaft D., eds. *Perspectives on Sexual Orientation and Diversity. The Gender Affirmative Model: An Interdisciplinary Approach to Supporting Transgender and Gender Expansive Children*. Washington, DC: American Psychological Association; 2018.
27. Zosuls KM, Ruble DN, Tamis-Lemonda CS, Shrout PE, Bornstein MH, Greulich FK. The acquisition of gender labels in infancy: implications for gender-typed play. *Develop Psychol*. 2009;45(3):688–701.
28. Grossman AH, D'Augelli AR. Transgender youth: invisible and vulnerable. *J Homosexual*. 2006;51(1):111–128.
29. Croll JK, Neumark-Sztainer D, Story M, Ireland M. Prevalence and risk and protective factors related to disordered eating

behaviors among adolescents: relationship to gender and ethnicity. *J Adolesc Health.* 2002;31(2):166–175.

30. Witcomb GL, Bouman WP, Brewin N, Richards C, Fernandez-Aranda F, Arcelus J. Body image dissatisfaction and eating-related psychopathology in trans individuals: a matched control study. *Eur Eat Disord Rev.* 2015;23:287–293.

31. Ackard DM, Peterson CB. Association between puberty and disordered eating, body image, and other psychological variables. *Int J Eat Disord.* 2001;29(2):187–194.

32. Coelho JS, Suen J, Clark BA, Marshall SK, Geller J, Lam PY. Eating disorder diagnoses and symptom presentation in transgender youth: a scoping review. *Curr Psychiat Rep.* 2019;21(11):107.

33. Merikangas KR, He JP, Burstein M, et al. Lifetime prevalence of mental disorders in U.S. adolescents: results from the National Comorbidity Survey Replication–Adolescent Supplement (NCS-A). *J Am Acad Child Adolesc Psychiatry.* 2010;49(10):980–989.

34. Hudson JI, Hiripi E, Pope HG, Kessler RC. The prevalence and correlates of eating disorders in the national comorbidity survey replication. *Biologic Psychiat J Psychiatr Neurosci Therap.* 2007;61(3):348–358.

35. Mustelin L, Lehtokari VL, Keski-Rahkonen A. Other specified and unspecified feeding or eating disorders among women in the community. *Int J Eat Disord.* 2016;49(11):1010–1017.

36. Jones BA, Haycraft E, Murjan S, Arcelus J. Body dissatisfaction and disordered eating in trans people: a systematic review of the literature. *Int Rev Psychiatr.* 2016;28(1):81–94.

37. Duffy ME, Henkel KE, Earnshaw VA. Transgender patients' experiences of eating disorder treatment. *J LGBT Issues Counsel.* 2016;10(3):136–149.

38. Ålgars M, Alanko K, Santtila, P, Sandnabba NK. Disordered eating and gender identity disorder: a qualitative study. *Eat Disord.* 2012;20:300–311.

39. Gordon AR, Austin SB, Krieger N, White Hughto JM, Reisner S. I have to constantly prove to myself, to people, that I fit the bill: Perspectives on weight and shape control behaviors among low-income, ethnically diverse young transgender women. *Soc Sci Med.* 2016;165:141–149.

40. McGuire JK, Doty JL, Catalpa JM, Ola C. Body image in transgender young people: findings from a qualitative, community based study. *Body Image.* 2016;18:96–107.

41. Hendricks ML, Testa RJ. A conceptual framework for clinical work with transgender and gender nonconforming patients: an adaptation of the minority stress model. *Prof Psychol Res Pract.* 2012;43(5):460–467.

42. Meyer IH. Minority stress and mental health in gay men. J Health Social Behav. 1995:38-56. https://www.jstor.org/stable/2137286?seq=1

43. Jäggi T, Jellestad L, Corbisiero S, et al. Gender minority stress and depressive symptoms in transitioned Swiss transpersons. *Biomed Res Int.* 2018;2018:8639263.

44. Donaldson AA, Hall A, Neukirch J, et al. Multidisciplinary care considerations for gender nonconforming adolescents with eating disorders: a case series. *Int J Eat Disord.* 2018;51:475–479.

45. Briere J, Scott C. Assessment of trauma symptoms in eating-disordered populations. *Eat Disord.* 2007;15(4):347–358.

46. Castellini G, Lo Sauro C, Ricca V, Rellini AH. Body esteem as a common factor of a tendency toward binge eating and sexual

47. Brewerton TD. Eating disorders, trauma, and comorbidity: focus on PTSD. *Eat Disord.* 2007;15(4):285–304.

48. Palmisano BT, Zhu L, Eckel RH, Stafford JM. Sex differences in lipid and lipoprotein metabolism. *Mol Metab.* 2018;15:45–55.

49. Adams J, Mrug S, Knight DC. Characteristics of child physical and sexual abuse as predictors of psychopathology. *Child Abuse Neglect.* 2018;86:167–177.

50. Mazzeo SE, Espelage DL. Association between childhood physical and emotional abuse and disordered eating behaviors in female undergraduates: an investigation of the mediating role of alexithymia and depression. *J Counsel Psychol.* 2002;49(1):86–100.

51. Harris C, Harris J, Oseroff K. Considerations to enhance the plate-by-plate approach for adolescents undergoing family-based treatment for eating disorders. *J Acad Nutr Dietet.* 2020;120(1):21–22.

52. Grant JM, Mottet LA, Tanis J, Harrison J, Herman JL, Keisling M. *Injustice at Every Turn: A Report of the National Transgender Discrimination Survey.* Washington, DC: National Center for Transgender Equality and National Gay and Lesbian Task Force; 2011.

53. Van der Kolk B. *The Body Keeps the Score: Brain, Mind, and Body in the Healing of Trauma.* New York: Penguin Books; 2015.

54. Bacon L. *Health at Every Size.* Dallas, TX: BenBella Books; 2010.

55. Linehan MM. *DBT Skills Training Manual.* 2nd ed. New York: Guilford Press; 2014.

56. Ardito RB, Rabellino D. Therapeutic alliance and outcome of psychotherapy: historical excursus, measurements, and prospects for research. *Front Psychol.* 2011;2:270.

57. Miller JB, Stiver IP. *The Healing Connection: How Women Form Relationships in Therapy and in Life.* Boston, MA: Beacon Press; 1997.

58. Winnicott DW. *Playing and Reality.* London: Tavistock; 1993.

59. Monge MC, Loh M. Medical complications of eating disorders in pediatric patients. *Pediatr Ann.* 2018;47(6):e238–e243.

60. Substance Abuse and Mental Health Services Administration (SAMHSA) Trauma-Informed Care in Behavioral Health Services. Treatment Improvement Protocol (TIP) Series 57. Rockville, MD: Substance Abuse and Mental Health Services Administration; 2014.

61. Rothschild B. *The Body Remembers.* New York: Norton and Company; 2016.

62. Kimber M, McTavish JR, Couturier J, et al. Consequences of child emotional abuse, emotional neglect and exposure to intimate partner violence for eating disorders: a systematic critical review. *BMC Psychol.* 2017:5–33.

63. Tribole E, Resch E. *Intuitive Eating.* New York: St. Martin's Griffin; 2012.

64. Bruch H. *Eating Disorders: Obesity, Anorexia and the Person Within.* New York: Persus Books; 1979.

65. Craig AD. How do you feel—now? The anterior insula and human awareness. *Nat Rev Neurosci.* 2009;10(1):59–70.

66. Neff KD, Germer CK. A pilot study and randomized controlled trial of the mindful self-compassion program. *J Clin Psychol.* 2013;69(1):28–44.

67. Arcelus J. Risk factors for non-suicidal self-injury among trans youth. *J Sex Med.* 2016;13(3):402–412.

68. Piran N, Neumark-Sztainer D. Yoga and the experience of embodiment: a discussion of possible links. *Eat Disord.* 2020;28(4):330–348.

69. Kimberly LL, McBride Folkers K, Friesen P, et al. Ethical issues in gender-affirming care for youth. *Pediatrics.* 2018;142(6): e20181537.

70. Dutton L, Koenig K, Fennie K. Gynecologic care of the female-to-male transgender man. *J Midwifery Womens Health [Internet].* 2008;53(4):331–337.

71. El-Hadi H, Stone J, Temple-Oberle C, Harrop AR. Gender-affirming surgery for transgender individuals: perceived satisfaction and barriers to care. *Plastic Surgery.* 2018;26(4):263–268.

72. Bergmeier HJ, Morris H, Mundell N, Skouteris H. What role can accredited exercise physiologists play in the treatment of eating disorders? A descriptive study. *Eat Disord.* 2019:1–19.

Screening and Prevention of HIV and Sexually Transmitted Infections

16

Asa Radix
Zil G. Goldstein

INTRODUCTION

Transgender and gender diverse (TGD) people have disparate rates of HIV infection and sexually transmitted infections (STIs) compared with **cisgender** populations, and they are often reluctant or unable to access health services that can provide treatment and preventive care. Although there are many reasons why TGD patients may not readily engage in health care, including sexual and reproductive health services, pervasive structural, interpersonal, and individual-level stigma is prominent.[1] TGD people often face discrimination in health care settings, including denial of medical care and health care professionals who lack relevant clinical knowledge and cultural responsiveness. In addition, they may also experience financial barriers that limit access to sexual health screenings and evidence-based prevention interventions.[2,3] This chapter discusses how clinicians can provide individualized screening recommendations, risk-reduction counseling, and biomedical interventions that enable the provision of gender-affirming and welcoming health care for TGD patients.

BACKGROUND

Approximately 1 million, or 0.4% of adults in the United States, identify as transgender, i.e., with a **gender identity** that differs from the sex they were assigned at birth.[4–6] A higher proportion of youth (about 2% of high-school-aged individuals) identify as transgender.[7] Although there are no population-based estimates for the prevalence of gender **nonbinary** people (those who identify outside the gender binary of boy/man or girl/woman), 35% of the respondents of the 2015 U.S. Transgender Survey (USTS) identified as gender nonbinary.[2] Some TGD individuals may seek gender-affirming interventions, such as medical (hormonal, surgical, or both), social (changing pronouns, gender presentation), or legal interventions.[6,8] Over the past decade, the incidence

of gender-affirming surgeries, especially genital surgeries, has increased in the United States.[9]

EPIDEMIOLOGY OF HIV INFECTION AND STIs IN THE TRANSGENDER POPULATION

The risk of HIV transmission is influenced by the type of sexual exposure (e.g., whether anal, vaginal, or oral) and the presence of coexisting STIs, genital inflammation, or mucous membrane tears. Condomless anal receptive sex carries the highest risk of HIV transmission.[10] Health care professionals must understand the demographics of their patients' sexual partners and potential sexual exposures to assess their risk of becoming infected with HIV. TGD people may have diverse sexual partners who may be cisgender, transgender, or gender diverse. Sexual orientation identity is similarly diverse; in the USTS, transgender respondents identified as queer (21%), pansexual (18%), gay/lesbian/same gender loving (16%), bisexual (14%), and asexual (10%).[2] Several studies have also indicated that the sexual orientation identity of some TGD people may shift over time, potentially altering their risk for HIV and STIs.[11]

A recent systematic review of HIV infection among transgender women in the United States estimated the prevalence of HIV to be 14% among transgender women, with the highest rates among Black (44%) and Hispanic/Latinx (26%) transgender women.[12] Similar elevated rates of HIV infection are seen in international settings, with approximately one in five transgender women living with HIV globally.[13] Fewer studies have been conducted in transgender men; however, research indicates an HIV prevalence of approximately 3%.[12] The elevated HIV prevalence in transgender populations is due to a combination of structural, individual, interpersonal, biologic, and network factors.[14] High rates of societal stigma and discrimination lead to social exclusion and psychological stress, unemployment, poverty, and reduced access to health care. Stigma is also associated with condomless anal sex, early sexual debut, sex work, and high numbers of predominately cisgender male sexual partners.[15–24]

There are few data on the prevalence of other STIs among transgender people, mainly due to inconsistent collection and reporting of gender identity data across U.S. jurisdictions that contribute to STI surveillance.[24] Both international and U.S. studies, however, have reported elevated incidence and prevalence of rectal and pharyngeal (extragenital) *Neisseria gonorrhoeae* and *Chlamydia trachomatis*, syphilis, and hepatitis B and C infections among transgender women. The rates of these infections in transgender women are similar to and frequently exceed the rates in cisgender men who have sex with men (MSM).[24–33] Among transgender men, the highest STI and HIV rates are among those who have sex with cisgender men.[34,35] Some studies have shown rates of gonorrhea, chlamydia, and hepatitis B and C among transgender men that are similar to those of transgender women.[36–38] Data from the Sexually Transmitted Disease (STD) Surveillance Network investigated STI prevalence among transgender people attending STD clinics in 25 jurisdictions across the United States and found high rates of STIs in both transgender men and women. Extragenital chlamydia and gonorrhea infections occurred in 16.8% and 15% of transgender women and 14.3% and 12.1% of transgender men, respectively, similar to rates in cisgender MSM. The rates of urogenital infections due to chlamydia and gonorrhea were higher among transgender men compared with transgender women, 4.1% and 7.1% versus 0.2% and 2.8%, respectively.[39] Few studies have investigated rates of STIs among gender nonbinary people; however, two recent studies found rates of bacterial STIs that were comparable to those of cisgender MSM and transgender women.[40,41]

Gender Affirmation and Risk of STIs

One of the gaps in the literature is that studies have not included information about **gender affirmation** and STIs. This information is important, because a person's history of genital surgery will influence STI screening recommendations and risk. Most transgender people have not undergone gender-affirming genital surgeries; thus, the majority of transgender women still have a penis, and the majority of transgender men still have a vagina. About 12% of transgender women in the United States have had surgery to create a vagina (**vaginoplasty**), most commonly using penile tissue[42,43] but occasionally using intestinal tissue (colo- or intestinal vaginoplasty). New procedures include the use of peritoneal or urethral mucosal grafts in the penile-inversion vaginoplasty to help improve natural lubrication.[44–46] Neovaginal STIs have infrequently been reported in the literature and include genital warts, herpes simplex infection, gonorrhea, and most recently, chlamydia in women with peritoneal or urethral grafts.[47–57]

To date, there are no case reports or other data regarding STIs among transgender men who have had gender-affirming genital surgeries such as **phalloplasty** or **metoidioplasty**.

Rates of HIV and STI Screening

Despite having a higher risk for HIV, transgender women and men who have sex with cisgender men are only half as likely to be screened for HIV compared with cisgender MSM.[55] Many factors contribute to lower screening rates in these populations, including avoidance of preventive care due to fear (real or anticipated) of discrimination, lack of access to transgender-affirming services, higher rates of substance use, concerns about confidentiality, HIV-related stigma, cost, homelessness, behavioral health comorbidities, and internalized transphobia.[2,56,57] Transgender women may also be focused on other health needs, such as finding housing or hormone care, and less concerned about HIV screening.[57,58] Data focusing on transgender women suggest that health care professionals may be less likely to offer HIV testing compared to cisgender people. One study shows that only 8% of surveyed transgender women in Brazil were offered HIV testing by a medical professional.[57]

Available data suggest that transgender MSM share many of the same barriers to HIV screening as cisgender MSM, such as HIV stigma, low perceived risk, and concerns about confidentiality, but also experience unique barriers in finding skilled clinicians and navigating sex-segregated services that are not inclusive of transgender MSM.

SEXUAL HEALTH ASSESSMENT

Screening for STIs in transgender populations should start with a comprehensive sexual health history, as this information will further define the risk as well as the sites potentially exposed to STIs. Because many TGD patients have avoided medical care, health care professionals should plan an extended visit to establish rapport and explain procedures before proceeding to the physical examination.

When obtaining a sexual health assessment, clinicians should be aware that many TGD patients have experienced sexual trauma, both in childhood and as adults.[59–61] Using a **trauma-informed care (TIC)** approach is essential to all patient interactions. TIC aims to understand, address, and alleviate the trauma burden faced by patients by recognizing the impact of trauma and enacting policies and procedures that aim to resist retraumatization. Examples include ensuring that the physical space is welcoming; making exits easily accessible; explicitly discussing confidentiality; explaining the reasons for asking sexual health questions; and obtaining permission before performing a history or any physical exam maneuver. Medical professionals should ask patients what terms they use for body parts, as some TGD patients may prefer terms that better align with their gender identity. Using nongendered terms, such as genitals or internal parts, is often acceptable to patients. Chapters 11, "Basic Principles of Trauma-Informed and Gender-Affirming Care" and 13, "Performing a Trauma-Informed Physical Examination" give additional details on how to conduct a patient encounter in a trauma-informed manner.

Chapter 12, "Obtaining a Gender-Affirming Sexual History," provides detailed information about the components of the sexual health history and how to conduct this type of health history using TIC strategies and gender-affirming practices. In general, all gender-affirming interventions, such as the use of hormones, both prescribed within and obtained outside of medical settings, should be documented. Any surgeries should be noted and an **anatomical inventory** taken of existing body parts, e.g., whether a person assigned female sex at birth still has a vagina, uterus, or ovaries, and whether they have undergone gender-affirming surgeries such as metoidioplasty. It is also important to record the use of soft tissue fillers, since these materials can be associated with medical complications, such as skin and soft tissue infections, silicone migration, granulomas, and vasculitis.[62-65] Skin-related complications from silicone use, such as ulceration and rash, may be difficult to distinguish from STIs, and clinicians should consider this in the differential diagnosis of skin lesions.

The sexual health history should also elicit information about the gender of sexual partners, without making assumptions that they are cisgender; sexual behaviors, including sex work; protection from STIs (condoms, postexposure prophylaxis [PEP], preexposure prophylaxis [PrEP]); past history of STI screening and results; and plans for pregnancy or contraception needs. The sexual health history is a good opportunity to discuss family planning options with transgender men, who may be unaware that they can get pregnant while on testosterone.

STI SCREENING AFTER GENDER-AFFIRMING GENITAL SURGERY

There are no national guidelines that provide details on how to conduct STI screening in individuals who have undergone gender-affirming surgeries. The Centers for Disease Control and Prevention (CDC) states that STI- and HIV-related risks should be assessed based on current anatomy and sexual behaviors.[66] Therefore, clinicians should have a detailed understanding of the types of surgeries that patients have undertaken to help guide decision making. STI screening for transgender people should also include screening for HIV, syphilis, and hepatitis C. Patients should be offered immunizations against hepatitis A and B and HPV. Although the frequency of STI screening for transgender people has not been determined by the CDC, a risk-based approach may be feasible, e.g., every 3–6 months if a person engages in higher-risk sexual behaviors, including condomless sex, having multiple partners or anonymous partners,

having sex under the influence of alcohol or drugs, and a history of STIs.

Transgender women who have had a vaginoplasty and who partner with cisgender men or other transgender women often continue to have receptive anal sex and should undergo screening for gonorrhea and chlamydia at extragenital sites. A visual inspection to look for genital lesions is important and can be performed during a pelvic exam using a small speculum or anoscope. It is not known whether urine samples or neovaginal swabs for gonorrhea and chlamydia are superior for screening.

Transgender men who have undergone metoidioplasty still have a vagina, uterus, and ovaries and should be screened for STIs accordingly. Extragenital testing should be done in all patients who engage in oral or anal receptive sex. Patients who have had a phalloplasty or metoidioplasty with urethral lengthening may still have a vagina; therefore, screening for gonorrhea and chlamydia requires a vaginal swab, since a urine sample is not sufficient to diagnose a vaginal infection. Transgender men who are taking testosterone can have atrophic vaginitis resulting in discomfort during pelvic exams. The current best practice is to use a small speculum and water-based lubricant. Some clinicians have reported benefits to prescribing vaginal estrogen 2 weeks prior to the exam.[67]

▶ Strategies to Improve HIV and STI Screening Rates

Several strategies have been evaluated to increase access to HIV and STI screening for TGD people. Screening can be facilitated by integrating sexual health services with gender-affirming care practices and by training health care professionals in the unique health care needs of the TGD population.[68]

There are many ways to create gender-affirming health care settings for TGD people. Being openly and visibly welcoming by displaying nondiscrimination policies, LGBTQIA+ flags or symbols, artwork, brochures, and magazines that are inclusive of gender diversity and having unisex or all-gender restrooms help convey an accepting and welcoming office environment. Even more important is to have clinic staff who are respectful and trained in how to address patients without assumptions about gender identity, such as avoiding the use of gendered pronouns or gendered language (e.g., ma'am, sir) unless one has specifically asked what terms a patient uses. All clinics should have registration forms that allow people to document their gender identity as well as sex assigned at birth.[69] Health care professionals should be knowledgeable about the specific preventive health care needs of TGD patients and the effects of gender-affirming hormone therapy. Office staff should also be prepared to troubleshoot the problems that inevitably arise with insurance companies, pharmacies, and laboratory services when a patient's gender identity is not congruent with insurance documentation (Table 16-1).

Specific tools to improve HIV screening include the use of rapid, point-of-care testing, i.e., testing done at the time and place of patient care with results immediately available. Point-of-care testing has been shown to increase HIV testing uptake among cisgender and sexual minority men. It is especially important when offering HIV testing to transgender women, since they are less likely than other populations to return to a clinic to obtain test results.[57] The use of mobile medical units has been a successful strategy to engage transgender women in sexual health services, particularly those exchanging sex for money, as they may be reluctant to engage in clinic-based services.[70] Many transgender women report being more interested in HIV testing if it is conducted by a peer rather than a health care professional.[57] This strategy is

consistent with data showing that both online and in-person social supports can improve HIV testing rates.[71] HIV self-testing may also increase screening rates among cisgender MSM and transgender women.[72] Emerging data, however, show that this strategy may result in lower rates of linkage to care than traditional tests administered by a clinician or trained HIV tester.[72–74]

Self-collection of specimens for gonorrhea and chlamydia testing has been shown to be feasible and equivalent compared to clinician-collected specimens.[75] Self-collection of specimens at home is preferred by many patients over collection in the clinic[76] and provides an acceptable alternative for TGD patients who may be reluctant to use clinic restrooms.

PREVENTION STRATEGIES

▶ HIV Prevention

Since the start of the HIV/AIDS pandemic, considerable progress has been made in understanding HIV transmission and prevention, yet staggering rates of new HIV infections continue to occur daily worldwide.[77] The HIV/AIDS pandemic occurs within a complex social environment where HIV transmission is impacted by a constellation of social norms.[78,79] Examples include specific sexual practices such as receptive anal intercourse, patterns of sexual partnering including multiple sexual partners, contextual influences such as engaging in sex in public venues, sexual networks, sex inequality, sex work, contraceptive choices, recreational use of substances that decrease sexual inhibitions and increase the risk of sharing drug paraphernalia, and a pernicious stigma that continues to restrict access to health care for many high-risk and infected individuals.[78,79]

Prevention of sexual HIV transmission has been a significant priority since the start of the HIV epidemic, and no single prevention intervention has proven to be completely effective.[78] The most potent intervention to reduce vertical and horizontal sexual transmission of HIV is ART for HIV-infected individuals, or "treatment as prevention."[78] Although imperfect, consistent use of barrier protection in the form of latex condoms or dental dams can decrease the transmission of HIV by 90–95%.[80] One of the most successful approaches for HIV prevention is **PrEP** with a daily, oral, fixed-dose combination of tenofovir disoproxil fumarate (TDF) and emtricitabine (FTC).

HIV PrEP using a fixed-dose combination of tenofovir disoproxil fumarate and emtricitabine (TDF/FTC) has been recommended by the CDC since 2011.[81] A second agent, tenofovir alafenamide and emtricitabine (TAF/FTC), was approved in 2019. The use of TDF/FTC is recommended for all persons at risk of acquiring HIV sexually,[82] while TAF/FTC is only approved for cisgender men and transgender women.

After starting TDF/FTC, protection against HIV acquisition via rectal exposure is thought to occur after 7 days. For genital and blood exposure, it is thought that drug

Table 16–1. How to Create a Gender-Affirming Clinical Setting

Action	Rationale
Prominently display transgender-inclusive posters, policies, and literature	Signal to TGD people that you have considered the best way to serve them
Using gender-inclusive language at all times to address all patients	You cannot tell someone's gender identity by looking at them, and this practice avoids the possibility of inadvertently misgendering someone
Gender-inclusive signage on all patient-accessible rest rooms	TGD people often have anxiety around being harassed because of their TGD status while using restrooms, and all-gender restrooms assure TGD people that they are welcome
Hire TGD staff	TGD staff will help contribute to a welcoming environment for transgender patients as well as create more exposure to transgender issues in the office
Delay physical exams that require disrobing until a patient–clinician relationship is well established	TGD patients will feel more comfortable having their bodies if they have a trusting relationship with the clinician
Ask for sex assigned at birth and current gender identity separately on intake forms	These questions gather all medical information and allow for TGD people to express the correct gender while also providing relevant information about their organs present at birth

TGD, transgender and gender-diverse.

concentrations reach optimal protective levels after 20 days of treatment, although protection may occur earlier. Because of the lag between starting PrEP and onset of protection, transgender men and nonbinary individuals having vaginal/frontal sex should be counseled about using condoms during this time.

Some small studies have suggested that the combination of estrogen hormone therapy with TDF/FTC may result in lower plasma tenofovir levels[83] and changes in the ratios of tenofovir metabolites in rectal tissue. These reductions, however, have not been shown to reduce the efficacy of PrEP in transgender women.[84] In both studies, estradiol levels were not affected by the presence of oral PrEP.[83,85] In fact, studies to date show that PrEP appears to be effective in transgender women who take it regularly. Drug concentrations in the iPrEx (Preexposure Prophylaxis Initiative) clinical trial correlated with PrEP protection, with no HIV infections occurring in transgender women who had drug concentrations equivalent to taking four or more tablets per week.[86,87] The greatest risk to PrEP efficacy in transgender individuals is lack of PrEP awareness and the fact that many have not been offered PrEP. Clinicians should assess all patients for PrEP eligibility, discuss risks and benefits of treatment, and facilitate access to patient assistance programs if finances are a barrier (Table 16-2.) It is important to emphasize to patients that PrEP does not decrease hormone levels since this fear may prevent transgender women from initiating treatment.[88,89] An alternative way of dosing PrEP with TDF/FTC is to take it on demand instead of daily, with two TDF/FTC tablets 2–24 hours before sex and one additional tablet at 24 and 48 hours after sex.[90] However, this dosing schedule is not recommended for transgender women receiving estrogen or for people who have vaginal/frontal sex, as it has only been studied in cisgender men.

There are other agents in the pipeline, including long-acting injectable PrEP (cabotegravir), and several agents with different mechanisms of action and modes of delivery (e.g., islatravir, vaginal rings, vaginal and rectal microbicides, and broadly neutralizing monoclonal antibodies, drug implants and transdermal devices).[91] Unfortunately, clinical trials to date have included few, if any, TGD people, so we know little about their treatment preferences. Transgender women have expressed interest in long-acting injectables due to perceived easier adherence; however, community concerns about the logistics of receiving treatment and possible drug interactions need to be addressed.[92]

Lastly, there remains hope on the horizon in the form of ongoing research on an effective HIV vaccine. Primary challenges to the development of an effective HIV vaccine include the need to protect against globally diverse virus strains and unclear immune correlates of protection.[93]

▶ STI Prevention

Interventions for STI prevention have traditionally focused on delaying sexual debut, improving rates of condom use, facilitating condom negotiation, reducing the number of sexual partners, and reducing the frequency of sexual intercourse.[94,95] There are only a few clinical trials that have focused on reduction of sexual risk among transgender people. One study that used a culturally specific and empowerment-based group HIV prevention intervention resulted in a significant 40% reduction in condomless anal sex among young transgender women.[96]

Biomedical interventions are currently being investigated in cisgender MSM populations to reduce bacterial STIs. In one small study, taking 200 mg of doxycycline within 24 hours of having condomless anal or oral sex reduced the incidence of syphilis and chlamydia.[97] In another small study, the use of 100 mg of doxycycline reduced gonorrhea, chlamydia, and syphilis incidence.[98] The long-term effects of doxycycline prophylaxis on antimicrobial resistance, however, are not known, and this approach has not been studied in transgender populations. Currently, doxycycline is not approved by the CDC or U.S. Food and Drug Administration for STI prophylaxis.

Another preventive strategy is vaccination. Currently, vaccines are available for hepatitis B and human papillomavirus. Guidelines for adult vaccinations are available at the CDC website (https://www.cdc.gov/vaccines/schedules/hcp/imz/adult.html).

SUMMARY

- TGD people, especially transgender Black and Hispanic/Latinx transgender women, experience high rates of HIV and STIs.

- Health care professionals play an important role in discussing HIV and STI prevention strategies with patients.

- A comprehensive sexual health history that includes details of all gender-affirming procedures should be obtained to provide individualized STI and HIV screening recommendations and risk-reduction counseling.

- HIV PrEP with emtricitabine/tenofovir disoproxil fumarate is an important biomedical intervention to reduce HIV acquisition for transgender people at risk for HIV infection.

Table 16–2. Preexposure Prophylaxis (PrEP) Resources

Program	Weblink
Ready, Set, PrEP Program	https://www.getyourprep.com/
The Advancing Access Co-Pay Coupon Program	https://www.gileadadvancingaccess.com/
The Advancing Access Medication Assistance Program	https://www.gileadadvancingaccess.com/

CASE STUDY: Esther

Esther is a 32-year-old transgender woman presenting for a routine health maintenance exam. She started gender-affirming hormone therapy at age 24 and currently takes oral estradiol 4 mg daily and spironolactone 300 mg daily. She has not had any gender-affirming surgeries but underwent silicone injection into her hips several years ago. Six months ago, she ended a long-term relationship with a cisgender man and has started dating again using online apps. She always uses condoms for anal sex with new partners, although she had not done so consistently with her ex-boyfriend. She is asymptomatic today. Findings from the routine examination are within normal limits. Screening for STIs includes a rapid HIV screen, anal and oropharyngeal swabs, a urine specimen for gonorrhea and chlamydia, and blood testing for syphilis and hepatitis C. She is known to be immune to hepatitis A and B. Results of the rapid HIV screening test are negative. Results the following day are positive for oral gonorrhea and syphilis RPR 1:32 (the last test 6 months ago was nonreactive). Esther is alarmed and states that she did not think that she was at risk for STIs because she always uses condoms with her new sexual partners. After discussing the results, she is treated with ceftriaxone, azithromycin, and benzathine penicillin G. Since she has been newly diagnosed with an STI, she meets criteria for HIV PrEP with oral emtricitabine/tenofovir disoproxil fumarate. This option is discussed with her. Esther says that she has heard of PrEP but never thought of herself as being at risk for HIV. She is interested but concerned about possible interactions with her hormone therapy as well as other adverse effects. She states that she wants to do some research on her own first but agrees to meeting with a PrEP peer navigator later in the week. An appointment is made in 3 days to meet with the PrEP navigator, and another appointment is made in 3 months for repeat STI screening. Esther is sent home with information about PrEP to discuss at the PrEP navigation visit. However, she fails to keep this first scheduled appointment.

▶ Discussion Questions

- What strategies can health professionals use to improve rates of STI screening among TGD patients?

- How might a health care professional address concerns about the efficacy and safety of HIV PrEP with a transgender woman who is concerned about the effects on her hormone regimen?

- How would you approach STI screening in a transgender man who has sex with cisgender men both before and after his gender-affirming surgery (metoidioplasty)?

- How would you counsel a nonbinary individual who was assigned female at birth, a transgender woman, and a transgender man about their options for HIV prevention?

- How should clinicians approach individuals who present with recurrent STIs over time and do not want to engage in preventive measures such as PrEP?

- What are best practices for obtaining sexual health histories in transgender individuals who have experienced trauma?

- What community resources are available to provide financial support to patients unable to pay for PrEP?

REFERENCES

1. White Hughto JM, Reisner SL, Pachankis JE. Transgender stigma and health: a critical review of stigma determinants, mechanisms, and interventions. *Soc Sci Med.* 2015;147:222–231.
2. James SE, Herman JL, Rankin S, Keisling M, Mottet L, Anafi M. The Report of the 2015 U.S. Transgender Survey. National Center for Transgender Equality. Published online 2016.
3. Reisner SL, Hughto JMW, Dunham EE, et al. Legal protections in public accommodations settings: a critical public health issue for transgender and gender-nonconforming people. *Milbank Q.* 2015;93(3):484–515.
4. Meerwijk EL, Sevelius JM. Transgender population size in the United States: a meta-regression of population-based probability samples. *Am J Public Health.* 2017;107(2):e1–e8.
5. Winter S, Diamond M, Green J, et al. Transgender people: health at the margins of society. *Lancet.* 2016;388(10042):390–400.
6. Coleman E, Bockting W, Botzer M, et al. Standards of care for the health of transsexual, transgender, and gender-nonconforming people, Version 7. *Int J Transgend.* 2012;13(4):165–232.
7. Johns MM, Lowry R, Andrzejewski J, et al. Transgender identity and experiences of violence victimization, substance use, suicide risk, and sexual risk behaviors among high school students —19 states and large urban school districts, 2017. *MMWR Morbid Mortal Weekly Rep.* 2019;68(3):67–71.
8. Reisner SL, Radix A, Deutsch MB. Integrated and gender-affirming transgender clinical care and research. *J Acquir Immune Defic Syndr.* 2016;72(Suppl 3):S235–S242.
9. Canner JK, Harfouch O, Kodadek LM, et al. Temporal trends in gender-affirming surgery among transgender patients in the United States. *JAMA Surgery.* 2018;153(7):609–616.
10. Patel P, Borkowf CB, Brooks JT, Lasry A, Lansky A, Mermin J. Estimating per-act HIV transmission risk: a systematic review. *AIDS.* 2014;28(10):1509–1519.
11. Fein LA, Salgado CJ, Sputova K, Estes CM, Medina CA. Sexual preferences and partnerships of transgender persons mid- or post-transition. *J Homosexual.* 2018;65(5):659–671.
12. Becasen JS, Denard CL, Mullins MM, Higa DH, Sipe TA. Estimating the prevalence of HIV and sexual behaviors among the US transgender population: a systematic review and meta-analysis, 2006–2017. *Am J Public Health.* 2019;109(1):e1–e8.
13. Baral SD, Poteat T, Strömdahl S, Wirtz AL, Guadamuz TE, Beyrer C. Worldwide burden of HIV in transgender women: a systematic review and meta-analysis. *Lancet Infect Dis.* 2013; 13(3):214–222.
14. Poteat T, Scheim A, Xavier J, Reisner S, Baral S. Global epidemiology of HIV infection and related syndemics affecting transgender people. *J Acquir Immune Deficiency Syndr (1999).* 2016;72(Suppl 3):S210–219.

15. Wansom T, Guadamuz TE, Vasan S. Transgender populations and HIV: unique risks, challenges and opportunities. *J Virus Erad*. 2(2):87–93.

16. Sevelius JM. Gender affirmation: a framework for conceptualizing risk behavior among transgender women of color. *Sex Roles*. 2013;68(11-12):675–689.

17. Nuttbrock L, Bockting W, Rosenblum A, et al. Gender abuse and major depression among transgender women: a prospective study of vulnerability and resilience. *Am J Public Health*. 2014;104(11):2191–2198.

18. Reback CJ, Fletcher JB. HIV prevalence, substance use, and sexual risk behaviors among transgender women recruited through outreach. *AIDS Behav*. 2014;18(7):1359–1367.

19. Reback CJ, Clark K, Holloway IW, Fletcher JB. Health disparities, risk behaviors and healthcare utilization among transgender women in Los Angeles County: a comparison from 1998–1999 to 2015–2016. *AIDS Behav*. 2018;22(8):2524–2533.

20. Herbst JH, Jacobs ED, Finlayson TJ, et al. Estimating HIV prevalence and risk behaviors of transgender persons in the United States: a systematic review. *AIDS Behav*. 2008;12(1):1–17.

21. Ongwandee S, Lertpiriyasuwat C, Khawcharoenporn T, et al. Implementation of a test, treat, and prevent HIV program among men who have sex with men and transgender women in Thailand, 2015–2016. *PLoS One*. 2018;13(7):e0201171.

22. Beckwith CG, Kuo I, Fredericksen RJ, et al. Risk behaviors and HIV care continuum outcomes among criminal justice-involved HIV-infected transgender women and cisgender men: data from the Seek, Test, Treat, and Retain Harmonization Initiative. *PLoS One*. 2018;13(5):e0197730.

23. Somia IKA, Teeratakulpisarn N, Jeo WS, et al. Prevalence of and risk factors for anal high-risk HPV among HIV-negative and HIV-positive MSM and transgender women in three countries at South-East Asia. *Medicine*. 2018;97(10):e9898.

24. Kojima N, Park H, Konda KA, et al. The PICASSO Cohort: baseline characteristics of a cohort of men who have sex with men and male-to-female transgender women at high risk for syphilis infection in Lima, Peru. *BMC Infect Dis*. 2017;17. https://www.ncbi.nlm.nih.gov/pmc/articles/PMC5387233/.

25. Allan-Blitz L-T, Konda KA, Calvo GM, et al. High incidence of extra-genital gonorrheal and chlamydial infections among high-risk men who have sex with men and transgender women in Peru. *Int J STD AIDS*. 2018;29(6):568–576.

26. Hiransuthikul A, Janamnuaysook R, Sungsing T, et al. High burden of chlamydia and gonorrhoea in pharyngeal, rectal and urethral sites among Thai transgender women: implications for anatomical site selection for the screening of STI. *Sex Transm Infect*. 2019;95(7):534–539.

27. Crosby RA, Salazar LF, Hill B, Mena L. A comparison of HIV-risk behaviors between young black cisgender men who have sex with men and young black transgender women who have sex with men. *Int J STD AIDS*. 2018;29(7):665–672.

28. Moriarty KE, Segura ER, Gonzales W, Lake JE, Cabello R, Clark JL. Assessing sexually transmitted infections and HIV risk among transgender women in Lima, Peru: beyond behavior. *LGBT Health*. 2019;6(7):370–376.

29. Fernandes FRP, Zanini PB, Rezende GR, et al. Syphilis infection, sexual practices and bisexual behaviour among men who have sex with men and transgender women: a cross-sectional study. *Sex Transm Infect*. 2015;91(2):142–149.

30. Sahastrabuddhe S, Gupta A, Stuart E, et al. Sexually transmitted infections and risk behaviors among transgender persons (Hijras) of Pune, India. *J Acquir Immune Defic Syndr (1999)*. 2012;59(1):72–78.

31. Dos Ramos Farías MS, Garcia MN, Reynaga E, et al. First report on sexually transmitted infections among trans (male to female transvestites, transsexuals, or transgender) and male sex workers in Argentina: high HIV, HPV, HBV, and syphilis prevalence. *Int J Infect Dis*. 2011;15(9):e635–e640.

32. Carobene M, Bolcic F, Farías MSDR, Quarleri J, Ávila MM. HIV, HBV, and HCV molecular epidemiology among trans (transvestites, transsexuals, and transgender) sex workers in Argentina. *J Med Virol*. 2014;86(1):64–70.

33. Callander D, Cook T, Read P, et al. Sexually transmissible infections among transgender men and women attending Australian sexual health clinics. *Med J Austr*. 2019;211(9):406–411.

34. Reisner SL, Hughto JMW, Pardee D, Sevelius J. Syndemics and gender affirmation: HIV sexual risk in female-to-male trans masculine adults reporting sexual contact with cisgender males. *Int J STD AIDS*. 2016;27(11):955–966.

35. Reisner SL, Moore CS, Asquith A, et al. High risk and low uptake of pre-exposure prophylaxis to prevent HIV acquisition in a national online sample of transgender men who have sex with men in the United States. *J Int AIDS Soc*. 2019;22(9):e25391.

36. Reisner SL, White JM, Mayer KH, Mimiaga MJ. Sexual risk behaviors and psychosocial health concerns of female-to-male transgender men screening for STDs at an urban community health center. *AIDS Care*. 2014;26(7):857–864.

37. Stephens SC, Bernstein KT, Philip SS. Male to female and female to male transgender persons have different sexual risk behaviors yet similar rates of STDs and HIV. *AIDS Behav*. 2011;15(3):683–686.

38. Prevalence of Human Immunodeficiency Virus, Hepatitis B Virus, and Hepatitis C Virus Infections Among Transgender Persons Referred to an Italian Center for Total Sex Reassignment Surgery—PubMed. https://pubmed.ncbi.nlm.nih.gov/27322038/.

39. Pitasi MA, Kerani RP, Kohn R, et al. Chlamydia, gonorrhea, and human immunodeficiency virus infection among transgender women and transgender men attending clinics that provide sexually transmitted disease services in six US cities: results from the Sexually Transmitted Disease Surveillance Network. *Sex Transm Dis*. 2019;46(2):112–117.

40. Shover CL, DeVost MA, Beymer MR, Gorbach PM, Flynn RP, Bolan RK. Using sexual orientation and gender identity to monitor disparities in HIV, sexually transmitted infections, and viral hepatitis. *Am J Public Health*. 2018;108(S4):S277–S283.

41. Tordoff DM, Morgan J, Dombrowski JC, Golden MR, Barbee LA. Increased ascertainment of transgender and non-binary patients using a 2-step versus 1-step gender identity intake question in an STD clinic setting. *Sex Transm Dis*. 2019;46(4):254–259.

42. Salim A, Poh M. Gender-affirming penile inversion vaginoplasty. *Clin Plastic Surg*. 2018;45(3):343–350.

43. Schechter LS. Gender confirmation surgery: an update for the primary care provider. *Transgend Health*. 2016;1(1):32–40.

44. Salgado CJ, Nugent A, Kuhn J, Janette M, Bahna H. Primary sigmoid vaginoplasty in transwomen: technique and outcomes. *BioMed Res Int*. Published May 10, 2018. https://www.hindawi.com/journals/bmri/2018/4907208/.

45. Safa B, Lin WC, Salim AM, Deschamps-Braly JC, Poh MM. Current concepts in feminizing gender surgery. *Plast Reconstr Surg*. 2019;143(5):1081e–1091e.

46. Slater MW, Vinaja X, Aly I, Loukas M, Terrell M, Schober J. Neovaginal construction with pelvic peritoneum: reviewing an old approach for a new application. *Clin Anat (New York, NY)*. 2017;31(2):175–180.

47. Elfering L, van der Sluis WB, Mermans JF, Buncamper ME. Herpes neolabialis: herpes simplex virus type 1 infection of the neolabia in a transgender woman. *Int J STD AIDS*. 2017; 28(8):841–843.

48. Fiumara NJ, Di Mattia A. Gonorrhoea and condyloma acuminata in a male transsexual. *Br J Vener Dis*. 1973;49(5):478–479.

49. Bodsworth NJ, Price R, Davies SC. Gonococcal infection of the neovagina in a male-to-female transsexual. *Sex Transm Dis*. 1994;21(4):211–212.

50. Liguori G, Trombetta C, Bucci S, et al. Condylomata acuminata of the neovagina in a HIV-seropositive male-to-female transsexual. *UIN*. 2004;73(1):87–88.

51. Buscema J, Rosenshein NB, Shah K. Condylomata acuminata arising in a neovagina. *Obstet Gynecol*. 1987;69(3 Pt 2): 528–530.

52. Yang C, Liu S, Xu K, Xiang Q, Yang S, Zhang X. Condylomata gigantea in a male transsexual. *Int J STD AIDS*. 2009;20(3):211–212.

53. Labanca T, Mañero I. Vulvar condylomatosis after sex reassignment surgery in a male-to-female transsexual: complete response to imiquimod cream. *Gynecologic Oncol Rep*. 2017;20:75–77.

54. Radix AE, Harris AB, Belkind U, Ting J, Goldstein ZG. Chlamydia trachomatis infection of the neovagina in transgender women. *Open Forum Infect Dis*. 2019;6(11):ofz470.

55. Pitasi MA. HIV testing among transgender women and men— 27 states and Guam, 2014–2015. *MMWR Morb Mortal Wkly Rep*. 2017;66(33):883–887.

56. Reback CJ, Ferlito D, Kisler KA, Fletcher JB. Recruiting, linking, and retaining high-risk transgender women into HIV prevention and care services: an overview of barriers, strategies, and lessons learned. *Int J Transgend*. 2015;16(4):209–221.

57. Vaitses Fontanari AM, Zanella GI, Feijó M, Churchill S, Rodrigues Lobato MI, Costa AB. HIV-related care for transgender people: a systematic review of studies from around the world. *Soc Sci Med*. 2019;230:280–294.

58. Sevelius JM, Patouhas E, Keatley JG, Johnson MO. Barriers and facilitators to engagement and retention in care among transgender women living with human immunodeficiency virus. *Ann Behav Med*. 2014;47(1):5–16.

59. Newcomb ME, Hill R, Buehler K, Ryan DT, Whitton SW, Mustanski B. High burden of mental health problems, substance use, violence, and related psychosocial factors in transgender, non-binary, and gender diverse youth and young adults. *Arch Sex Behav*. 2020;49(2):645–659.

60. Murchison GR, Agénor M, Reisner SL, Watson RJ. School restroom and locker room restrictions and sexual assault risk among transgender youth. *Pediatrics*. 2019;143(6). https://pediatrics.aappublications.org/content/143/6/e20182902.

61. Griner SB, Vamos CA, Thompson EL, Logan R, Vázquez-Otero C, Daley EM. The intersection of gender identity and violence: victimization experienced by transgender college students. *J Interpers Viol*. 2020;35(23–24):5704–5725.

62. Lungu E, Thibault-Lemyre A, Dominguez JM, Trudel D, Bureau NJ. A case of recurrent leg necrotic ulcers secondary to silicone migration in a transgender patient: radiographic, ultrasound and MRI findings. *BJR Case Rep*. 2016;2(1):20150309.

63. Leonardi NR, Compoginis JM, Luce EA. Illicit cosmetic silicone injection: a recent reiteration of history. *Ann Plast Surg*. 2016;77(4):485–490.

64. Agrawal N, Altiner S, Mezitis NHE, Helbig S. Silicone-induced granuloma after injection for cosmetic purposes: a rare entity of calcitriol-mediated hypercalcemia. *Case Rep Med*. 2013;2013. https://www.ncbi.nlm.nih.gov/pmc/articles/PMC3864076/.

65. Soeroso NN, Rhinsilva E, Soeroso L. Acute pneumonitis following breast silicone liquid injection. *Respirol Case Rep*. 2018;6(6). https://www.ncbi.nlm.nih.gov/pmc/articles/PMC5987833/.

66. Workowski KA, Bolan G. *Sexually Transmitted Diseases Treatment Guidelines*; 2015. https://www.cdc.gov/mmwr/preview/mmwrhtml/rr6403a1.htm. Accessed October 26, 2020.

67. UCSF Transgender Care, Department of Family and Community Medicine, University of California San Francisco. Guidelines for the Primary and Gender-Affirming Care of Transgender and Gender Nonbinary People | Transgender Care. Published 2016. https://transcare.ucsf.edu/guidelines.

68. Scheim AI, Travers R. Barriers and facilitators to HIV and sexually transmitted infections testing for gay, bisexual, and other transgender men who have sex with men. *AIDS Care*. 2017;29(8):990–995.

69. Cahill S, Singal R, Grasso C, et al. Do ask, do tell: high levels of acceptability by patients of routine collection of sexual orientation and gender identity data in four diverse American community health centers. *PLoS One*. 2014;9(9):e107104.

70. Lipsitz MC, Segura ER, Castro JL, et al. Bringing testing to the people—benefits of mobile unit HIV/syphilis testing in Lima, Peru, 2007-2009. *Int J STD AIDS*. 2014;25(5):325–331.

71. Lelutiu-Weinberger C, Wilton L, Koblin BA, et al. The role of social support in HIV testing and PrEP awareness among young black men and transgender women who have sex with men or transgender women. *J Urban Health Bull New York Acad Med*. 2020;97(5):715–727.

72. Phanuphak N, Jantarapakde J, Himmad L, et al. Linkages to HIV confirmatory testing and antiretroviral therapy after online, supervised, HIV self-testing among Thai men who have sex with men and transgender women. *J Int AIDS Soc*. 2020;23(1):e25448.

73. Bustamante MJ, Konda KA, Joseph Davey D, et al. HIV self-testing in Peru: questionable availability, high acceptability but potential low linkage to care among men who have sex with men and transgender women. *Int J STD AIDS*. 2017;28(2): 133–137.

74. Katz DA, Golden MR, Hughes JP, Farquhar C, Stekler JD. HIV self-testing increases HIV testing frequency in high-risk men who have sex with men: a randomized controlled trial. *J Acquir Immune Defic Syndr (1999)*. 2018;78(5):505–512.

75. Lunny C, Taylor D, Hoang L, et al. Self-collected versus clinician-collected sampling for chlamydia and gonorrhea screening: a systemic review and meta-analysis. *PLoS One*. 2015;10(7):e0132776.

76. Shih SL, Graseck AS, Secura GM, Peipert JF. Screening for sexually transmitted infections at home or in the clinic? *Curr Opin Infect Dis*. 2011;24(1):78–84.

77. Piot P, Bartos M, Larson H, Zewdie D, Mane P. Coming to terms with complexity: a call to action for HIV prevention. *Lancet*. 2008;372(9641):845–859.

78. Maartens G, Celum C, Lewin SR. HIV infection: epidemiology, pathogenesis, treatment, and prevention. *Lancet*. 2014;384(9939):258–271.

79. Miner MH, Peterson JL, Welles SL, Jacoby SM, Rosser BRS. How do social norms impact HIV sexual risk behavior in HIV-positive men who have sex with men?: Multiple mediator effects. *J Health Psychol*. 2009;14(6):761–770.

80. Sd P, Dr H, Fr B. Postexposure treatment of HIV. *N Engl J Med*. 1997;337(7):500–501.

81. Interim Guidance: Preexposure Prophylaxis for the Prevention of HIV Infection in Men Who Have Sex with Men. https://www.cdc.gov/mmwr/preview/mmwrhtml/mm6003a1.htm.

82. US Preventive Services Task Force, Owens DK, Davidson KW, et al. Preexposure prophylaxis for the prevention of HIV infection: US Preventive Services Task Force recommendation statement. *JAMA*. 2019;321(22):2203–2213.

83. Hiransuthikul A, Janamnuaysook R, Himmad K, et al. Drug-drug interactions between feminizing hormone therapy and pre-exposure prophylaxis among transgender women: the iFACT study. *J Int AIDS Soc*. 2019;22(7):e25338.

84. Cottrell ML, Prince HMA, Schauer AP, et al. Decreased tenofovir diphosphate concentrations in a transgender female cohort: implications for human immunodeficiency virus preexposure prophylaxis. *Clin Infect Dis*. 2019;69(12):2201–2204.

85. Shieh E, Marzinke MA, Fuchs EJ, et al. Transgender women on oral HIV pre-exposure prophylaxis have significantly lower tenofovir and emtricitabine concentrations when also taking oestrogen when compared to cisgender men. *J Int AIDS Soc*. 2019;22(11):e25405.

86. Buchbinder SP, Glidden DV, Liu AY, et al. HIV pre-exposure prophylaxis in men who have sex with men and transgender women: a secondary analysis of a phase 3 randomised controlled efficacy trial. *Lancet Infect Dis*. 2014;14(6):468–475.

87. Grant RM, Anderson PL, McMahan V, et al. Uptake of pre-exposure prophylaxis, sexual practices, and HIV incidence in men and transgender women who have sex with men: a cohort study. *Lancet Infect Dis*. 2014;14(9):820–829.

88. Wood SM, Lee S, Barg FK, Castillo M, Dowshen N. Young transgender women's attitudes toward HIV pre-exposure prophylaxis. *J Adolesc Health Off Publ Soc Adolesc Med*. 2017;60(5):549–555.

89. Rael CT, Martinez M, Giguere R, et al. Barriers and facilitators to oral PrEP use among transgender women in New York City. *AIDS Behav*. 2018;22(11):3627–3636.

90. Molina J-M, Capitant C, Spire B, et al. On-demand preexposure prophylaxis in men at high risk for HIV-1 infection. *N Engl J Med*. 2015;373(23):2237–2246.

91. Coelho LE, Torres TS, Veloso VG, Landovitz RJ, Grinsztejn B. Pre-exposure prophylaxis 2.0: new drugs and technologies in the pipeline. *Lancet HIV*. 2019;6(11):e788–e799.

92. Rael CT, Martinez M, Giguere R, et al. Transgender women's concerns and preferences on potential future long-acting biomedical HIV prevention strategies: the case of injections and implanted medication delivery devices (IMDDs). *AIDS Behav*. 2020;24(5):1452–1462.

93. Barouch DH. A step forward for HIV vaccines. *Lancet HIV*. 2018;5(7):e338–e339.

94. Petrova D, Garcia-Retamero R. Effective evidence-based programs for preventing sexually-transmitted infections: a meta-analysis. *Curr HIV Res*. 2015;13(5):432–438.

95. Kalamar AM, Bayer AM, Hindin MJ. Interventions to prevent sexually transmitted infections, including HIV, among young people in low- and middle-income countries: a systematic review of the published and gray literature. *J Adolesc Health Off Publ Soc Adolesc Med*. 2016;59(3 Suppl):S22–S31.

96. Garofalo R, Kuhns LM, Reisner SL, Biello K, Mimiaga MJ. Efficacy of an empowerment-based, group-delivered HIV prevention intervention for young transgender women: the project lifeskills randomized clinical trial. *JAMA Pediatr*. 2018;172(10):916–923.

97. Molina J-M, Charreau I, Chidiac C, et al. Post-exposure prophylaxis with doxycycline to prevent sexually transmitted infections in men who have sex with men: an open-label randomised substudy of the ANRS IPERGAY trial. *Lancet Infect Dis*. 2018;18(3):308–317.

98. Bolan RK, Beymer MR, Weiss RE, Flynn RP, Leibowitz AA, Klausner JD. Doxycycline prophylaxis to reduce incident syphilis among HIV-infected men who have sex with men who continue to engage in high-risk sex: a randomized, controlled pilot study. *Sex Transm Dis*. 2015;42(2):98–103.

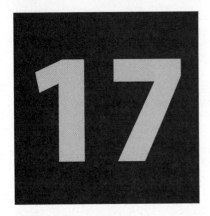

Treatment of HIV and Sexually Transmitted Infections

Ami Multani

INTRODUCTION

Sexually transmitted infections (STIs) represent a significant public health concern. In 2018, the CDC reported that combined cases of syphilis, gonorrhea, and chlamydia reached an all-time high in the United States. Especially concerning was the notable increase in cases of congenital syphilis.[1] Approximately 20 million new STI cases are diagnosed each year, with an estimated annual cost to the U.S. health care system of $16 billion. Almost one-half of these new cases occur in adolescents and young adults.

Few research studies have been conducted about STI prevalence in **transgender and gender diverse (TGD)** patients compared with the overall population; however, there is evidence suggesting an increased risk of rectal STIs among transgender women, particularly those who engage in transactional sex.[2,3] Due to the diversity of TGD individuals with regards to gender-affirming surgical procedures, hormone use, and sexual practices, clinicians should regularly assess for STI risk based on their patients' current anatomy and sexual health and sexual risk behaviors.[4,5] Moreover, it is crucial to obtain a clear understanding of what body parts a patient has used during sexual encounters with their partner(s) to know which sites to test during a screening evaluation. Clinicians must also discuss STI screening options with their patients, including self-swabbing, which may improve comfort and thereby willingness to complete STI screening.[6] The recommendations below are adapted from the 2015 *CDC Sexually Transmitted Disease Treatment Guidelines.*[4]

GENITAL ULCER DISEASES

Infectious genital ulcers, often due to an STI, can be classified as painless ulcers (syphilis, lymphogranuloma venereum [LGV], granuloma inguinale) or painful ulcers (herpes simplex virus [HSV], chancroid). In the United States, genital ulcers in sexually active patients are most likely to be due to HSV or syphilis and can represent multiple concurrent infections. A complete diagnostic workup should be obtained with attention to diseases that may be more common based on geography or the sexual community.[4] Since genital herpes infection, syphilis, and chancroid are all associated with an increased risk of HIV acquisition, HIV testing should also be included in the evaluation.[4,7] Despite complete diagnostic efforts, approximately one-fourth of patients with genital ulcers have no identified etiology.[4,7]

▶ Syphilis

Syphilis is a chronic bacterial infection caused by *Treponema pallidum*, renowned for its invasiveness and its ability to evade the immune system.[8] The infection is characterized by three stages: primary (chancre or ulcer), secondary (rash, lymphadenopathy), and tertiary (cardiac involvement, gummatous lesions). Latent syphilis, or asymptomatic infection diagnosed by serologic testing, can be further categorized as "early latent infection" if acquired in the past year, or "late latent infection" if acquired more than a year ago or if the duration of infection is unknown. While late latent syphilis is no longer contagious, treatment prevents further complications from infection and transmission to the fetus in pregnant persons.[4,8] Neurosyphilis, *T. pallidum* infection of the central nervous system, can occur at any stage of infection and can present with neurologic manifestations 30 years after the initial infection. Antibiotic management for patients with syphilis varies by stage of infection.

Management of syphilis requires early detection of disease, prompt treatment with effective antibiotics, and treatment of the index patient's sexual partners.[8] The preferred treatment for syphilis, regardless of infection stage, is parenterally administered Penicillin G. Preparation, dosage, and duration of treatment, however, are determined by the clinical manifestations and disease stage (Table 17-1). A single

Table 17-1. Treatment Recommendations for Syphilis[4]

Primary and secondary syphilis	Benzathine penicillin G 2.4 million units IM once
Primary and secondary syphilis with a penicillin allergy	Doxycycline 100 mg by mouth (PO) twice daily for 14 days OR Tetracycline 500 mg PO four times daily for 14 days
Tertiary syphilis with normal CSF studies	Benzathine penicillin G 2.4 million units intramuscularly (IM) once per week for 3 weeks
Neurosyphilis or ocular syphilis	Aqueous crystalline penicillin G 3–4 million units intravenously (IV) every 4 hours (or continuous infusion) for 10–14 days OR Procaine penicillin G 2.4 million units IM once daily PLUS probenecid 500 mg PO four times daily both for 10–14 days
Early latent syphilis	Benzathine penicillin G 2.4 million units IM once
Late latent syphilis or latent syphilis of unknown duration	Benzathine penicillin G 2.4 million units IM once per week for 3 weeks
Latent syphilis with a penicillin allergy (* considered an alternative regimen)	Doxycycline 100 mg PO twice daily for 28 days OR * Tetracycline 500 mg PO four times daily for 28 days

dose of benzathine penicillin G maintains penicillin levels in the blood above the minimum inhibitory concentration (MIC) for at least 10 days and is recommended for specific stages of syphilis.[8] Pregnant individuals who are allergic to penicillin should be desensitized and treated with penicillin. Treatment of syphilis may result in a Jarisch-Herxheimer reaction, an acute self-limited febrile response often accompanied by headache, myalgia, and fever, more commonly seen in patients with early syphilis. This response to treatment typically occurs within the first 24 hours and is managed with hydration and antipyretics.[4,8]

Following appropriate antibiotic treatment, clinical and serological evaluation should be performed at 6 and 12 months for all patients diagnosed with any stage of syphilis to document a fourfold decline in nontreponemal titers.[4] In patients who have recurrent symptoms or who fail to improve with at least a fourfold increase in nontreponemal titer, the clinician should consider either reinfection with syphilis or treatment failure. Repeat treatment should be administered with benzathine penicillin G 2.4 million units

IM once weekly for 3 weeks.[4] If the patient does not achieve a fourfold decrease in their nontreponemal testing 1 year after treatment, optimal management is unclear. These patients should continue to be monitored closely and evaluated for HIV infection.[4]

For patients with latent syphilis who miss one of their weekly doses of penicillin, an interval of 10–14 days between doses may be acceptable prior to the need to restart the 3-week series of weekly injections.[4] Patients with no evidence of neurosyphilis who have been reinfected or for whom treatment has failed should receive weekly injections of 2.4 million units benzathine penicillin G for 3 weeks.[4]

There is no microbiologic test of cure following treatment of neurosyphilis; successful treatment is based on the resolution of presenting neurologic symptoms and by normalization of the cerebrospinal fluid (CSF) white blood cell count.[9] It is advised that a CSF exam be performed every 3 to 6 months posttreatment and every 6 months thereafter until the CSF-VDRL (venereal disease research laboratory) is nonreactive and the CSF white blood cell count has normalized.[9] Administration of 2.4 million units of benzathine penicillin G IM once weekly for 3 weeks can be considered after completion of a neurosyphilis treatment regimen to provide a total treatment course length that is comparable to that used for latent syphilis.[4]

Persons who report sexual contact with a person recently diagnosed with syphilis should be evaluated clinically and serologically.[4] If a person reports sexual contact with a person who was diagnosed with primary, secondary, or early latent syphilis within the 90 days preceding diagnosis, they should be treated presumptively for early syphilis even if the serologic testing result is negative.[4] If the sexual contact occurred greater than 90 days before the diagnosis, the patient should be treated presumptively for early syphilis, and serologic testing should be performed. If results are negative, treatment should be stopped.[4]

▶ Herpes Simplex Virus (HSV)

Genital herpes simplex is a common and chronic life-long viral infection that is caused by either HSV-1 or HSV-2.[4] The majority of cases of recurrent genital herpes are caused by HSV-2; however, the incidence of anogenital infection caused by HSV-1 is increasing.[10] Although systemic antiviral therapy offers the benefit of reducing disease severity and shedding, it does not eradicate latent virus.[4,11,12] Topical antiviral therapy has no clinical benefit and is not indicated in the management of genital HSV infection.[4] Treatment for the initial clinical episode of genital herpes is listed in Table 17-2. If healing of the herpetic lesions is incomplete, treatment can be extended.[4]

Patients with recurrent genital herpes may benefit from suppressive therapy, which reduces the frequency of outbreaks by 70–80% and has been associated with improved

Table 17-2. Treatment Recommendations for Genital Herpes[4]

Treatment for initial clinical episode of genital herpes	Acyclovir 400 mg by mouth (PO) three times daily for 7–10 days OR Acyclovir 200 mg PO five times daily for 7–10 days OR Valacyclovir 1 g PO twice daily for 7–10 days OR Famciclovir 250 mg PO three times daily for 7–10 days
Suppressive treatment for recurrent genital herpes	Acyclovir 400 mg PO twice daily OR Valacyclovir 500 mg PO once daily OR Valacyclovir 1 g PO once daily OR Famciclovir 250 mg PO twice daily
Episodic treatment for recurrent genital herpes	Acyclovir 400 mg PO three times daily for 5 days OR Acyclovir 800 mg PO twice daily for 5 days OR Acyclovir 800 mg PO three times daily for 2 days OR Valacyclovir 500 mg PO twice daily for 3 days OR Valacyclovir 1 g PO daily for 5 days OR Famciclovir 125 mg PO twice daily for 5 days OR Famciclovir 1 g PO twice daily for 1 day OR Famciclovir 500 mg PO once, followed by 250 mg PO twice daily for 2 days

Table 17-3. Treatment Recommendations for LGV[4]

Recommended treatment	Doxycycline 100 mg by mouth (PO) twice daily for 21 days
Alternative treatment	Erythromycin base 500 mg PO four times daily for 21 days

Table 17-4. Treatment Recommendations for Chancroid[4]

Recommended treatment	Azithromycin 1 g by mouth (PO) once OR Ceftriaxone 250 mg intramuscularly (IM) once OR Ciprofloxacin 500 mg PO twice daily for 3 days OR Erythromycin base 500 mg PO three times daily for 7 days

quality of life.[13,14] For patients who prefer episodic therapy for treatment of recurrent genital herpes, therapy should be initiated during the prodrome that can precede the outbreak or within one day of the onset of herpetic lesions.[4] If a patient presents with severe HSV disease, disseminated disease, or central nervous system complications, they should be referred for intravenous (IV) acyclovir therapy.[4] If HSV lesions persist or recur despite appropriate treatment, evaluation for HSV resistance should be performed using a representative sample submitted for sensitivity testing.[15]

Lymphogranuloma Venereum (LGV)

Lymphogranuloma venereum (LGV), a disease of lymphatic tissue, is caused by the L1, L2, and L3 invasive serovars of *Chlamydia trachomatis*.[8] Manifestations include a transient genital ulcer, discrete inflammatory reaction at the site of inoculation, tender unilateral inguinal lymphadenopathy, or proctocolitis.[16,17] Untreated, the infection can lead to significant long-term complications such as deep tissue abscess, fissures, strictures, and chronic pain.[17,18] Persons presenting with clinical symptoms consistent with those described should be treated presumptively for LGV with one of the regimens listed in Table 17-3.

Patients should be followed until their initial symptoms have resolved and should be tested for other STIs as appropriate. Persons who report sexual contact with a patient diagnosed with LGV within 60 days of the onset of the patient's symptoms should be tested for chlamydial infection at all anatomic sites of exposure and presumptively treated with azithromycin 1 g orally once or doxycycline 100 mg orally twice a day for 7 days.[4]

Chancroid

Chancroid, a less common STI caused by *Haemophilus ducreyi*, presents with both a painful genital ulcer and tender suppurative inguinal lymphadenopathy. Chancroid is a clinical diagnosis made after the exclusion of syphilis and HSV.[4,19] The recommended treatment is listed in Table 17-4. Patients should be examined 3–7 days after treatment to assess for improvement in genital ulcers. If the ulcers have not improved, additional evaluation should be completed.[4] Sexual partners of patients with chancroid should be examined and treated if they report sexual contact with the patient during the 10 days before the onset of symptoms.[4]

Table 17-5. Treatment Recommendations for Granuloma inguinale (Donovanosis)[4]

Recommended treatment	Azithromycin 1 g by mouth (PO) once weekly or 500 mg PO daily for at least 3 weeks
Alternative treatment	Doxycycline 100 mg PO twice daily for at least 3 weeks OR Ciprofloxacin 750 mg PO twice daily for at least 3 weeks Erythromycin base 500 mg PO four times daily for at least 3 weeks OR Trimethoprim-sulfamethoxazole, one double-strength (160 mg/800 mg) tablet PO twice daily for at least 3 weeks

Table 17-6. Treatment Recommendations for Chlamydia Infection[4]

Recommended treatment	Azithromycin 1 g by mouth (PO) once OR Doxycycline 100 mg PO twice daily for 7 days
Alternative treatment	Erythromycin base 500 mg PO four times daily for 7 days OR Erythromycin ethylsuccinate 800 mg PO four times daily for 7 days OR Levofloxacin 500 mg PO daily for 7 days OR Ofloxacin 300 mg PO twice daily for 7 days

▶ Granuloma Inguinale (Donovanosis)

Granuloma inguinale, another less common STI caused by *Klebsiella granulomatis*, presents with painless, indolent, highly vascular, and progressing ulcerative lesions without associated lymphadenopathy.[4,19] Recommended treatment regimens are listed in Table 17-5. Treatment should be continued until all lesions have completely healed.[4] Sexual partners of patients with granuloma inguinale should be examined and offered treatment if they report sexual contact within 60 days prior to the onset of symptoms.[4]

CHLAMYDIA

C. trachomatis, an obligate intracellular bacterium, is the most common cause of bacterial STI.[18,20] It is often asymptomatic. Infection can result in significant sequelae, including urethritis, cervicitis, proctitis, epididymitis, ectopic pregnancy, pelvic inflammatory disease, and infertility. Early diagnosis and treatment are of utmost importance in preventing these complications.[4] Recommended treatment is detailed in Table 17-6. Sexual partners should be evaluated, screened, and presumptively treated if they have had sexual contact with the partner 60 days prior to the patient's chlamydia diagnosis or onset of symptoms.[4] Once treated, patients should be advised to abstain from all sexual activity for 7 days to decrease the risk of sexual transmission to their sexual partners.[4]

Growing evidence suggests that the efficacy of treatment with oral doxycycline is superior to that of oral azithromycin for oropharyngeal or rectal chlamydia .[21] Although the *CDC 2015 Treatment Guidelines* do not recommend routine oropharyngeal chlamydia screening, data suggest that oropharyngeal infection can be transmitted to genital sites and that, therefore, if detected, these infections should be treated appropriately.[4,22,23] If a patient has been treated with a recommended or alternative regimen with full adherence, a test of cure is not recommended.[4] It is advised that patients treated for chlamydia should be retested approximately 3 months after treatment due to concern for reinfection.[24,25]

GONORRHEA

Neisseria gonorrhea infection is the second most commonly reported STI.[26] Gonorrheal infection can lead to complications of urethritis, cervicitis, epididymitis, proctitis, ectopic pregnancy, disseminated disease, pelvic inflammatory disease, and infertility, and thus expedited detection and treatment are essential.[4,27] The treatment of gonorrhea is complicated by the organism's ability to develop antimicrobial resistance and concern that it is actively evolving into a "superbug" with resistance to most classes of available antibiotics.[4,27] It is due to this concern that the CDC 2015 Treatment Guidelines recommend dual therapy to treat gonorrhea with two different antimicrobials with two different mechanisms of action[4] (Table 17-7).

Once treated, patients should be advised to avoid all sexual activities for 7 days to decrease sexual transmission to their sexual partners and until all sex partners are adequately treated.[4] Any partners who report sexual contact with the patient in the 60 days prior to the onset of symptoms or formal diagnosis should be evaluated, tested, and presumptively treated with dual treatment.[4] If a patient has received treatment with a recommended or alternative regimen for an uncomplicated urogenital or rectal gonorrhea infection, a test of cure is not needed.[4]

An additional treatment consideration is treatment of pharyngeal gonorrhea (see Table 17-7). These infections tend to be more difficult to eradicate than infections at urogenital or anorectal sites.[28] If a patient with pharyngeal gonorrhea was treated with an alternative regimen, they should return

Table 17-7. Treatment Recommendations for Gonorrhea Infection[4]

Recommended treatment[a]	Ceftriaxone 250 mg intramuscularly (IM) once PLUS Azithromycin 1 g by mouth (PO) once
Alternative treatment (if ceftriaxone is not available)[a]	Cefixime 400 mg PO once PLUS Azithromycin 1 g PO once
Recommended pharyngeal gonorrhea treatment[a]	Ceftriaxone 250 mg IM once PLUS Azithromycin 1 g PO once

[a]Administered together on the same day.

Table 17-8. Treatment Recommendations for Nongonococcal Urethritis[4]

Recommended treatment	Azithromycin 1 g by mouth (PO) once OR Doxycycline 100 mg PO twice daily for 7 days
Alternative treatment	Erythromycin base 500 mg PO four times daily for 7 days OR Erythromycin ethylsuccinate 800 mg PO four times daily for 7 days OR Levofloxacin 500 mg PO daily for 7 days OR Ofloxacin 300 mg PO twice daily for 7 days

14 days after therapy for a test of cure.[4] If test results are positive in this case, a confirmatory culture should be obtained and screened for antimicrobial resistance.[4]

NONGONOCOCCAL URETHRITIS

Urethritis, or urethral inflammation, can result from a number of both infectious and noninfectious causes and often presents with urethral discharge and dysuria.[4] The most common cause of nongonococcal urethritis (NGU) is chlamydia, followed by *Mycoplasma genitalium;* however, approximately one-half of all cases have no distinct etiology, as causative organisms can be difficult to identify with currently available testing.[4,29] Treatment for NGU is often presumptive (Table 17-8).

If a diagnosis of *M. genitalium* is confirmed, treatment with azithromycin may have better efficacy than doxycycline, although cure rates with azithromycin appear to be declining.[30] Once treated, patients should refrain from all sexual activities for 7 days after both they and their partner(s) have been appropriately treated.[4] If symptoms recur or persist despite treatment with full adherence, further evaluation with testing should be completed prior to considering additional antibiotic treatment.[4] All sexual partners of patients with NGU who report sexual activity within the prior 60 days should be evaluated, tested, and treated presumptively with a regimen with activity against chlamydia.[4]

PELVIC INFLAMMATORY DISEASE

Pelvic inflammatory disease (PID) refers to an infection-induced inflammation of the upper female genital tract structures involving the uterus, fallopian tubes, and ovaries as well as risk to adjacent pelvic organs.[4,31,32] Etiologies may include gonorrhea, chlamydia, *M. genitalium*, and organisms that comprise vaginal flora or enteric organisms.[4,33,34] Treatment of PID should provide broad empiric coverage of likely pathogens. Severe infections may require inpatient management.[4] Treatment should be expedited as soon as the presumptive diagnosis has been determined to prevent long-term sequelae such as ectopic pregnancy and infertility.[4,35]

Patients with severe PID who are hospitalized should receive parenteral therapy.[31] Patients can often be transitioned from parenteral to oral therapy after 24 hours of improvement in symptoms[31] (Table 17-9). It should be noted that oral and IV administration of doxycycline provide similar bioavailability and that doxycycline administered via IV is associated with increased pain.[4] If using parenteral regimens with cefotetan or cefoxitin, doxycycline 100 mg orally twice daily can be used 24–48 hours after clinical improvement to complete a 14-day course of therapy.[4] If employing a clindamycin/gentamicin regimen, oral therapy with clindamycin 450 mg orally four times daily or doxycycline 100 mg twice daily can be used to complete the 14-day course of therapy. Lastly, if a tubo-ovarian abscess is present, clindamycin 450 mg orally four times daily or metronidazole 500 mg twice daily should be used to complete at least 14 days of therapy with doxycycline.[4]

For patients with mild to moderately severe PID, oral or intramuscular treatment can be considered, with transition to parenteral treatment if there is a lack of response to therapy within 72 hours (Table 17-9).[4]

Patients should be advised to abstain from all sexual activities until therapy is completed, their symptoms have resolved, and their partners have been appropriately treated.[4] Most patients will experience improvement in their symptoms within 72 hours of initiation of therapy, and if not, further evaluation or escalation in care may be appropriate.[4] If the patient has confirmed chlamydial or gonococcal PID, they should be retested 3 months after the completion of PID therapy.[24] Additionally, all sexual partners of the patient within the 60 days prior to the onset of their symptoms should be evaluated, tested, and presumptively treated for chlamydia and gonorrhea regardless of the patient's STI results.[4]

Table 17-9. Treatment Recommendations for Pelvic Inflammatory Disease[4]

Recommended parenteral treatment	Cefotetan 2 g intravenously (IV) every 12 hours PLUS Doxycycline 100 mg by mouth (PO) or IV every 12 hours OR Cefoxitin 2 g IV every 6 hours PLUS Doxycycline 100 mg PO or IV every 12 hours OR Clindamycin 900 mg IV every 8 hours PLUS Gentamicin loading dose IV or intramuscularly (IM) (2 mg/kg), followed by a maintenance dose (1.5 mg/kg) every 8 hours
Alternative parenteral treatment	Ampicillin/Sulbactam 3 g IV every 6 hours PLUS Doxycycline 100 mg PO or IV every 12 hours
Recommended intramuscular/oral treatment	Ceftriaxone 250 mg IM once PLUS Doxycycline 100 mg PO twice daily for 14 days WITH OR WITHOUT Metronidazole 500 mg PO twice daily for 14 days OR Cefoxitin 2 g IM once and Probenecid 1 g once PLUS Doxycycline 100 mg PO twice daily for 14 days WITH OR WITHOUT Metronidazole 500 mg PO twice daily for 14 days OR Other parenteral third-generation cephalosporin (e.g., ceftizoxime or cefotaxime) PLUS Doxycycline 100 mg PO twice daily for 14 days WITH OR WITHOUT Metronidazole 500 mg PO twice daily for 14 days

Table 17-10. Recommended Treatment for Epididymitis[4]

Recommended treatment for acute epididymitis likely caused by sexually transmitted chlamydia and gonorrhea	Ceftriaxone 250 mg intramuscularly (IM) once PLUS Doxycycline 100 mg by mouth (PO) twice daily for 10 days
Recommended treatment for acute epididymitis caused by sexually transmitted chlamydia and gonorrhea and enteric organisms (men who practice insertive anal sex)	Ceftriaxone 250 mg IM once PLUS Levofloxacin 500 mg PO once daily for 10 days OR Ofloxacin 300 mg PO twice daily for 10 days
Recommended treatment for acute epididymitis most likely caused by enteric organisms	Levofloxacin 500 mg PO daily for 10 days OR Ofloxacin 300 mg PO twice daily for 10 days

EPIDIDYMITIS

Epididymitis is the most common cause of scrotal pain in adults in the outpatient setting and presents with a triad of symptoms that consists of swelling, testicular pain, and inflammation of the epididymis.[36,37] Among sexually active men younger than 35 years, acute epididymitis is most often caused by either *N. gonorrhea* or *C. trachomatis* infection, although sexually transmitted enteric bacteria should also be considered for patients who report insertive anal intercourse.[4] Among men aged 35 years and older who do not report insertive anal intercourse, sexually transmitted etiologies are less common; instead, bacteria associated with obstructive uropathy should be considered.[38] Patients should be fully evaluated and empiric therapy prescribed to prevent

transmission of STIs and sequelae (including chronic pain and infertility) while lab results are pending[39] (Table 17-10).

If the patient has confirmed or suspected infection with gonorrhea or chlamydia, they should be advised to refrain from all sexual intercourse until both they and their partners have been appropriately treated and symptoms have resolved.[4] All sexual partners of these patients within the prior 60 days preceding the onset of epididymitis symptoms that are suspected or confirmed to be caused by gonorrhea or chlamydia should be appropriately tested and treated presumptively.[4] If the patient's symptoms fail to improve within 72 hours of treatment, they should have further evaluation with their clinician.[4]

VAGINAL DISCHARGE SYNDROMES

Patients with a vagina may experience a vaginal infection with vaginal discharge, pruritus, odor, or discomfort at some point during their lifetime.[4,39] A detailed history, physical exam, microscopy, and laboratory testing are essential to determine the etiology of symptoms and appropriate treatment.[4,38] The three most common diseases associated with vaginal discharge are bacterial vaginosis, trichomoniasis, and vulvovaginal candidiasis.[4]

▶ Bacterial Vaginosis

Bacterial vaginosis (BV) is a clinical condition characterized by a shift in vaginal flora. Lactobacillus species and instead replaced with more diverse bacterial species, including anaerobic bacteria that cause an increase in vaginal pH.[4,40] Table 17-11 lists recommended treatment regimens.

Table 17-11. Treatment Recommendations for Bacterial Vaginosis[4]

Recommended treatment	Metronidazole 500 mg by mouth (PO) twice daily for 7 days OR Metronidazole gel 0.75%, one full applicator (5 g) intravaginally, daily for 5 days OR Clindamycin cream 2%, one full applicator (5 g) intravaginally nightly for 7 days
Alternative treatment	Tinidazole 2 g PO daily for 2 days OR Tinidazole 1 g PO daily for 5 days OR Clindamycin 300 mg PO twice daily for 7 days OR Clindamycin ovules 100 mg intravaginally once nightly for 3 days

Table 17-12. Treatment Recommendations for Trichomoniasis[4]

Recommended treatment	Metronidazole 2 g by mouth (PO) once OR Tinidazole 2 g PO once
Alternative treatment	Metronidazole 500 mg PO twice daily for 7 days

Treatment efficacy is comparable between metronidazole and clindamycin, regardless of delivery route. Both result in a high rate of clinical cure.[40] Of note, there are no studies that support the use of probiotics for the treatment of BV.[41] Follow-up is not necessary if symptoms resolve with appropriate treatment.[4]

▶ Trichomoniasis

Trichomoniasis is a genitourinary infection caused by the protozoan parasite *Trichomonas vaginalis* and is the most common nonviral sexually transmitted disease both in the United States and worldwide.[42] Treatment is advised for both symptomatic and asymptomatic individuals to ameliorate symptoms, reduce the prevalence of *T. vaginalis* carriage in the population, and decrease the risk of sequelae, including both the acquisition and transmission of HIV[4] (Table 17-12). Patients should be advised to abstain from all sexual activities until both they and their sexual partners have been treated. Patients should be retested 3 months following appropriate treatment, given the high rates of reinfection.[4]

▶ Vulvovaginal Candidiasis

Vulvovaginal candidiasis is most often caused by *Candida albicans* and presents with a variety of symptoms, including vaginal discharge, pruritus, dysuria, vaginal pain, and dyspareunia.[4] Treatment is determined based on whether the patient has mild, uncomplicated, or severe disease. The latter is defined as either recurrent disease, disease in an immunocompromised host, or an infection with a nonalbicans candida species.[42] Many topical and oral treatments are available for the treatment of uncomplicated vulvovaginal candidiasis that achieve similar cure rates[42] (Table 17-13). In general,

Table 17-13. Treatment Recommendations for Vulvovaginal Candidiasis[4]

Recommended treatment for mild, uncomplicated disease (over-the-counter intravaginal agents)	Clotrimazole 1% cream 5 g intravaginally daily for 7–14 days OR Clotrimazole 2% cream 5 g intravaginally daily for 3 days OR Miconazole 2% cream 5 g intravaginally daily for 7 days Miconazole 4% cream 5 g intravaginally daily for 3 days OR Miconazole 100 mg vaginal suppository, one suppository daily for 7 days OR Miconazole 200 mg vaginal suppository, one suppository for 3 days OR Miconazole 1200 mg vaginal suppository, one suppository for 1 day OR Tioconazole 6.5% ointment 5 g intravaginally in one application
Recommended treatment for mild-to-moderate uncomplicated disease (prescription intravaginal agents)	Butoconazole 2% cream, 5 g intravaginally in one application OR Terconazole 0.4% cream 5 g intravaginally daily for 7 days Terconazole 0.8% cream 5 g intravaginally for 3 days OR Terconazole 80 mg vaginal suppository, one suppository daily for 3 days
Recommended treatment for mild-to-moderate uncomplicated disease (prescription oral agent)	Fluconazole 150 mg by mouth (PO) once

follow-up after appropriate therapy is not necessary unless the patient experiences persistent or recurrent symptoms.[42]

ANOGENITAL WARTS

Anogenital warts occur on the penis, groin, scrotum, vulva, perineum, external anus, and perianus and are caused by human papillomavirus. Over 90% of anogenital warts are caused by nononcogenic HPV types 6 and 11.[43] HPV types 16, 18, 31, 33, and 35 can also be found in anogenital warts and may be associated with foci of high-grade squamous intraepithelial lesions (HSIL), especially in patients with HIV infection. Highly effective HPV vaccines are available that offer protection against multiple strains of HPV that cause genital warts and genital cancers and provide benefit to all eligible patients, including transgender patients.[4]

Most anogenital warts are asymptomatic; however, some patients can find them to be pruritic or painful and the appearance to be stigmatizing.[4] Treatment of anogenital warts is focused on wart removal but not necessarily eradication of HPV. The decision for treatment is based on several factors, including the location, size, and number of warts; patient preference; cost of treatment; treatment reactions; and provider experience.[4,44] Recommended treatment of warts is listed in Table 17-14.

Another consideration for patients with external anal warts is to consider further evaluation for internal anal warts with either digital rectal examination, standard anoscopy, or high-resolution anoscopy.[4] The majority of anogenital warts will respond to treatment within 3 months of therapy and if not, an alternate treatment modality should be considered.[4] Patients can also be counseled that HPV infections associated with genital warts in immunocompetent patients typically clear within 2 years.[45]

Table 17-14. Treatment Recommendations for External Anogenital Warts[4]

Patient-applied	Imiquimod 3.75% or 5% cream OR Podofilox 0.5% solution or gel OR Sinecatechins 15% ointment
Provider-administered	Cryotherapy with liquid nitrogen or cryoprobe OR Surgical removal by tangential scissor excision, tangential shave excision, curettage, laser, or electrosurgery OR Trichloroacetic acid (TCA) or bichloroacetic acid (BCA) 80%–90% solution

CASE STUDY 1

A 23-year-old White trans woman presents to the outpatient clinic with 10 days of low-grade fever, rectal pain, and alternating diarrhea and constipation. She has not had upper respiratory symptoms, nausea, vomiting, abdominal pain, dysuria, or penile discharge. She has had no recent travel, ill contacts, or ingestion of raw or undercooked foods. She is sexually active with male partners and reports unprotected receptive anal intercourse. Her medications include emtricitabine/tenofovir disoproxil for PrEP, estradiol 6 mg PO daily, and spironolactone 100 mg PO daily, all of which she takes as prescribed. On physical examination, she has rectal tenderness and inflammation with cloudy rectal discharge noted at the perianus; no ulcers are noted. No inguinal lymphadenopathy is noted. Laboratory test results reveal a benign complete blood count (CBC) and comprehensive metabolic panel (CMP), and stool studies are negative for salmonella, shigella, campylobacter, and ova and parasites. She is immune to hepatitis A. A full STI panel is negative for syphilis, HIV, and hepatitis C; anal swab is negative for HSV; oropharyngeal swab is negative for gonorrhea; and urine testing is negative for both gonorrhea and chlamydia. NAAT testing on a rectal swab is positive for chlamydia. She is treated with azithromycin 1 g orally. She presents again 1 week later and reports that her symptoms improved transiently for 3 to 4 days following treatment but recurred thereafter, and she now has increased rectal pain and profuse rectal discharge. She has remained abstinent since her prior office visit and denies current sexual activity.

Discussion questions

1. Why did the patient only have transient improvement in her symptoms after appropriate treatment of chlamydia infection and reported sexual abstinence?

2. What additional diagnostic tests should be ordered for this patient?

Resolution: An LGV serologic panel is ordered and *C. trachomatis* L1 IgM is positive with a titer of >1.256. The patient is prescribed doxycycline 100 mg PO twice daily for 21 days. The patient reported full resolution of her symptoms after completion of antibiotics.

When evaluating rectal pain and diarrhea, it is important to complete a thorough sexual history and examination. LGV can be difficult to diagnose and should be considered in the patient with positive rectal chlamydia testing that does not respond to appropriate treatment. This patient experienced transient improvement in her symptoms after she received azithromycin because her LGV was partially but not fully treated on this regimen. It is important to order additional testing in this scenario with an LGV panel to help distinguish between chlamydia and LGV.

HIV

In the late 1990s, potent combination antiretroviral therapy (ART) regimens were developed that suppress viral replication and transformed HIV from a progressive, fatal illness to a manageable chronic disease.[46] Currently, there are over 30 FDA-approved antiretroviral therapies that provide clinicians with ample options to tailor therapy for their HIV patients.[47] The availability of ART has been associated with an astounding reduction in morbidity and mortality regardless of gender, race, ethnicity, or sexual transmission risk factors.[48] Despite these advances, mortality rates remain inordinately high, and HIV suppression rates remain low in populations with poor access to health care, such as communities of color, transgender women, young adults, and those living in poor inner-city and rural neighborhoods who are often unaware of their HIV infection, may not be linked to care, or who initiate medical care with late AIDS-related opportunistic.[49-51] Within the transgender population, transgender women living with HIV are less likely than cisgender men to receive ART, follow ART recommendations, and achieve viral suppression.[52-54] It is important to recognize that transgender people report increased exposure to violence, discrimination, and other trauma, which have been associated with poor HIV outcomes, including ART failure.[55,56] Incorporation of trauma-informed principles throughout all aspects of care is of paramount importance. For more information on trauma-informed care, see Chapter 11, "Basic Principles of Trauma-Informed and Gender-Affirming Care."

Current ART regimens are less toxic, highly effective, have a decreased pill burden, and are dosed less frequently than prior protease inhibitor-based regimens.[46] After initiation of ART, the plasma viral load decreases to concentrations below the lower limit of detection with available commercial assays within 3 months in most patients.[46] In contrast, the recovery of CD4 T-cells in patients on ART can be variable and often is impacted by multiple factors, including host factors such as older age, lower CD4 cell nadir and higher baseline HIV viral load, and viral factors including coinfection with cytomegalovirus or hepatitis C virus.[46,57]

Basics of ART

The discovery of the multistep replication life cycle of HIV in CD4 T-cells led to the identification of potential drug targets to block or slow the replication process, which resulted in extraordinary progress in the development of ART.[47] Patients can be infected with "wild-type" HIV (the original parent virus without mutations) or a resistant strain of HIV; in the latter case, resistance testing can help guide effective ART treatment decision.[51] There are now seven classes of medications available for the treatment of HIV infection: nucleoside reverse transcriptase inhibitors (NRTIs), non-nucleoside reverse transcriptase inhibitors (NNRTIs), integrase strand inhibitors (InSTIs), protease inhibitors (PIs), fusion inhibitors (FIs), CCR5 receptor antagonists, and CD4 T-lymphocyte postattachment inhibitors.

NRTIs were the first class of ART drugs approved for use in the United States and remain an integral component of most combination regimens.[47] NRTIs are phosphorylated intracellularly to their active metabolites, which then inhibit the enzymatic action of HIV reverse transcriptase by incorporating into the nucleotide analogue; this, in turn, causes DNA chain termination, which terminates the conversion of viral RNA into double-stranded DNA.[47] Currently, the most commonly used NRTIs are tenofovir disoproxil fumarate (TDF), tenofovir alafenamide (TAF), abacavir, emtricitabine, and lamivudine.[47] Regarding tenofovir formulations, TAF is an oral prodrug of TDF. Administration of TAF results in higher concentrations of tenofovir in tissues but lower concentrations in plasma than does administration with TDF—the clinical significance of which continues to be studied. Before starting an abacavir-containing regimen, the patient must be screened for HLA B*5701, and if positive, use of this drug is contraindicated as the patient would be at risk for developing an abacavir hypersensitivity reaction.

NNRTIs differ from NRTIs, in that they do not require intracellular phosphorylation and reduce viral replication via noncompetitive inhibition of reverse transcriptase.[47] The most commonly used NNRTIs are efavirenz, etravirine, rilpivirine, and doravirine. NNRTIs are excellent ART drugs; however, their use is limited by drug interactions based on their metabolization by CYP450, overall low threshold for the emergence of HIV drug resistance, and reported side effects.[47] It is important to consider the fact that efavirenz, etravirine, and nevirapine may decrease concentrations of estradiol, dutasteride, finasteride, and testosterone; therefore, it may be necessary to increase the dosages of these drugs to achieve desired serum hormone concentrations and corresponding physical effects.[51]

InSTIs block the integrase enzyme from catalyzing the formation of covalent bonds between the host and viral DNA, preventing the viral DNA from incorporating itself into the host genome.[47] The most commonly used InSTIs include dolutegravir, bictegravir, elvitegravir, and raltegravir. InSTIs are extremely potent and well tolerated, and both dolutegravir and bictegravir have a high barrier to resistance.[47] Of note, all InSTIs can bind to polyvalent cations and have the potential for interactions with magnesium, calcium, aluminum, and iron.[47] In addition, neural tube defects have been reported in patients who received dolutegravir immediately before and during early pregnancy, and this must be discussed with all patients with childbearing potential.[51] Data remain forthcoming regarding InSTI use and weight gain.[51]

PIs bind to HIV proteases and prevent these enzymes from working properly, resulting in the inability to produce mature, infectious HIV virions.[47] PIs are prescribed in conjunction with a pharmacokinetic (PK) enhancer or "booster" drug consisting of either ritonavir or cobicistat. Commonly used PIs include darunavir, atazanavir, and lopinavir. PIs remain an important mainstay in treatment due to their high barrier to resistance, although attention must be paid to a multitude of potential drug interactions.[47] Boosted PIs may increase drug levels of dutasteride, finasteride, and testosterone and decrease the drug level of estradiol. Therefore, patients taking these medications for gender-affirming hormone therapy should be monitored closely.[51] Interactions between cobicistat and estradiol remain unclear; therefore, patients receiving this combination should have their estradiol dosage titrated to achieve desired serum hormone levels and corresponding physical effects.[51]

FIs interfere with the fusion process by binding to components of the viral envelope glycoprotein gp41, preventing fusion of the viral and CD4 cellular membrane.[47] Enfuvirtide is currently the only FI available for use. CD4 T-lymphocyte postattachment inhibitors are humanized monoclonal antibodies that attach to the host CD4 receptor, thereby blocking entry of the virus to host cells.[51] Currently, the only available drug in this class is ibalizumab, which is administered parenterally.

Lastly, CCR5 receptor antagonists, or entry inhibitors, selectively bind to the host CCR5 receptor and block the interaction of HIV gp120 and the host CCR5 receptor for CCR5-tropic virus. Before beginning an entry inhibitor, it is imperative to test for the presence of CXCR-tropic HIV, in the presence of which these drugs are ineffective.[47] The only available drug in this class is maraviroc. These three classes of drugs—FIs, CD4 T-lymphocyte postattachment inhibitors, and CCR5 receptor antagonists—tend to be most valuable when included as part of a salvage regimen in ART-experienced individuals.

The goals of ART are to achieve and maintain HIV viral suppression and increase CD4 T-cell count, thereby improving overall immune function; reduce HIV-associated morbidity; prolong survival; and reduce the risk of HIV transmission both to sexual partners and, in pregnant individuals, reduce vertical transmission.[47,58] Recent data show that early initiation of ART to persistently suppress HIV viral loads <200 copies/mL reduces the rate of sexual transmission of HIV, now widely supported as "treatment as prevention" and "U=U" ("Undetectable = Untransmittable").[58,59] Standard ART regimens should consist of preferably three (but at least two) active drugs that usually combine two NRTIs plus either an InSTI, an NNRTI, or a PI with a PK enhancer.[46,47] It is also important to note that despite the potency of current ART, residual HIV remains in different sanctuary reservoirs, and thus even a short lapse in treatment can result in viral rebound in a majority of patients, and can result in drug resistance mutations.[47,51,60] Hence, patients must maintain adherence to ART in order to achieve sustained viral suppression.[47]

Current guidelines for the use of antiretroviral agents in HIV-1-infected adults and adolescents from the U.S.

Department of Health and Human Services includes the following three-drug InSTI-based options as initial regimens for most people with HIV[51,58]: bictegravir/TAF/emtricitabine; dolutegravir/abacavir/lamivudine (in patients who are negative for HLA-B*5701); dolutegravir plus tenofovir (TAF/TDF)/emtricitabine (or lamivudine); and raltegravir plus tenofovir (TAF/TDF)/emtricitabine (or lamivudine). In December 2019, the two-drug regimen of dolutegravir plus lamivudine was added to the list of recommended initial regimens for most people with HIV, except for individuals with a pretreatment HIV viral load >500,000 copies/mL, who are known to have active hepatitis B coinfection, or who are starting ART prior to receiving results of HIV genotyping or HBV testing.[51]

Historically, expert advice and opinion on when to start ART have varied according to CD4 count, the presence or absence of an AIDS-defining event, and concerns regarding potential adverse effects of treatment.[61-63] Current recommendations advise ART for nearly all HIV-infected patients as soon as possible after HIV diagnosis, regardless of CD4 count, including immediate (same day) and rapid (within days to weeks of diagnosis) initiation of ART when possible.[51,61] Multiple studies have demonstrated that the deferral of ART is associated with increased mortality compared with early initiation of therapy. Patients who start therapy early have lower levels of T-cell activation (which can cause chronic inflammation), smaller HIV reservoir size, and increased ART uptake and engagement in care.[51,63,64] Individuals with acute HIV infection (acute retroviral syndrome) should also be evaluated for immediate therapy as soon as possible following diagnosis to reduce their potential for transmission to others during their period of highest viremia.[59,65] In 2017, the WHO endorsed ART initiation within 7 days of new diagnosis (including same-day start) due to improved viral suppression.[66] Current recommendations advise starting an immediate ART regime consisting of dolutegravir/tenofovir (TDF/TAF)/emtricitabine (or lamivudine); bictegravir/TAF/emtricitabine; or tenofovir (TDF/TAF)/emtricitabine with boosted darunavir.[51] These immediate recommendations differ from those advised as initial regimens, as immediate ART regimens are safe to start while still awaiting HIV resistance data.

Some individuals may be at an increased risk for HIV-associated morbidity and mortality, including patients who are pregnant, coinfected with Hepatitis B or C virus, and patients who have already developed complications from HIV. These patients may require more urgent and subspecialized evaluation. Other important considerations with choosing an optimal ART regimen for a patient include patient preference; cost; access to medications; the regimen's barrier to resistance; drug interactions; and underlying health conditions such as renal disease, liver disease, cardiovascular disease (CVD), dyslipidemia, psychiatric illness, and conditions associated with bone mineral density loss such as osteopenia and osteoporosis.[51]

Transgender people may have an elevated CVD risk due to both traditional factors (such as increased tobacco use) and risk factors associated with hormone use.[51] Studies have shown that transgender women have an increased risk of venous thromboembolism and ischemic stroke, which may be associated with the duration of estrogen use, although long-term data are needed.[51] Dyslipidemia also should be considered when selecting appropriate ART and gender-affirming hormone therapy regimens, as transgender women taking estrogen may have elevated serum triglycerides and HDL and decreased LDL, while transgender men on exogenous testosterone may have increased LDL and decreased HDL. For transgender people at elevated CVD risk or with a personal history of prior cardiovascular events, ART options that are associated with CVD risk, such as abacavir and boosted darunavir, should be avoided.[51]

There remains a lack of research on ART and bone health among transgender patients; however, there is concern that transgender women have higher rates of osteopenia before initiating hormone therapy, and that transgender men who are receiving testosterone therapy appear to sustain adequate bone mineral density.[67,68] The risk for osteoporosis increases after gonadectomy for both transgender men and transgender women. Therefore, particularly in the setting of hormone therapy cessation, providers should consider early bone density screening.[51]

When counseling transgender patients about ART, it is imperative to discuss ART in relation to gender-affirming hormone therapy and perceived side effects, such as changes in body image and appearance, to ensure maximum ART adherence.[69-71] Currently, the majority of research that has studied exogenous estrogens and ART has focused on oral contraceptive use in cisgender women; results of studies in TGD patients are awaited eagerly.[72]

Caution is advised when initiating ART in the setting of opportunistic infections. Current recommendations advise that ART be started within the first 2 weeks of diagnosis for most opportunistic infections.[51] In the setting of tuberculosis or cryptococcal meningitis, infectious disease consultation should be considered to ensure safe and expeditious care in these complex cases with potentially fatal outcomes in the absence of appropriate care.

Monitoring and Adherence

CD4 T-cell (CD4) count and HIV RNA viral load are the two laboratory markers of HIV disease progression and immune response to ART and remain the gold standard for surveillance of HIV infection.[51] On initiation of ART therapy, patients should have a CD4 count, HIV viral load, CBC, CMP, lipid profile, and urinalysis performed. Within 2–4 weeks, but no later than 8 weeks after starting ART, the patient should be reassessed with an HIV viral load and queried regarding adherence, tolerance, and side effects[51] (Table

17-15). The goal of therapy is to achieve a viral load <50, indicating sufficient initial virologic response to ART, an appropriate ART regimen, and patient adherence to therapy.[51] Once the HIV viral load is <50 copies/mL, monitoring is recommended every 3–4 months until suppression has been achieved for 2 years, at which time monitoring can be extended to every 6 months if the patient remains adherent to therapy.[51] For most patients on ART, the CD4 count will rise by 50–150 cells/mm^3 during the first year of therapy, and then approximately 50–100 cells/mm^3 per year subsequently until a steady state is reached.[73] A CD4 count can be checked every 3–6 months for the first 2 years following ART initiation and then annually once the CD4 level has been consistently between 300 and 500 cells/mm^3 for at least 2 years. Once the CD4 is consistently >500 cells/mm^3 for at least 2 years, checking a CD4 count is optional.[51] If the patient develops a rising HIV viral load L above 50 copies/mL, adherence and tolerability should be reassessed.[51]

When monitoring lab test results, if the HIV viral load increases above 200 copies/mL on at least two consecutive laboratory screens, virologic failure is likely, and resistance testing should be pursued as discussed below.[51] The clinician must remain constantly aware of the potential for interactions between hormone therapy and ART and adjust laboratory monitoring accordingly.[72]

Adherence to ART is complex, and a patient can face multiple barriers that impede their ability to take their medication regularly. Examples of these obstacles include cost, inadequate housing, food insecurity, active substance use, psychiatric disorders, medication side effects, interruptions in patient access to medication, and pill burden. Regular medication use can be optimized by individualizing care to meet each unique patient's needs and utilizing a multidisciplinary approach to care when possible.[51] It has been established that transgender women on ART are less likely to take their medications regularly compared to nontransgender patients, report feeling less confident in their ability to remain consistent in taking their ART daily, and experience fewer positive interactions with their health care team.[69] These observations emphasize the need to provide increased support to these patients in the form of gender-affirming health care, which includes integration of HIV care, hormone therapy, and behavioral health services within primary care along with increased navigation and outreach.[74]

HIV Resistance Testing and ART Modification

The effectiveness of ART can be limited due to many factors, including not taking medications as instructed, medication interactions that decrease medication effectiveness, medication intolerance, and antiretroviral resistance.[75] ART taken in the presence of ongoing viral replication results in the selection of subpopulations of HIV with mutations conferring

Table 17-15. Diagnostic Laboratory Testing for Initial Evaluation and Monitoring of HIV Infection[51,83]

Laboratory Test	Rationale	Suggested Monitoring Interval
Quantitative HIV RNA PCR (HIV viral load)	Monitoring of HIV replication activity Monitoring antiretroviral therapy efficacy	Baseline At the time of ART initiation or ART modification Repeat 2–8 weeks after ART initiation, then every 4–8 weeks until viral load <50 Every 3–4 months during the first 2 years of ART, then every 6 months for patients with consistently suppressed viral load ≥ 2 years
CD4 count	Evaluation of degree of immunosuppression Monitoring ART efficacy	Baseline Every 3–6 months if not on ART Every 3–6 months during the first 2 years of ART Every 12 months after 2 years of ART with suppressed viral load and CD4 300–500 cells/mm^3 Optional after 2 years of suppressed viral load and CD4 >500 cells/mm^3
HIV genotyping	Evaluation for mutations associated with resistance to ART To guide changes in ART management	Baseline At time of ART initiation or modification At time of virologic failure
Complete blood count	Monitoring for underlying hematologic abnormalities Evaluate for hematotoxicity of ART	Baseline At the time of ART initiation or modification Every 3–6 months if not on ART or as clinically indicated Every 12 months when no longer monitoring CD4 count
Chemistry labs (including serum electrolytes, BUN and creatinine, ALT, AST, total bilirubin)	Evaluation of baseline renal and liver function Monitoring for drug toxicities	Baseline At 2–8 weeks after ART initiation or modification Every 6 months More frequently in patients as clinically indicated Every 6–12 months if not on ART
Lipid profile	Monitoring for baseline metabolic abnormalities Monitoring for drug toxicities	Baseline At the time of ART initiation or modification Every 6 months if abnormal Every 12 months if benign
Random or fasting glucose	Monitoring for baseline metabolic abnormalities Monitoring for drug toxicities	Baseline At the time of ART initiation or modification Every 6 months if abnormal Every 12 months if benign
HLA B*5701	Assess genetic risk of hypersensitivity reaction to abacavir	Prior to initiation of abacavir as part of an ART regimen
Urinalysis and creatinine clearance	Evaluation for the risk of nephropathy and prior to using potentially nephrotoxic therapy	Baseline Prior to initiation or modification of ART Every 6 months if on a tenofovir (TDF)-containing ART regimen, otherwise every 12 months
Hepatitis profile (hepatitis A, B, and C)	Diagnosis of viral hepatitis Evaluation for prior vaccination and immunity to Hepatitis A and B	Baseline During potential acute infection

Abbreviations: ALT, alanine transaminase; ART, antiretroviral therapy; AST, aspartate transaminase; BUN, blood-urea-nitrogen; PCR, polymerase chain reaction.

resistance to specific antiretroviral therapies.[46] Not taking medications regularly is a major factor associated with the development of resistance.[75] Antiretroviral drugs differ in their ability to select for resistant mutations.[46] The main factors associated with class-specific adherence resistance include antiretroviral potency, HIV viral fitness and whether the infectious strain possesses antiretroviral resistance mutations, and the antiretroviral agents' genetic barrier to resistance.[75] Some antiretroviral drugs (e.g., efavirenz, emtricitabine, lamivudine, nevirapine, raltegravir) rapidly select for one mutation conferring high-level resistance, whereas most other antiretrovirals select for resistance mutations slowly and require multiple resistant mutations before the drug loses effectiveness.[46] Patients who develop antiretroviral resistance can transmit the resistant virus.[46] Transmission of drug-resistant HIV has been recognized in most countries where ART is available.[58] The prevalence of antiretroviral resistance in treatment-naïve patients in high-income countries reached a plateau of 10–17% with resistance to one or more antiretroviral drugs in 2014, whereas the prevalence is steadily increasing in low-income and middle-income countries, estimated to be between 3.2 and 11% in 2016.[46,76]

Due to increasing and widespread ART resistance, resistance testing has become indispensable in the management of patients with detectable HIV viral load, in instances of treatment failure, and, in some scenarios, when modifying an ART regimen.[58] Drug resistance has been demonstrated to lead to a delay in virologic suppression and an increased risk of earlier virologic failure.[77,78] The two types of resistance assays that are widely available for use in clinical practice are genotypic assays and phenotypic assays.[58] Genotypic assays, which are more commonly used, sequence HIV to detect mutations that confer drug resistance; phenotypic assays assess cell-cultured HIV in the presence of serial dilutions of one or more ART drugs.[58] Appropriate interpretation of drug resistance testing and resultant ART modification remains challenging and should be addressed with care and infectious disease consultation when necessary.

Short-Term Complications

Immune reconstitution disease (IRD), also referred to as immune reconstitution inflammatory syndrome (IRIS), is an immunopathological response resulting from the rapid restoration of pathogen-specific immune responses to preexisting antigens combined with immune dysregulation, which occurs soon after initiation of ART.[46,79,80]

Complications related to IRIS include uncovering previously subclinical infections and paradoxical worsening of treated opportunistic infections, and inflammatory reactions in HIV-1-infected persons after initiation of highly active antiretroviral. Most often, the antigens triggering IRIS are from opportunistic infections, notably tuberculosis, cryptococcal meningitis, mycobacterium avium complex,

and cytomegalovirus retinitis. IRIS occurs more frequently when ART is started in patients with low CD4 T-cell counts or soon after starting treatment for an opportunistic infection.[46] Approaches to reduce IRIS include initiation of ART at high CD4 counts, delayed initiation of ART in patients with an infection (with special care if the infection involves the central nervous system), and screening for and prevention of opportunistic infections before initiation of ART.[79] The treatment of IRIS is not well established; however, the use of anti-inflammatory agents, such as nonsteroidal drugs and local or systemic steroids, shows promise in halting the cascade of inflammatory damage associated with IRIS.[80]

Long-Term Complications

HIV infection is characterized by a significant increase in immune activation of both the adaptive and innate immune systems.[81] Evidence of residual inflammation or increased immune reactivation persists in HIV patients despite CD4 T-cell restoration on ART.[46] Markers of residual inflammation in patients with HIV on ART have been significantly associated with CVD, neurological disease, cancer, liver disease, and mortality,[46] suggesting that low-level HIV replication may contribute to persistent inflammation.[46] This possibility highlights the importance of regular primary care follow-up and ongoing monitoring for complications in these HIV patients who now have life expectancies approaching those of the general population.[82]

CASE STUDY 2

A 35-year-old trans woman presents to the outpatient clinic for follow-up. She was diagnosed with HIV infection 1 month ago when she presented to the emergency room with a rash on her left leg that proved to be herpes zoster and had a positive rapid HIV antibody test result. She initiated care with you 3 weeks ago but was not yet ready to initiate ART, as she had concerns that it would interact with her hormone therapy regimen. She has a stable job and lives with one roommate. Initial laboratory results at her first visit included a CBC showing mild lymphopenia, benign chemistry labs, normal lipids, normal urinalysis, and negative hepatitis B and C and STI screening. Her CD4 count was 423 cells/mm^3, and her HIV viral load was noted to be 40,000 copies/mL. An HIV genotype was negative for any significant mutations. At the current visit, she notes that she is starting to come to terms with her new diagnosis and is now ready to start ART. Her current medications include estradiol valerate (20 mg/mL) 0.5 mL IM every 2 weeks and micronized progesterone 100 mg daily that she has been taking for 2 years and orders via the internet. On further questioning, you find that she also drinks a tea that her family sends her from the Dominican Republic that helps her mood. She is concerned that starting ART will decrease her estrogen levels and cause her to lose weight and change her appearance.

▶ **Discussion Questions**

1. Is this patient ready to start ART?

2. How can you help this patient take her ART medications regularly?

3. Do you have any concerns regarding medication interactions?

Next steps: You review the importance of taking ART medications regularly to manage her HIV infection and long-term health, tell her that none of the currently recommended initial ART regimens has been shown to interact with her hormone therapy, and assess her readiness to start ART. You also advise against the use of herbal supplements and teas that could have ingredients that may potentially impair the metabolization of her ART and hormone therapy. Lastly, you engage the patient with your case management team and ensure that she has support and is able to afford her ART and attend scheduled visits at your clinic.

Highlights: It is important to review readiness to start ART with the patient before prescribing ART by assessing patient attitude, concerns regarding side effects, and ability to consistently afford and obtain ART. It is also advised to review both prescribed and over-the-counter medications and supplements with the patient before starting ART to avoid potential interactions that could decrease ART effectiveness and increase the risk of developing mutations. Lastly, it is imperative to discuss any perceived interactions between hormone therapy and ART to ensure effective HIV treatment in transgender patients.

SUMMARY

- Clinicians should regularly assess for STI risk based on their patients' current anatomy and sexual health and sexual risk behaviors. It is also crucial to know the patient's body parts involved during sexual encounters with their partner(s) to ascertain the sites to test during a screening evaluation.

- Recommendations for STI treatment are based on the 2015 *CDC Sexually Transmitted Disease Treatment Guidelines*.

- Infectious genital ulcers, often due to STI, can be classified as painless ulcers (syphilis, lymphogranuloma venereum, granuloma inguinale) or painful ulcers (herpes simplex virus [HSV], chancroid). Because all are associated with increased risk of HIV acquisition, HIV testing should be included in the evaluation.

- Dual therapy is recommended to treat gonorrheal infections because of the causative organism's ability to develop microbial resistance. Pharyngeal gonorrhea is more difficult to eradicate that urogenital or anorectal infections; a test of cure is recommended after 14 days of treatment.

- The most common cause of nongonococcal urethritis (NGU) is chlamydia, followed by *Mycoplasma genitalium*; however, in approximately one-half of all cases, no distinct etiology is identified. Treatment is therefore often presumptive.

- Pelvic inflammatory disease (PID) refers to an infection-induced inflammation of the upper female genital tract structures. Causes include gonorrhea, chlamydia, *M. genitalium*, and organisms that comprise vaginal flora or enteric organisms. Prompt treatment is necessary to prevent long-term complications, such as ectopic pregnancy and infertility.

- Patients with epididymitis should be fully evaluated and empiric therapy prescribed to prevent transmission of STIs and sequelae (including chronic pain and infertility).

- *Trichomonas vaginalis* is the most common nonviral sexually transmitted disease both in the United States and worldwide. Because of the high rates of reinfection, patients should be retested 3 months after appropriate treatment.

- Anogenital warts are caused by HPV. Treatment (removal of warts) may be necessary in some cases. A vaccine is available that protects against the most common nononcogenic and oncogenic strains of HPV.

- Antiretroviral therapy (ART) regimens for HIV include nucleoside reverse transcriptase inhibitors (NRTIs), non-nucleoside reverse transcriptase inhibitors (NNRTIs), integrase strand inhibitors (InSTIs), protease inhibitors (PIs), fusion inhibitors (FIs), CCR5 receptor antagonists, and CD4 T-lymphocyte postattachment inhibitors.

- Counseling for transgender patients about ART should include a discussion about ART in relation to gender-affirming hormone therapy and perceived side effects, such as changes in body image and appearance, to ensure maximum ART adherence.

- Adherence to ART is complex, and a patient can face multiple barriers that impede their ability to take their medication regularly.

REFERENCES

1. STDs Continue to Rise in the U.S. Press Release | CDC. Published October 7, 2019. https://www.cdc.gov/nchhstp/newsroom/2019/2018-STD-surveillance-report-press-release.html.

2. Prabawanti C, Bollen L, Palupy R, et al. HIV, sexually transmitted infections, and sexual risk behavior among transgenders in Indonesia. *AIDS Behav*. 2011;15(3):663–673.

3. Reisner SL, White JM, Mayer KH, Mimiaga MJ. Sexual risk behaviors and psychosocial health concerns of female-to-male transgender men screening for STDs at an urban community health center. *AIDS Care*. 2014;26(7):857–864.

4. Workowski KA, Bolan G. Sexually Transmitted Diseases Treatment Guidelines, 2015. https://www.cdc.gov/mmwr/preview/mmwrhtml/rr6403a1.htm. Accessed October 26, 2020.

5. Reisner SL, Murchison GR. A global research synthesis of HIV and STI biobehavioural risks in female-to-male transgender adults. *Glob Public Health.* 2016;11(7-8):866–887.

6. Reisner SL, Poteat T, Keatley J, et al. Global health burden and needs of transgender populations: a review. *Lancet Lond Engl.* 2016;388(10042):412–436.

7. Schmid GP. Approach to the patient with genital ulcer disease. *Med Clin North Am.* 1990;74(6):1559–1572.

8. Peeling RW, Mabey D, Kamb ML, Chen X-S, Radolf JD, Benzaken AS. Syphilis. *Nat Rev Dis Primer.* 2017;3(1):1–21.

9. Marra CM, Maxwell CL, Tantalo LC, Sahi SK, Lukehart SA. Normalization of serum rapid plasma reagin titer predicts normalization of cerebrospinal fluid and clinical abnormalities after treatment of neurosyphilis. *Clin Infect Dis Off Publ Infect Dis Soc Am.* 2008;47(7):893–899.

10. Ryder N, Jin F, McNulty AM, Grulich AE, Donovan B. Increasing role of herpes simplex virus type 1 in first-episode anogenital herpes in heterosexual women and younger men who have sex with men, 1992–2006. *Sex Transm Infect.* 2009;85(6):416–419.

11. Mertz GJ, Critchlow CW, Benedetti J, et al. Double-blind placebo-controlled trial of oral acyclovir in first-episode genital herpes simplex virus infection. *JAMA.* 1984;252(9):1147–1151.

12. Bryson YJ, Dillon M, Lovett M, et al. Treatment of first episodes of genital herpes simplex virus infection with oral acyclovir. A randomized double-blind controlled trial in normal subjects. *N Engl J Med.* 1983;308(16):916–921.

13. Mertz GJ, Loveless MO, Levin MJ, et al. Oral famciclovir for suppression of recurrent genital herpes simplex virus infection in women. A multicenter, double-blind, placebo-controlled trial. Collaborative Famciclovir Genital Herpes Research Group. *Arch Intern Med.* 1997;157(3):343–349.

14. Bartlett BL, Tyring SK, Fife K, et al. Famciclovir treatment options for patients with frequent outbreaks of recurrent genital herpes: the RELIEF trial. *J Clin Virol Off Publ Pan Am Soc Clin Virol.* 2008;43(2):190–195.

15. Reyes M, Shaik NS, Graber JM, et al. Acyclovir-resistant genital herpes among persons attending sexually transmitted disease and human immunodeficiency virus clinics. *Arch Intern Med.* 2003;163(1):76–80.

16. Ward H, Martin I, Macdonald N, et al. Lymphogranuloma venereum in the United kingdom. *Clin Infect Dis Off Publ Infect Dis Soc Am.* 2007;44(1):26–32.

17. Stoner BP, Cohen SE. Lymphogranuloma venereum 2015: clinical presentation, diagnosis, and treatment. *Clin Infect Dis Off Publ Infect Dis Soc Am.* 2015;61(Suppl 8):S865–S873.

18. Stamm WE. Lymphogranuloma venereum. In: Holmes KK, Sparling PF, Stamm WE, et al. eds. *Sexually Transmitted Diseases.* 4th ed. New York: McGraw-Hill Professional; 2007:595–606.

19. O'Farrell N. Donovanosis: an update. *Int J STD AIDS.* 2001;12(7):423–427.

20. Stamm WE. Chlamydia trachomatis infections of the adult. In: Holmes KK, Sparling PF, Mardh PA, et al. eds. *Sexually Transmitted Diseases.* 4th ed. New York: McGraw-Hill; 2008:575.

21. Lau A, Kong F, Fairley CK, et al. Treatment efficacy of azithromycin 1 g single dose versus doxycycline 100 mg twice daily for 7 days for the treatment of rectal chlamydia among men who have sex with men: a double-blind randomised controlled trial protocol. *BMC Infect Dis.* 2017;17(1):35.

22. Bernstein KT, Stephens SC, Barry PM, et al. *Chlamydia trachomatis* and *Neisseria gonorrhoeae* transmission from the oropharynx to the urethra among men who have sex with men. *Clin Infect Dis Off Publ Infect Dis Soc Am.* 2009;49(12):1793–1797.

23. Marcus JL, Kohn RP, Barry PM, Philip SS, Bernstein KT. *Chlamydia trachomatis* and *Neisseria gonorrhoeae* transmission from the female oropharynx to the male urethra. *Sex Transm Dis.* 2011;38(5):372–373.

24. Hosenfeld CB, Workowski KA, Berman S, et al. Repeat infection with Chlamydia and gonorrhea among females: a systematic review of the literature. *Sex Transm Dis.* 2009;36(8):478–489.

25. Fung M, Scott KC, Kent CK, Klausner JD. Chlamydial and gonococcal reinfection among men: a systematic review of data to evaluate the need for retesting. *Sex Transm Infect.* 2007;83(4):304–309.

26. CDC Division of STD Prevention. Sexually Transmitted Disease Surveillance 2013; 2014. https://wonder.cdc.gov/wonder/help/STD/STDSurv2013.pdf.

27. Unemo M, Shafer WM. Antimicrobial resistance in Neisseria gonorrhoeae in the 21st century: past, evolution, and future. *Clin Microbiol Rev.* 2014;27(3):587–613.

28. Ota KV, Fisman DN, Tamari IE, et al. Incidence and treatment outcomes of pharyngeal Neisseria gonorrhoeae and Chlamydia trachomatis infections in men who have sex with men: a 13-year retrospective cohort study. *Clin Infect Dis Off Publ Infect Dis Soc Am.* 2009;48(9):1237–1243.

29. Sarier M, Kukul E. Classification of non-gonococcal urethritis: a review. *Int Urol Nephrol.* 2019;51(6):901–907.

30. Read TRH, Fairley CK, Tabrizi SN, et al. Azithromycin 1.5g over 5 days compared to 1g single dose in urethral mycoplasma genitalium: impact on treatment outcome and resistance. *Clin Infect Dis Off Publ Infect Dis Soc Am.* 2017;64(3):250–256.

31. Wiesenfeld H. Pelvic inflammatory disease: treatment in adults and adolescents. UpToDate. Published 2019. https://www.uptodate.com/contents/pelvic-inflammatory-disease-treatment-in-adults-and-adolescents. Accessed October 26, 2020.

32. Brunham RC, Gottlieb SL, Paavonen J. Pelvic Inflammatory Disease. *N Engl J Med.* 2015;372(21):2039–2048.

33. Wiesenfeld HC, Hillier SL, Meyn L, et al. Mycoplasma genitalium—is it a pathogen in acute pelvic inflammatory disease (PID)? *Sex Transm Infect.* 2013;89(Suppl 1):A34–A34.

34. Ness RB, Kip KE, Hillier SL, et al. A cluster analysis of bacterial vaginosis-associated microflora and pelvic inflammatory disease. *Am J Epidemiol.* 2005;162(6):585–590.

35. Smith KJ, Ness RB, Wiesenfeld HC, Roberts MS. Cost-effectiveness of alternative outpatient pelvic inflammatory disease treatment strategies. *Sex Transm Dis.* 2007;34(12):960–966.

36. Trojian T, Lishnak TS, Heiman DL. Epididymitis and orchitis: an overview. *Am Fam Physician.* 2009;79(7):583–587.

37. Tracy CR, Steers WD, Costabile R. Diagnosis and management of epididymitis. *Urol Clin North Am.* 2008;35(1):101–108; vii.

38. Sobel JD. Approach to females with symptoms of vaginitis. UpToDate. Published 2019. https://www.uptodate.com/contents/approach-to-females-with-symptoms-of-vaginitis.

39. Sobel JD. Bacterial vaginosis: clinical manifestations and diagnosis. UpToDate. https://www.uptodate.com/contents/bacterial-vaginosis-clinical-manifestations-and-diagnosis. Accessed October 27, 2020.

40. Sobel JD. Bacterial vaginosis: treatment. UpToDate. https://www.uptodate.com/contents/bacterial-vaginosis-treatment.

41. Senok AC, Verstraelen H, Temmerman M, Botta GA. Probiotics for the treatment of bacterial vaginosis. *Cochrane Database Syst Rev.* 2009;(4):CD006289.

42. Sobel JD. Candida vulvovaginitis: treatment. UpToDate. Published 2019. https://www.uptodate.com/contents/candida-vulvovaginitis-treatment.

43. Garland SM, Steben M, Sings HL, et al. Natural history of genital warts: analysis of the placebo arm of 2 randomized phase III trials of a quadrivalent human papillomavirus (types 6, 11, 16, and 18) vaccine. *J Infect Dis.* 2009;199(6):805–814.

44. Ferenczy A, Mitao M, Nagai N, Silverstein SJ, Crum CP. Latent papillomavirus and recurring genital warts. *N Engl J Med.* 1985;313(13):784–788.

45. Sycuro LK, Xi LF, Hughes JP, et al. Persistence of genital human papillomavirus infection in a long-term follow-up study of female university students. *J Infect Dis.* 2008;198(7):971–978.

46. Maartens G, Celum C, Lewin SR. HIV infection: epidemiology, pathogenesis, treatment, and prevention. *Lancet Lond Engl.* 2014;384(9939):258–271.

47. Pau AK, George JM. Antiretroviral therapy: current drugs. *Infect Dis Clin North Am.* 2014;28(3):371–402.

48. Palella FJ, Delaney KM, Moorman AC, et al. Declining morbidity and mortality among patients with advanced human immunodeficiency virus infection. HIV Outpatient Study Investigators. *N Engl J Med.* 1998;338(13):853–860.

49. Zolopa A, Andersen J, Powderly W, et al. Early antiretroviral therapy reduces AIDS progression/death in individuals with acute opportunistic infections: a multicenter randomized strategy trial. *PLoS One.* 2009;4(5):e5575.

50. Baral SD, Poteat T, Strömdahl S, Wirtz AL, Guadamuz TE, Beyrer C. Worldwide burden of HIV in transgender women: a systematic review and meta-analysis. *Lancet Infect Dis.* 2013;13(3):214–222.

51. Saag MS, Benson CA, Gandhi RT, et al. Antiretroviral drugs for treatment and prevention of HIV infection in adults: 2018 recommendations of the International Antiviral Society-USA Panel. *JAMA.* 2018;320(4):379–396.

52. Beckwith CG, Kuo I, Fredericksen RJ, et al. Risk behaviors and HIV care continuum outcomes among criminal justice-involved HIV-infected transgender women and cisgender men: data from the Seek, Test, Treat, and Retain Harmonization Initiative. *PLoS One.* 2018;13(5):e0197730.

53. Poteat T, Aids for the NAACCOR and D of the IED to E, Hanna DB, et al. Characterizing the human immunodeficiency virus care continuum among transgender women and cisgender women and men in clinical care: a retrospective time-series analysis. *Clin Infect Dis.* 2020;70(6):1131–1138.

54. Kalichman SC, Hernandez D, Finneran S, Price D, Driver R. Transgender women and HIV-related health disparities: falling off the HIV treatment cascade. *Sex Health.* 2017;14(5):469–476.

55. James SE, Herman JL, Rankin S, Keisling M, Mottet L, Anafi M. The Report of the 2015 U.S. Transgender Survey. Natl Cent Transgender Equal. Published online 2016.

56. Machtinger EL, Haberer JE, Wilson TC, Weiss DS. Recent trauma is associated with antiretroviral failure and HIV transmission risk behavior among HIV-positive women and female-identified transgenders. *AIDS Behav.* 2012;16(8): 2160–2170.

57. Rajasuriar R, Gouillou M, Spelman T, et al. Clinical predictors of immune reconstitution following combination antiretroviral therapy in patients from the Australian HIV Observational Database. *PLoS One.* 2011;6(6):e20713.

58. Hirsch MS, Günthard HF, Schapiro JM, et al. Antiretroviral drug resistance testing in adult HIV-1 infection: 2008 recommendations of an International AIDS Society-USA panel. *Clin Infect Dis Off Publ Infect Dis Soc Am.* 2008;47(2):266–285.

59. Cohen MS, Chen YQ, McCauley M, et al. Prevention of HIV-1 infection with early antiretroviral therapy. *N Engl J Med.* 2011;365(6):493–505.

60. Davey RT, Bhat N, Yoder C, et al. HIV-1 and T cell dynamics after interruption of highly active antiretroviral therapy (HAART) in patients with a history of sustained viral suppression. *Proc Natl Acad Sci U S A.* 1999;96(26):15109–15114.

61. INSIGHT START Study Group, Lundgren JD, Babiker AG, et al. Initiation of Antiretroviral Therapy in Early Asymptomatic HIV Infection. *N Engl J Med.* 2015;373(9):795–807.

62. When To Start Consortium, Sterne JAC, May M, et al. Timing of initiation of antiretroviral therapy in AIDS-free HIV-1-infected patients: a collaborative analysis of 18 HIV cohort studies. *Lancet Lond Engl.* 2009;373(9672):1352–1363.

63. Kitahata MM, Gange SJ, Abraham AG, et al. Effect of early versus deferred antiretroviral therapy for HIV on survival. *N Engl J Med.* 2009;360(18):1815–1826.

64. Jain V, Hartogensis W, Bacchetti P, et al. Antiretroviral therapy initiated within 6 months of HIV infection is associated with lower T-cell activation and smaller HIV reservoir size. *J Infect Dis.* 2013;208(8):1202–1211.

65. Pilcher CD, Tien HC, Eron JJ, et al. Brief but efficient: acute HIV infection and the sexual transmission of HIV. *J Infect Dis.* 2004;189(10):1785–1792.

66. WHO | Guidelines for medico-legal care for victims of sexual violence. WHO. https://www.who.int/violence_injury_prevention/publications/violence/med_leg_guidelines/en/. Accessed October 23, 2020.

67. Wierckx K, Mueller S, Weyers S, et al. Long-term evaluation of cross-sex hormone treatment in transsexual persons. *J Sex Med.* 2012;9(10):2641–2651.

68. Van Caenegem E, Wierckx K, Taes Y, et al. Bone mass, bone geometry, and body composition in female-to-male transsexual persons after long-term cross-sex hormonal therapy. *J Clin Endocrinol Metab.* 2012;97(7):2503–2511.

69. Sevelius JM, Patouhas E, Keatley JG, Johnson MO. Barriers and facilitators to engagement and retention in care among transgender women living with human immunodeficiency virus. *Ann Behav Med Publ Soc Behav Med.* 2014;47(1):5–16.

70. Braun HM, Candelario J, Hanlon CL, et al. Transgender women living with HIV frequently take antiretroviral therapy and/or feminizing hormone therapy differently than prescribed due to drug-drug interaction concerns. *LGBT Health.* 2017;4(5):371–375.

71. Jaspal R, Kennedy L, Tariq S. Human immunodeficiency virus and trans women: a literature review. *Transgender Health.* 2018;3(1):239–250.

72. Radix A, Sevelius J, Deutsch MB. Transgender women, hormonal therapy and HIV treatment: a comprehensive review of the literature and recommendations for best practices. *J Int AIDS Soc.* 2016;19(3 Suppl 2):20810.

73. Kaufmann GR, Perrin L, Pantaleo G, et al. CD4 T-lymphocyte recovery in individuals with advanced HIV-1 infection receiving potent antiretroviral therapy for 4 years: the Swiss HIV Cohort Study. *Arch Intern Med.* 2003;163(18):2187–2195.

74. Sevelius JM, Carrico A, Johnson MO. Antiretroviral therapy adherence among transgender women living with HIV. *J Assoc Nurses AIDS Care JANAC.* 2010;21(3):256–264.

75. Gardner EM, Burman WJ, Steiner JF, Anderson PL, Bangsberg DR. Antiretroviral medication adherence and the development of class-specific antiretroviral resistance. *AIDS Lond Engl.* 2009;23(9):1035–1046.

76. Hamers RL, de Wit TFR, Holmes CB. HIV drug resistance in low-income and middle-income countries. *Lancet HIV*. 2018;5(10):e588–e596.

77. Little SJ, Holte S, Routy J-P, et al. Antiretroviral-drug resistance among patients recently infected with HIV. *N Engl J Med*. 2002;347(6):385–394.

78. Kuritzkes DR, Lalama CM, Ribaudo HJ, et al. Preexisting resistance to nonnucleoside reverse-transcriptase inhibitors predicts virologic failure of an efavirenz-based regimen in treatment-naive HIV-1-infected subjects. *J Infect Dis*. 2008;197(6):867–870.

79. Lawn SD, Meintjes G. Pathogenesis and prevention of immune reconstitution disease during antiretroviral therapy. *Expert Rev Anti Infect Ther*. 2011;9(4):415–430.

80. Cheng VC, Yuen KY, Chan WM, Wong SS, Ma ES, Chan RM. Immunorestitution disease involving the innate and adaptive response. *Clin Infect Dis Off Publ Infect Dis Soc Am*. 2000;30(6):882–892.

81. Lichtfuss GF, Hoy J, Rajasuriar R, Kramski M, Crowe SM, Lewin SR. Biomarkers of immune dysfunction following combination antiretroviral therapy for HIV infection. *Biomark Med*. 2011;5(2):171–186.

82. Samji H, Cescon A, Hogg RS, et al. Closing the gap: increases in life expectancy among treated HIV-positive individuals in the United States and Canada. *PLoS One*. 2013;8(12).

83. Multani A, Padival S. Human immunodeficiency virus II: clinical presentation, opportunistic infections, treatment and prevention. In: Domachowske J, ed. *Introduction to Clinical Infectious Diseases*. Springer; 2019:425–436.

Screening for Cancer and Cardiovascular Disease

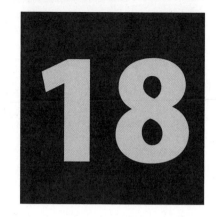

Alex Gonzalez

INTRODUCTION

Heart disease and cancer are the two leading causes of death in the general population in the United States,[1] but their impact on **transgender and gender diverse** (TGD) people is poorly understood. **Gender-affirming hormone therapy** (GAHT) can play a role in the development of certain cancers, and may worsen some risk factors for cardiovascular disease. Societal and health care sector marginalization of TGD people—via economic disenfranchisement, increased risky behavior, decreased access to care, decreased patient willingness to seek care, and increased stigma—can contribute to higher oncologic and cardiovascular risk as well. This chapter will review what we know about cancer and cardiovascular disease epidemiology in TGD people as well as how to approach screening for these diseases in a primary care setting.

CANCER IN TRANSGENDER AND GENDER DIVERSE ADULTS

▶ Epidemiology

Cancer rates and risks for TGD people remain unclear, even though research on this population has grown exponentially in the past decade.[2] There are multiple reasons for this. First, most studies on TGD people focus primarily on other topics such as behavioral health and substance use, sexual health, and sexually transmitted infections. Second, research and health registry methodologies for identifying and classifying TGD people vary, leading to sampling errors and a lack of uniformity in data collection.[3] Third, very few large-scale prospective studies of any kind about TGD people exist, and recruitment for these can often be exceedingly difficult.[2]

Despite these challenges, several TGD population cohort studies have been conducted over the past four decades. The earliest of these started in the Netherlands in 1972 with 425 patients (71% AMAB=**assigned male sex at birth**, 29%

AFAB=**assigned female sex at birth**), more than tripling in size by 2007. In 2011, Djhene and colleagues published a retrospective cohort study assessing cancer mortality of 324 Swedish transgender people (59% AMAB, 41% AFAB) between 1973 and 2003. Two different cohorts from Ghent University Hospital in Belgium have been studied; the earlier cohort consisted of 100 transgender people (50% AMAB, 50% AFAB), while the later cohort looked at 352 individuals (61% AMAB, 39% AFAB). All of these European studies had too small a sample size, not statistical power, and too few incident cases to be effective at analyzing links between certain malignancies and gender dysphoria, its treatments, or a person's transgender status.[2]

In the United States, Brown and colleagues have recently studied a cohort of 5135 transgender patients—over half of whom had been prescribed GAHT—within the Veterans Affairs system. Cancer mortality was only one of several variables studied, and cohort members' gender identities were not accurately categorized, leading to results that were difficult to interpret.[2] In 2017, Silverberg and colleagues looked at cancer risk among a cohort of 4889 transgender people (57% AMAB, 43% AFAB) from three large regional subsidiaries within the Kaiser Permanente (a large non-for-profit health consortium) system.[4] They evaluated all cancers combined, individual cancer sites with at least five cases, and grouped categories of cancers with shared risk factors such as smoking, viral (HIV, human papillomavirus [HPV], hepatitis C virus [HCV], Epstein-Barr virus [EBV], human herpesvirus-8 [HHV-8]) infection, and presence of an effective screening test. Like the previous cohort studies mentioned above, this study was limited by its small sample size and the relatively few events observed. Nevertheless, the study did indicate all of the following statistically significant findings:

- Overall cancer incidence rates for transgender people did not differ from those of **cisgender** people in the matching reference populations.

- AMAB TGD people on GAHT had a lower risk of prostate cancer (adjusted hazard ratio [AHR], 0.4; 95% CI, 0.2,0.9) versus reference cisgender men.

- AMAB TGD people on GAHT had a higher risk of endocrine (thyroid, adrenal, pituitary, pineal) gland cancer (AHR, 5.2; CI, 1.8,15.1) versus reference cisgender men.

- AMAB TGD people on GAHT had a higher risk of viral infection-induced (cervical, anal, head/neck, liver, Kaposi sarcoma, non-Hodgkin or Hodgkin lymphoma) cancer (AHR, 2.0; CI, 1.0,3.9) versus reference cisgender men.

- AMAB TGD people on GAHT had a higher risk of lymphatic and hematopoietic cancers (AHR, 3.0; CI, 1.4,6.3) versus reference cisgender women.

- AFAB TGD people on GAHT had a higher risk of breast cancer (AHR, 82; CI = 10,673) versus reference cisgender men.

- AFAB TGD people on GAHT had a higher risk of smoking-related (lung, esophagus, head/neck, cervix, stomach, pancreas, urinary bladder, kidney) cancer (AHR, 2.7; CI, 1.3,5.6).

It is hoped that the Kaiser Permanente cohort will continue to be followed, leading to a more comprehensive profile of cancer risk in the years to come.[4]

▶ Screening Rates

Breast, cervical, and colon cancer screening rates in the overall U.S. population in 2015 were 71.7%, 81.3%, and 63.4%, respectively.[5] It is likely that these rates are significantly lower among TGD people, but limited information is available. The 2015 U.S. Transgender Survey of over 27,000 TGD respondents showed that only 27% of AFAB TGD survey participants had received a Pap test in the previous 12 months, and 13% of all TGD survey participants had been denied coverage for services such as gender-specific cancer screenings.[6] A cross-sectional study at a major hospital system in Canada in 2019 compared breast, cervical, and colon cancer screening rates among TGD and cisgender patients and found significantly lower screening rates for each of these as well as for all of them combined; even after adjusting for age, income quintile, and number of visits, TGD patients had significantly lower odds of being screened for breast (adjusted odds ratio [AOR], 0.27; CI, 0.12,0.59), cervical (AOR, 0.39; CI, 0.25,0.62), and colon (AHR, 0.50; CI, 0.26,0.99) cancer when compared to cisgender counterparts.[7] Various barriers to accessing cancer screening exist for TGD people (Box 18-1).[6,7]

▶ Screening Recommendations

The United States Preventive Services Task Force (USPSTF) develops national recommendations for clinical preventive services but lacks specific recommendations for TGD people. The University of California San Francisco (UCSF)

Transgender Care and Treatment Guidelines state, "As a rule, if an individual has a particular body part or organ and otherwise meets criteria for screening based on risk factors or symptoms, screening should proceed regardless of hormone use."[8] Table 18-1 lists the most recent consensus guidelines for cancer screening in TGD people, in comparison with existing USPSTF screening recommendations.[8-13]

▶ Approach to Cancer Screening for TGD Adults

It is important for health care professionals to ensure that TGD patients receive comprehensive health care, including cancer screening. **Trauma-informed care** is an approach to health care that aims to understand, address, and alleviate the trauma burden faced by patients. Positive communication with patients can begin before an office visit even takes place by posting nondiscrimination statements on the practice's literature and website. Practices can create welcoming environments in their waiting rooms by having all-gender restrooms and by offering diverse reading materials including trans-friendly health brochures. Phone, registration, and check-in staff specially trained in transgender cultural competency can also decrease patient apprehension around seeking care in general. In the exam room, a provider can be trans-affirming by meeting with the patient before asking them to disrobe for examination, always using the patient's affirmed name and pronouns, and explaining why potentially difficult parts of an office visit conversation (such as a sexual history or **anatomical inventory**) are necessary. Preparing patients for examinations and cancer screening procedures may require multiple visits so that providers can educate patients about the following:

- Why certain examinations or procedures are needed

- Their right to make the informed decision to defer or decline the examination or procedure and to revisit these decisions at a future visit

- Risks associated with deferring/declining the exam or procedure

- Ways to make the examination or procedure more tolerable

TGD patients should also be encouraged to ask questions about cancer screening. See Chapters 11 (Basic Principles of Trauma-Informed and Gender-Affirming Care) and 13 (Performing a Trauma-Informed Physical Examination) for more details about conducting care in a trauma-informed manner.[8,14-16]

Resources:
1. National LGBT Cancer Network. https://cancer-network.org/
2. UCSF Transgender Care. https://transcare.ucsf.edu/
3. American College of Cardiology Foundation ASCVD Risk Estimator Plus. http://tools.acc.org/ASCVD-Risk-Estimator-Plus/#!/calculate/estimate/

BOX 18–1 Barriers to Accessing Cancer Screening for TGD People

Lack of adequate insurance coverage
- High deductibles or copayments for care
- Grandfathered plans not required to comply with Affordable Care Act mandate to offer free preventive care
- Decreased access to employer-based health insurance (due to higher rates of unemployment and underemployment among TGD people)

Mistreatment by insurers
- Insurer refuses to change patient's name and/or gender on insurance record
- Insurer refuses to cover gender-specific care when a gender mismatch is perceived (e.g. cervical cytology for AFAB TGD person whose sex is listed as "male" on insurance record)
- Insurer refuses to cover gender affirmative care

Mistreatment by health care providers
- Misnaming/misgendering by health care providers, support staff, and information systems
- Health care provider or staff ask invasive/unnecessary questions about being transgender
- Health care provider or staff refuse to provide gender affirmative care

Health care providers' discomfort/inexperience with treating TGD people
- Lack of gender identity/sex at birth/organ inventory information capture by health care providers
- Lack of clinical or cultural competency training in TGD care for health care providers and support staff

Inability of population health efforts to detect care gaps among TGD people
- Cancer screening initiatives relying largely on gender recorded in patient's health record to determine screening eligibility might inadvertently exclude TGD patients who have changed their gender marker from their sex assigned at birth
- Information systems may not detect TGD status of patients who have requested that such a status not be entered into the health record, or of patients whose health care providers have not correctly entered this status into the health record

Risk of increased gender dysphoria caused by the actual cancer screening experience
- Waiting room not welcoming to TGD people
- Removal of clothing for procedure that will be conducted by health care staff a TGD person has never met
- Cancer screening test can be physically and/or emotionally painful, especially if TGD patient has a history of sexual trauma, vaginal atrophy, or nulliparity

Lack of knowledge by TGD patient about impact of gender-affirmative surgical care on cancer screening
- AMAB TGD patients: prostate is not removed during vaginoplasty; breast implants can obscure mammogram images
- AFAB TGD patients: cervix (rarely) may not be removed during hysterectomy; vaginal cytology still required in post-hysterectomy patient with history of cervical dysplasia; breast tissue still remains after top surgery

Distance required to see health care providers for clinically and culturally competent care

Lack of TGD-specific health education about the importance of cancer screening

CARDIOVASCULAR DISEASE IN TRANSGENDER AND GENDER DIVERSE ADULTS

▶ Epidemiology

Several recent retrospective, electronic record-based cohort studies help describe the occurrence of acute cardiovascular events—including stroke, myocardial infarction, and venous thromboembolism—among TGD people receiving GAHT. Nota and colleagues reviewed the medical records of 2517 AMAB and 1358 AFAB TGD individuals who had visited a Dutch gender clinic between 1972 and 2015 and reported the following statistically significant findings[17]:

- Higher incidence of strokes in AMAB TGD individuals receiving GAHT compared with both cisgender women (standardized incidence ratio SIR = 2.42; 95% confidence

Table 18-1. Cancer Screening Recommendations for TGD Adults

Organ	USPSTF Recommendation	AFAB Recommendation	AMAB Recommendation
Breasts	Screening mammography every 2 years for cisgender women aged 50–74 years	Same as USPSTF Notes • In AFAB persons aged 50–74 years who have undergone bilateral mastectomy, consider chest wall exam followed by ultrasound or magnetic resonance imaging only if any palpable lesions present	Screening mammography every 2 years for AMAB persons on feminizing GAHT at age 50 years, or 5 years after onset of feminizing GAHT, whichever is later
Cervix	Cervical cytology screening alone every 3 years for cisgender women aged 21–29 years High-risk HPV screening with or without cytology screening every 5 years for women aged 30–65 years	Same as USPSTF	Not applicable for almost all AMAB persons Same as USPSTF *only* for AMAB persons who have undergone vaginoplasty using glans penis tissue to create a neocervix (rare)
Colon	Screening every year up to every 10 years depending on screening test for adults aged 50–75 years	Same as USPSTF	Same as USPSTF
Lung	Annual screening with low-dose computed tomography (LDCT) in adults aged 55–80 years who have a 30 pack-year smoking history and currently smoke or have quit within the past 15 years	Same as USPSTF	Same as USPSTF
Prostate	Provider-patient discussion followed by individual decision to screen with periodic PSA testing for cisgender men aged 55–69 years	Not applicable	Same as USPSTF Notes • In AMAB persons on GAHT: Upper limit of normal for PSA is 1.0 ng/mL • In AMB persons who have undergone vaginoplasty, consider digital neovaginal *and* rectal exam

Abbreviations: AFAB, assigned female sex at birth; AMAB, assigned male sex at birth; GAHT, gender-affirming hormone therapy; PSA, prostate-specific antigen; USPSTF, United States Preventive Services Task Force.
Data from Deutsch MB, ed. *Guidelines for the primary and gender-affirming care of transgender and gender nonbinary people.* San Francisco: UCSF, 2016. https://transcare.ucsf.edu/guidelines; U.S. Preventive Services Task Force. Screening for breast cancer: U.S. Preventive Services Task Force recommendation statement. *Ann Intern Med.* 2016;164:279-296; U.S. Preventive Services Task Force. Screening for cervical cancer: U.S. Preventive Services Task Force recommendation statement. *JAMA.* 2018;320(7):674-686; U.S. Preventive Services Task Force. Screening for colorectal cancer: U.S. Preventive Services Task Force recommendation statement. *JAMA.* 2016;315(23):2564-2575; U.S. Preventive Services Task Force. Screening for lung cancer: U.S. Preventive Services Task Force recommendation statement. *Ann. Intern. Med.* 2014;160:330-338; U.S. Preventive Services Task Force. Screening for prostate cancer: U.S. Preventive Services Task Force recommendation statement. *JAMA.* 2018;319(18):1901-1913.

interval CI = 1.65, 3.42) and cisgender men (SIR = 1.80; CI = 1.23, 2.56)

• Higher incidence of venous thromboembolism in AMAB TGD individuals receiving GAHT compared with both cisgender women (SIR = 5.52; CI = 4.36, 6.90) and cisgender men (SIR = 4.55; CI = 3.59, 5.69)

• Higher incidence of myocardial infarction in AMAB TGD individuals receiving GAHT compared with cisgender women (SIR = 2.64; CI = 1.81, 3.72)

• Higher incidence of myocardial infarction in AFAB TGD individuals receiving GAHT compared with cisgender women (SIR = 3.69; CI = 1.94, 6.42)

Getahun and colleagues reviewed the medical records of 2842 AMAB and 2118 AFAB TGD individuals who received care at Kaiser Permanente clinics in Georgia and California between 2006 and 2016 and reported similar findings[18]:

- Higher incidence of strokes in AMAB TGD individuals receiving GAHT compared with both cisgender women (adjusted hazard ratio [AHR] = 2.9; 95% confidence interval CI = 1.5, 5.5) and cisgender men (AHR = 2.3; CI = 1.2, 4.3)

- Higher incidence of venous thromboembolism in AMAB TGD individuals receiving GAHT compared with both cisgender women (AHR = 2.5; CI = 1.2, 5.0) and cisgender men (AHR = 3.2; CI = 1.5, 6.5)

- Higher incidence of myocardial infarction in AMAB TGD individuals overall compared with cisgender women (AHR = 1.8; CI = 1.1, 2.9)

- In contrast to the Dutch study, there was no finding of higher incidence of myocardial infarction in AFAB TGD individuals receiving GAHT compared with cisgender women

While these studies suggest that GAHT in both transgender men and women can lead to an increased risk of certain cardiovascular events, it is important to note their limitations. Both studies did not adjust for psychosocial stressors and HIV infection, and the Dutch study did not adjust for smoking; these are three potential confounders with historically high prevalence rates among TGD people.[17-19] Moreover, the AFAB TGD patients in both cohorts tended to be younger, whereas cardiovascular events tend to occur later in life, so it is possible that a longer observation period will yield different results. Neither study could fully ascertain variations in GAHT type, GAHT dosing, and prestudy period GAHT lifetime use among the TGD people studied; all of these are factors that could possibly adversely affect a TGD person's cardiovascular risk. Lastly, the cardiovascular risks of GAHT must be weighed against the known overall benefits of GAHT, specifically with respect to reducing morbidity and mortality from depression, suicidality, and substance use disorders, all known to have very high prevalence rates among TGD people.[19]

Screening Rates

Data are lacking for cardiovascular disease screening rates among TGD people in the United States, but these rates are likely low compared to the general population. In the Getahun cohort mentioned above, 20% of TGD patients studied did not have blood cholesterol levels listed in their medical records and 8% did not have a body mass index (BMI) recorded.[18] The 2015 U.S. Transgender Survey reported that one in three TGD people surveyed had at least one negative health care experience in the past year, and that almost a quarter of respondents did not seek medical care when they needed it because of fear of being mistreated as a TGD

person.[6] TGD people of color, particularly American Indian, Black, and Latinx people—all racial/ethnic groups at higher risk of developing cardiovascular disease and/or diabetes—are more likely to be uninsured than the general population.[6] These barriers likely prevent or delay timely and appropriate cardiovascular screening among TGD populations.

Screening Recommendations

The USPSTF lists several measures related to cardiovascular disease screening and prevention; listed below are those with a Grade A or B recommendation:

- Screening for high blood pressure in adults aged 18 years or older[20]

- Universal lipid screening in adults aged 40–75 years, with initiation of a statin drug and/or a low-dose aspirin in adults meeting certain additional criteria based on the Atherosclerotic Cardiovascular Disease (ASCVD) Risk Estimator Plus calculator, which takes natal sex into account[8,21,22]

- Screening for abnormal blood glucose in overweight or obese adults aged 40–70 years[23]

- A one-time screening for abdominal aortic aneurysm with ultrasonography in cisgender men aged 65–75 years who have ever smoked[24]

- Referral to intensive, multicomponent behavioral interventions for adults with a BMI of 30 or higher[25]

- Screening for tobacco use in all adults, advising all tobacco users to stop using tobacco, and providing all tobacco users with behavioral interventions and pharmacotherapy for cessation[26]

The UCSF Transgender Care and Treatment Guidelines predate the release of the Nota and Getahun cohort studies and recommend the following[8]:

- Check lipid panel based on USPSTF guidelines; check lipid panel at baseline and as needed thereafter only if clinician discretion deems it necessary.

- Depending on the age at which hormone therapy is started and total length of exposure, clinicians may choose to use the risk calculator for the natal sex, the affirmed gender, or an average of the two.

- Check hemoglobin A1c or blood glucose levels based on USPSTF guidelines; check hemoglobin A1c or blood glucose levels at baseline and as needed thereafter if clinician discretion deems it necessary.

- Low-dose aspirin can be considered as an additional preventive measure in AMAB TGD patients on GAHT.

- Transdermal estrogen is the preferred form of GAHT to minimize risk in AMAB TGD patients who use tobacco or have cardiovascular risk factors or known cardiovascular disease.

Table 18-2. Cardiovascular Disease Screening Recommendations for TGD Adults

Cardiovascular Event or Condition	USPSTF Recommendation	AFAB Recommendation	AMAB Recommendation
Hypertension	Screen for high blood pressure in adults aged 18 years or older • Check blood pressure annually in adults aged 40 years or older OR adults aged 18 years or older with increased risk for high blood pressure • Check blood pressure every 3–5 years in adults aged 18–39 years without risk factors • Risk factors: • High-to-normal blood pressure (130–139 / 85–89 mm Hg) • Being overweight or obese • African American background	Same as USPSTF Notes • Consider checking blood pressure at baseline visit and at least annually thereafter	Same as USPSTF Notes • Consider checking blood pressure at baseline visit and at least annually thereafter
Hyperlipidemia, myocardial infarction, and stroke	Universal lipid screening in adults aged 40–75 years, with initiation of a statin drug and/or a low-dose aspirin in adults meeting certain additional criteria, using the ASCVD Risk Estimator Plus calculator, which takes natal sex into account. Recheck lipid levels every 5 years	• Same as USPSTF • Consider universal lipid screening at baseline visit in all adults regardless of age, and every 1–5 years thereafter based on patient's history of GAHT use and their other risk factors • Use the ASCVD Risk Estimator Plus risk score for the patient's natal gender, affirmed gender, or an average of both of these, depending on the patient's history of GAHT use and their other risk factors	• Same as USPSTF • Consider universal lipid screening at baseline visit in all adults regardless of age, and every 1–5 years thereafter based on patient's history of GAHT use and their other risk factors • Use the ASCVD Risk Estimator Plus risk score for the patient's natal gender, affirmed gender, or an average of both of these, depending on the patient's history of GAHT use and their other risk factors
Diabetes mellitus	Screening for abnormal blood glucose (with hemoglobin A1c, fasting plasma glucose, or oral glucose tolerance test) in overweight or obese adults aged 40–70 years. Recheck every 3 years	• Same as USPSTF • Consider universal abnormal glucose screening at baseline visit in all adults regardless of age, and annually thereafter in patients with diabetes risk factors	• Same as USPSTF • Consider universal abnormal glucose screening at baseline visit in all adults regardless of age, and annually thereafter in patients with diabetes risk factors
Abdominal aortic aneurysm	A one-time screening for abdominal aortic aneurysm with ultrasonography in cisgender men aged 65–75 years who have ever smoked	• Same as USPSTF • Consider screening based on the patient's history of GAHT use and their other risk factors	Same as USPSTF
Obesity	Referral to intensive, multicomponent behavioral interventions for adults with a BMI of 30 or higher	Same as USPSTF	Same as USPSTF
Tobacco use disorder	Screening for tobacco use in all adults, advising all tobacco users to stop using tobacco, and providing all tobacco users with behavioral interventions and pharmacotherapy for cessation	Same as USPSTF	Same as USPSTF

(Continued)

Table 18-2. Cardiovascular Disease Screening Recommendations for TGD Adults *(Continued)*

Abbreviations: AFAB, assigned female sex at birth; AMAB, assigned male sex at birth; ASCVD, atherosclerotic cardiovascular disease; BMI, body mass index; GAHT, gender-affirming hormone therapy; USPSTF, United States Preventive Services Task Force.
Data from Cavanaugh T, Hopwood R, Gonzalez A, et al. *The Medical Care of Transgender Persons*. Boston, MA: Fenway Health; 2015; Hembree WC, Cohen-Kettenis PT, Gooren L, et al. Endocrine treatment of gender-dysphoric/gender-incongruent persons: an Endocrine Society clinical practice guideline. *J Clin Endocrinol Metab*. 2017;102(11):3869-3903; Radix A, Meacher P, Vavasis A, et al. *Protocols for the Provision of Hormone Therapy*. New York City: Callen Lorde Community Health Center; 2016; U.S. Preventive Services Task Force. Aspirin use for the primary prevention of cardiovascular disease and colorectal cancer: U.S. Preventive Services Task Force recommendation statement. *Ann Intern Med*. 2016;164(12):836-845; U.S. Preventive Services Task Force. Behavioral and pharmacotherapy interventions for tobacco smoking cessation in adults, including pregnant women: U.S. Preventive Services Task Force recommendation statement. *Ann Intern Med*. 2015;163(8):622-635; U.S. Preventive Services Task Force. Behavioral weight loss interventions to prevent obesity-related morbidity and mortality in adults: U.S. Preventive Services Task Force recommendation statement. *JAMA*. 2018;320(11):1163-1171; U.S. Preventive Services Task Force. Screening for abdominal aortic aneurysm: U.S. Preventive Services Task Force recommendation statement. *JAMA*. 2019;322(22):2211-2218; U.S. Preventive Services Task Force. Screening for abnormal blood glucose and type 2 diabetes mellitus: U.S. Preventive Services Task Force recommendation statement. *Ann Intern Med*. 2015;163(11):861-869; U.S. Preventive Services Task Force. Screening for high blood pressure in adults: U.S. Preventive Services Task Force recommendation statement. *Ann Intern Med*. 2015;163(10):778-787; U.S. Preventive Services Task Force. Statin use for the primary prevention of cardiovascular disease in adults: U.S. Preventive Services Task Force recommendation statement. *JAMA*. 2016;316(19):1997-2007.

- Routine universal venous thromboembolism prophylaxis with aspirin in transgender populations is not recommended.

Other guidelines, such as those of Fenway Health, Callen-Lorde Community Health Center, and the Endocrine Society, also predate the Nota and Getahun cohort studies but differ from the UCSF guidelines, in that they recommend baseline lipid panel testing in all TGD patients prior to initiating GAHT and then at regular intervals (such as annually), as well as baseline and subsequent annual blood glucose or hemoglobin A1c testing in TGD patients with risk factors for diabetes.[27-29] Table 18-2 lists these proposed screening guidelines that consider the most recent data in comparison with existing USPSTF screening recommendations.[17,18,20-29]

▶ **Approach to Cardiovascular Disease Screening for TGD Adults**

As with cisgender people, counseling about the prevention of cardiovascular disease among TGD people should focus on smoking cessation, healthy eating, increased physical activity, and regular primary care visits. Because AFAB TGD people may find testosterone-related weight gain and AMAB TGD people may find estrogen-related subcutaneous fat redistribution desirable, clinicians should focus less on BMI or weight goals and more on individual goal setting centered on adopting healthy behaviors or stopping/reducing less healthy ones.[30] Gender-affirming surgeries often have BMI limits, exclude active smokers, and require patients with cardiovascular disease or diabetes to have adequate blood pressure, blood sugar, and symptom control. Clinicians can assist TGD patients who are motivated in

pursuing these procedures, including prescribing of GAHT, which can reduce anxiety and depression and improve social functioning, thereby facilitating any needed behavior changes.[8] Given that so many TGD people have a history of mistreatment or discrimination in health care, it is very important to engage in shared decision-making with TGD patients, including the use of **harm reduction** approaches that prevent the restriction or denial of GAHT to patients whenever possible.

SUMMARY

- Cancer rates and risks for TGD people remain unclear. Overall cancer incidence rates for transgender people do not seem to differ from those of cisgender people, but more research is needed on this issue.

- Cancer screening should be based on a TGD person's anatomy and not their gender identity; if they have it, check it.

- Recent studies suggest that GAHT in both AFAB and AMAB TGD adults can lead to an increased risk of certain cardiovascular events. Specifically, AMAB TGD adults have higher risks of stroke, venous thromboembolism, and myocardial infarction compared with cisgender adults, and AFAB TGD adults have a higher risk of myocardial infarction compared with cisgender women.

- The cardiovascular risks of GAHT must be weighed against the known overall benefits of GAHT, specifically with respect to reducing morbidity and mortality from depression, suicidality, and substance use disorders, all known to have very high prevalence rates among TGD people.

CASE STUDY 1: BLAS

Blas is a 45-year-old Latino transgender male (AFAB) whose status is post-cervix-sparing hysterectomy, bilateral salpingo-oophorectomy, and bilateral chest reconstruction and he has been on testosterone for the past 20 years. Blas now presents for his annual physical. He has a male gender marker on both his insurance and your clinic's medical record. He has no previous abnormal cervical cytology results, and he is a nonsmoker.

▶ Discussion Questions

1. What cancer screening tests should you perform?
2. What cardiovascular disease screening tests should you perform?

▶ Discussion

1. Cancer Screening
   - Cervical Cancer: You perform a cervical cytology and HPV testing on Blas since there is still a cervix present, noting on your lab requisition that Blas is AFAB, on testosterone therapy, and amenorrheic. Your additional comments allow both the receiving laboratory to process the submitted specimen efficiently and the lab's pathologist to accurately interpret the specimen. The result is negative for intraepithelial lesion or malignancy, and HPV cotesting is negative as well.

2. Cardiovascular Screening
   - Hypertension: You check Blas's blood pressure at least annually; today's reading is 110/72 mm Hg, which is normal.
   - Hyperlipidemia, myocardial infarction, and stroke: You check Blas's total, low-density lipoprotein (LDL), and high-density lipoprotein (HDL) cholesterol levels as well as his triglyceride level at least once every 5 years and enter his results into the ASCVD Risk Estimate Plus calculator. His ASCVD 10-year risk is 1% using his affirmed gender of male and 0.4% using his sex assigned at birth, which was female. Both of these results are low and do not require him to start a statin or a low-dose aspirin.
   - Diabetes mellitus: Blas's baseline glucose testing many years ago was normal, and his BMI is in the normal range and he has no diabetes risk factors, so you do not perform glucose testing.
   - Other: You counsel Blas at his annual physical about the importance of healthy behaviors in preventing cardiovascular events; these behaviors include healthy eating, increased physical activity, and not smoking.

CASE STUDY 2: SUKI

Suki is a 62-year-old Black transgender female (AMAB) with a previous history of major depressive disorder and tobacco use disorder. She presents to your clinic requesting initiation of gender-affirming hormone therapy and primary care.

▶ Discussion Questions

1. What cancer screening tests should you perform?
2. What cardiovascular disease screening tests should you perform?

▶ Discussion

1. Cancer Screening
   - Breast cancer: Suki has not been on GAHT for more than 5 years, so she does not need to initiate screening mammograms at this point.
   - Colon cancer: You educate Suki about her multiple screening options (guaiac fecal occult blood test, fecal immunohistochemical test, fecal immunohistochemical test with DNA testing, flexible sigmoidoscopy, colonoscopy, CT colonography). She opts for fecal immunohistochemical testing, which shows no abnormalities.
   - Lung cancer: You educate Suki about lung cancer screening, and she agrees to undergo low-dose computed tomography screening, which shows scattered, small pulmonary nodules that are not suspicious for malignancy.
   - Prostate cancer: You have a shared decision-making discussion with Suki about prostate cancer screening. Suki decides to undergo PSA testing as well as a digital rectal examination, given that Black people with prostates are at increased risk of prostate cancer. Her PSA comes back as a Stage 1, Gleason score 6 prostate adenocarcinoma. You are able to refer Suki to a trans-competent urologist and oncologist who formulate a treatment plan consisting of active surveillance for now.

2. Cardiovascular Screening
   - Hypertension: You check Suki's blood pressure at her baseline visit. Her blood pressure is 163/92 mm Hg. You counsel Suki on lifestyle changes, including smoking cessation, healthy eating, and increased physical activity, which can reduce her blood pressure. You also discuss hypertension pharmacotherapy options with Suki. After confirming that her renal function is normal, you determine that spironolactone will be an optimal first-line agent because it will lower her blood pressure and her testosterone levels.
   - Hyperlipidemia, myocardial infarction, and stroke: You check Suki's total, LDL, and HDL cholesterol levels as well as her triglyceride level at baseline and enter her results into the ASCVD Risk Estimator Plus calculator. Her ASCVD 10-year risk is over 10% regardless of the gender used in the calculator, and Suki agrees to start both a high-dose statin and low-dose aspirin.

- Diabetes mellitus: Suki's baseline glucose testing is normal. Given her cardiovascular risk factors, you let Suki know it would be helpful to check her glucose levels test at least annually.

- Abdominal aortic aneurysm: You counsel Suki about reports of aneurysm risk in cisgender male smokers, and she agrees to undergo screening with an abdominal ultrasound, which is normal.

- Tobacco use disorder: You advise Suki to stop using tobacco and educate her about her smoking cessation options. Suki expresses ambivalence about quitting smoking and fears that she won't be allowed to start GAHT if she continues to smoke. You reassure Suki that you are her partner in her care and will continue to work with her on smoking cessation efforts in the future if she is not ready now. You recommend that she set other health-related goals that may be more of a priority for her. You also reassure her that you will prescribe GAHT despite her tobacco use as long as she understands the risks of continuing to smoke and is willing to start with a low-dose of transdermal or sublingual estrogen regimen, which is thought to be safer from a cardiovascular perspective.

REFERENCES

1. Murphy SL, Xu JQ, Kochanek KD, et al. Mortality in the United States, 2017. NCHS Data Brief, no 328. Hyattsville, MD: National Center for Health Statistics; 2018.
2. Braun H, Nash R, Tangpricha V, et al. Cancer in transgender people: evidence and methodological considerations. *Epidemiol Rev*. 2017;39:93-107.
3. Reisner SL, Deutsch MB, Goodman M. Advancing methods for U.S transgender health research. *Curr Opin Endocrinol Diabetes Obes*. 2016;23(2):198-207.
4. Silverberg MJ, Nash R, Becerra-Culqui TA, et al. Cohort study of cancer risk among insured transgender people. *Ann Epidemiol*. 2017;27:499-501.
5. Hall IJ, Tangka FK, Sabatino SA, et al. Patterns and trends in cancer screening in the United States. *Prev Chronic Dis*. 2018;15:170465.
6. James SE, Herman JL, Rankin S, et al. *The Report of the 2015 U.S. Transgender Survey*. Washington, DC: National Center for Transgender Equality; 2016.
7. Kiran T, Davie S, Singh D, et al. Cancer screening rates among transgender adults. *Canadian Family Physician*. 2019;65:e30-e37.
8. Deutsch MB, ed. *Guidelines for the Primary and Gender-Affirming Care of Transgender and Gender Nonbinary People*. San Francisco, CA: UCSF; 2016. https://transcare.ucsf.edu/guidelines.
9. U.S. Preventive Services Task Force. Screening for breast cancer: U.S. Preventive Services Task Force recommendation statement. *Ann Intern Med*. 2016;164:279-296.
10. U.S. Preventive Services Task Force. Screening for cervical cancer: U.S. Preventive Services Task Force recommendation statement. *JAMA*. 2018;320(7):674-686.
11. U.S. Preventive Services Task Force. Screening for colorectal cancer: U.S. Preventive Services Task Force recommendation statement. *JAMA*. 2016;315(23):2564-2575.
12. U.S. Preventive Services Task Force. Screening for lung cancer: U.S. Preventive Services Task Force recommendation statement. *Ann Intern Med*. 2014;160:330-338.
13. U.S. Preventive Services Task Force. Screening for prostate cancer: U.S. Preventive Services Task Force recommendation statement. *JAMA*. 2018;319(18):1901-1913.
14. Nelson B. A cancer screening crisis for transgender patients. *Cancer Cytopathol*. 2019;127(7):421-422.
15. Rollston R. *Promoting Cervical Cancer Screening among Female-to-Male Transmasculine Patients*. Boston, MA: The Fenway Institute; 2019.
16. Puechl AM, Russell K, Gray BA. Care and cancer screening of the transgender population. *J Women's Health*. 2019;28(6):761-768.
17. Nota NM, Wiepjes CM, de Blok CJM, et al. Occurrence of acute cardiovascular events in transgender individuals receiving hormone therapy: results from a large cohort study. *Circulation*. 2019;139:1461-1462.
18. Getahun D, Nash R, Flanders WD, et al. Cross-sex hormones and acute cardiovascular events in transgender persons: a cohort study. *Ann Intern Med*. 2018;169(4):205-214.
19. Goldstein Z, Streed C, Resiman T, et al. Cross-Sex hormones and acute cardiovascular events in transgender persons: a cohort study [letter]. *Ann Intern Med*. 2019;170(2):142-143.
20. U.S. Preventive Services Task Force. Screening for high blood pressure in adults: U.S. Preventive Services Task Force recommendation statement. *Ann Intern Med*. 2015;163(10):778-787.
21. U.S. Preventive Services Task Force. Statin use for the primary prevention of cardiovascular disease in adults: U.S. Preventive Services Task Force recommendation statement. *JAMA*. 2016;316(19):1997-2007.
22. U.S. Preventive Services Task Force. Aspirin use for the primary prevention of cardiovascular disease and colorectal cancer: U.S. Preventive Services Task Force recommendation statement. *Ann Intern Med*. 2016;164(12):836-845.
23. U.S. Preventive Services Task Force. Screening for abnormal blood glucose and type 2 diabetes mellitus: U.S. Preventive Services Task Force recommendation statement. *Ann Intern Med*. 2015;163(11):861-869.
24. U.S. Preventive Services Task Force. Screening for abdominal aortic aneurysm: U.S. Preventive Services Task Force recommendation statement. *JAMA*. 2019;322(22):2211-2218.
25. U.S. Preventive Services Task Force. Behavioral weight loss interventions to prevent obesity-related morbidity and mortality in adults: U.S. Preventive Services Task Force recommendation statement. *JAMA*. 2018;320(11):1163-1171.
26. U.S. Preventive Services Task Force. Behavioral and pharmacotherapy interventions for tobacco smoking cessation in adults, including pregnant women: U.S. Preventive Services Task Force recommendation statement. *Ann Intern Med*. 2015;163(8):622-635.
27. Cavanaugh T, Hopwood R, Gonzalez A, et al. *The Medical Care of Transgender Persons*. Boston, MA: Fenway Health; 2015.
28. Radix A, Meacher P, Vavasis A, et al. *Protocols for the Provision of Hormone Therapy*. New York City: Callen Lorde Community Health Center; 2016.
29. Hembree WC, Cohen-Kettenis PT, Gooren L, et al. Endocrine treatment of gender-dysphoric/gender-incongruent persons: an Endocrine Society clinical practice guideline. *J Clin Endocrinol Metab*. 2017;102(11):3869-3903.
30. Morris C. *Supporting Clients to Make Healthy Food Choices and Increase Physical Activity*. Rockville, MD: Substance Abuse and Mental Health Services Administration; 2014.

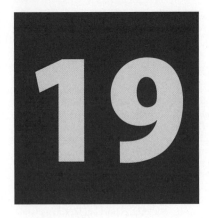

Reproductive Health, Obstetric Care, and Family Building

Mason J. Dunn
Samuel C. Pang
Rebekah P. Viloria

This chapter focuses on the reproductive and obstetric aspects of health that are specific to **transgender and gender diverse (TGD)** populations. Sexual health, including prevention of HIV and sexually transmitted infections (STIs), is covered elsewhere in this book (see Chapter 16, "Screening and Prevention of HIV and Sexually Transmitted Infections" and Chapter 17, "Treatment of HIV and Sexually Transmitted Infections"). This chapter also discusses legal and financial aspects of family building for TGD individuals and provides resources for patients who are exploring ways to build a family.

REPRODUCTIVE HEALTH

The term **reproductive health** refers to the condition of the human reproductive systems during all life stages. The World Health Organization (WHO) expands this definition to include "complete physical, mental and social well-being, and not merely the absence of disease or infirmity" and states that reproductive health implies that "people are able to have a satisfying and safe sex life and that they have the capability to reproduce and the freedom to decide if, when, and how often to do so."[1] Reproductive health care includes contraception counseling, screening for and treatment of STIs, cancer screening, and discussion of a reproductive plan. For those who wish to become pregnant, prepregnancy counseling provides the opportunity to achieve optimal health before pregnancy and address modifiable risk factors to improve obstetric outcomes.[2] For TGD individuals, additional reproductive health issues may include education about how **gender-affirming hormone therapy (GAHT)** and surgeries may affect fertility and reproductive planning and consequent fertility treatment and preservation. Many of these services, especially those related to preventive health care, can be provided by clinicians who do not have specific expertise in TGD care. Other services, such as GAHT and

gender-affirming surgery, may be best managed in consultation with experts who specialize in the care and treatment of TGD individuals.[3]

BARRIERS TO REPRODUCTIVE HEALTH

Many TGD people report barriers to accessing reproductive health care while at the same time acknowledging their need for such health care and their interest in addressing various reproductive health concerns, including cervical cancer screening, STI testing and prevention, and contraception. TGD patients seek information about gender-affirming care, including the impact of GAHT on pregnancy, how to preserve future fertility when pursuing gender-affirming treatments, and the use of GAHT following gender-affirming surgery.[4]

Barriers to reproductive care include structural barriers, such as the failure of health insurance plans to cover mental health services and gender-affirming care. Social and economic marginalizations constitute another barrier to consistent, quality health care. **Discrimination** and **stigma** often discourage TGD individuals from seeking professional health care due to the lack of education and acceptance among health care professionals about TGD health needs. In one study, TGD people **assigned female sex at birth (AFAB)** point to the association of reproductive health care with "women's health" as a major barrier to addressing reproductive health issues and describe the discomfort and anxiety of seeking such care.[3] The lack of specificity about gender on intake forms not only creates an unwelcoming environment but also limits a patient's ability to accurately communicate about reproductive health care needs. Being unable to report one's sexual behavior, gender identity, and sexual orientation on intake forms or to practice staff can significantly impact whether an individual receives recommended cervical cancer screening and STI infection screening tests. Clinician assumptions or lack of awareness regarding the types of sexual behavior and activity among TGD individuals also impact the types of reproductive health care services these patients receive. Asking only the standard question, "Are you sexually active?" and assuming that this question applies exclusively to penis-in-vagina sex limits the focus to pregnancy and STI acquisition via only one route and ignores the multiplicity of TGD sexual experiences.[4]

Clinicians must recognize these unique needs and take steps to educate themselves about obtaining an individual's sexual and social history, conducting an **anatomical inventory**, and discussing future reproductive plans for all patients, including TGD patients. These best practices not only ensure that all patients receive the health care interventions that are appropriate to their sexual behavior and anatomy but also help relieve patient anxiety and promote partnership with the health care system. Chapters 11 (Basic Principles of Trauma-Informed and Gender-Affirming Care) and 13 (Performing a Trauma-Informed Physical Examination) provide detailed information about gender-affirming health care practices.

▶ Contraception

Contraception counseling should be provided to all individuals of reproductive age who are sexually active and able to achieve pregnancy or to make someone else pregnant, including TGD individuals. TGD individuals who require contraceptive counseling include AFAB persons with a uterus and ovaries who engage in sexual activity that may result in pregnancy with a sperm-producing partner and persons **assigned male sex at birth (AMAB)** who produce sperm and who engage in sexual activity that may result in pregnancy with a partner who has a uterus and ovaries.

Existing data reveal significant room for clinical improvement in providing contraceptive counseling for TGD patient populations. For example, in a study of 26 TGD AFAB individuals presenting to a clinic for sex workers, 13 were at risk for pregnancy. Of those desiring to avoid pregnancy ($n = 11$), few used highly effective contraception, and many used no contraception.[5] Other studies indicate that up to 31% of TGD AFAB individuals believe that testosterone therapy is an effective contraceptive method.[6] Unintended pregnancy rates among TGD men are comparable to those of the general population. In one small study of transgender men who had been pregnant and delivered a neonate, almost one-half of the participants who were not using testosterone and one-fourth of those using testosterone reported that their pregnancy had not been planned.[7]

Special Considerations for TGD Individuals

GAHT does not render a person completely infertile and should not be relied on to provide contraception. It is important to educate all TGD individuals on GAHT about the potential for pregnancy. Although estrogen therapy among trans feminine people decreases spermatogenesis and causes testicular atrophy, and testosterone therapy among trans masculine people alters ovarian histology and suppresses ovulation, these effects are incomplete.[8] Furthermore, the extent to which fertility is affected can be different for different people. And although menstruation ceases in most trans masculine people on testosterone, lack of menstruation is not a reliable indicator of lack of fertility, as ovulation may continue to occur.[9] These patients should be counseled that contraception is necessary to prevent pregnancy if they engage in sexual activity that could result in pregnancy.

Conversely, the fertility-reducing effects of testosterone may boost the effectiveness of contraceptive methods. Although no studies have been performed to investigate this question, it is thought that testosterone may have greater efficacy in trans masculine people on testosterone therapy compared with cisgender women. The Society for Family Planning recommends that patients be counseled about the additional effect of testosterone on the efficacy of both hormonal and nonhormonal methods of contraception.[10]

Contraceptive Options

Data from the 2015–2017 National Survey of Family Growth showed that 64.9% of women (ages 15–49) in the United States were using contraception. Female sterilization (18.6%) was the most commonly used method, followed by oral contraceptive pills (12.6%), long-acting reversible contraception (10.3%), and the **external condom** (8.7%).[11] In a recent study of 197 TGD people assigned female sex at birth aged 18–45, 60% reported using contraception, with condoms and pills most commonly utilized. Methods of contraception did not differ between testosterone and nontestosterone users except for hormonal intrauterine devices (IUDs; 20% using T vs. 7% non-T).

All forms of contraception that are offered routinely to cisgender women should be offered to TGD AFAB people who are at risk for pregnancy. Among the reversible methods (those that can be stopped at any time if pregnancy is desired), the IUD and the contraceptive implant are most effective in preventing unintended pregnancy (Table 19-1). Sterilization is a highly effective permanent method of contraception. Barrier methods such as external and **internal condoms** can reduce the risk of infections transmitted through sexual activity, including HIV, hepatitis B and C, Zika, and Ebola.

In addition to preventing pregnancy, hormonal methods of contraception have noncontraceptive effects that may be desirable. Continuous combined hormonal contraception, depot medroxyprogesterone acetate (DMPA), and the levonorgestrel IUDs provide long-term reduction or suppression of menstrual-related bleeding or pain[12] and reduction in testosterone-related bleeding. Combined hormonal contraception improves acne and hirsutism and provides

Table 19-1. Contraceptive Failure Rates

Method	% of Patients Experiencing an Unintended Pregnancy During the First Year of Typical Use[a] of Contraception
No method	85
Spermicides	21
Internal condom	21
Withdrawal	20
Diaphragm	17
Sponge (parous, nulliparous)	24, 14
Fertility awareness-based methods	15
External condom	13
Combined pill and progestin-only pill	7
Contraceptive patch	7
Contraceptive ring	7
Depot medroxyprogesterone acetate	4
Intrauterine device (copper, levonorgestrel)	0.8, 0.1–0.4
Contraceptive implant	0.1
Sterilization (vasectomy and tubal ligation)	0.5, 0.15

[a]Typical use is defined as the actual use of a method that includes inconsistent or incorrect use.
Data from Hatcher RA, Nelson AL, Trussell J, et al: *Contraceptive Technology*, 21st ed. New York, NY: Ayer Company Publishers, Inc: 2018.

risk reduction for endometrial and ovarian cancer. These effects should be considered when choosing a contraceptive method. It is important to counsel patients that these effects may not occur immediately upon starting these methods and that some methods may cause irregular bleeding and unpredictable spotting for the first months of use.[8,12]

For patients interested in hormonal contraceptive methods, there is little research about whether testosterone contributes to or mitigates the known risks associated with hormonal contraception. The known risk profiles of progestin-only methods, such as the levonorgestrel IUD, DMPA, contraceptive implant, and progestin-only pills, make these reasonable options for TGD patients on

testosterone therapy.[6,13] Combined hormonal methods can also be used with testosterone. While no studies are available, there is a theoretical risk that estrogen can interfere with the clinical masculinizing effects of testosterone, and there are anecdotal reports of glandular breast tissue development in some individuals using contraceptive methods containing estrogen.[13] In addition, the three- to fivefold increase in the risk of venous thromboembolism associated with combined hormonal contraception may theoretically be higher with concurrent testosterone use.[14] Finally, some trans masculine people may wish to avoid estrogen because they perceive it to be gender discordant. Given the lack of data about potential risks, patients and clinicians may want to consider other forms of contraception until safety data are available for the use of combined hormonal methods with trans masculine people on testosterone therapy.[13]

▶ Patient Choice and Contraceptive Counseling

Choosing a specific method depends on multiple factors, including effectiveness, ease of use, invisibility to a partner, noncontraceptive effects (e.g., control of menses), and the presence of risk factors for a particular method.[15] When helping a patient choose a contraceptive method, these factors should be explored in a shared decision-making context that allows the patient to weigh each method's risks and benefits.[16] Patient preferences can be elicited with the question, "What is most important to you in a contraceptive method?" Depending on the patient's answer, a variety of methods should be presented to the patient. Health care professionals must be careful to avoid coercion and bias when counseling about contraception. Keeping some methods "off the table" because the clinician does not think they are appropriate for a patient is a form of contraceptive bias; similarly, encouraging a patient to use a method they do not want to use based on what the clinician thinks is best for that patient is also a form of bias and is coercive.[17]

▶ Use of the *U.S. Medical Eligibility Criteria for Contraceptive Use*

Many patients have risk factors that make some methods of contraception less desirable or even contraindicated due to the risk of serious complications. For example, use of combined contraceptives (those containing both estrogen and progesterone, such as the pill, patch, and ring) in patients with known genetic thrombogenic conditions (e.g., Factor V Leiden, prothrombin mutation, and protein S, C, and antithrombin deficiencies) increases the risk of thrombosis by 2- to 20-fold. The Centers for Disease Control and Prevention's *U.S. Medical Eligibility Criteria for Contraceptive Use* (CDC MEC)[18] provides comprehensive recommendations for using specific contraceptive methods by individuals with certain characteristics or medical conditions. The CDC uses a 4-point scale to categorize its recommendations by characteristic or risk factor for the various contraceptive methods:

1—No restriction (method can be used)

2—Advantages generally outweigh theoretical or proven risks

3—Theoretical or proven risks usually outweigh the advantages

4—Unacceptable health risk (method not to be used)

It is important to note that the CDC-MEC was developed based on studies of cisgender women and binary gender identities. And although the CDC MEC is intended to be used as guidance to aid the selection of a contraceptive method, health care professionals should also consider a patient's individual circumstances seeking contraception. The CDC MEC is available as a chart, wheel, and an app on the CDC website (https://www.cdc.gov/reproductivehealth/contraception/mmwr/mec/summary.html).

Emergency Contraception

Emergency contraception (EC) is indicated when sexual activity occurs without contraception or if a birth control method fails (e.g., condom breaks) and is not intended to be a regular method of contraception. EC is most effective in preventing unintended pregnancy when taken as soon as possible after condomless sex. EC does not cause abortion; rather, it prevents ovulation. All data about EC are based on studies of cisgender women; no studies are available about the use of EC in transgender men. The following methods of EC are available in the United States[14]:

- Copper IUD. Insertion of a copper IUD within 5 days of condomless sex is the most effective form of EC, reducing the risk of pregnancy following condomless intercourse by 99%.

- Emergency contraceptive pills. EC pills are taken up to 5 days after condomless sex. Three different types of pills are available, some of which are available over the counter:

  - Ulipristal acetate (UPA): This method is the most effective EC oral medication; it has been shown to reduce the risk of pregnancy by 62–85%.

  - Levonorgestrel: This EC method has been shown to reduce the risk of pregnancy by 52–100%.

  - Combined oral estrogen and levonorgestrel contraceptive pills (Yuzpe method): The Yuzpe method can be an effective alternative when combined hormonal contraceptives using 100 μg of ethinyl estradiol and 0.5 mg of LNG (or the equivalent) are available. Repeat dosing in 12 hours is required. It is the least effective EC method, reducing the risk of pregnancy by about 50%.

Abortion

TGD people who are assigned female sex at birth and capable of pregnancy may need abortion care. Despite this need, very little research has been published regarding how many TGD people seek abortion care, and little is known about their experiences of abortion care. One study estimated that there were between 462 and 530 TGD abortion patients in the United States in 2017, although this estimate is likely to be low.[19] Another survey of 450 TGD adults assigned female sex at birth found that 6% had an unplanned pregnancy, and of these, 32% had an abortion.[20] There are no data that describe the types of abortions (i.e., medical vs. surgical) that TGD individuals have had or the gestational ages at which the abortion was performed.[21]

Abortion care can be provided by hospitals and nonhospital clinic facilities. A study of nonhospital abortion facilities found that although many (85%) provide abortion services for TGD people, most of these facilities (73%) did not provide TGD-specific health care for patients.[22] These findings suggest that although abortion care is a necessary part of TGD health care, few facilities provide relevant gender-affirming and trauma-informed care.

Despite the lack of data surrounding abortion and TGD populations, some research has been performed in this area, and some key findings are beginning to emerge. A survey of 1694 TGD individuals assigned female sex or intersex at birth revealed the following information about abortion preferences[23]:

- 42% of participants stated their preference for a medication abortion rather than surgical (13%) or an unlisted method (2%) abortion.

- Reasons given for preferring a medical abortion were that it was the least invasive method; that it afforded the most privacy; and that it did not require anesthesia.

- Reasons given for preferring a surgical abortion were that it would be performed in the presence of medical personnel; it was the fastest method; and that it avoided the hormones necessary for a medical abortion.

- 30% of participants did not know which method they would prefer.

- Despite a strong preference for medical abortion, twice as many survey respondents who had abortions reported having a surgical abortion. The reasons for this preponderance do not appear to be due to gestational age limits, as most respondents reported obtaining an abortion before 10 weeks of pregnancy.

- Respondents who had abortions ($n = 67$) were asked to provide recommendations about the abortion care they received to improve the experience for TGD patients. Responses included:

  - Clinics should adopt intake forms that are gender-inclusive and gender-affirming of sexual orientation.

- Staff should use gender-inclusive language.
- Gender-affirming abortion care should be more accessible.

Future research is needed to explore these findings in more detail so that the preferences of TGD patients can be operationalized in facilities that provide abortion care.

REPRODUCTIVE HEALTH AND OPTIONS

The desire to become a parent is compelling for many people, regardless of sexual orientation or gender identity. Several studies have demonstrated that TGD people do desire parenthood, or at least wish to preserve that possibility.[24,25] Interestingly, more transgender women preferred to build families through adoption, while more transgender men desired biological offspring, and in fact would prefer to build families through sexual intercourse or by carrying a pregnancy.[26]

Many TGD people use **assisted reproductive technologies (ART)** to have genetically related children.[27] TGD individuals who want to have genetically related children may need to plan ahead, as some of the hormonal and surgical procedures employed in their gender affirmation may render them incapable of having genetically related children. Reproductive options for TGD people depend on where in the gender-affirming process they are and whether they are ready to have children immediately or are planning to have children in the future (Box 19-1). It is recommended that all TGD people receive counseling about reproductive options and the effects that GAHT and surgical procedures may have on future fertility prior to initiating such treatment.[28]

BOX 19-1   Reproductive Options

Reproductive Options for Transgender and Gender Diverse People Assigned Male Sex at Birth

Sperm cryopreservation for fertility preservation
Intrauterine insemination (IUI)
In vitro fertilization (IVF)
  Partner's oocytes and uterus
  Donor oocytes
  Gestational surrogacy

Reproductive Options for Transgender and Gender Diverse People Assigned Female Sex at Birth

Oocyte cryopreservation for fertility preservation
Intrauterine insemination (IUI)
  Partner's sperm or donor sperm
In vitro fertilization (IVF)
  Partner's sperm or donor sperm
  Gestational surrogacy

▶ Fertility Preservation

Fertility preservation is an option for TGD people who are not ready to have children prior to or at the time of their medical or surgical gender affirmation. While the ability to cryopreserve human sperm has been available for decades, effective and reliable cryopreservation of unfertilized human oocytes has only recently become available with the development of vitrification technology.[29] Fertilization and pregnancy rates are similar to in vitro fertilization (IVF) with fresh oocytes when previously vitrified oocytes from young women are used in IVF.[30] Although data are limited, no increase in chromosomal abnormalities, birth defects, and developmental deficits has been reported in the offspring born from vitrified oocytes compared to pregnancies from conventional IVF and the general population.[31,32] In 2013, the American Society for Reproductive Medicine (ASRM) stated that vitrification of mature oocytes should not be considered experimental.[33] Vitrification of mature oocytes is the technology currently being used for frozen donor egg banks, as well as for the purpose of fertility preservation in young women who have been diagnosed with cancer. This same technology is now being used for fertility preservation with trans masculine people.[34-37]

Sperm and oocyte cryopreservation can only be accomplished in people who are postpubertal, so this is not an option that may be offered to prepubertal children, or those who have had puberty intentionally suppressed with gonadotropin-releasing hormone (GnRH) agonists prior to GAHT. While cryopreservation of ovarian tissue or immature testicular tissue has been suggested and attempted,[38,39] these procedures are considered experimental because successful birth outcomes from cryopreservation of ovarian or immature testicular tissue have not been demonstrated.

Fertility Preservation for Transgender and Gender Diverse People Assigned Female Sex at Birth

TGD AFAB people who have mature functional ovaries may cryopreserve their oocytes for potential use in the future.[35-37] Ideally, cryopreservation should be done prior to the initiation of testosterone therapy. However, TGD AFAB people who have initiated testosterone therapy may also undergo oocyte cryopreservation.[35] Historically, these patients have been instructed to discontinue testosterone therapy temporarily in order to undergo the oocyte cryopreservation process, after which they would then resume testosterone therapy. Recently, there has been some discussion regarding the possibility of proceeding with the oocyte cryopreservation process in TGD AFAB people without discontinuation of testosterone therapy. The rationale for this approach is based on experience with use of androgens in IVF protocols for infertility patients who respond poorly to gonadotropin stimulation. Low doses of testosterone added to ovarian stimulation protocols have the theoretical benefit of increasing levels of ovarian follicle-stimulating hormone (FSH) receptors. Because androgens are substrates in estradiol biosynthesis, estradiol production may be higher when androgens are added to the ovarian stimulation protocol, and some studies have reported an increase in the mean number of oocytes retrieved.[40] However, the continuation of testosterone therapy during the oocyte cryopreservation process in TGD AFAB people is experimental, as it is unclear what impact, if any, exposure to supraphysiological levels of testosterone may have on developing oocytes and resultant offspring conceived from these oocytes.

The process for oocyte cryopreservation is identical to the process that cisgender women undergo during IVF for treatment of infertility. The process requires controlled ovarian stimulation with daily gonadotropin injections for an average of 10–12 days. Monitoring of ovarian follicular development is done with periodic **frontal canal** ultrasound and measurements of blood estradiol levels until it is determined that the ovarian follicles are mature and the oocytes are ready for harvesting. Oocyte retrieval is performed under anesthesia. More than one oocyte cryopreservation cycle may be done, depending on how many oocytes are desired to be banked.

Fertility Preservation for Transgender and Gender Diverse People Assigned Male Sex at Birth

TGD AMAB people who have mature functional testicles may cryopreserve their sperm for potential future use. Because estrogen suppresses spermatogenesis, sperm cryopreservation should be done prior to initiation of estrogen therapy, although some experts contend that it can be done after discontinuation of estrogen for an indeterminate amount of time until spermatogenesis returns to normal levels.[41] However, before initiating such therapy, patients should be informed that the suppressive effects of estrogen therapy on spermatogenesis may not be reversible. Banking of sperm can be done conveniently at any commercial sperm bank. Banking of multiple specimens is recommended.

▶ Assisted Reproductive Technologies

Multiple **assisted reproductive technologies (ART)** have been progressively developed since the late 1970s. Although these technologies were originally developed to treat people with infertility, all of these technologies may also be used by TGD people who wish to have genetically related children.

Intrauterine Insemination (IUI)

Sperm that has been specially prepared to remove seminal fluid is injected into the uterine cavity. Sperm that has been freshly ejaculated or sperm that has previously been frozen and thawed may be used. The insemination procedure is done on the day of ovulation. The appropriate day for IUI may be determined using urinary ovulation predictor kits or by testing the blood for the luteinizing hormone (LH) surge. In patients with ovulatory dysfunction or anovulation, induction of ovulation may be achieved using clomiphene citrate, letrozole, or injectable gonadotropins.

In Vitro Fertilization (IVF)

Oocytes are retrieved from the ovaries and inseminated with sperm outside the body in a petri dish. Following ovarian stimulation with gonadotropins for an average of 10–12 days, the oocyte retrieval procedure is performed under anesthesia. IVF may be done with either freshly retrieved oocytes or oocytes that have previously been cryopreserved and thawed. Sperm used for IVF may either be from a freshly ejaculated semen specimen or sperm that has previously been cryopreserved and thawed. Conventional insemination involves overnight incubation of oocytes and sperm in a microdrop of culture medium in a petri dish in a highly specialized incubator, after which the oocytes are then inspected to determine whether fertilization has occurred. An alternative method of insemination is intracytoplasmic sperm injection (ICSI), a procedure whereby a single sperm is injected into each oocyte using a microscopic needle under microscopic guidance by a specially trained and highly skilled embryologist. ICSI is typically used in situations where there is poor semen quality or a history of low or no fertilization with regular insemination in a prior IVF cycle. ICSI is also recommended when inseminating previously vitrified oocytes.

Oocytes that appear to be normally fertilized are incubated in a culture medium for another 4–5 days until they reach the blastocyst stage. Blastocysts may either be transferred to the uterus or cryopreserved for future transfer. In the past, two to three blastocysts were transferred to the uterus, which often resulted in a high rate of multiple pregnancies and carries significant risk to both the gestating parent and fetuses. Currently, the ASRM recommends single-embryo transfer for the majority of patients because of its enhanced rate of success and reduced risk of morbidity and mortality.[42]

The source of oocytes for IVF may be either from intended parents or egg donors. Similarly, the source of sperm for IVF may be either from intended parents or sperm donors. Embryo transfer may be either to the uterus of the intended parent or the uterus of a designated **gestational surrogate**.

Donor Sperm

Donors who donate sperm to a commercial sperm bank have been tested for a standard list of infectious diseases mandated by the Food and Drug Administration (FDA), which has published regulations regarding donation of human tissues.[43] These regulations mandate testing of all donors for infectious diseases that may potentially be transmitted in semen prior to collecting semen specimens intended for donation. Sperm specimens are frozen and quarantined for 6 months, after which the donor is retested for infectious diseases. If the repeat test results are negative, the quarantined frozen sperm specimens may then be released by the sperm bank for donation. If any test for infectious diseases is positive, the quarantined sperm specimens cannot be donated and must be discarded.

Some patients may choose to use sperm from a known (or directed) donor, typically a friend or acquaintance. Family building with sperm from a known donor has significant psychosocial and legal ramifications; therefore, psychosocial and legal counseling, as well as legal contracts, is strongly recommended. The counseling and legal contracts address the questions of who owns the donor sperm specimens and controls their use, parental rights and obligations of the intended parent(s), as well as the lack of parental rights and obligations of the donor. If a patient wishes to use sperm from a known donor, the most efficient process is for the desired donor to bank sperm at a commercial sperm bank and specifically designate the banked sperm specimens for use by the recipient. There are FDA regulations specifically governing the use of sperm from a known/directed donor if a clinician is performing the insemination in a medical facility.[43] If any test result for infectious diseases is positive, the recipient must be counseled regarding the potential risk of infection. If they knowingly choose to use the potentially infectious frozen donor sperm specimens for insemination, they must sign a waiver acknowledging that they have been counseled regarding the risks.

Donor Eggs

Donors recruited by egg donor agencies are typically healthy young people who are ideally between the ages of 21 and 29 years. However, known egg donors, typically a friend or acquaintance of the intended parent(s), may be in their mid- to late 30s and may be acceptable as egg donors if they are healthy and have good ovarian reserve.

Donors recruited and matched through an egg donor agency are compensated for their time, effort, inconvenience, time off from work, and pain of undergoing a surgical egg retrieval procedure under anesthesia. Donors are compensated with a fixed agreed-upon amount per donation cycle, regardless of the number of oocytes retrieved. A legal contract is mandatory between the egg donor and the intended parents, who must be represented by separate attorneys.

IVF cycles using donor eggs may be synchronized with the person who is carrying the pregnancy to ensure that a fresh embryo is transferred, and any untransferred embryos are cryopreserved for potential future use. More recently, the ability to cryopreserve unfertilized human oocytes successfully has resulted in the development of frozen donor egg banks, which have become an alternative source of donor

oocytes. Following extensive evaluation, donors to frozen donor egg banks undergo gonadotropin stimulation oocyte retrieval via the frontal canal. The resulting mature oocytes are then cryopreserved. Donors' detailed profiles are posted on the website of the frozen donor egg bank. Intended parents may choose to use frozen donor eggs instead of searching for a donor through an egg donor agency. The cost of using frozen donor oocytes is significantly lower than that of using donor oocytes from a donor recruited and matched through an egg donor agency. However, the major advantage of a fresh donor egg cycle is the higher probability of having excess untransferred embryos cryopreserved for potential future use. Frozen donor egg cycles are typically allotted six to eight eggs per treatment cycle, whereas with fresh donor egg cycles, the intended parents receive all of the oocytes retrieved from their designated donor.

Gestational Surrogacy

A gestational surrogate (or gestational carrier) may be a family member or friend, or a person recruited and matched through a surrogacy agency. Psychosocial and legal counseling for all parties and a legal contract between the surrogate and intended parents are necessary. Legal counseling should be provided by an attorney (or law firm), preferably one that specializes in reproductive law (see discussion of legal requirements later in this chapter).

Once the prospective surrogate has been selected, they undergo extensive evaluation, including psychological testing, medical testing, and screening for infectious diseases. After a comprehensive evaluation, the surrogate's menstrual cycle is synchronized with that of the intended parent or oocyte donor using medications. On rare occasions, due to unanticipated events, synchronization is unachievable, in which case all the embryos created are cryopreserved for a frozen embryo transfer. Synchronization is unnecessary if frozen donor oocytes are used or if all embryos created are intentionally cryopreserved for a tandem frozen embryo transfer. However, in either case, estradiol and progesterone hormones are used to prepare the surrogate's endometrium for implantation when the embryo is ready for transfer.

Recently, the option to screen embryos using preimplantation genetic testing for aneuploidy (PGT-A) has become available. Many intended parents choose PGT-A, after which the embryos are cryopreserved for future frozen embryo transfer to their gestational surrogate. This strategy results in more efficient utilization of their gestational surrogate's time and decreases the risk of a negative pregnancy test or spontaneous abortion due to aneuploidy of the embryo or the unfortunate situation of pregnancy with an aneuploid fetus.

▶ Reproductive Options

Any of the above elements of ART may be adapted for use by TGD people to have genetically related children. Specialists who assist people in becoming parents include general obstetrician-gynecologists as well as reproductive endocrinologists, who are obstetrician-gynecologists with specialty training in fertility and reproductive technologies.

Reproductive Options for Transgender and Gender Diverse People Assigned Female Sex at Birth

TGD AFAB people who have had the opportunity to cryopreserve oocytes may use their cryopreserved oocytes to have children when they are ready to do so. Their cryopreserved oocytes may be thawed for IVF. Intracytoplasmic sperm injection (ICSI) is strongly recommended when previously vitrified oocytes are being used for IVF, as the fertilization rate with regular conventional microdrop insemination may be very low. The source of sperm depends on personal preferences and reproductive capabilities:

- If a TGD AFAB person is in a relationship with someone who has functioning testicles and can provide sperm, they may use their partner's sperm to inseminate their oocytes in an IVF cycle. The TGD AFAB person may choose to carry the pregnancy or use a gestational surrogate to carry their pregnancy.

- If a TGD AFAB person is in a relationship with someone who has a functioning uterus, they may use donor sperm to inseminate their oocytes in an IVF cycle, and their partner may gestate the pregnancy.

If a trans masculine AFAB person has not had surgery to remove their ovaries and/or uterus and has not cryopreserved their oocytes, they may choose to discontinue testosterone therapy to have a child. There are several possible choices about the method by which pregnancy can be achieved in this scenario[7]:

- If a TGD AFAB person is in a relationship with a partner who has functioning testicles and can provide sperm, they may use their partner's sperm to have children. If a TGD AFAB person is in a relationship with someone who does not have functioning testicles, or if they are single, they may use donor sperm for IUI or IVF.

- If a TGD AFAB person chooses to carry the pregnancy, they may become pregnant by having sex with their partner who has functioning testicles.

- If infertility or other factors are present that prevent spontaneous pregnancy with sexual activity, IUI or IVF may be used. With IVF, the TGD AFAB person may choose to carry the pregnancy themselves if they wish, or the embryos resulting from their IVF treatment may be transferred into the uterus of another person to gestate the pregnancy, such as a gestational surrogate.

TGD AFAB people who intend to gestate the pregnancy themselves should discontinue testosterone therapy to avoid exposure of the fetus to testosterone in utero. In other animal species, testosterone exposure in utero during early pregnancy causes changes in the development of sexual organs in fetuses, as well as differences in play and sexual response behavior. In other animal species, there may also be effects on fetal growth and litter size[44,45]; it is unknown whether similar consequences may occur in humans. It is important to recognize that stopping testosterone may cause or exacerbate gender dysphoria among TGD AFAB people, and anticipatory guidance about the psychological impact of testosterone cessation should be provided.[7,46] Psychosocial support should be available to these patients if they experience gender dysphoria.

Reproductive Options for Transgender and Gender Diverse People Assigned Male Sex at Birth

TGD AMAB people who have cryopreserved sperm may return to use their frozen sperm to have children when they are ready to do so. The source of oocytes and the person who carries the pregnancy also depend on the relationship status of the TGD AMAB person at the time they decide to use their cryopreserved sperm. If the TGD AMAB person is in a relationship with a person who has functional ovaries and uterus, previously cryopreserved sperm may be thawed for either IUI or IVF, depending on the quantity of cryopreserved sperm available. If the TGD AMAB person is in a relationship with a person who does not have functional ovaries and uterus, previously cryopreserved sperm may be thawed for IVF using donor oocytes, and the resulting embryos transferred into a gestational surrogate.

TGD AMAB people who have not cryopreserved sperm may or may not be able to have genetically related children, depending on whether they have undergone any gender-affirming surgical procedures that would render them infertile (such as bilateral orchiectomy). Even if they have retained one or both testicles, estrogen therapy suppresses spermatogenesis to the point of azoospermia (total absence of sperm in the ejaculate) or severe oligozoospermia (presence of very few sperm in the ejaculate). Spermatogenesis may not resume after estrogen therapy is discontinued. To date, there are no published studies evaluating recovery of spermatogenesis among TGD AMAB people after discontinuation of estrogen therapy. Even if spermatogenesis resumes following discontinuation of estrogen therapy, the sperm numbers may be extremely low, eliminating IUI as a treatment option. Instead, IVF would need to be performed with ICSI.

▶ Prepregnancy Counseling

Prepregnancy counseling should be provided for anyone planning to become pregnant, including TGD people. The goal of prepregnancy counseling is to decrease the risk of adverse outcomes for the pregnant person, fetus, and newborn by optimizing health before pregnancy, identifying and addressing modifiable risk factors, and educating about diet, exercise, substance use, and other elements of a healthy pregnancy. Components of prepregnancy counseling should include the following[47]:

- Health history including current medications, use of alcohol and tobacco, and use of nonprescribed drugs
- Immunization status
- Identification of any underlying health conditions, including diabetes, hypertension, and mental illness, which may affect pregnancy outcomes, and planning of interventions to manage these conditions before pregnancy
- Education about genetic testing and screening, including prepregnancy carrier screening, along with a discussion about the risks and benefits of each option and the implications of positive and negative testing results
- Assessment of risk factors for sexually transmitted infections to determine the need for screening prior to pregnancy
- Discussion about the benefits of starting folic acid supplementation before pregnancy to reduce the risk of neural tube defects
- Screening for intimate partner violence
- Screening for depression
- Anticipatory guidance about the physical and psychological effects of testosterone cessation

▶ Obstetric Care

Routine prenatal care has been shown to decrease morbidity and mortality for both the pregnant individual and the neonate. Specific aspects of care should include anticipated physical changes of pregnancy, standard antepartum testing, childbirth and parenting education and peer support options, and discussion about the modes of delivery, infant-feeding choices, and newborn care. Contraceptive counseling, if applicable, should also be offered during pregnancy.[48]

TGD AFAB people may experience a range of emotional and physical changes during pregnancy. Despite the acceptance of pregnancy as a necessary step in building a family, many TGD AFAB people who become pregnant report feelings of loneliness and isolation.[7,49] Supportive resources aimed at this pregnant population are scarce or nonexistent. Pregnancy can also cause or increase the intensity of gender dysphoria, particularly as the pregnancy progresses and becomes more physically obvious (Light).[7] Some TGD AFAB people do not experience gender dysphoria as a result of body changes caused by pregnancy but do experience distress when others misgender them due to pregnancy changes, particularly due to the growth of breast tissue, which can occur even in people who have had top surgery that does not include removal of the mammary glands.[50]

The mode of delivery for childbirth may also trigger dysphoria stemming from a patient's concerns about the birth process. Some people prefer to deliver their baby through the frontal canal, while others prefer a cesarean delivery. More research is needed in this area to determine best practices about the mode of delivery for this patient population (Ellis). Current recommendations surrounding elective cesarean delivery (defined as a cesarean delivery in the absence of a medical indication) include discussion and consideration of the patient's specific risk factors, such as age, BMI, and general health, that may impact the patient's risk of developing complications as well as the reasons for requesting the cesarean delivery. Patients should be counseled that multiple cesarean deliveries are associated with an increased risk of complications in later pregnancies, including placenta accrete spectrum and placenta previa. If a patient elects cesarean delivery, the American College of Obstetricians and Gynecologists states that delivery should not be performed before 39 weeks of gestation.[51]

Gender-affirming care may help minimize these feelings of isolation in TGD AFAB people, demonstrate support and encouragement from the health care system, and mitigate discrimination and bias. Gender-affirming care includes inquiring about and using a patient's affirmed name and pronouns; using gender-inclusive language, such as "carrier," "father," and "gestational parent" in accordance with the birthing parent's wishes; and educating office staff, nurses, and other health care workers in principles of gender-affirming care.[48] More information about gender-affirming care can be found in Chapter 11, "Basic Principles of Trauma-Informed and Gender-Affirming Care."

▶ Postpartum Care

Many aspects of postpartum care will be the same as the care offered to cisgender women. However, some postpartum care principles should be modified to meet the unique needs and concerns of TGD people, such as lactation and infant-feeding choices, resumption of gender-affirming hormone therapy, postpartum contraception and counseling, and postpartum depression.

Education about Postdelivery Warning Signs

Postpartum people are at increased risk for several complications, such as postpartum hemorrhage, deep vein thrombosis and pulmonary embolism, postpartum depression, preeclampsia, and infection. Almost one in three cases of preeclampsia occur after childbirth, and of these late-onset cases, most occur within 7 days of delivery, although it can occur up to 6 weeks later.[52] All individuals should be counseled about postpartum warning signs prior to discharge from the hospital and instructed to go to the emergency room if they experience any of the following:[53]

- Headache that persists or worsens over time
- Dizziness or fainting
- Thoughts about hurting oneself or the baby

- Fever
- Trouble breathing
- Chest pain or fast heartbeat
- Persistent, severe abdominal pain
- Severe nausea
- Swelling, redness, or pain in the leg
- Extreme swelling of the face or hands
- Severe vaginal bleeding or fluid leakage
- Overwhelming fatigue

▶ Lactation and Breast/Chestfeeding

Human milk provides optimal nutrition for infants as well as protective antibodies that help protect against certain health conditions. Current guidelines from the American Academy of Pediatrics recommend exclusive breast/chest-feeding for the first 6 months of life followed by continued breast/chestfeeding while introducing food until the child is 1 year old.[54,1] Most TGD people are physiologically able to breast/chestfeed. TGD AFAB people who have had mammary gland-sparing top surgery are still capable of milk production and may be able to pump their milk or feed their infants from the chest.[55] TGD AMAB people may be able to induce lactation with hormones and preparation of the chest with pumping and massage. A reproductive endocrinologist or board-certified lactation consultant can provide expert guidance about achieving lactation in a nongestational parent.[56] Another option is to use a nursing supplementer, a device that delivers milk from a bottle through tubing that loops around a parent's neck; the opening of the tube can be placed at or near a parent's nipple so that the infant can feed. A supplementer may be used to help stimulate milk production or can be used to exclusively breast/chestfeed.[57]

Not all parents wish to feed their infants from the breast/chest, and this decision should be supported. TGD AFAB people who affirm their gender identity with GAHT may avoid testosterone while breastfeeding/chestfeeding in order to ensure a steady milk supply; however, this can cause a decrease in masculine **secondary sex characteristics** and a concomitant increase in feminine secondary sex characteristics. The growth of breast tissue during pregnancy and the activity of breastfeeding/chestfeeding can feel misaligned with a TGD AFAB person's gender identity. All of these effects may lead to or intensify gender dysphoria. Those who do not wish to breastfeed/chestfeed can suppress lactation with medication or by natural means and bottlefeed their infants with donor milk or formula.

---

[1]Some TGD community members use the terms *breast* and *breast-feeding*, while some use the terms *chest* and *chestfeeding*. It is important to first ask each patient how they refer to their body parts and to reflect their own language back with them.

Postpartum Contraception Counseling and Gender-Affirming Hormone Therapy

TGD AFAB people wishing to resume testosterone therapy may believe that they do not need to use postpartum contraception. However, testosterone therapy does not provide complete protection against pregnancy. Postpartum contraception will ensure adequate pregnancy spacing and family planning.[58] Although data about the optimal time to restart testosterone therapy are limited, some studies suggest that restarting testosterone 4–6 weeks following delivery is appropriate. This is the same timeframe that is recommended for restarting hormonal contraception.[46]

▶ Postpartum Depression

Postpartum depression is a common complication following childbirth, affecting approximately one in eight cisgender women. It is characterized by intense feelings of sadness and hopelessness that can last for months or even years. Postpartum depression can interfere with bonding and may cause problems with sleeping, eating, and behavior for the infant. Although research is lacking, TGD AFAB people may be at higher risk for postpartum depression than cisgender women due to increased gender dysphoria that may result from the misgendering experiences of pregnancy and childbirth. All individuals should be screened for postpartum depression during the postpartum period and treatment initiated for those who screen positive.[59] Treatment includes counseling for mild to moderate depression and a combination of counseling and antidepressant medications for moderate to severe depression. Although all antidepressant medications pass into the parent's milk, those recommended as first-line agents for postpartum depression—citalopram, nortriptyline, sertraline, and paroxetine—have the lowest rates of transmission and are associated with low-to-undetectable concentrations in the parent's milk.[60,61] Additional or non-SSRI/SNRI medications can be used in consultation with behavioral health and pediatric input.

LEGAL CONSIDERATIONS

There are several legal considerations for TGD people and their clinicians to consider when building a family. It should be noted that this area of law is regularly expanding and changing. TGD people and their clinicians should consult with an attorney in their state to determine the status of policy or ahead of signing any agreements.

▶ Insurance Coverage of Fertility Preservation Procedures

Predictably, insurance coverage for TGD health care varies widely across providers and geography.[62] Fertility preservation procedures, while widely available, are costly and not often covered by insurance.[63] Currently, ten states have passed laws compelling insurers to cover fertility preservation procedures where iatrogenic infertility is likely (CA, CO, CT, DE, IL, MD, NH, NJ, NY, RI).[64] Other states are actively pursuing legislation on the matter. However, it is unclear if these laws can or will apply to TGD people, as the definitions of "infertility" are largely heteronormative and cis-normative in their language. Future litigation and/or advocacy will likely see progress made through the legal system, as courts weigh in on the definitions of "interfertility," "medically necessary," and other terms often utilized in fertility preservation legislation.

▶ Adoption, Foster Care, and Adoption/Parentage Judgments

Much like fertility preservation laws, states vary widely in the legal rights provided to TGD people seeking to adopt or foster children. Currently, 25 states prohibit discrimination based on gender identity in adoption or foster care. Conversely, 11 states permit state-licensed child welfare agencies to refuse placement with LGBTQIA+ people (which includes the TGD population) if doing so conflicts with their "religious beliefs."[65]

Prospective parents have several options when adopting: public agency adoption, private agency adoption, open independent adoption, or international adoption. Each of these options has unique processes that vary based on the state or country the parents are adopting from. Like states, some countries may prohibit or allow discrimination against a prospective TGD parent based on gender identity.

Adoption and/or parentage judgments are important documents that protect the rights of TGD parents facing immediate or future legal challenges. Adoption judgments create the legal relationship between the child and parent(s), and are commonly sought when an individual is adopting a child that is legally related to their spouse, or where a child is adopted by a biologically unrelated individual. A parentage judgment is a court order recognizing the parental rights of an individual not listed on a child's birth certificate or who may not be otherwise acknowledged as a legal parent through marriage. These judgments can protect a TGD parent from future disagreements when traveling to states that may not recognize their legal relationship to a child or in the face of other challenges to their parenting status.

▶ Gestational Surrogacy

As with previously discussed legal matters, statutes and case law pertaining to surrogacy vary across state lines. In some states, gestational surrogacy is not permitted or heavily restricted, while in others, legal considerations have been weighed to protect the rights of both the intended parents and the surrogate. At the time of writing, compensated surrogacy is prohibited under state statute or case law in Louisiana,[2] Michigan,[3] Nebraska,[4] and New York (until 2/15/2021).[5] In Arizona and Indiana, surrogacy is permitted, but surrogacy contracts are void and unenforceable.[66,67]

The gestational carrier contract defines the rights of and duties of the parties involved in a gestational surrogacy. This agreement is between the intended parents and the gestational carrier (and the carrier's spouse, if the carrier is married). It outlines the rights, duties, and expectations of the involved parties. As with any contract, attorneys for all parties should participate in its drafting and negotiation. A gestational carrier contract should lay out details relevant to have control over medical decisions, location for delivery, insurance considerations, payment of medical bills, and compensation (if relevant and/or permitted under state law).

▶ Birth Certificates

Accurate and affirming recognition of a parent on a child's birth certificate can be a unique challenge for TGD parents. Whether a person is a gestational parent, adopted parent, or parent via surrogacy can change how a state might recognize them on a birth certificate. Additionally, making amendments or alterations to a birth certificate after birth can be challenging or altogether impossible depending on state policy.

To change or amend a child's birth certificate, a parent should contact their state or local vital records office to determine the requirements. Some states may require a motion through a local probate court to allow changes to a child's birth certificate. Some states may require documentation from a physician to affirm a petitioner's gender identity. In January 2020, a transgender couple in Chicago had to petition the Illinois Department of Public Health to be listed correctly on their child's birth certificate.[68] According to state officials, this was "the first time" the state had been informed or petitioned for such a request. Other states, such as Idaho[69] and Tennessee,[70] make it illegal to alter a birth certificate for TGD people, presumptively both in cases of a TGD child or TGD parents, though changing a parent's information has not been litigated.

---

[2]Louisiana Bill 1102 (2016) restricts gestational surrogacy to heterosexual married couples (unclear if or how gender identity may complicate the reading of this law). The law also requires the intended parents use their own gametes and forbids compensation.
[3]Michigan Surrogate Parenting Act MCL Section 722.851: " A surrogate parentage contract is void and unenforceable as contrary to public policy."
[4]R.R.S. Neb. 25-21, 200 (2007): "A surrogate parenthood contract entered into shall be void and unenforceable."
[5]Domestic Relations Laws § 122, The Child Parent Security Act "CPSA" signed April 3, 2020, goes into effect February 15, 2021. This legislation permits gestational surrogacy and lays out a Surrogates' Bill of Rights.

Parentage Fitness Challenges

The majority of policy pertaining to this topic comes from case law, and decisions vary widely by state. Where a TGD person is a party in a custody dispute, there may be attempts to use their gender identity as a basis to limit or deny custody or visitation to the children in question. Courts generally evaluate what is in the "best interest of the child" in these cases and take into account elements such as the relationship between the child and TGD parent, the willingness of one parent to support a relationship with the other parent, the stability of the child's homelife, and the ability of the parent in question to provide for the child's overall well-being. If a child is deemed mature enough, the court will also consider the desires of the child.

If the fitness of a TGD parent is challenged in a custody disagreement, the testimony of expert witnesses, such as doctors, psychologists, or guardians *ad litem*, can be crucial in helping the court understand the circumstances and determine what is in the best interest of the child. Courts that were provided expert testimony in these cases were more likely to clarify that a parent's gender identity, expression, or affirmation should not be a factor when analyzing what is in the best interest of the child.[71]

SUMMARY

- Many TGD people report barriers to accessing reproductive health care services while acknowledging their need for such health care and their interest in addressing reproductive health concerns.

- Barriers to reproductive care include social and economic discrimination and stigma, lack of education and acceptance among health care providers professionals, and failure of health insurance to cover needed services.

- Best practices include obtaining an inclusive sexual and social history, conducting an **anatomical inventory**, discussing future reproductive plans and options, and providing appropriate counseling and preventive health services.

- Contraception counseling should be offered to all TGD people of reproductive age who are sexually active and do not wish to achieve pregnancy or make someone else pregnant.

- As many TGD people desire future parenthood, fertility preservation, reproductive options, and alternative parenting methods should be discussed routinely.

CASE STUDIES

Case Study 1: Shannon

Shannon is a 23-year-old trans man who initiated GAHT approximately one year ago. Currently he is having casual frontal sex with both cisgender men and trans feminine people.

1. What counseling would you provide regarding contraception?

2. What counseling would you provide regarding fertility preservation?

3. If Shannon wants to become pregnant in the future, what are his options?

Case Study 2: Ronelle

Ronelle is a 32-year-old trans feminine person who has been in a long-term relationship with a primary partner who is a cisgender woman. The couple has an open relationship; Ronelle enjoys oral and penis-in-vagina sex with her primary partner and occasionally has receptive anal sex with cisgender men. She and her primary partner want to have genetically related children together in a few years. Ronelle is eager to initiate GAHT but wants to make sure that she preserves her fertility options.

1. What counseling would you provide regarding contraception?

2. What counseling would you provide regarding fertility preservation?

3. What reproductive options can Ronelle and her primary partner pursue when they are ready to try to achieve pregnancy?

REFERENCES

1. World Health Organization. Reproductive Health. https://www.who.int/westernpacific/health-topics/reproductive-health. Accessed November 10, 2020.
2. ACOG Committee Opinion No. 762: Prepregnancy counseling. *Obstet Gynecol*. 2019;133(1):e78-e89.
3. American College of Obstetricians and Gynecologists. ACOG Committee Opinion No. 512: health care for transgender individuals. *Obstet Gynecol*. 2011;118:1454-1458.
4. Wingo E, Ingraham N, Roberts SCM. Reproductive health care priorities and barriers to effective care for LGBTQ people assigned female at birth: a qualitative study. *Womens Health Issues*. 2018;28(4):350-357.
5. Cipres D, Seidman D, Cloniger C 3rd, Nova C, O'Shea A, Obedin-Maliver J. Contraceptive use and pregnancy intentions among transgender men presenting to a clinic for sex workers and their families in San Francisco. *Contraception*. 2017;95(2):186-189.
6. Krempasky C, Harris M, Abern L, Grimstad F. Contraception across the transmasculine spectrum. *Am J Obstet Gynecol*. 2020;222(2):134-143.
7. Light AD, Obedin-Maliver J, Sevelius JM, Kerns JL. Transgender men who experienced pregnancy after female-to-male gender transitioning. *Obstet Gynecol*. 2014;124(6):1120-1127.
8. Beckwith N, Reisner SL, Zaslow S, Mayer KH, Keuroghlian AS. Factors associated with gender-affirming surgery and

age of hormone therapy initiation among transgender adults. *Transgend Health.* 2017;2(1):156-164.

9. Irwig MS. Testosterone therapy for transgender men. *Lancet Diabetes Endocrinol.* 2017;5(4):301-311.

10. Bonnington A, Dianat S, Kerns J, et al. Society of Family Planning clinical recommendations: contraceptive counseling for transgender and gender diverse people who were female sex assigned at birth. *Contraception.* 2020;102(2):70-82.

11. Daniels K, Abma JC. *Current Contraceptive Status among Women Aged 15-49.* Hyattsville, MD: National Center for Health Statistics; 2018.

12. American College of Obstetricians and Gynecologists. ACOG Practice Bulletin No. 110: noncontraceptive uses of hormonal contraceptives. *Obstet Gynecol.* 2010;115(1):206-218.

13. Boudreau D, Mukerjee R. Contraception care for transmasculine individuals on testosterone therapy. *J Midwifery Womens Health.* 2019;64(4):395-402.

14. Hatcher R, Nelson A, Trussell J, et al. *Contraceptive Technology.* 21 ed. New York, NY: Ayer Publishers, Inc.; 2018.

15. Dehlendorf C, Diedrich J, Drey E, Postone A, Steinauer J. Preferences for decision-making about contraception and general health care among reproductive age women at an abortion clinic. *Patient Educ Couns.* 2010;81(3):343-348.

16. Dehlendorf C, Grumbach K, Schmittdiel JA, Steinauer J. Shared decision making in contraceptive counseling. *Contraception.* 2017;95(5):452-455.

17. Elwyn G, Frosch D, Thomson R, et al. Shared decision making: a model for clinical practice. *J Gen Intern Med.* 2012;27(10):1361-1367.

18. U S. Medical Eligibility Criteria for Contraceptive Use, 2010. *MMWR Recomm Rep.* 2010;59(Rr-4):1-86.

19. Jones RK, Jerman J. Abortion incidence and service availability in the United States, 2014. *Perspect Sex Reprod Health.* 2017;49(1):17-27.

20. Light A, Wang LF, Zeymo A, Gomez-Lobo V. Family planning and contraception use in transgender men. *Contraception.* 2018;98(4):266-269.

21. Moseson H, Zazanis N, Goldberg E, et al. The imperative for transgender and gender nonbinary inclusion: beyond women's health. *Obstet Gynecol.* 2020;135(5):1059-1068.

22. Jones RK, Witwer E, Jerman J. Transgender abortion patients and the provision of transgender-specific care at non-hospital facilities that provide abortions. *Contracept X.* 2020;2:100019.

23. Moseson H, Fix L, Ragosta S, et al. Abortion experiences and preferences of transgender, nonbinary, and gender-expansive people in the United States. *Am J Obstet Gynecol.* 2020.

24. Wierckx K, Van Caenegem E, Pennings G, et al. Reproductive wish in transsexual men. *Hum Reprod.* 2012;27(2):483-487.

25. Auer MK, Fuss J, Nieder TO, et al. Desire to have children among transgender people in Germany: a cross-sectional multi-center study. *J Sex Med.* 2018;15(5):757-767.

26. Tornello SL, Bos H. Parenting intentions among transgender individuals. *LGBT Health.* 2017;4(2):115-120.

27. James-Abra S, Tarasoff LA, Green D, et al. Trans people's experiences with assisted reproduction services: a qualitative study. *Hum Reprod.* 2015;30(6):1365-1374.

28. Amato P. Fertility options for transgender people. Guidelines for the Primary and Gender-Affirming Care of Transgender and Gender Nonbinary People Web site. https://transcare.ucsf.edu/guidelines. Published 2016. Accessed November 22, 2020.

29. Smith GD, Serafini PC, Fioravanti J, et al. Prospective randomized comparison of human oocyte cryopreservation with slow-rate freezing or vitrification. *Fertil Steril.* 2010;94(6):2088-2095.

30. Cobo A, Kuwayama M, Perez S, Ruiz A, Pellicer A, Remohi J. Comparison of concomitant outcome achieved with fresh and cryopreserved donor oocytes vitrified by the Cryotop method. *Fertil Steril.* 2008;89(6):1657-1664.

31. Cobo A, Rubio C, Gerli S, Ruiz A, Pellicer A, Remohí J. Use of fluorescence in situ hybridization to assess the chromosomal status of embryos obtained from cryopreserved oocytes. *Fertil Steril.* 2001;75(2):354-360.

32. Noyes N, Porcu E, Borini A. Over 900 oocyte cryopreservation babies born with no apparent increase in congenital anomalies. *Reprod Biomed Online.* 2009;18(6):769-776.

33. American Society for Reproductive Medicine and the Society for Assisted Reproductive Technology. Mature oocyte cryopreservation: a guideline. *Fertil Steril.* 2013;99(1):37-43.

34. De Roo C, Tilleman K, T'Sjoen G, De Sutter P. Fertility options in transgender people. *Int Rev Psychiatry.* 2016;28(1):112-119.

35. Leung A, Sakkas D, Pang S, Thornton K, Resetkova N. Assisted reproductive technology outcomes in female-to-male transgender patients compared with cisgender patients: a new frontier in reproductive medicine. *Fertil Steril.* 2019;112(5):858-865.

36. Maxwell S, Noyes N, Keefe D, Berkeley AS, Goldman KN. Pregnancy outcomes after fertility preservation in transgender men. *Obstet Gynecol.* 2017;129(6):1031-1034.

37. Wallace SA, Blough KL, Kondapalli LA. Fertility preservation in the transgender patient: expanding oncofertility care beyond cancer. *Gynecol Endocrinol.* 2014;30(12):868-871.

38. Onofre J, Baert Y, Faes K, Goossens E. Cryopreservation of testicular tissue or testicular cell suspensions: a pivotal step in fertility preservation. *Hum Reprod Update.* 2016;22(6):744-761.

39. Vuković P, Kasum M, Orešković D, et al. Importance of ovarian tissue cryopreservation in fertility preservation and anti-aging treatment. *Gynecol Endocrinol.* 2019;35(11):919-923.

40. Saharkhiz N, Zademodares S, Salehpour S, Hosseini S, Nazari L, Tehrani HG. The effect of testosterone gel on fertility outcomes in women with a poor response in vitro fertilization cycles: a pilot randomized clinical trial. *J Res Med Sci.* 2018;23:3.

41. Liu W, Schulster ML, Alukal JP, Najari BB. Fertility preservation in male to female transgender patients. *Urol Clin North Am.* 2019;46(4):487-493.

42. Guidance on the limits to the number of embryos to transfer: a committee opinion. *Fertil Steril.* 2017;107(4):901-903.

43. Food, Drug Administration HHS. Eligibility determination for donors of human cells, tissues, and cellular and tissue-based products. Final rule. *Fed Regist.* 2004;69(101):29785-29834.

44. Dean A, Smith LB, Macpherson S, Sharpe RM. The effect of dihydrotestosterone exposure during or prior to the masculinization programming window on reproductive development in male and female rats. *Int J Androl.* 2012;35(3):330-339.

45. Carlsen SM, Jacobsen G, Romundstad P. Maternal testosterone levels during pregnancy are associated with offspring size at birth. *Eur J Endocrinol.* 2006;155(2):365-370.

46. Brandt JS, Patel AJ, Marshall I, Bachmann GA. Transgender men, pregnancy, and the "new" advanced paternal age: a review of the literature. *Maturitas.* 2019;128:17-21.

47. American College of Obstetricians and Gynecologists. ACOG Committee Opinion No. 762: Prepregnancy Counseling. *Obstet Gynecol.* 2019;133(1):e78-e89.

48. Hahn M, Sheran N, Weber S, Cohan D, Obedin-Maliver J. Providing patient-centered perinatal care for transgender men and gender-diverse individuals: a collaborative multidisciplinary team approach. *Obstet Gynecol.* 2019;134(5):959-963.

49. Ellis SA, Wojnar DM, Pettinato M. Conception, pregnancy, and birth experiences of male and gender variant gestational parents: it's how we could have a family. *J Midwifery Womens Health.* 2015;60(1):62-69.

50. MacDonald T, Noel-Weiss J, West D, et al. Transmasculine individuals' experiences with lactation, chestfeeding, and gender identity: a qualitative study. *BMC Pregnancy Childbirth.* 2016;16:106.

51. ACOG Committee Opinion No. 761: cesarean delivery on maternal request. *Obstet Gynecol.* 2019;133(1):e73-e77.

52. Al-Safi Z, Imudia AN, Filetti LC, Hobson DT, Bahado-Singh RO, Awonuga AO. Delayed postpartum preeclampsia and eclampsia: demographics, clinical course, and complications. *Obstet Gynecol.* 2011;118(5):1102-1107.

53. Council on Patient Safety in Women's Health Care. Urgent maternal warning signs. American College of Obstetricians and Gynecologists. https://safehealthcareforeverywoman.org/council/patient-safety-tools/urgent-maternal-signs/. Published 2020. Accessed November 28, 2020.

54. Breastfeeding and the use of human milk. *Pediatrics.* 2012;129(3):e827-841.

55. International LLL. Support for transgender and non-binary parents. https://www.llli.org/breastfeeding-info/transgender-non-binary-parents/#:~:text=If%20you%20have%20had%20chest,have%20been%20damaged%20in%20surgery. Accessed November 29, 2020.

56. Schell AS. Breastfeeding without giving birth. La Leche League International. https://www.llli.org/breastfeeding-without-giving-birth-2/. Published 2020. Accessed November 29, 2020.

57. La Leche League GB. Nursing supplementers. https://www.laleche.org.uk/nursing-supplementers/. Published 2016. Accessed November 29, 2020.

58. Schummers L, Hutcheon JA, Hernandez-Diaz S, et al. Association of short interpregnancy interval with pregnancy outcomes according to maternal age. *JAMA Intern Med.* 2018;178(12):1661-1670.

59. ACOG Committee Opinion No. 757: Screening for Perinatal Depression. *Obstet Gynecol.* 2018;132(5):e208-e212.

60. Davanzo R, Copertino M, De Cunto A, Minen F, Amaddeo A. Antidepressant drugs and breastfeeding: a review of the literature. *Breastfeed Med.* 2011;6(2):89-98.

61. American College of Obstetricians and Gynecologists. ACOG Practice Bulletin No. 92: Use of psychiatric medications during pregnancy and lactation. *Obstet Gynecol.* 2008;111(4):1001-1020.

62. Learmonth C, Viloria R, Lambert C, Goldhammer H, Keuroghlian AS. Barriers to insurance coverage for transgender patients. *Am J Obstet Gynecol.* 2018;219(3):272 e271-272 e274.

63. Kyweluk MA, Reinecke J, Chen D. Fertility Preservation Legislation in the United States: potential implications for transgender individuals. *LGBT Health.* 2019;6(7):331-334.

64. Alliance for Fertility Preservation. Fertility Preservation State Laws & Legislation. https://www.allianceforfertilitypreservation.org/advocacy/state-legislation. Published 2020. Accessed December 31, 2020.

65. Movement Advancement Project. Foster and Adoption Laws. https://www.lgbtmap.org/equality-maps/foster_and_adoption_laws. Published 2020. Accessed.

66. Surrogate parentage contracts; prohibition; custody; definition, AZ Rev Stat § 25-218 (2011).

67. Surrogate Agreements, IN Code § 31 20-1-1(2006).

68. Schoenberg N. In a first for Illinois, transgender man who gave birth will be listed as the father on his baby's birth certificate. *Chicago Tribune.* Jan 14, 2020.

69. Idaho Vital Statistics Act, Idaho 39 § 240(2020).

70. Amendment of records, Tenn. Code Ann. § 68-3-203(2010).

71. Cooper L. American Civil Liberties Union. Protecting the rights of transgender parents and their children: a guide for parents and lawyers. 2013. https://www.aclu.org/report/protecting-rights-transgender-parents-and-their-children. Accessed December 31, 2020.

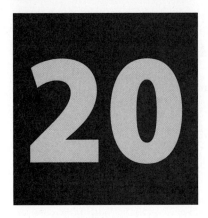

Case Studies in Transgender and Gender Diverse Primary Care

Jennifer Reske-Nielsen

INTRODUCTION

This chapter comprises clinical case scenarios based on common clinical presentations encountered in primary care. These cases can be used by individuals for self-study or by groups of learners to foster discussion. The goal of these cases is to highlight key aspects of primary care provision for **transgender and gender diverse (TGD)** individuals and to offer possible ways to approach the scenarios.

CASE STUDY 1: Mandy

Mandy is a 60-year-old transgender woman who presents for her annual physical. She has been seeing you as her primary care provider for years. She began oral estradiol therapy 15 years ago and switched to transdermal patches 10 years ago. She underwent **vaginoplasty** and breast augmentation surgery 5 and 7 years ago, respectively. She has a 30-pack-year history of smoking but quit before having the surgeries; she states that she has just started social tobacco smoking when out with friends (approximately 10 cigarettes per week). She drinks alcohol socially. There is no family history of breast cancer or lung cancer. Her father died of prostate cancer at age 55. Mandy has not had a mammogram since she had her breast augmentation surgery, as she is worried about her breast implants "popping" when she gets the mammogram. She is up to date on colon cancer screening with colonoscopy.

▶ Discussion Questions

1. Is Mandy due for breast cancer screening? If so, what modality should be used if she has breast implants?

   It is recommended that transgender women on feminizing hormones start breast cancer screening at age 50 or earlier if they have a family history of breast cancer[1] (see Chapter 18, "Screening for Cancer and Cardiovascular Disease"). A study of 2260 transgender women in the Netherlands found higher rates of breast cancer in this population compared with **cisgender** men but lower rates compared with cisgender women.[1] Individuals with either silicone or saline breast implants still need mammography for breast cancer screening. Although many women worry about breast implants "popping" during a mammogram due to the compression used, this event happens very rarely. Individuals should notify the mammographer that they have implants so that the appropriate views are obtained.

2. If she had injected silicone into her breasts (also known colloquially as "pumping"), would that change which breast cancer screening modality is appropriate?

   Mammograms are less accurate for breast cancer screening in the presence of injected silicone or other free particulates as they obscure breast tissue. Contrast-enhanced magnetic resonance imaging of the breast is the imaging modality of choice in this situation.[4]

3. Is Mandy eligible for any additional health screenings because of her history of smoking? How would you counsel her on the risks of restarting smoking socially at this time?

   a. Mandy meets the United States Preventive Services Task Force (USPSTF) criteria for lung cancer screening: she is an adult between the ages of 55 and 80 years old with a 30-pack-year history of smoking, and she is currently smoking.[2] Additionally, the USPSTF recommends one-time screening ultrasound of the abdominal aorta for men aged 65–75 years who smoke or who used to smoke. Since Mandy was assigned male sex at birth and exposed to testosterone for most of her life, it would be reasonable for her to follow aortic aneurysm screening guidelines for cisgender men when she turns 65.[3]

   b. Because Mandy has restarted smoking socially, she should be counseled regarding the increased risk of cardiovascular disease and blood clots associated with combining smoking and estradiol use. As Mandy had previously quit smoking, it would be important to explore why she started smoking again and how she had quit previously in a motivational interviewing approach.

4. Is it appropriate to screen Mandy for prostate cancer? If so, how would you counsel her? How would you screen her?

Mandy may still need prostate cancer screening. Despite having had a vaginoplasty and orchiectomy, she still has a prostate (located anterior to the neovagina).[5] Although lowering her testosterone levels will have reduced her risk of prostate cancer, this risk is not completely eliminated.[6] The USPSTF recommends that prostate cancer screening with periodic prostate-specific antigen (PSA) measurement be individualized for men aged 55–69 years based on a discussion of the risks and benefits. Since Mandy retains a prostate, it would be reasonable to engage her in a similar shared decision-making process. Of note, if palpation of the prostate is clinically indicated, for example, to evaluate a patient like Mandy for possible prostatitis, perform a vaginal exam (palpating anteriorly) in addition to a rectal exam as the prostate is located anterior to the neovagina and may be better assessed through a vaginal approach.

CASE STUDY 2: Adam

Adam is a 33-year-old transgender man who presents for his yearly physical exam. He has been on intramuscular testosterone for more than 5 years and has undergone chest masculinization surgery. He is sexually active with his wife only. He is a social drinker, does not use tobacco, and has no chronic medical conditions. He has never had testing for sexually transmitted infections or a pelvic exam. He has heard that he does not need to have cervical cancer screening because he has never had receptive vaginal sex with a penis. He has not received the human papillomavirus (HPV) vaccine.

▶ **Discussion Questions**

1. Is Adam at risk for cervical cancer? How would you counsel him on this?

Anyone with a cervix is at potential risk for cervical cancer regardless of the type of sexual contact. The USPSTF guidelines recommend cervical cancer screening for anyone aged 21–65 years who has a cervix.[7] The specific recommendation for Adam's age group (30–65 years) is screening with cervical cytology (Pap test) alone every 3 years, screening with high-risk HPV testing alone every 5 years, or cotesting with cervical cytology plus high-risk HPV screening every 5 years. Studies have shown that **trans masculine** people are less likely to have cervical cancer screening than cisgender women because of patient-level and clinician-level barriers to care.[8]

2. What anatomical changes might you see on a pelvic exam as a result of Adam's testosterone treatment? Could any of these changes affect his cervical cytology results?

An external genital exam may reveal clitoromegaly due to testosterone use. On internal exam, the vaginal walls typically appear similar to those of postmenopausal women (i.e., pale pink and without a lot of lubrication) due to decreased levels of circulating estrogen. The cervical transformation zone, from which the sample for cervical cytology should be collected, is also likely to have migrated into the cervical os; thus, it is important to use the correct sampling instrument (e.g., cytobrush) in order to obtain a satisfactory specimen. If the clinician is unable to obtain a sufficient sample with this technique, vaginal estrogen application for 1 week prior to performing repeat cytological testing test may be helpful and will not interfere with testosterone therapy.[8]

3. How would you conduct the pelvic exam in a trauma-informed manner?

Given the high prevalence of trauma in TGD patients and the history of health care discrimination against TGD people, **trauma-informed care (TIC)** is a vital approach for all clinicians working with TGD patients. **Gender dysphoria** surrounding discordance of body parts with one's gender identity may also make the genital exam especially distressing for TGD patients. All pelvic exams should be performed in a trauma-informed manner. Information about how to incorporate a trauma-informed approach into the physical examination is presented in Chapter 13, "Professional Communication of Drug Information," and is summarized in Table 20-1.

CASE STUDY 3: Elliott

Elliot is a 28-year-old transgender man who presents with vaginal bleeding. Elliot has been on testosterone for 5 years. His menses had stopped when he started testosterone, and he did not have any bleeding until 6 months ago. Currently, he is experiencing monthly bleeding. He denies fever, chills, vaginal discharge, pelvic pain, or urinary symptoms and has had no bleeding from other sites. He wants to stop the bleeding because it is upsetting to him.

▶ **Discussion Questions**

1. What additional questions should you ask to explore the possible reasons for his bleeding?

a. To determine whether the bleeding could be related to changes in testosterone exposure, you should ask whether he has missed any doses of testosterone (either topical or injectable). Has he had any trouble getting the medication? Has he had any problems with injections? How much is he drawing up? Using too much testosterone can cause its aromatization in adipose

Table 20-1. Performing a Trauma-Informed Pelvic Examination

Timing	Trauma-Informed Care Components
Before the exam	• Ask patient what terms they use to refer to their anatomy. • Explain the reasons for doing the exam and what it will involve. • Ask about prior experience with pelvic exams. • Discuss options to optimize comfort. • Explain that they will be in control of the exam at all times. • Obtain explicit consent before proceeding.
During the exam	• Provide anticipatory guidance prior to performing each exam maneuver. • Use non carbomer-containing lubricant during the speculum placement to ease insertion. • Check in with the patient periodically to see how they are doing. • Stop immediately if the patient manifests distress or asks you to stop. • Assist distressed patients by utilizing grounding and other self-soothing techniques.
After the exam	• Give the patient time to dress before discussing exam findings and next steps. • Assist distressed patients by helping them formulate a self-care plan for after the encounter. • Provide resources for connection to TGD-sensitive trauma recovery services.

tissue, which then increases estrogen levels and can lead to resumption of menses.

b. To determine whether the bleeding could also be related to vaginal mucosal atrophy, you should ask questions such as: When do you notice the bleeding? Does it occur spontaneously? Or only after stimulation (e.g., penetration)? Mucosal atrophy can be treated with topical estrogen.

c. Bleeding could also be caused by other abnormalities, such as cervical or endometrial polyps or cervical cancer. It is important to ask about Elliott's cervical cancer screening history and determine when his last screening was performed. Abnormal bleeding should always be worked up even if a patient is up-to-date with screening.

2. What would the next steps be in the diagnostic work-up (e.g., exams or testing)?

a. Bloodwork: A good first step is to check the blood total testosterone level. If the level of testosterone is too low or too high, the dose can be adjusted accordingly.

b. Examination: If the testosterone level is in the normal range, then the next step is a pelvic exam to ensure there is no vaginal mucosal or cervical abnormality.

c. Imaging: If the pelvic exam is normal, the next step would be a pelvic ultrasound to check the endometrial lining and rule out uterine or adnexal masses. This workup is similar to that performed to evaluate postmenopausal bleeding.

d. Referral: A referral to a gender-affirming gynecologist is the last step if the bleeding persists to determine whether an endometrial biopsy is warranted.

3. If the bleeding continues with a negative workup, what options could you consider to stop the bleeding?

a. Progestin-only pills can be used to stop menses. They can also be used to stop menses prior to starting on testosterone or in conjunction with starting testosterone therapy. A progesterone implant, depot medroxyprogesterone acetate, or a hormonal IUD is another long-acting reversible option that can be used. For this case, Elliot still has a uterus but does not engage in any penis-in-vagina (PIV) sex; however, individuals who do engage in PIV sex and who still have a uterus continue to require contraception even if they are on testosterone. Pregnancy is still possible, and testosterone is teratogenic. The above methods have the dual benefit of providing contraception as well as menses control.

CASE STUDY 4: Max

Max is a 28-year-old, **genderfluid** person who was assigned male sex at birth and presents for rectal pain and discharge. Symptoms started a week ago. They are sexually active with one male partner. They report fevers, pain with bowel movements, and rectal discharge. They have no history of sexually transmitted infections (STIs), and their last testing was 2 years ago. Their only medications are estradiol and spironolactone. They are concerned that they could have an STI. When you ask about their relationship with their partner, they shrug and look away. You follow up by asking if they feel safe in the relationship, and they answer that they are not sure.

▶ Discussion Questions

1. What other questions could you ask that would help determine Max's risks for acquiring an STI?

a. "What types of sex do you have?" It is important to know if they engage in insertive anal sex, receptive anal sex, or oral sex, as this information will inform where they may have contracted an STI and which anatomical sites that you need to test. Asking in an open-ended manner and using the plural ("types") lets the patient know that any answer is acceptable.

b. "Do you use condoms sometimes, always, or never?" Including the options "sometimes" or "never" makes it more likely that the patient will be forthcoming and provides important information that can then be addressed during counseling.

c. "How many partners have you had in the past few months? Do you know them well, kind of well, are they anonymous, or a mix?"

d. "Do you use any substances or alcohol when engaging in sex?" Being aware of how well a patient knows their partners can indicate their possible risk level as well as their likelihood to be informed if a partner tests positive for an STI.

Max informs you that they engage in condomless receptive anal intercourse, insertive anal intercourse, and oral sex and that they know their partners well.

2. What types of STI testing would be appropriate for Max?[9]

a. Blood testing for HIV and syphilis.

b. Urine testing for chlamydia and gonorrhea.

c. Throat swab for gonorrhea.

d. Rectal swab for chlamydia and gonorrhea.

e. Lymphogranuloma venereum (LGV) testing could also be warranted. LGV presents with proctitis symptoms and swollen inguinal lymph nodes. Max has tenesmus, fever, and rectal discharge. If Max also has swollen lymph nodes, it would be appropriate to perform LGV testing.[9]

3. What counseling should you provide regarding safer sex practices? Are there any other options for STI prevention that you should discuss with them?

a. Use of condoms to prevent STIs.

b. (For patients with more than one partner): Limiting partners or talking with partners about their testing prior to engaging in sex.

c. It would also be appropriate to offer HIV preexposure prophylaxis.

4. What is a more comprehensive way to inquire about IPV than asking if Max feels safe in their relationship? If Max discloses IPV after more detailed questioning, what TGD-sensitive violence prevention and recovery resources could you provide?

There are many forms of IPV that Max could be experiencing, including physical, emotional, or sexual abuse. The Fenway screening questions for IPV aim to cover each of these areas to facilitate a complete risk assessment:

In the past year, did a current or former partner…

…make you feel cut off from others, trapped, or controlled in a way that you did not like?"

…make you feel afraid that they might try to hurt you in some way?"

… pressure or force you to do something sexual that you didn't want to do?"

…hit, kick, punch, slap, shove, or otherwise physically hurt you?"

For TGD people, abuse can be in the form of intimidation, preventing access to hormones, threatening to "out" someone, or socially isolating the abused partner. When asking questions about IPV it is also important to be prepared to direct survivors to TGD-responsive services and treatment, including legal aid, shelters, and counseling. Because IPV is more prevalent among TGD populations, regular screening has been recommended.[10] See Chapter 14, "Recognizing and Addressing Intimate Partner Violence," for more information about IPV.

CASE STUDY 5: Phil

Phil is a 45-year-old transgender man. He has been on topical testosterone for 15 years, has had top surgery, and feels good about these gender-affirming interventions. He has a family history of cardiovascular disease (CVD): his father had a heart attack at age 45, and his brother has coronary artery disease that required a stent at age 48. His body mass index (BMI) is 40. He works as a construction worker. He drinks 12 alcoholic beverages per week, smokes 1 pack of cigarettes per day, and does not use any substances. During his annual physical exam, he asks if he should be worried about his heart.

▶ Discussion Questions

1. What are Phil's risk factors for heart disease? Which of these are modifiable?

Phil smokes tobacco, has an elevated BMI, and has a family history of early CVD. His modifiable risk factors are tobacco use and elevated BMI. Although results of his lipid panel are not available, modification of his cholesterol levels may also be needed. His nonmodifiable risk factor is his family history of early coronary artery disease. His testosterone therapy is not necessarily a "modifiable" risk factor because it is important for his gender affirmation.

2. Is Phil at higher risk of a heart attack because he is taking testosterone?

Testosterone use is associated with an increase in BMI and a decrease in high-density lipoprotein (HDL) cholesterol, which are both known to increase CVD risk. It is not clear whether these changes correlate with a higher risk of adverse CVD outcomes among TGD persons using testosterone, as no long-term studies have been done.

3. How can Phil decrease his risk of CVD?

Counsel him to quit smoking and assess his cholesterol levels to determine if he meets criteria for a lipid-lowering medication. Given that he is taking testosterone, it is currently unclear whether his CVD risk assessment should be based on his sex assigned at birth (female) or his gender identity (man) (Connelly et al 2019). One approach is to assess his risk based on guidelines for both females and males using the Atherosclerotic Cardiovascular Disease (ASCVD) Risk Estimator Plus risk calculator and average the results. Phil should also be counseled about healthy eating and physical activity. He does not need to stop his testosterone, but it is appropriate to check testosterone levels to ensure they do not exceed the normal range described for cisgender men.

REFERENCES

1. de Blok CJM, Wiepjes CM, Nota NM, et al. Breast cancer risk in transgender people receiving hormone treatment: nationwide cohort study in the Netherlands. *BMJ*. 2019;365:l1652.
2. Moyer VA. Screening for lung cancer: U.S. Preventive Services Task Force recommendation statement. *Ann Intern Med*. 2014;160(5):330-338.
3. Guirguis-Blake JM, Beil TL, Senger CA, Coppola EL. Primary care screening for abdominal aortic aneurysm: updated evidence report and systematic review for the US Preventive Services Task Force. *JAMA*. 2019;322(22):2219-2238.
4. Sonnenblick EB, Shah AD, Goldstein Z, Reisman T. Breast imaging of transgender individuals: a review. *Curr Radiol Rep*. 2018;6(1):1.
5. Weyers S, De Sutter P, Hoebeke S, et al. Gynaecological aspects of the treatment and follow-up of transsexual men and women. *Facts Views Vis Obgyn*. 2010;2(1):35-54.
6. Braun H, Nash R, Tangpricha V, Brockman J, Ward K, Goodman M. Cancer in transgender people: evidence and methodological considerations. *Epidemiol Rev*. 2017;39(1):93-107.
7. Curry SJ, Krist AH, Owens DK, et al. Screening for cervical cancer: US Preventive Services Task Force Recommendation Statement. *JAMA*. 2018;320(7):674-686.
8. Peitzmeier SM, Khullar K, Reisner SL, Potter J. Pap test use is lower among female-to-male patients than non-transgender women. *Am J Prev Med*. 2014;47(6):808-812.
9. Workowski KA, Bolan GA. Sexually transmitted diseases treatment guidelines, 2015. *MMWR Recomm Rep*. 2015;64 (Rr-03): 1-137.
10. Valentine SE, Peitzmeier SM, King DS, et al. Disparities in exposure to intimate partner violence among transgender/gender nonconforming and sexual minority primary care patients. *LGBT Health*. 2017;4(4):260-267.

Transgender and Gender Diverse Populations

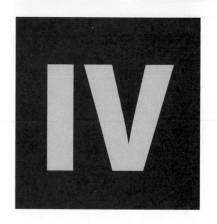

Transgender and Gender Diverse People Who Are Black, Indigenous, and People of Color

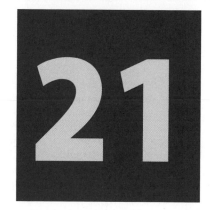

Vanessa Warri, Jack Bruno, Jenna J. Rapues,
JoAnne Keatley, Jae M. Sevelius

INTRODUCTION

Through the lens of **intersectionality**, this chapter illustrates how racism, transphobia, classism, and other social processes of privilege and oppression shape experiences of health care engagement among **transgender and gender diverse (TGD)** people who are Black, Indigenous, and People of Color (BIPOC). This chapter also explores how addressing **social determinants of health** outside of mainstream health care engagement, such as education and economic development, can complement mainstream health care engagement practices to be inclusive and improve overall health outcomes for BIPOC TGD communities. Outside of the context of the United States, there is significant diversity in concepts, definitions, and understandings of what constitutes health care, what are prioritized as social determinants of health, as well as sociocultural beliefs about gender. For the purpose of this chapter, we will focus on these elements within a North American context.

IDENTITY-RELATED CONCEPTS AND TERMINOLOGIES

A vast array of gender identities and expressions exist within BIPOC TGD communities, situated within their own socio-cultural and sociohistorical contexts. These terms can be highly specific, change over time and across generations, and carry different social, cultural, and political implications. Shared identities and language help community members develop a sense of belonging and strengthen relational ties. However, even within groups, there often exist many different ways that individuals choose to identify and describe themselves, and for many different reasons. For example, the term "queen" (also "femme queen," and "reyna" in Spanish) has been used by communities of Black and Latina transgender women to identify themselves and was widely used in the "ballroom scene" of the 1960s, although its use likely traces back much further. "Queen" has been commonly used to identify transgender women who participate in pageants and ballroom competitions. Contemporary adaptations of the term "queen" among some communities of Black transgender women (and "king" among Black transgender men) have expanded the use of the term in cultural alignment with Black empowerment movements as a means to increase social solidarity and elevate the experiences of its members amid the ongoing fight against racial injustice in the United States.

In addition, some Black transgender people identify as a "woman (or man) of transgender experience," emphasizing that some TGD people identify with the gender binary and regard their transgender experience as part of their history rather than their present identity. Individuals of transgender experience often do not identify with the terms "transgender man" (or "trans man") or "transgender woman" (or "trans woman") as others in the same community might and may reject medicalized or research-oriented categorizations of their experience. Two-step methodologies to collect demographic information about individuals from TGD communities that permit individuals to indicate their gender identity followed by a question about **sex assigned at birth** may prove more acceptable by some, but not all members of BIPOC TGD communities.

Within Latinx communities, the term "travesti" is commonly used throughout South America and has been widely reclaimed as a term of political empowerment and decolonization. In Mexico, particularly among the Indigenous Zapotec, the term "muxe" has been used to describe individuals who are assigned male at birth, embody many gender roles of womanhood, and have shamanic qualities akin to curanderas. Like the Indian "hijra," muxes embody a third gender status within their communities, rather than occupying male or female roles. Nonbinary gender identities, identities that exist outside and beyond the gender binary of female or male, are increasingly being reported and documented within and across diverse communities of color.

It is a common misconception that the term "Two-Spirit" simply refers to Native Americans who are members of the LGBTQIA+ community. However, Indigenous people who identify as Two-Spirit may or may not identify as a member of the LGBTQIA+ community. In addition, people may use a term specific to their tribal language to define themselves. Many Indigenous languages include terms for people who live outside of colonial constructs of binary gender identities. "Two-Spirit" was coined in the 1990s by Indigenous activists who sought to create a term that addressed traditional, Indigenous understandings of gender and sexuality, the resilience of Indigenous peoples in the face of genocide, and the development of pantribal political organization and community building.[1] Colloquially, a Two-Spirit person is considered someone who embodies both a female and male spirit, thus having two spirits. In common usage, an individual may consider their Two-Spirit identity to refer to their gender identity, sexual orientation, or both aspects of themselves.

Historically, many different tribal groups held space in their communities for people who occupied spiritual, occupational, political, familial, and ceremonial roles that included gender expressions outside of the Western construct of the gender binary. Individuals may be aware of, and connected to, their communities' traditional terms and utilize that language for themselves. Due to genocidal policies such as English-only boarding schools and the outlawing of religious practices, not all tribal communities were able to retain fluency in their languages. The persecution of those who lived outside of these imposed constructs disrupted the intergenerational transmission of these traditions. Tribal understandings of varied gender identities and sexualities went underground, became coded, or were renounced over the course of forced assimilation and cultural genocide. The development of "Two-Spirit" as an idea referring to sexuality and/or gender identity was an act of resistance that reclaimed the variety of ways in which Indigenous communities understand gender and sexuality, pushing back against the heterosexist, cissexist, and binary frameworks for conceptualizing gender that were brought to North America during European colonization.

The usage of the term "Two-Spirit" by people who are not Indigenous is considered cultural appropriation. The concept of a Two-Spirit identity as such was created in response to the ways in which colonialism has impacted Indigenous ways of understanding gender and sexuality. Therefore, it cannot apply to those who are not Indigenous. It is also used to acknowledge that many Two-Spirit people face racism and colonialism within the LGBTQIA+ community. In addition, people may signal their connection to their Indigenous communities by claiming a Two-Spirit identity, thereby aligning themselves with the political goals and culture of their nation or tribe.

INTERSECTIONALITY AND INTERSECTIONAL STIGMA

BIPOC TGD people disproportionately report negative experiences in health care and worse health outcomes compared to cisgender people and white people. These data, however, are often reported in terms of a single identity (e.g., transgender, racial, or ethnic identity). Recent data indicate that BIPOC TGD communities experience unique and often more profound disparities than those who belong to only one such minoritized group, such as white transgender people or BIPOC cisgender people.[2]

Intersectionality is a theoretical framework that emerged from Black feminism and has recently been increasingly applied to studies of health and health disparities.[3,4] Intersectionality elucidates how systems of power and oppression at the macro (structural) level impact the experiences of individuals based on the multiple social categories to which they belong.[4] As a critical theory, intersectionality posits that power relations construct our perspectives and experiences and seeks to inform the empowerment of individuals and groups that are negatively impacted by those power relations.[5] **Stigma** is a social process enacted through societal structures and interpersonal interactions that devalue human differences, marginalize stigmatized individuals, and create a social hierarchy that reinforces inequities.[6] Stigma is a fundamental cause of health disparities.[7] Globally, transgender women experience extreme social and economic marginalization due to intersectional stigma.[8–10] **Intersectional stigma** (Figure 21-1) occurs at the juncture of multiple stigmatizing forces that fall within or across several categories: (1) health-related stigma that affects people who have one or more coexisting health conditions such as HIV, mental illness, or substance use disorder; (2) stigma based on sociodemographic characteristics such as racism, transphobia, gender discrimination, sexual orientation, immigration status, the influence of settler-colonialism, xenophobia, etc.; and (3) stigma related to behaviors or experiences such as substance use and sex work.

Within BIPOC TGD communities, gender- and race-based stigma can intersect with experiences and social positions, such as engagement in sex work and substance use,[11,12] to generate a social context of increased vulnerability to multiple negative health outcomes.[13] Experiences of **enacted stigma** (i.e., being stigmatized or discriminated against) often lead to **anticipated stigma** (i.e., expectations of experiencing stigma), whereby BIPOC TGD people anticipate experiences of stigma from health care providers. Both enacted and anticipated stigma can lead to health care avoidance and **internalized stigma** (adopting stigmatizing attitudes toward oneself).[14] Consider the example of the *model minority myth*, which posits that all Asian-Americans are exceptionally more driven, successful, and assimilated than all other minority groups in the United States, and the impact this stereotype

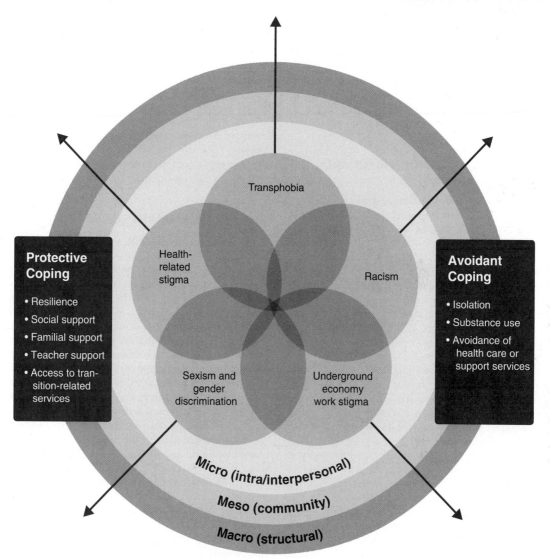

▲ **Figure 21–1.** Processes of intersectional stigma. (Reproduced with permission from Logie CH, James L, Tharao W, et al: HIV, gender, race, sexual orientation, and sex work: a qualitative study of intersectional stigma experienced by HIV-positive women in Ontario, Canada, *PLoS Med* 2011 Nov;8(11):e1001124.)

could potentially have on overall health outcomes of Asian and Pacific Islander (API) TGD people. Failure to perform to the idealized levels of functioning as dictated by the model minority stereotype can negatively impact an individual's mental health through internalization of the sanctions that are imposed on them, both by members of their own communities who navigate within the model minority context and by the dominant society that actively stigmatizes them.

To illustrate this further, consider the legacy of racialized stigma enacted against Black Americans in the United States and the stereotype of Black Americans as being *angry, loud, and prone to violence.* Experiencing the traumatic enactment of stigma across the lifespan, in turn, becomes internalized to the point where engaging with institutions such as health care becomes challenging due to the anticipation of experiencing stigma. In both examples, anticipated stigma has the potential to prevent an individual from seeking health services, and the stigma faced by TGD people increases the likelihood of disengagement with health care settings. Stigma **resilience** is the ability to cope with or challenge enacted stigma, seek health care despite anticipated stigma, and resist internalization of stigmatizing beliefs.[10,15,16] Stigma resilience can be described as being empowered in one's health care despite the context of stigma.[17]

HEALTH DISPARITIES AMONG BIPOC TGD PEOPLE

Racism, transphobia, sexism, poverty, immigration status, and other syndemic factors intersect to shape the health and health care experiences of BIPOC TGD people and marginalize these communities from access to full participation within society. These stressors, in turn, create challenges in accessing necessary health resources and maintaining regular health care engagement. As a result, BIPOC TGD communities face disproportionate rates of poor health outcomes. Additional factors such as mental health problems, substance use disorders, and incarceration increase the likelihood of decreased health management and primary care engagement.[18] The health disparities that BIPOC TGD persons face are directly related to gender- and race-based stigmas embedded within the structures of the United States, including health care settings. For example, policies and practices often reflect and reinforce Western binary concepts of gender that emphasize an individual's sex assigned at birth over their gender identity.[14]

Data from the *2015 US Transgender Survey* found that 33% of respondents reported having a negative experience with a health care provider, and 23% of respondents reported not seeing a doctor due to fear of being mistreated.[2] Negative experiences when seeking health care, such as being refused treatment, being assaulted sexually, physically, or verbally, or having to teach the provider about transgender people, were particularly common among American Indian and Alaskan Native respondents (50%).[19] Further, 17% of Latinx respondents, 20% of Black respondents, and 18% of American Indian and Alaska Native reported not having health insurance.[19,20] In addition to the structural barriers that stigma creates, it is important to note that each person carries biases that may be implicitly or explicitly expressed in health and social service settings.[21]

BIPOC TGD people, Black and Brown TGD people in particular, experience disproportionate levels of trauma, including systemic racism and anti-blackness, police brutality and incarceration, intimate partner violence, sexual abuse (both in childhood and as adults), survival sex work, family dysfunction, poverty, and homelessness.[22,23] Black and Brown transgender women, and Black and Latinx transgender women in particular, are disproportionately represented among the high rates of reported murders of transgender people worldwide. In 2020, as the Black Lives Matter movement gained unprecedented visibility and support in the wake of several killings of Black people by police and others, including a Black trans man, Tony McDade, and two Black trans women, Dominique Fells and Riah Milton, Black trans people mobilized with extraordinary momentum. However, structural violence against trans people, particularly Black trans people, is not new. The syndemics of discrimination, poverty, and incarceration serve to economically marginalize transgender people, creating systematic vulnerabilities that lead to increased exposure to violence, including police violence.

SOCIAL DETERMINANTS OF HEALTH

Social determinants of health are the social conditions that are necessary for optimal health. These conditions may be categorized as economics, environment, education, food, social context, and health care. Taken holistically, all of these social factors together influence and determine the overall health of an individual.[24]

Much of the current research on health disparities experienced by TGD communities documents the disproportionate impact of the HIV epidemic on BIPOC transgender women and emphasizes the development of interventions to improve health care engagement around HIV treatment and prevention.[25-27] From an intersectional perspective, improving the health outcomes of Black and Brown TGD people involves addressing the socioeconomic inequalities and injustices impacting these communities. Black, Latinx, and American Indian and Alaskan Native TGD individuals face rates of poverty at nearly 3.5 times the national average, with 42% of Black transgender people and 31% of Latinx transgender people experiencing homelessness in their lifetime.[2] American Indian and Alaska Native TGD people, in particular, are severely impacted by homelessness, with more than one-half (57%) experiencing homelessness at some point in their lives.[19]

Social determinants of health are interconnected and mutually reinforcing. For example, a person's living environment and socioeconomic status directly affect the level of access that they have to other vital resources, such as healthy food options. Further, if a person is experiencing homelessness, they likely face additional barriers to financial stability, which is crucial to obtaining stable housing. For Black and Brown TGD people who are already more likely than the general population to experience homelessness and poverty, this becomes a self-perpetuating cycle that requires specific investigation and intervention from community-based researchers, led and informed by people with these lived experiences.

Education is another example of a social determinant of health for BIPOC TGD people that requires additional intervention development. Creating more supportive educational pathways and opportunities for Black and Brown TGD people is critical to counteract the harassment and discrimination that often results in early school drop-out and low employment rates. Opportunities for secure employment and stable housing provide a space from which they can tend to other aspects of their holistic health. As highlighted by the case study later in this chapter, engaging Black and Brown TGD communities in peer-based health and social service work *as* a form of educational development can provide opportunities for these individuals to conceptualize futures that envision higher education as possible. An educational model of this kind can also serve to develop future generations of peer community leaders and researchers developed from *within* the community. Social support is an additional social determinant that has great potential to improve health outcomes among Black and Brown TGD communities. Developing more opportunities for social support within health services and interventions and creating more pathways for peer-facilitated social services within health-based agencies can prove useful in improving health care engagement, medication adherence, and overall quality of life and self-efficacy.[28]

COMMUNITY-BASED HEALTH CARE MODELS

In many TGD communities, especially in BIPOC communities, individuals who interact with the health care system are often not given the opportunity to influence the patient care environment or learn about gender-affirming care options. Hiring TGD staff and developing programs and services that are responsive to the expressed needs of TGD communities are critical steps toward successful TGD-affirming health care. In addition to the value of their lived expertise, TGD staff can best devise strategies for engaging TGD communities, build trust, and assist in translating critical health information into gender-affirming and accessible language for members of TGD communities.[29,30] It is essential that providers with the agency and position to lead these efforts do so in collaboration with TGD communities. Hiring TGD staff can also provide opportunities for economic empowerment and capacity building for those who have often been marginalized by traditional education and employment sectors. This also serves to benefit and attract TGD people who are more likely to engage with health and social services when they see themselves reflected among staff. Incorporating peer-led models within health and social services for TGD communities provides opportunities for health-related and other conversations to be had more comfortably. TGD people may be likelier to engage in sensitive discussions when providers and/or staff reflect diverse identities and experiences. Due to the marginalization that TGD communities continue to face, managers

and supervisors must be committed to taking the time to properly train TGD staff, provide opportunities for professional development, and continuously support their staff by providing adequate supervision.[31,32]

BIPOC TGD people can benefit tremendously from services using peer-based support and health navigation, which have been shown to increase engagement in care and address issues of mistrust of the medical system.[33,34] Peer staff, however, may experience vicarious trauma, or secondary traumatic stress, due to exposure to highly traumatic stories and situations experienced by their interactions with participants coupled with high levels of identification with participants based on their peer status.[35] Secondary traumatic stress is a pervasive experience among peer staff working with BIPOC TGD people due to extremely high levels of trauma experienced by this population. This phenomenon should be considered more explicitly in peer-based interventions to adequately support staff and prevent burnout. Considerations for preventing burnout and supporting staff include providing positive coping skills training, helping staff develop and maintain healthy boundaries with participants, debriefing traumatic content in supervision (both professional and clinical), and following up with staff to identify ongoing difficulties and early signs of burnout.[36]

Engaging a community advisory board (CAB) to help guide models of service provision can be a vital source of inspiration, insight, and expertise for engaging in TGD-affirming health care. The composition of a CAB should reflect the specific communities at the center of the health care services. If services are intended to focus on BIPOC transgender women, the CAB should be primarily comprised of BIPOC transgender women. It may also be appropriate to include representatives from community-based organizations that serve the community of interest, depending on what type of community expertise is needed. It is important to support the participation of TGD people on CABs by providing food, monetary compensation for their time, and/or transportation. It is also important to ensure that all participants feel supported in contributing to decision-making and feedback processes, especially in the context of a CAB where some participants may have more experience with providing feedback than others. Such support can be accomplished by setting a "take space/ make space" norm early in the formation of the CAB, and by incorporating capacity-building activities into the CAB meetings to provide opportunities for less experienced CAB members to learn about community-based health care models.[37] The CAB can also serve as a unique entry point for TGD people who are interested in learning more about how community-based services and research are developed, to take on a larger role and help facilitate an increased interest in community health, social services, and community-based research.

RESILIENCE AMONG BIPOC TGD PEOPLE

Despite facing exceptional challenges, BIPOC TGD people are extraordinarily resilient. Resilience is both an individual and collective process of navigating and overcoming adversity, such as experiencing stigma when seeking health care. Research on resilience among BIPOC transgender people, transgender women, and TGD people living with HIV emphasizes the importance of gender and racial/ethnic pride, recognizing and navigating stigma and oppression, accessing resources, and building community around advocacy.[38,39] Spirituality and social support from family and significant others have also been found to be important factors in resilience among TGD people.[38,40] Among American Indian and Alaska Native peoples, traditional healing practices, connectedness to ancestors, tribal language fluency, and perceived level of cultural continuity are protective cultural factors that can significantly contribute to the resilience of Two-Spirit people.[41-43] The Transgender Law Center has produced a community-led guide to advance a collective trans liberation agenda, which includes the leadership of Black trans women, respect for Indigenous cultural practices, the importance of intergenerational connectedness, self-definition, and freedom for all.[44]

SUMMARY

- Intersectionality elucidates how systems of power and oppression at the macro (structural) level impact the experiences of individuals based on the multiple social categories to which they belong.
- Stigma is a fundamental cause of health disparities. Intersectional stigma describes a multiplicity of stigmatizing forces based on health status, sociodemographic characteristics, and behaviors or experiences that create extreme social and economic marginalization.
- Racism, anti-Blackness, transphobia, sexism, poverty, immigration status, and other syndemic factors intersect to shape the health and health care experiences of BIPOC TGD people, creating challenges to accessing necessary health resources and disproportionate rates of poor health outcomes. Additional factors such as mental health problems, substance use disorders, and incarceration increase the likelihood of decreased health management and primary care engagement.
- Social determinants of health are the social conditions that are necessary for optimal health. Improving the health outcomes of BIPOC TGD people involves addressing the socioeconomic injustices that impact these communities.
- Involvement of TGD people who are also BIPOC within the health care system can help to foster trust and provide opportunities for economic and educational empowerment. Community Advisory Boards (CABs) are vital in providing the inspiration, insight, and expertise needed to codevelop TGD-affirming models of service provision.

CASE STUDY: GABRIELLE

Gabrielle, a young Black transgender woman in her early twenties, had been homeless after emancipating from the foster care system in her hometown several years prior. She acquired some work experience through various youth internships with a focus on civic engagement and community-building as a teenager. Aside from this, she did not have any professional work experience. Finding work was incredibly difficult for Gabrielle, who spent most of her days sleeping as a result of staying up all night to remain as safe as possible while living on the streets. With no permanent dwelling, stable living environment, or steady source of income, she never thought that a professional career or education was an achievable option for her, and she focused instead on survival sex work to meet her daily basic needs.

Being deeply connected with a community of local transgender women of color, Gabrielle soon learned of a community-based health and social services program that she could access in the neighborhood. She decided to visit and began engaging with the program regularly. She soon was able to secure a part-time position working as a program assistant. In this capacity, she was able to learn more about health education and the unique needs of her community, as well as become more connected to her community at large. Before long, she became an active member of an advocacy group working within local government for systemic and programmatic change for her community. Gabrielle was able to use her own experiences as well as the experiences that she had gleaned from her peers and fellow community members to effectively support efforts to secure much-needed funding for community programs and affect change within local policy regarding the safety and security of the transgender community.

It was in this capacity that she was approached by the principal investigator of a community-based research organization who was seeking to develop and test peer-based health interventions with transgender women of color and asked her to join the community advisory board for the project. Gabrielle was excited to see that her lived experiences were being validated and sought after as fundamental to the development of initiatives that could help her community, and that, as a member of her community, she was being seen as having some expertise in a professional capacity. Gabrielle would remain an active member of this community advisory board, engaged in a reciprocal relationship: providing feedback to inform intervention development, and in turn learning about the process and benefits of community-based research. Gabrielle was most interested in discovering the role that community-based research could play in fostering policy change and increasing the body of health care knowledge. Gabrielle began to understand through this interaction that her lived experiences, in combination with research experience, had the potential to position her such that she, as a member of her community, could influence great change. Gabrielle was eager for more opportunities to engage with community-based research.

Noticing her commitment to her community, the principal investigator approached Gabrielle and offered her a position facilitating the same intervention she had served on the community advisory board for. Gabrielle was very excited, and eagerly accepted the position. She would now begin to gain hands-on experience in conducting community-based research. The increase in hours and pay made it possible for Gabrielle to secure housing and get off the streets. With a stable home, a source of income, and an exciting new career prospect, she started thinking for the first time about the one thing she had always thought was out-of-reach: pursuing higher education. She enrolled in her local community college and began taking prerequisite courses for a social science major. In school, she discovered that she was quite gifted academically, and realized that her lived experiences in conjunction with the professional experiences she was gaining in social science research helped her to relate better to the material she was learning and excel in ways she previously had not thought possible.

Almost 4 years went by and Gabrielle, now in her late twenties, was ready to transfer to a 4-year bachelor's program. She had accumulated nearly a decade of experience working within her community, with almost four of those years being solely dedicated to community-based research. She had facilitated and supported four research projects and gained a wide variety of relevant research-related skills, from group-level interventions and one-on-one qualitative interviewing to data collection and analysis. Gabrielle felt ready to pursue the next phase of her academic journey and now believed it was well within reach, as she was prepared and supported by a team of community members and mentors who championed her endeavors.

▶ Discussion Questions

1. How does this case study demonstrate ways in which intentional inclusion and education about community health and social services, and hands-on involvement in a professional capacity can improve overall health?

2. From Gabrielle's story, how were social determinants of health addressed through her professional and educational journey?

3. This case study highlights opportunities for improved quality of life by engaging Black TGD communities in educationally and professionally innovative ways within community-based research. How might this empowerment-based model be implemented in other health and social service realms?

4. What are some main issues to consider when creating community-based health models that include education and professional development for BIPOC TGD communities as a part of their framework?

REFERENCES

1. Fewster PH. Two-spirit community. https://lgbtqhealth.ca/community/two-spirit.php. Published 2021. Accessed April 25, 2021.
2. James SE, Herman JL, Rankin S, Keisling M, Mottet L, Anafi M. *The Report of the 2015 U.S. Transgender Survey.* Washington, DC: National Center for Transgender Equality; 2016.
3. Crenshaw K. Demarginalizing the Intersection of Race and Sex: A Black Feminist Critique of Antidiscrimination Doctrine, Feminist Theory and Antiracist Politics. 1989.
4. Bowleg L. The problem with the phrase women and minorities: intersectionality-an important theoretical framework for public health. *Am J Public Health.* 2012;102(7):1267–1273.
5. Else-Quest NM, Hyde JS. Intersectionality in quantitative psychological research: I. Theoretical and epistemological issues. *Psychol Women Q.* 2016;40(2):155–170.
6. Herek GM. A nuanced view of stigma for understanding and addressing sexual and gender minority health disparities. *LGBT Health.* 2016 (2325-8306 (Electronic)).
7. Hatzenbuehler ML, Phelan JC, Link BG. Stigma as a fundamental cause of population health inequalities. *Am J Public Health.* 2013;103(5):813–821.
8. Baral SD, Poteat T, Stromdahl S, Wirtz AL, Guadamuz TE, Beyrer C. Worldwide burden of HIV in transgender women: a systematic review and meta-analysis. *Lancet Infect Dis.* 2013;13(3):214–222.
9. Sevelius J, Murray LR, Martinez Fernandes N, Veras MA, Grinsztejn B, Lippman SA. Optimising HIV programming for transgender women in Brazil. *Cult Health Sex.* 2018:1–15.
10. Perez-Brumer AG, Reisner SL, McLean SA, et al. Leveraging social capital: multilevel stigma, associated HIV vulnerabilities, and social resilience strategies among transgender women in Lima, Peru. *J Int AIDS Soc.* 2017;20(1):1–8.
11. Poteat T, Wirtz AL, Radix A, et al. HIV risk and preventive interventions in transgender women sex workers. *Lancet.* 2015;385(9964):274–286.
12. Avila MM, Dos Ramos Farias MS, Fazzi L, et al. High frequency of illegal drug use influences condom use among female transgender sex workers in Argentina: impact on HIV and syphilis infections. *AIDS Behav.* 2017;21(7):2059–2068.
13. Parsons JT, Antebi-Gruszka N, Millar BM, Cain D, Gurung S. Syndemic conditions, HIV transmission risk behavior, and transactional sex among transgender women. *AIDS Behav.* 2018;22(7):2056–2067.
14. White Hughto JM, Reisner SL, Pachankis JE. Transgender stigma and health: a critical review of stigma determinants, mechanisms, and interventions. *Soc Sci Med.* 2015;147:222–231.
15. Bockting WO, Miner MH, Swinburne Romine RE, Hamilton A, Coleman E. Stigma, mental health, and resilience in an online sample of the US transgender population. *Am J Public Health.* 2013;103(5):943–951.
16. Bockting W. Transgender identity and HIV: resilience in the face of stigma. *Focus Guide AIDS Res Counsel.* 2008;23(2):1–4.

17. Johnson MO. The shifting landscape of health care: toward a model of health care empowerment. *Am J Public Health.* 2011;101(2):265–270.

18. Safer JD, Coleman E, Feldman J, et al. Barriers to healthcare for transgender individuals. *Curr Opin Endocrinol Diab Obes.* 2016;23(2):168–171.

19. James S, Jackson T, Jim M. *2015 U.S. Transgender Survey: Report on the Experiences of American Indian and Alaska Native Respondents.* Washington, DC: National Center for Transgender Equality; 2017.

20. James SE, Brown C, Wilson I. *2015 U.S. Transgender Survey: Report on the Experiences of Black Respondents.* Washington, DC and Dallas, TX: National Center for Transgender Equality; 2017.

21. Nadal KL, Whitman CN, Davis LS, Erazo T, Davidoff KC. Microaggressions toward lesbian, gay, bisexual, transgender, queer, and genderqueer people: a review of the literature. *The J Sex Res.* 2016;53(4-5):488–508.

22. Valentine SE, Shipherd JC. A systematic review of social stress and mental health among transgender and gender nonconforming people in the United States. *Clin Psychol Rev.* 2018;66:24–38.

23. Machtinger E, Haberer J, Wilson T, Weiss D. Recent trauma is associated with antiretroviral Failure and HIV transmission risk behavior among HIV-positive women and female-identified transgenders. *AIDS Behav.* 2012;16(8):2160–2170.

24. Baah FO, Teitelman AM, Riegel B. Marginalization: conceptualizing patient vulnerabilities in the framework of social determinants of health—an integrative review. *Nurs Inq.* 2019;26(1):e12268.

25. Rebchook G, Keatley J, Contreras R, et al. The transgender women of color initiative: implementing and evaluating innovative interventions to enhance engagement and retention in HIV care. *Am J Public Health.* 2017;107(2):224–229.

26. Poteat T, Wirtz A, Malik M, et al. A gap between willingness and uptake: findings from mixed methods research on HIV prevention among Black and Latina transgender women. *J Acquir Immune Defic Syndr.* 2019;82(2):131–140.

27. Sevelius JM, Neilands TB, Dilworth S, Castro D, Johnson MO. Sheroes: feasibility and acceptability of a community-driven, group-level HIV Intervention Program for transgender women. *AIDS Behav.* 2020;24(5):1551–1559.

28. Kalichman SC, Hernandez D, Finneran S, Price D, Driver R. Transgender women and HIV-related health disparities: falling off the HIV treatment cascade. *Sexual Health.* 2017;14(5):469–476.

29. Giblon R, Bauer GR. Health care availability, quality, and unmet need: a comparison of transgender and cisgender residents of Ontario, Canada. *BMC Health Serv Res.* 2017;17(1):283.

30. Paxton K, Guentzel H, Trombacco K. Lessons learned in developing a research partnership with the transgender community. *Am J Commun Psychol.* 2006;37(3-4):349–356.

31. Israel T, Willging C, Ley D. Development and evaluation of training for rural LGBTQ mental health peer advocates. *Rural Mental Health.* 2016;40(1):40–62.

32. Benoit C, Jansson M, Millar A, Phillips R. Community-academic research on hard-to-reach populations: benefits and challenges. *Qual Health Res.* 2005;15(2):263–282.

33. Poteat T, Wirtz AL, Reisner S. Strategies for engaging transgender populations in HIV prevention and care. *Curr Opin HIV AIDS.* 2019;14(5):393–400.

34. Sevelius J, Patouhas E, Keatley J, Johnson M. Barriers and facilitators to engagement and retention in care among transgender women living with human immunodeficiency virus. *Ann Behav Med.* 2014;47(1):5–16.

35. Canfield J. Secondary traumatization, burnout, and vicarious traumatization. *Smith College Studies Social Work.* 2005;75(2):81–101.

36. Bercier ML, Maynard BR. Interventions for secondary traumatic stress with mental health workers: a systematic review. *Res Social Work Practice.* 2015;25(1):81–89.

37. Lee MY, Zaharlick A. *Culturally Competent Research : Using Ethnography as a Meta-Framework.* Oxford; New York, NY: Oxford University Press; 2013.

38. Singh AA, McKleroy VS. "Just Getting Out of Bed Is a Revolutionary Act": the resilience of transgender people of color who have survived traumatic life events. *Traumatology.* 2011;17(2):34–44.

39. Lacombe-Duncan A, Logie CH, Newman PA, Bauer GR, Kazemi M. A qualitative study of resilience among transgender women living with HIV in response to stigma in healthcare. *AIDS Care.* 2020;32(8):1008–1013.

40. Weinhardt LS, Xie H, Wesp LM, et al. The role of family, friend, and significant other support in well-being among transgender and non-binary youth. *J GLBT Family Studies.* 2019;15(4):311–325.

41. Angelino AC, Bell S, Roxby A, et al. Developing resources for American Indian/Alaska native transgender and two-spirit youth, their relatives, and healthcare providers. *Progress in Community Health Partnerships: Research, Education, and Action.* Johns Hopkins University Press. 2020;14(4).

42. Hallett D, Chandler MJ, Lalonde CE. Aboriginal language knowledge and youth suicide. *Cogn Dev.* 2007;22(3):392–399.

43. Chandler MJ, Lalonde C. Cultural continuity as a hedge against suicide in Canada's first nations. *Transcultural Psychiatry.* 1998;35(2):191–219.

44. Micky B, Stephens A. *Trans Agenda for Liberation.* Transgender Law Center.

Health Needs and Service Delivery Models for Transgender Communities in Low- and Middle-Income Countries

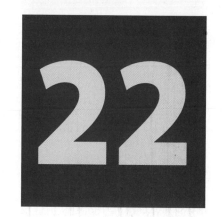

S. Wilson Beckham

Eli Sauerwalt

Katherine N. Elfer

Omar Harfouch

Stefan Baral

INTRODUCTION

This chapter focuses on **transgender and gender diverse** (TGD) communities in low- and middle-income countries (LMIC) and explores both key differences in the communities compared with higher resource areas as well as issues that are similar across settings. Data suggest there are no fewer TGD people in LMIC compared with higher resource countries, and their health care needs are similar. However, given pervasive and intersectional stigma, it is harder to conduct research about and provide health care to TGD in LMIC. Therefore, there are less data on TGD, their health, and effective service models in LMIC. Nevertheless, providers and implementers must consider stigma and discrimination when designing and delivering evidence-based and high-quality services. This chapter discusses some of the roles of intersectional stigma and violence, including stigma related to gender, sexual behavior, and HIV/AIDS; then highlights issues of sexual health, infectious disease, mental health, and substance use that are particular to TGD people in LMIC. The chapter then discusses service models for affirming health care for TGD people and concludes with a case study about TGD health care for individuals in Lebanon.

▶ Intersectional Stigma and Violence

Worldwide, TGD individuals are at a disproportionately high risk of experiencing discrimination and violence due to sexual- or gender-related stigma. **Stigma** is a decrease in social value as a result of deviation from the values and social norms of a community.[1] Members of society may stigmatize TGD people who do not conform to mainstream cis- and heteronormative standards, and may also commit discrimination or violence against TGD people. Health behaviors, such as seeking care or continuing a treatment plan, are also strongly influenced by the intersection of anticipated, perceived, and enacted stigma.[2] Health services can also be restricted due to discriminatory inclusion and exclusion policies.[3] Stigma generates discrimination and violence at the individual, interpersonal, and societal level. Stigma also influences physical and mental health outcomes and can disrupt or inhibit access to resources. Discrimination as a result of stigma can include name-calling and insults, such as accusations of sex work or HIV-positive status. It can also include being threatened, physically or socially, or harassed. Stigma and discrimination can be strong social determinants of health and effect one's psychological well-being through both self-esteem and interpersonal relationships.[4] As an example, in a study of Latin American transgender women, at least 50% of respondents reported being denied employment, housing, and access to restrooms; detained by law enforcement; and rejected by family members.[5] In this section, we discuss how TGD individuals in low- and middle-income countries are at risk of experiencing stigma due to **gender identity** and **gender expression**, sexual behavior, and actual or perceived HIV status.

Gender-Related Stigma

While gender identity is an aspect of the internal sense of self, gender expression, roles, and expectations are socially constructed. Expressions, roles, and expectations therefore vary across societal and cultural contexts, including the gender norms associated with occupation, familial roles, and societal values. Gender performance by TGD individuals may be perceived as a defiance of mainstream cisnormative expectations. Stigma can arise from either the perception of or the disclosure of gender expansive behaviors, presentations, and identities, including TGD identity,[6] whether or not it is labeled as such.

For example, in the Dominican Republic, transgender women faced stigma, discrimination, and abuse, low social support, and increased suicidality. They also experienced negative interpersonal interactions with family, friends, colleagues, and higher perceived transgender stigma. These social dynamics were associated with involvement in sex work, in which they experienced increased stigma and exposure to extreme gender-based physical and sexual violence, including attempted murder.[7,8] imilarly, in Brazil and India, where there are long histories of cultural roles of trans feminine people, TGD nevertheless report being treated poorly by strangers in public, as well as by classmates, family, and partner and clients for their gender presentations.[9]

Another example is the *hijra* community of the Indian subcontinent. The *hijra* community comprises individuals who were assigned male at birth, identify variously as women, feminine men, neither men nor women, transgender women, etc., and are recognized as third gender. This social category has existed for centuries; however, despite the fact that hijra play certain ceremonial roles (singers, dancers, blessers of weddings),[10] they have been historically excluded and stigmatized by mainstream cisheteronormative society and health systems, leading to vulnerabilities and socioeconomic insecurities. When adolescent *hijra* fail to portray stereotypical gender behaviors and fulfill familial expectations, they experience a higher risk of negligence, humiliation, and abusive incidents. *Hijra* are sometimes expected to assume two gender roles, a feminine role with age peers and outside the family, and a more "traditional" masculine role with relatives and family members,[11] placing an extra burden on their stress and mental health. An estimated one-third to two-thirds of *hijra* engage in sex work as a means of survival.[12]

Members of society can stigmatize and feel threatened by gender diversity, and sometimes enact sexual and intimate partner violence against TGD people. A Thailand-based study found a relationship between gender diversity and the prevalence of forced sex. Furthermore, TGD individuals in that study who experienced intimate partner violence feared secondary victimization due to social isolation and discrimination by law enforcement and support service providers.[13]

Sexual Behavior–Related Stigma

In addition to gender-related stigma, TGD people globally face sexual behavior–related stigma, whether that behavior is actual or presumed. Gender diversity is often interpreted as evidence of homosexual behavior, and in much of the world, gender identity is conflated with sexual orientation. Thus, it is often the sexual behavior that is *presumed* along with gender diversity that is stigmatized and policed by society, putting TGD people at risk of violence and discrimination. The vast majority of African TGD refugees in South Africa, for example, seek asylum for sexual orientation, rather than for gender identity.[14] In many cases, transgender women are seen as gay men, while transgender men are seen as lesbian women (and, conversely, gay men are stigmatized as "acting like women" or too feminine, and lesbian women as too masculine). Indeed, in sexual health research, transgender women (a proportion of whom have sex with **cisgender** women) are grouped erroneously with cisgender men who have sex with men, while transgender men (a proportion of whom have sex with cisgender men), are presumed to only have cisgender female sexual partners and thus are assumed to be at low risk for HIV and other sexually transmitted infections (STI).[6,15-17] Additionally, some TGD people may self-identify as gay rather than TGD, or use terms and labels, or a combination, that are unfamiliar to Westerners. Victor Mukasa, for example, an activist from Uganda who first sought asylum in South Africa and then the United States, labels himself as a "lesbian transgender man," and while recognizing that others may take issue with this term, feels that it encompasses his identity well.[14] Attention must be paid in clinical settings to understanding an individual's full sexual risk profile, rather than presuming TGD people's sexual orientation (which may be straight, gay, bisexual, queer, etc.), and gender or anatomy of their sexual partners (who may be cisgender or TGD, and also of any sexual orientation).

The psychosocial ramifications of stigma can result in low self-efficacy and negotiating power in sexual relationships to practice safer sex, making TGD individuals more vulnerable to sexual violence. There is some evidence that TGD individuals may also use sexual intercourse to reaffirm their gender identity and attractiveness among partners, which also may make them more vulnerable to exploitation and violence.[18,19] Studies in Lima, Peru found that transgender women are less likely to use condoms when they are not aware of their HIV status.[20] Another study found that transgender women are also more likely to feel pressured to take a receptive or insertive role in anal sex contrary to their preference compared with gay or bisexual men.[21] In a study of violence against TGD individuals in Lima, Peru, 65% of respondents had experienced violence.[22] Violence from law enforcement officers was often associated with survival sex work, especially as work conducted on the streets exposed workers to higher likelihood of police interactions. Institutional discrimination can reinforce this stigma as laws and policies that criminalize sex work and condone harassment by law enforcement can increase this population's vulnerability to violence.[23]

HIV-Related Stigma

Stigma related to HIV/AIDS status, whether actual or perceived, can result in social as well as health care–related discrimination. TGD individuals face constrained access to health care, which can affect the entire continuum of HIV prevention and care including access to preexposure prophylaxis (PrEP), antiretroviral postexposure prophylaxis, HIV testing, and maintaining antiretroviral therapy.[6] Additionally, stigma surrounding transgender women in particular affects both their risk perception and motivation to seek HIV testing and health services.[2] This stigma is predominantly enacted in places where TGD rights are not protected,[24] and where HIV service access is already burdened by HIV-related stigma and other structural barriers (distance, resource constraints, legal and policy environment).

Among Latinx respondents living with HIV, HIV/AIDS stigma has been linked to social isolation, low self-esteem, and negative psychological outcomes.[2] Evidence indicates that in many Latin American and Caribbean communities, people living with HIV/AIDS are considered deserving of their illness because of socially deviant behavior, such as engaging in "homosexual" relations (again, transgender women may be misread and mislabeled as homosexual men) or substance use disorders, and are therefore deemed untrustworthy. Even within the community (in this case, transgender women and cisgender men who have sex with men), "sero-sorting" (choosing partners based on HIV status) commonly occurs, in which HIV-negative individuals only associate with others who are HIV-negative.[25]

Similarly, discrimination and the fear of discrimination related to government-sponsored health services are prevalent in some settings. Accordingly, Brazilian transgender women seek health care from nongovernment organizations at a rate three times higher than from government-sponsored services.[26] Conversely, some governments recognize and include TGD populations in their official health policies. For example, the Laos government, recognizing that the *kathoey* (a trans feminine population) is a possible "bridge population" for STI transmission, included this group in the *National Strategy and Action Plan on HIV/AIDS/STI Control and Prevention 2006-2010*.[27] Ideally, the *kathoey* would be included as people at high risk of STI/HIV for their own sake, and not simply as a "bridge" to cisheteronormative people, which may further stigmatize and blame TGD. Providers and policymakers must take care to avoid perpetuating stigma against TGD people, particularly given the high risk of HIV among TGD populations, especially **trans feminine** people.

Sexual Health and Infectious Disease

Much of the data regarding TGD people's health comes from the United States and Canada, and much of the research from North America and especially around the world focuses on HIV in transgender women. Globally, transgender women are 48.8 times more likely to be HIV positive compared with all adults of reproductive age[28]; therefore, it is not surprising that much of the extant literature is HIV related. Much less is known about transgender men, nonbinary people, and non-HIV health conditions and needs of all TGD people.

A relatively small number of studies include data about transgender men's sexual health. The information that is available shows that TGD individuals **assigned female at birth (AFAB)** are at lower risk of becoming HIV positive than TGD individuals **assigned male at birth (AMAB)**, although both groups are at risk of HIV and other STIs when they have sex with cisgender men. TGD AFAB people can be at additional risk of unintended pregnancy[29] and reproductive conditions such as cervical cancer, while TGD AMAB people can be at risk of prostate as well as breast cancers. A review of studies available on HIV prevalence among TGD people in the United States estimates that 1.2–3.2% of transgender men and 14.2–21% of transgender women are living with HIV. However, 28.7% of transgender men and 21.1% of transgender women reported a history of STI,[30] indicating high risk in both groups, as well as an unmet need for safe and affirming sexual health services. A study assessing TGD patients who attend sexual health clinics in Australia illustrates how the progression of certain STI differs between transgender men and transgender women. A significant spike in the frequency of gonorrhea diagnoses among transgender women from 2013 to 2014 was not reflected in transgender men.[31] Transgender men, transgender women, and other TGD people face different sexual health risks and should not be viewed as a homogenous group by health care providers, but instead need to have health care services tailored to their unique needs.

As discussed above, stigma and discrimination impact the lives of TGD people to varying degrees. Anticipated stigma has been proven to impact a person's willingness to pursue sexual health resources.[32] Stigma and discrimination may lead to unemployment, social isolation, or homelessness, which necessitate sex work for many TGD people as a primary or secondary form of income. One study estimates that 31% of the TGD population in the United States has engaged in sex work. Transgender women are more likely than transgender men to engage in sex work, with 37.9% of the group reporting a history of sex work.[30] Although there are also transgender men who sell sex, almost no data exists about the experiences of these individuals. Globally, HIV prevalence is estimated to be 27.3% among transgender women engaging in sex work and 14.7% among those who do not.[28] The criminalization of and stigma against sex work increases the potential for dangerous partners and power dynamics, along with drug and alcohol use and coercive sex, including condomless sex.[33]

A qualitative study on PrEP in India provides an illustrative example of the health care barriers that TGD communities may face. This study included conversations with community leaders, local medical providers, and members of the *hijra* community. Many *hijra* experience unemployment and homelessness after rejection by family and society.[32] Most participants reacted positively to the possibility of PrEP, citing their belief that it would absolve some of the anxiety they felt when dealing with aggressive clients or untrustworthy law enforcement. However, fear of being publicly labeled as HIV positive remained a primary concern and unfortunately deterred a majority of participants from engaging with health care services. Participants also mentioned logistical barriers to accessing PrEP. Regularly traveling to a distribution location was anticipated to be difficult due to inconsistent but necessary work schedules. Participants and medical providers also mentioned concerns about unintended interactions with self-prescribed, unregulated hormones.[32]

Studies in Thailand and Cambodia on STI in transgender women demonstrate additional challenges encountered once TGD individuals enter into the health care setting. In a cohort of transgender women in Thailand, 37% tested positive for chlamydia or gonorrhea and 90% reported receptive anal intercourse with low prevalence of condom use. In a similar study conducted in Cambodia, having an STI dramatically increased the risk of contracting HIV.[34] Even if a TGD patient prioritizes HIV/STI testing, many diagnoses are missed if the anatomical sites tested are limited to sites of self-reported exposure.[35] Health care providers must be comfortable discussing TGD bodies in respectful and affirming ways. They must also be knowledgeable about and able to discuss high-risk behaviors in order to administer effective guidance and testing.

▶ Mental Health and Substance Use

Given the impacts of stigma, discrimination, and minority stress,[36–38] TGD people face higher rates of depression, suicidal ideation, and substance use disorders than cisgender people of any sexual orientation.[39] Early access to affirming mental health care may minimize rates of depression and anxiety among socially affirmed prepubescent TGD children. One study found that TGD children who are supported to live openly in their affirmed gender have the same rates of depression and only slightly elevated symptoms of anxiety when compared with cisgender children of the same age.[40] Many TGD people take steps to begin medical affirmation to alleviate psychological stress associated with gender dysphoria. Gender-affirming hormone therapy may be accompanied by surgery to align sex characteristics with a person's expressed gender. Hormone therapy has been linked to reduced depression, anxiety, and improved overall quality of life.[41] Both hormone therapy and gender-affirming surgeries (GAS), are essential for the mental health and physical safety of many TGD people, but access to treatment is often restricted by medical providers and income, especially in LMIC.[42,43]

TGD people in many LMIC experience high prevalence of depression and suicidal ideation, high rates of discrimination, and limited access to affirming healthcare. A 2019 survey found that 66.8% of Chinese participants would not accept their own child as TGD.[44] Many TGD people living in China are able to pursue an education and find employment, but the prevalence of depression remains high. In a 2019 national population survey in China, 80% of the TGD population was actively seeking hormone therapy.[45] A study on the challenges TGD people face in Pakistan also recounted widespread stigma and limited access to health care. The cultural emphasis on familial structures in Pakistan often results in isolation from the biological family and necessitates independent sources of income. Most participants lack a formal education, struggle with homelessness, and regularly engage in sex work to support themselves and their communities.[46] Comparatively, none of those challenges are listed as contributing factors in the U.S. or Chinese studies on mental health among TGD people; nevertheless, the rate of suicidal ideation falls between 54% and 57% for all three populations, with high rates of perceived stigma and minimal access to affirming medical treatment.

Affirming medical treatment is provided by a variety of different health care professionals. Those who resist or do not understand the needs of TGD patients make care inaccessible. Thoughtless and destructive encounters with mental health, general care, or surgical providers may further hinder a person's willingness to pursue better care.[47] A study found that transgender women in the United States struggling with depression and suicidal ideation were more likely to be afraid of seeking health care and avoid health care services.[48]

Nonbinary and other individuals who do not identify as either transgender women or transgender men are significantly less likely to have providers who know of and respect their identities and may be more likely to be misgendered than their binary TGD peers.[47] While data distinguishing between types of TGD individuals are sparse, some studies have identified varying rates of mental health challenges among binary and nonbinary TGD people that were assigned the same sex at birth.[49] A provider who is unaware of the distinctions between binary and nonbinary TGD people, as well as all the variations of gender diversity across different cultures and geographies, may hinder a person's ability to access appropriate care.

High rates of depression and social isolation experienced by TGD people contribute to disproportionate rates of substance use disorders. TGD people are two to four times more likely to abuse alcohol or drugs than cisgender people.[50] Drugs and alcohol may be used to cope with gender dysphoria or chronic pain as well as symptoms of depression and anxiety.[51] TGD people engaging in sex work are more likely to abuse a combination of drugs and alcohol to facilitate their work. Among TGD sex workers in China, for example, the highest rates of combination drug and alcohol use before transactional sex were observed in those with low self-esteem, loneliness, and depression.[52] Similarly, increased mental health distress was associated with greater use of amphetamine-like stimulants among TGD sex workers in Cambodia.[53] Depression and dysphoria are consistent factors throughout studies on substance abuse involving TGD people, no matter the frequency of sex work among participants. It is therefore paramount to include mental health services in models of care for TGD populations.

SERVICE MODELS FOR TRANSGENDER AND GENDER DIVERSE COMMUNITIES IN LMIC

Increasing coverage of culturally and clinically responsive services remains critical across the world, including in LMIC. Broadly, there are three categories of service delivery models for TGD health care. These include the following: (1) *mainstream models* where TGD people are served clinically in the context of health care services which also support cisgender people; (2) *integrated services* where the same physical spaces are used as in mainstream models but services are provided separately; and finally, (3) *stand-alone services* where the care for TGD clients is provided in physical spaces independent from other health care services. There is also a move toward the provision of general health services for TGD people in the context of primary care clinics, as long as there has been sufficient training among providers and efforts to improve the nonstigmatizing delivery of these services.[54,55]

To achieve high-quality mainstream or integrated services, there are critical areas to consider, such as modifying both the delivery and content of existing services. For delivery, the use of chosen names and personal pronouns, and the use of electronic health record systems that can record names on official documentation and chosen names, sex recorded at birth, current sex and gender identity on official documentation, and pronouns are paramount (see Chapter 4, "Harnassing Information Technology to Improve Clinical Care"). Moreover, modifications to the space are important, including all-inclusive restrooms and celebratory, affirming posters and artwork, in addition to ensuring training to support positive approaches to the celebration of gender identity in all engagements with clients.

Regarding content, best practices have been published by the Human Rights Campaign for service providers to better address the needs of TGD people. To work toward achieving health equity for TGD patients, organizations can utilize the Health Care Equality Index (HEI), a tool that focuses on nondiscrimination, equal visitation, employment nondiscrimination, and training in trans-affirming, patient-centered care. An additional tool developed by the Joint Commission (TJC) is the "Advancing Effective Communication, Cultural Competence Field Guide" that can be used to support improved service provision for TGD people.[56] Integration of training on gender-affirmative health care is a crucial ingredient of health practitioner training and should be done collaboratively with TGD community organizations. Evidence from these training curricula support the inclusion of gender-affirmative care early in clinical service training.[57,58]

Stand-alone services have been introduced at two extremes. At one end of the spectrum, stand-alone services operate in settings where stigma and criminalization limit the utility of mainstream or integrated services. These more nascent models are often created by community groups working to increase any gender-affirmative services in partnership with providers. At the other end of the spectrum, services have evolved into more comprehensive services for TGD people, but that are difficult to operationalize within the existing health care landscape. The Gender Units in Spain provide an example of comprehensive stand-alone services for TGD clients, and include leadership by the TGD community in partnership with clinics.[59]

SUMMARY

- Despite the fact that the majority of studies on the health and health care needs of TGD people to date have been performed in North America, TGD people exist in LMIC around the world, endure identity-based stigma and discrimination, and face higher risk of negative health outcomes, including but not limited to HIV, STIs, physical and sexual violence, mental health issues, and substance use disorders.

- Gender diversity and TGD identities vary widely across different cultures and geographies and are called many different names and do not have one-to-one equivalent constructs across cultures. These differences and nuances should be celebrated and studied to better understand their impacts on engagement in health care and health care outcomes.

- In designing and delivering interventions and health care services for TGD people, providers, policymakers, and implementers should be knowledgeable about the local situation around TGD issues, and not further perpetuate stigma against TGD people, especially in locations where TGD populations face stigma and discrimination from various quarters, including health and service providers.

- Transgender women, transgender men, nonbinary, and other gender diverse people face disparate health risks and needs and should have health care services tailored to their different needs. While certain TGD may be more visible than others in a given location (i.e., *hijra*, *kathoey*), a full spectrum of gender diversity exists everywhere, and each group deserves attention to their health needs and priorities.

- Health care professionals must also be competent and comfortable to discuss TGD bodies in respectful and affirming ways, and knowledgeable about their various health risks to initiate appropriate guidance, screening, and testing. This necessitates sensitivity training adapted to address local gender diversity, terminology, and availability of transition-related care.

- Whether health services are provided in mainstream models, integrated, stand-alone, or primary care services, all health care for TGD should prioritize nondiscrimination and training in trans-competent, patient-centered care. Choice of model must be informed by local legal and social conditions, with extra attention paid to privacy and confidentiality, and care taken to not further exacerbate stigma and discrimination.

CASE STUDY

In Lebanon, TGD people face intersectional stigma across many facets of life. According to the most recent Pew survey, more than 80% of Lebanese people support a strictly binary gendered society, and a majority believe that it is important to adhere to the concept of sex as opposed to a flexible interpretation of gender. A study of social support and gender affirmation in the Middle East found that one-third of the TGD Lebanese participants have engaged in sex work, and less than one-half have ever been tested for HIV or other STIs. Most participants reported experiencing physical violence, and half of the participants had experienced sexual assault. At least 10% of the trans feminine population is estimated to be living with HIV.[60] This estimate is likely low, but the rate surpasses that of any other key population in Lebanon, including the 1.5–3.6% prevalence among cisgender men who have sex with men.[61] Local efforts have found a lack of knowledge among health care providers in the country regarding TGD health[62] and have focused on providing a list of affirming providers to work with TGD individuals.[63]

Imagine you work as a clinical provider in a queer- and gender-affirming clinic in the United States. You are hired as a consultant to provide technical assistance to a grassroots organization in Beirut, Lebanon that wants to expand into clinical HIV services. During a site visit, the organization hosts a listening session with some of their clientele for you to attend. In the room are clients of various gender expressions and presentations, and participants variously introduce themselves as men, women, transgender, gay, "she male," and with local terminology that does not translate well to English. As the session proceeds, the facilitator has

the participants discuss HIV prevention and treatment services, but the conversation also turns to other topics: drunk, violent clients in the sex work industry; hormone therapy; storage and disposal of used syringes; tobacco and alcohol use; dependence on, but stigma from and rejection by family; religious stigma about homosexuality; and discrimination from care providers. As these topics arise, the facilitator politely acknowledges them, expresses sympathy, then steers the discussion back to HIV prevention and treatment. The session indicates there is some interest in PrEP, interest in free condoms despite inconsistent use, and good knowledge of HIV, but variable self-awareness of HIV vulnerability. One participant reveals she is living with the virus and feels embarrassed and ashamed when she accesses care, because she has to pretend that she is male, which is her sex assigned at birth and the designation on her identification. Another traveled 3 hours on two different buses to arrive at the meeting in Beirut.

▶ Discussion Questions

- What assumptions did you make about the participants' gender identities? How do these differ from and challenge your definitions of sexual orientation and gender identity?

- What considerations are important in cross-cultural clinical work with regard to terminology, differing cultural values and beliefs, and religion?

- What assumptions did you make about people's sexual risks with the descriptions above? Who is at risk of acquiring or transmitting HIV? Who is not? How do you know? Who is at risk of pregnancy? Who is not? How do you know?

- After the listening session, what issues do you want to discuss with the organization's leadership on expanding HIV services?

- What key issues will you recommend the providers need to be trained on, including and beyond HIV-related care?

- What barriers do you anticipate the target clientele will face in accessing the clinic in Lebanon? In adherence to and persistence on PrEP/antiretroviral therapy?

- In addition to HIV clinical services, what, if any, other services do you recommend the organization provide that might support and affirm the clients?

REFERENCES

1. Goffman E. *Stigma*. London: Penguin; 1963.
2. Magno L, Silva L, Veras MA, Pereira-Santos M, Dourado I. Stigma and discrimination related to gender identity and vulnerability to HIV/AIDS among transgender women: a systematic review. *Cad Saude Publica*. 2019;35(4):e00112718.

3. Poteat T, German D, Kerrigan D. Managing uncertainty: a grounded theory of stigma in transgender health care encounters. *Soc Sci Med*. 2013;84:22-29.

4. Bouman WP, Davey A, Meyer C, Witcomb GL, Arcelus J. Predictors of psychological well-being among treatment seeking transgender individuals. *Sex Relation Ther*. 2016:1-17.

5. Bazargan M, Galvan F. Perceived discrimination and depression among low-income Latina male-to-female transgender women. *BMC Public Health*. 2012;12(663).

6. Poteat T, German D, Flynn C. The conflation of gender and sex: Gaps and opportunities in HIV data among transgender women and MSM. *Glob Public Health*. 2016;11(7-8):835-848.

7. Budhwani H, Hearld KR, Milner AN, et al. Transgender women's experiences with stigma, trauma, and attempted suicide in the Dominican Republic. *Suicide Life-Threatening Behav*. 2018;48(6):788-796.

8. Milner AN, Hearld KR, Abreau N, Budhwani H, Mayra Rodriguez-Lauzurique R, Paulino-Ramirez R. Sex work, social support, and stigma: Experiences of transgender women in the Dominican Republic. *Int J Transgend*. 2019;20(4):403-412.

9. Gomes de Jesus J, Belden CM, Huynh HV, et al. Mental health and challenges of transgender women: a qualitative study in Brazil and India. *Int J Transg Health*. 2020;21(4):418-430.

10. Chakrapani V. *Hijras/Transgender Women in India: HIV, Human Rights and Social Exclusion*. India: UNDP; 2010.

11. Rodriquez Madera SL. *TRANSGender: Moving Through the Gray Zones*. San Juan, Puerto Rico: Terranova; 2009.

12. National AIDS Control Organization (NACO). *National Integrated Biological and Behavioral Surveillance 2014-15 Hijras/Transgender People*. Ministry of Health and Family Welfare, Government of India; 2016.

13. Guadamuz TE, Wimonsate W, Varangrat A, et al. Correlates of forced sex among populations of men who have sex with men in Thailand. *Arch Sex Behav*. 2011;40(2):259-266.

14. Camminga B. *Transgender Refugees and the Imagined South Africa: Bodies Over Borders and Borders Over Bodies*. London: Palgrave Macmillan; 2018.

15. Stephenson R, Riley E, Rogers E, et al. The sexual health of transgender men: a scoping review. *J Sex Res*. 2017;54(4-5):424-445.

16. Reisner SL, Moore CS, Asquith A, et al. High risk and low uptake of pre-exposure prophylaxis to prevent HIV acquisition in a national online sample of transgender men who have sex with men in the United States. *J Int AIDS Soc*. 2019;22(9).

17. Scheim AI, Santos G-M, Arreola S, et al. Inequities in access to HIV prevention services for transgender men: results of a global survey of men who have sex with men. 2016;19 (3 Suppl 2).

18. Sevelius JM. Gender affirmation: a framework for conceptualizing risk behavior among transgender women of color. *Sex Roles*. 2013;68(11-12):675-689.

19. Reisner SL, Perkovich B, Mimiaga MJ. A mixed methods study of the sexual health needs of New England transmen who have sex with nontransgender men. *AIDS Patient Care STDs*. 2010;24(8):501-513.

20. Satcher MF, Segura ER, Silva-Santisteban A, Sanchez J, Lama JR, Clark JL. Partner-level factors associated with insertive and receptive condomless anal intercourse among transgender women in Lima, Peru. *AIDS Behav*. 2017;21(8):2439-2451.

21. Satcher M, Segura ER, Silva-Santisteban A, Reisner SL, Lama JR, Clark JL. Exploring contextual differences for receptive and

22. Murphy EC, Segura ER, Lake JE, et al. Intimate partner violence against transgender women: prevalence and correlates in Lima, Peru (2016-2018). *AIDS Behav*. 2019.

insertive role strain among transgender women and men who have sex with men in Lima, Peru. *Sex Transm Inf*. 2015;91.

23. Delgado JB, Castro MC. Construction and validation of a subjective scale of stigma and discrimination (SISD) for the gay men and transgender women population in Chile. *Sexual Res Social Policy*. 2014;11(3):187-198.

24. International Lesbian G, Bisexual, Trans and Intersex Association, Chiam Z, Duffy S, Mtilda GG. *Trans Legal Mapping Report: Recognition before the Law*. Geneva: ILGA; November 2017.

25. Ramirez-Valles J, Molina Y, Dirkes J. Stigma towards PLWHA: the role of internalized homosexual stigma in Latino gay/bisexual male and transgender communities. *AIDS Educ Prev*. 2013;25(3):179-189.

26. Pinheiro Junior FM, Kendall C, Martins TA, et al. Risk factors associated with resistance to HIV testing among transwomen in Brazil. *AIDS Care*. 2016;28(1):92-97.

27. Longfield K, Panyanouvong X, Chen J, Kays MB. Increasing safer sexual behavior among Lao kathoy through an integrated social marketing approach. *BMC Public Health*. 2011;11:872.

28. Baral S, Poteat T, Stromdahl S, Wirtz A, Guadamuz T, Beyrer C. Worldwide burden of HIV in transgender women: a systematic review and meta-analysis. *Lancet Infect Dis*. 2013;13:214-222.

29. Hoffkling A, Obedin-Maliver J, Sevelius J. From erasure to opportunity: a qualitative study of the experiences of transgender men around pregnancy and recommendations for providers. *BMC Pregnancy Childbirth*. 2017;17(suppl 2):332.

30. Becasen JS, Denard CL, Mullins MM, Higa DH, Sipe TA. Estimating the prevalence of HIV and sexual behaviors among the US transgender population: a systematic review and meta-analysis, 2006-2017. *Am J Public Health*. 2018:e1-e8.

31. Callander D, Cook T, Read P, et al. Sexually transmissible infections among transgender men and women attending Australian sexual health clinics. *Med J Aust*. 2019;211(9):406-411.

32. Chakrapani V, Shunmugam M, Rawat S, Baruah D, Nelson R, Newman PA. Acceptability of HIV pre-exposure prophylaxis among transgender women in India: a qualitative investigation. *AIDS Patient Care STDS*. 2020;34(2):92-98.

33. UNAIDS. UNAIDS Data 2018. UNAIDS. https://www.unaids.org/sites/default/files/media_asset/unaids-data-2018_en.pdf. Published 2018. Accessed December 2019.

34. Chhim S, Ngin C, Chhoun P, et al. HIV prevalence and factors associated with HIV infection among transgender women in Cambodia: results from a national Integrated Biological and Behavioral Survey. *BMJ Open*. 2017;7(8):e015390.

35. Hiransuthikul A, Janamnuaysook R, Sungsing T, et al. High burden of chlamydia and gonorrhea in pharyngeal, rectal and urethral sites among Thai transgender women: implications for anatomical site selection for the screening of STI. *Sex Transm Infect*. 2019;95(7):534-539.

36. Testa RJ, Habarth J, Peta J, Balsam K, Bockting W. Development of the gender minority stress and resilience measure. *Psychol Sexual Orient Gender Diversity*. 2015;2(1):65-77.

37. Brooks V. *Minority Stress and Lesbian Women*. Lexington, MA: Lexington Books; 1981.

38. Meyer IH. Prejudice, social stress, and mental health in lesbian, gay, and bisexual populations: conceptual issues and research evidence. *Psychol Bull*. 2003;129(5):674-697.

39. Price-Feeney M, Green AE, Dorison S. Understanding the mental health of transgender and nonbinary youth. *J Adolesc Health.* 2020.

40. Olson KR, Durwood L, DeMeules M, McLaughlin KA. Mental health of transgender children who are supported in their identities. *Pediatrics.* 2016;137(3):e20153223.

41. Nguyen HB, Chavez AM, Lipner E, et al. Gender-affirming hormone use in transgender individuals: impact on behavioral health and cognition. *Curr Psychiatry Rep.* 2018;20(12):110.

42. Rowniak S, Bolt L, Sharifi C. Effect of cross-sex hormones on the quality of life, depression and anxiety of transgender individuals: a quantitative systematic review. *JBI Database System Rev Implement Rep.* 2019;17(9):1826-1854.

43. Wernick JA, Busa S, Matouk K, Nicholson J, Janssen A. A systematic review of the psychological benefits of gender-affirming surgery. *Urol Clin North Am.* 2019;46(4):475-486.

44. Wang Y, Hu Z, Peng K, et al. Discrimination against LGBT populations in China. *Lancet Public Health.* 2019;4(9):e440-e441.

45. Chen R, Zhu X, Wright L, et al. Suicidal ideation and attempted suicide amongst Chinese transgender persons: National population study. *J Affect Disord.* 2019;245:1126-1134.

46. Shah HBU, Rashid F, Atif I, et al. Challenges faced by marginalized communities such as transgenders in Pakistan. *Pan Afr Med J.* 2018;30:96.

47. Kattari SK, Bakko M, Hecht HK, Kattari L. Correlations between healthcare provider interactions and mental health among transgender and nonbinary adults. *SSM Popul Health.* 2020;10:100525.

48. Maksut JL, Sanchez TH, Wiginton JM, et al. Gender identity and sexual behavior stigmas, severe psychological distress, and suicidality in an online sample of transgender women in the United States. *Ann Epidemiol.* 2020;52:15-22.

49. Newcomb ME, Hill R, Buehler K, Ryan DT, Whitton SW, Mustanski B. High burden of mental health problems, substance use, violence, and related psychosocial factors in transgender, non-binary, and gender diverse youth and young adults. *Arch Sex Behav.* 2020;49(2):645-659.

50. Day JK, Fish JN, Perez-Brumer A, Hatzenbuehler ML, Russell ST. Transgender youth substance use disparities: results from a population-based sample. *J Adolesc Health.* 2017;61(6):729-735.

51. Carmel TC, Erickson-Schroth L. Mental health and the transgender population. *J Psychosoc Nurs Ment Health Serv.* 2016;54(12):44-48.

52. Wang Q, Chang R, Wang Y, et al. Correlates of alcohol and illicit drug use before commercial sex among transgender women with a history of sex work in China. *Sex Health.* 2019.

53. Mburu G, Tuot S, Mun P, Chhoun P, Chann N, Yi S. Prevalence and correlates of amphetamine-type stimulant use among transgender women in Cambodia. *Int J Drug Policy.* 2019;74:136-143.

54. Safer JD, Tangpricha V. Care of the transgender patient. *Ann Intern Med.* 2019;171(1):Itc1-itc16.

55. Creating respectful health care for trans patients. *The Lancet.* 2019;394(10192).

56. The Joint Commission. *Advancing Effective Communication, Cultural Competence, and Patient- and Family-Centered Care for the Lesbian, Gay, Bisexual, and Transgender (LGBT) Community: A Field Guide.* Oak Brook, IL: The Joint Commission; 2011.

57. Dowshen N, Nguyen GT, Gilbert K, Feiler A, Margo KL. Improving transgender health education for future doctors. *Am J Public Health.* 2014;104(7):e5-6.

58. Safer JD, Pearce EN. A simple curriculum content change increased medical student comfort with transgender medicine. *Endocr Pract.* 2013;19(4):633-637.

59. Esteva de Antonio I, Gómez-Gil E. Coordination of healthcare for transsexual persons: a multidisciplinary approach. *Curr Opin Endocrinol Diabetes Obes.* 2013;20(6):585-591.

60. Kaplan RL, McGowan J, Wagner GJ. HIV prevalence and demographic determinants of condomless receptive anal intercourse among trans feminine individuals in Beirut, Lebanon. *J Int AIDS Soc.* 2016;19(3 suppl 2):20787.

61. Wagner GJ, Tohme J, Hoover M, et al. HIV prevalence and demographic determinants of unprotected anal sex and HIV testing among men who have sex with men in Beirut, Lebanon. *Arch Sex Behav.* 2014;43(4):779-788.

62. Wright K, Peplinksi B, Abboud S, Harfouch O. *A Stakeholder Analysis of the Current Lebanese Context for Transgender Healthcare: The Perspectives of Non-Governmental Organizations.* Beirut, Lebanon: Lebanese Medical Association for Sexual Health Johns: Hopkins Bloomberg School of Public Health; 2017.

63. Naal H, Abboud S, Mahmoud H. Developing an LGBT-affirming healthcare provider directory in Lebanon. *J Gay Lesbian Mental Health.* 2018;23(1):107-110.

Transgender and Gender Diverse People and Incarceration

23

Jaclyn White Hughto

Kirsty A. Clark

INTRODUCTION

Although there are currently no systematic efforts to document the number of **transgender and gender diverse** (TGD) people in U.S. jails and prisons, research finds that TGD people are disproportionately incarcerated in the United States relative to the general population.[1] Some evidence suggests that 16% of the estimated 1.4 million transgender adults in the United States[2] have been incarcerated in their lifetime,[3] compared with just 3% of the general U.S. population.[4] Although both **trans feminine** people and **trans masculine** people are at disproportionate risk for incarceration, the incarceration rate is particularly elevated among trans feminine people, with lifetime estimates of incarceration ranging from 19% to 65% across studies.[3,5–7]

One of the main drivers behind the high burden of incarceration among TGD people is **stigma.** Stigma is the social process of labeling, stereotyping, and rejecting human difference as a form of social control.[8,9] Stigma restricts access to resources for TGD people, including employment and housing, leading some TGD people to turn to street economies, such as survival sex work or substance use to cope with mistreatment, which places them at higher risk for arrest and incarceration.[3,6,10,11] Biased policing and sentencing practices also contribute to high rates of incarceration among TGD people.[3,12]

Once incarcerated, TGD people are typically housed in sex-segregated facilities according to their genitalia. Thus, TGD people who have not had genital construction surgery are typically placed in facilities that do not match their **gender identity** or expression; for example, trans feminine people are typically incarcerated in men's prisons. Once incarcerated, TGD people are at high risk for experiencing verbal, physical, and sexual assault.[3,13,14] Victimization of TGD people may be perpetrated by other inmates as well as jail and prison staff.[3,13,15] These risks are particularly elevated for trans feminine people in men's facilities, where femininity is not only devalued but routinely punished.[16–18] Notably,

experiencing victimization in correctional facilities has been shown to contribute to poor physical and mental health for TGD people.[14,19–22]

Like all detainees, incarcerated TGD people may need to access physical and mental health services to meet their preventative, chronic, and urgent health care needs; some TGD people may also require medical care to affirm their gender. Medically affirming one's gender can include the use of exogenous hormone therapy (e.g., estrogen for trans feminine people, testosterone for trans masculine people) or surgery (e.g., genital construction surgery) to feminize or masculinize the body. Hormone therapy may be the first or only form of medical gender affirmation intervention sought.[23] Given that TGD people may require a variety of health services while incarcerated, access to supportive health care professionals who are knowledgeable about TGD people and their needs is essential to ensuring the health of incarcerated TGD people.

This chapter uses the **ecological (or ecosocial) model** of transgender stigma[20] to outline the structural (institutions, culture, policies) and interpersonal (interactions with others) factors that influence the health of incarcerated TGD people at the individual or person level (see Figure 3-2). This chapter also documents the resilience of incarcerated TGD people and the ways in which TGD people fight back against systems of oppression within correctional environments. Factors impacting incarcerated TGD people's health are described using a combination of empirical research and case studies drawn from empirical research. Steps that correctional health care professionals (e.g., physicians, nurses, mental health professionals) can take to combat stigmatizing forces in jails and prisons are outlined. Also described are the ways in which correctional health care professionals can intervene to address health outcomes for TGD people and provide specific recommendations about changes that are needed in correctional facilities to improve the health of incarcerated TGD people.

STRUCTURAL FACTORS THAT INFLUENCE THE HEALTH OF INCARCERATED TGD PEOPLE

Structured according to sex, and more specifically, to genitalia, jails and prisons are among the most gender-binary institutions that exist in the United States. Within this **binary** system, having a gender identity or expression that aligns based on traditional expectations with one's physical sex characteristics is seen as normative, while TGD people are seen as the "other."[24,25] It is the very structure of correctional environments that legitimatizes social norms regarding what it means to be a man or woman and bestows the **cisgender** majority (e.g., cisgender inmates, correctional officers, health care professionals, and administrators) with the power and privilege to control and subjugate incarcerated TGD people.[24,25] In addition to the environmental conditions of correctional facilities, **structural stigma** toward TGD people in jails and prisons is manifested through policies and practices that restrict access to health-promoting resources and limit the opportunities, health, and well-being of incarcerated TGD people.[16] This section highlights three primary structural forces that impact the health of incarcerated TGD people: correctional housing policies and practices, correctional health care policies, and correctional policies dictating gender expression.

▶ Correctional Housing Policies and Practices

Incarcerated TGD people who have not had gender-affirming genital construction surgery are generally housed according to their genitalia.[26-29] Housing is assigned regardless of a person's appearance, legal changes in gender markers, or whether they have had feminizing or masculinizing hormones or surgical gender affirmation (e.g., breast augmentation for trans feminine people or chest construction surgery for trans masculine people).[16] Due to the potential for victimization, genitalia-based housing classification is often associated with adverse health outcomes for incarcerated TGD people, especially for trans feminine people incarcerated in men's facilities. Moreover, under the guise of protection, many TGD people are placed in segregated housing units (e.g., solitary confinement), which can result in psychological distress and self-harm.[16]

Because of the threats of violence and victimization faced by incarcerated TGD people, many choose to enter or are forced to enter a segregated housing unit (SHU) or "protective custody," for example, housing an inmate away from the general population due to risk of violence.[15,16,18] In contrast, some trans masculine people in women's facilities are forced to enter SHU due to administrators' fears that they will make cisgender inmates feel uncomfortable or commit violence against cisgender inmates.[30] SHUs are reserved for inmates who are considered to be more likely to commit violence

against others or those who are at a higher risk of victimization by inmates in the general population, including political figures, child sex offenders, or gang members.[31] In many SHUs, inmates are confined to their cell for 23 hours per day, 7 days a week, and have no access to educational, vocational, or rehabilitative programs afforded to the general population.[32,33] The adverse mental health effects associated with long-term correctional isolation are well established, including symptoms of depression, psychosis, and posttraumatic stress disorder, along with higher rates of self-harm and suicide compared with the general prison population.[34] TGD people who enter SHUs report feelings of isolation, rejection, and fears of discrimination from the general inmate population.[33,35]

▶ Correctional Policies Dictating Gender Expression

Prison rules, regulations, and practices encourage prison officials and correctional officers to express commitment to hegemonic gender norms, including traditional notions of femininity and masculinity.[16,33,36] For instance, TGD people are often misgendered in jails and prisons even after having a legal name change (e.g., trans feminine people whose pronouns are she/her are housed in men's facilities and often referred to with he/him pronouns).[33] Furthermore, TGD people are often subject to gendered dress codes.[16,33] For instance, in the California correctional system's Department Operations Manuals (DOM), people incarcerated in women's facilities are permitted to wear earrings, makeup, clear nail polish, and have access to women's undergarments; in contrast, people incarcerated in men's facilities are denied these expressions of femininity.[33] Additionally, grooming standards often require trans feminine people in men's facilities to keep their hair short and stereotypically masculine, with many facilities forcing inmates to cut their hair short upon intake. Similarly, research conducted with transgender women who were housed in men's facilities in New England found that transgender women were prevented from wearing makeup and wearing their hair in a ponytail while incarcerated.[16] In many men's facilities, a transgender person discovered with designated female commissary items is punished for possession of "contraband," often leading to solitary confinement as a form of punishment.[16,29,31] Although less is known about the experiences of trans masculine people incarcerated in women's facilities, masculinity is valued in all correctional environments, and thus expressions of masculinity are common among both incarcerated cisgender men and trans masculine people.[30]

Efforts to control the gender expression of trans feminine people housed in men's facilities have been linked to poor mental health in this population. A qualitative study of transgender women in New England found that policies and practices that restricted and even punished transgender women for having a feminine gender expression led transgender women to feel controlled, belittled, and demoralized as a result.[16] In another study of transgender women incarcerated in men's facilities in New York, participants described feeling depressed and reported the need for counseling in order to prevent them from harming themselves.[31] This research demonstrates how the presence and enforcement of rules and regulations that inhibit TGD people's gender expression while incarcerated can ultimately influence the development of depression and suicidality in this population.

Correctional Health Care Policies

Because of the health disparities faced by TGD people relative to the general U.S. population,[37,38] TGD people are likely to enter the correctional system with health care needs.[39,40] Incarcerated TGD people also require medical care to meet their general and gender identity-related health care needs, including gender-affirming interventions such as hormone therapy or surgical procedures.[23] Many TGD people meet the diagnostic criteria for **gender dysphoria**.[41] An established body of medical research demonstrates the clinical value of access to gender-affirming mental health care, hormone therapy, and surgery as efficacious treatments for gender dysphoria.[23,42,43] For incarcerated TGD people, however, gender dysphoria is often ignored by correctional staff, and medically necessary treatment is frequently prohibited. Notably, failure to treat gender dysphoria can result in clinically significant psychological distress, depression, anxiety, suicidal thoughts and behaviors, and autocastration attempts among incarcerated TGD people.[23,27,28]

Efforts have been made to help ensure the safety and protection of incarcerated TGD people at the federal and state levels, with varied results. One such change is the Prison Rape Elimination Act (PREA). Enacted in 2002, PREA is a federal mandate to document instances of prison rape in Federal, State, and local jurisdictions and to provide recommendations to protect individuals from prison rape.[44] PREA recognizes transgender people as a vulnerable population and provides guidelines on their health care and housing in U.S. prisons.[45] However, there are limited data regarding oversight of this policy in practice, and reports from incarcerated transgender women cite lack of enforcement of the PREA guidelines, except when utilized punitively, such as prison administrators using PREA to justify housing transgender women involuntarily in segregated housing units.[32,46]

At the state level, correctional health care policies pertaining to incarcerated TGD people vary considerably in length, depth, cultural responsiveness, and enforcement.[26,27] One study from 2009 employed the Freedom of Information Act to request state-level transgender health care policies from U.S. Departments of Correction (DOC).[26] Overall, 6 states refused to respond; 19 states reported they had zero guidelines, policies, or directives on managing the health of incarcerated transgender people; and the remaining 25 states varied considerably in the length, breadth, and level of cultural responsiveness of policies and guidelines specific to gender-affirming medical care. A more recent content analysis from 2015 examined state-level statutes and DOC policies from all 50 states on incarcerated transgender people's medical care.[27] Similar to the investigation from 2009, policies varied widely from state to state and treatment to treatment, with 10 states having no policies available on medical care for incarcerated transgender people; 28 states denying access to all gender-affirming treatments (e.g., hormone therapy, surgery); 21 states allowing for the continuation of hormone therapy if prescribed prior to incarceration; 13 states allowing for initiation of hormone therapy while incarcerated; and just 7 states allowing for gender-affirming surgery.[27]

Because of the wide variability in policies across states and lack of oversight or enforcement of such policies, the potential for harm associated with the delivery of gender-affirming medical care (or lack thereof) in prisons and jails is immense. One clear example of such harm is the abrupt cessation of medically necessary hormone therapy upon incarceration. Hormone therapy is an essential component of health care for some TGD people, as it alleviates the psychological distress of gender dysphoria[23,47] and has been linked to improved mental health outcomes (e.g., reduced depression and anxiety) and quality of life.[43,48] Even in states where there is a policy in place allowing TGD people to continue hormone therapy, policies often stipulate that once incarcerated, the inmate must procure a letter from a physician or provide a prescription proving that they were accessing hormones prior to incarceration.[16,29,49,50] TGD people report experiencing significant barriers to accessing medical care prior to incarceration, including refusal of health care, harassment, and violence in medical settings,[20,51] as well as the high rates of poverty, unemployment, and homelessness among TGD populations.[13,20] Many TGD people who are not incarcerated are forced to procure hormones from nonmedical sources, including friends, community members, and "street" vendors, to alleviate their gender dysphoria.[52,53] As a result, TGD people who are accessing hormones from nonmedical sources, and later become incarcerated, are unable to provide the documentation required to continue hormone therapy while in jail or prison.[3,13] When hormone therapy is stopped abruptly upon entering incarceration, TGD people can face severe adverse health outcomes, including nausea, severe itching, depression, and genital self-mutilation.[27] Indeed, one study investigating the health care experiences of incarcerated transgender women showed that 5% reported attempted (2%) or completed (3%) autocastration, with one incarcerated transgender woman noting that the department of corrections refused to treat her gender dysphoria and therefore she removed her testicles herself as a means to block the source of testosterone in her body.[50,54]

Together, these structural factors highlight the urgent need to revise restrictive policies that isolate incarcerated TGD people, minimize gender expression, and restrict access to medically necessary, gender-affirming care for incarcerated TGD people.

▶ Recommended Changes at the Structural Level

The following is a list of recommended changes that can be implemented at the structural level to support TGD people in navigating system-level barriers to health and well-being while incarcerated, including recommendations specific to housing, gender expression, and health care policies. These recommendations are drawn from research documenting structural barriers to health for incarcerated TGD people with correctional health care professionals, administrators, formerly incarcerated TGD people, criminal justice advocates, and transgender health scholars in the United States and globally[15,28,29,55,56]:

- Institute a case-by-case housing policy whereby TGD people are assessed individually for their housing assignment, taking into consideration the individual's gender identity and personal housing preference, in conjunction with the individual's overall safety and security.

- Reassess housing policies at least twice per year to assure that housing circumstances are appropriate and that the inmate has not faced abuse or harm based on the housing assignment, including being placed in "protective custody."

- Provide the option, where relevant and desired by both parties, for a TGD person to be housed in the same cell or unit as another TGD or LGBTQIA+ person.

- Establish standards of health care for incarcerated TGD people in consultation with correctional health care professionals, experts in TGD health, and current standards of care for the provision of gender-affirming medical and mental health care for TGD populations.

- Provide general and gender-affirming health care (e.g., hormone therapy) for all incarcerated TGD people who require it, regardless of an individual's ability to document prior medical care or prescriptions.

- Create clear policies that provide incarcerated TGD people with access to gender-affirming mental health care, including individual and group talk therapy with other transgender or LGBTQIA+ inmates, as recommended by mental health clinicians.

- Allow TGD people to access gender-specific clothing, grooming, hygiene, and commissary items, including undergarments consistent with their gender identity.

- Ensure all correctional facility staff adopt incarcerated TGD people's correct name and pronouns, in accordance with each inmate's wishes.

▶ What Health Care Professionals Can Do to Address Structural Factors that Influence the Health of Incarcerated TGD People

Although health care professionals in correctional settings often report feeling confined by the structural factors that negatively impact the health of incarcerated TGD people,[49] there are many ways in which they can navigate structural barriers to improve the health and well-being of incarcerated TGD people. For instance, health care professionals can take the initiative to understand the housing, health care, and gender expression policies in place at their institution. Because of the wide variability in policies from state to state and institution to institution, it is pertinent that health care professionals investigate and become knowledgeable about the gender identity- and gender expression-related policies specific to their institution. Additionally, correctional health care professionals can advocate for the creation of gender-affirming policies and practices within their institutions. For example, in correctional settings in which a TGD person's housing is decided on a case-by-case basis (e.g., the decision to place a TGD inmate in "protective custody" or general population at intake), health care professionals might ask to participate in housing discussions to provide informed medical consultation on the impact of housing decisions on TGD inmates' safety and health. Health care professionals should also educate their peers on the harms of denying access to medically necessary hormones and encourage their colleagues to advocate for initiating or continuing hormone therapy for TGD people who require these treatments. By becoming educated on the current policies and guidelines related to TGD medical care in their state and at their institution, and advocating for the well-being of TGD people regarding correctional housing, health care, and gender expression policies, correctional health care professionals can play a critical role in advancing the health of incarcerated TGD people.

INTERPERSONAL FACTORS THAT INFLUENCE THE HEALTH OF INCARCERATED TGD PEOPLE

Given their stigmatized identity inside and outside of incarceration settings, TGD people are prone to experiencing interpersonal stigma, which refers to the unfair treatment of a stigmatized person by a nonstigmatized person,[57] with actions ranging from exclusion to verbal abuse to violent attacks.[20] In correctional settings, interpersonal stigma toward TGD people manifests in the form of verbal, physical, and sexual assaults, and violence from other incarcerated people and staff, including correctional health care professionals.[18,28,36,56,58]

▶ Interpersonal Stigma from Inmates and Prison Staff

Reports of cisgender inmates verbally abusing incarcerated TGD people are common and include name-calling, referring to TGD people with homophobic and transphobic slurs, and stating that TGD people have a "mental disease" or would be better off dead.[31,36,59] Reports of harassment and mistreatment coming from correctional officers (COs) are also common and include severe verbal harassment[49,50] and purposeful humiliation through targeted gender-based discrimination (e.g., hanging up a transgender woman's undergarments for the men's unit to see).[31,36]

Incarcerated TGD people are also at risk for physical assault and harassment by COs and other inmates. Physical assault by COs is often enacted in the form of aggressive means of subduing an inmate or violent forms of punishment, for example, slamming a TGD inmate against a wall, causing bodily harm.[31,60] A U.S. study of 6450 transgender individuals found that among the 749 transgender women in the sample who had been incarcerated, 38% had been harassed, and 9% had been physically assaulted by prison staff.[61] Physical assaults by other inmates are also highly prevalent in incarceration settings, especially in men's prison facilities, where hypermasculinity drives violence against trans feminine people. Physical assaults by other inmates have included acts of violence toward incarcerated TGD people, ranging from slapping and punching to acts of violence, causing grave bodily injury.[36,62]

Sexual assault in the U.S. prison system is also widespread. The National Inmate Survey (NIS), conducted between 2011 and 2012, highlights that an estimated 4% of state and federal prison inmates report sexual assault by prisoners or staff while incarcerated.[63] Although TGD people were likely miscategorized as female or male in the National Inmate Survey, the current literature suggests that sexual victimization of incarcerated TGD people, especially trans feminine people, is disproportionately high. In a sample of inmates in California, 59% of incarcerated TGD people reported experiencing sexual assault while incarcerated, which is 13 times higher than the prevalence of sexual assault experienced among the general prison population.[17] In the California-based sample, 75% of the transgender inmates reported being sexually assaulted on multiple occasions. Qualitative research also highlights sexual assault against incarcerated trans feminine people, including unwanted sexual touching, unwarranted strip searches and pat-downs, and forcible oral and anal penetrative sex by inmates and COs.[16,31,33,36,59,64,65]

The adverse health effects of interpersonal stigma through verbal, physical, and sexual abuse are severe. In addition to the direct bodily harm resultant from physical and sexual violence, incarcerated TGD people who have experienced assault report feelings of depression, anxiety, suicidal ideation and attempt, and self-harm.[29,31,50] Death by suicide as a result of sexual assault against incarcerated transgender women has also been reported.[59]

▶ Interpersonal Stigma and Support from Correctional Health Care Professionals

Access to health care in prisons and jails is also fraught with interpersonal stigma. TGD people experience gender-based discrimination from correctional health care professionals, which is often due to professionals' lack of gender identity-related cultural responsiveness and clinical skills.[16,49] Indeed, qualitative research has shown that some correctional health care professionals misgender their transgender patients, are unsure of how to provide medical care to transgender patients, conflate gender dysphoria with mental illness, and withhold gender-affirming hormone therapy from transgender inmates as a form of punishment.[49] All of these actions are forms of interpersonal stigma that have been corroborated by formerly incarcerated transgender women.[16]

Interpersonal stigma from health care professionals is associated with delaying or avoiding necessary medical care among TGD people.[66] Moreover, correctional health care professionals with limited training on gender-affirming health care report being unaware of how to adequately monitor hormone therapy.[49] Additionally, correctional health care professionals might be unaware of the need to provide medically necessary preventative health care for TGD people (e.g., prostate exams for trans feminine people; cervical cancer screening for trans masculine people), which can put patients at greater risk of disease.[67] Further, incarcerated TGD people are particularly vulnerable to the adverse health effects of interpersonal stigma from correctional health care professionals due to their poorer health upon incarceration compared with the general prison population.[13,20] Because interpersonal stigma from correctional health care professionals can lead to deleterious health outcomes among incarcerated TGD people, health care professionals can also create "safe spaces" in their correctional clinics to affirm TGD inmates' identities and promote their overall health and well-being.

▶ Recommended Changes at the Interpersonal Level

The following recommended interpersonal-level changes can be implemented to limit harms such as verbal, physical, sexual, and health care-related abuse that TGD inmates disproportionately face in prisons and jails. These recommendations are drawn from empirical research with correctional health care professionals, formerly incarcerated TGD people, criminal justice advocates, and transgender health scholars in the United States and globally.[15,28,29,55,56]

- Swiftly and thoroughly investigate all allegations of bullying, harassment, sexual violence, and assault (by correctional staff or other incarcerated people).

- Ensure that there are multiple, clear, and safe means by which TGD people can report abuse, free from the fear of retaliation by other incarcerated people and correctional staff.

- Create and enforce appropriate repercussions for perpetrators who verbally, physically, and sexually abuse incarcerated TGD people in accordance with human rights recommendations.

- Utilize the incarcerated TGD person's correct pronouns and name if safe to do so.

- Avoid language that misgenders incarcerated TGD people.

- Mandate culture humility training for all staff, including corrections officers, prison staff, and health care professionals.

- Ensure that correctional health care professionals are properly trained and capable of providing culturally responsive and clinically skilled care for TGD patients.

What Health Care Professionals Can Do to Address Interpersonal Factors That Influence the Health of Incarcerated TGD People

Correctional health care professionals play a critical role in responding to and reducing the interpersonal stigma experienced by incarcerated TGD people. First, correctional health care professionals have a duty to report instances of verbal, physical, or sexual victimization experienced by their TGD patients via the necessary administrative channels, and to follow up on these reports to ensure action is taken against the perpetrator. Second, correctional health care professionals can affirm their TGD patient's gender identities by creating "safe spaces" in clinical settings, for example, by using their patients' correct pronouns and affirming each patient's desired gender expression (see Case Study 3). In especially stigmatizing correctional environments where using a TGD inmate's correct pronouns or name might put them or their patients at risk, correctional health care professionals can instead refer to an inmate by their last name. Using last names is a nongendered, normative method for referring to inmates that allows professionals to treat their transgender patients with respect while circumventing restrictive policies or practices. Third, correctional health care professionals have a duty to increase their cultural responsiveness and clinical skills around providing health care for TGD inmates. Correctional health care professionals can advocate for institutionally supported training on TGD health care. If training is unavailable, correctional health care professionals have a duty to review available online self-directed learning resources, such as those developed by The Fenway Institute's National LGBT Health Education Center,[68] the University of California's Primary Care Protocols,[69] and current clinical standards of care on adequately providing health care

for TGD patients.[23] Depending on their specific health care role, professionals should become knowledgeable about the current standards of care regarding provision of gender-affirming health care, including hormone therapy, mental health care, and primary and preventative health care (e.g., a trans masculine person might still require cervical cancer screening[70]; see the pertinent chapters in this textbook). By taking steps to reduce interpersonal stigmatization by other inmates and correctional staff, and increase cultural responsiveness and clinical skill, correctional health care professionals can greatly improve the health and well-being of incarcerated TGD people.

Transgender Resilience at the Individual Level

Despite the binary gender system and rigid policies that reinforce gender norms and create environments in which TGD people are routinely victimized, many incarcerated TGD people are highly resilient, utilizing various strategies to protect their physical and emotional well-being. **Resilience** is the use of coping strategies that enable individuals and communities to thrive despite adversity.

Managing Victimization

In the face of structural and interpersonal forms of stigma, many incarcerated TGD people learn to navigate stigmatizing correctional environments to prevent or cope with experiences of victimization. One primary way in which TGD people manage victimization is through their gender presentation. Consistent with prior research in noncorrectional settings,[11] some TGD people choose to conceal or minimize their discordant gender expression (e.g., femininity in men's prisons) to prevent victimization. TGD people's ability to conceal their gender identity while incarcerated often hinges on their gender expression and the extent to which they are able to blend in visually as a cisgender woman or man. For example, one qualitative study found that some transgender women incarcerated in men's prisons did not disclose their transgender status and walked and talked "like a man" so that other people could not tell they were transgender.[16] Despite the difficulty of concealing one's authentic self, many incarcerated TGD people consider it to be necessary to survive the correctional environment. For other incarcerated TGD people, the very act of concealing one's true self is not only physically impossible but, in many cases, emotionally prohibitive. For example, in the same qualitative study, some transgender women reported being unable to conceal their femininity because they had developed breasts through gender-affirming medical care; others indicated that they simply could not go back into the closet no matter what the costs were, and they chose to live as women in a men's correctional facility despite the potential risks to their personal safety.[16] For these incarcerated transgender women, the decision to safeguard their mental health by being out in the correctional environment took precedence over the potential for future victimization.

Access to Hormone Therapy

Because of restrictive policies, many TGD people must persistently lobby for, and in some cases obtain legal support, to gain access to medically necessary care. In one qualitative study, transgender women incarcerated in men's prisons described how the bureaucracy within the jail system and lack of urgency on the part of professionals created delays in accessing hormone therapy, leading them to challenge those in power to access medically necessary hormones.[16] Several transgender women reported obtaining legal counsel to circumvent restrictive policies and practices and gain access to gender-affirming hormones. Legal and media reports dating back to the 1990s highlight similar instances of TGD inmates who challenged bureaucratic and legal restrictions to access the medical care necessary to live authentically while incarcerated (see legal reviews by Arkles, and Jenness and Smyth).[58,71] In this way, the very act of accessing hormone therapy in a sex-segregated correctional facility challenges institutional efforts that force TGD people to conform to the gender norms of the institution and provides those who challenge restrictive policies with a sense of empowerment that enables them to survive the stigmatizing correctional environment.[16]

Identifying Sources of Social Support

In a high-stress correctional environment, identifying sources of social support is critical to ensuring well-being and survival. In some cases, TGD people can identify sources of social support within the correctional environment; for many, however, sources of support come from beyond the prison walls.

In the face of stigma, accessing social support from other inmates can be a challenge for many TGD people, who make up a small proportion of the overall inmate population.[13,15,16] Research finds that for incarcerated TGD people, access to supportive peers can vary according to how much exposure a TGD person has had to the correctional system throughout their lives. For example, one qualitative study found that TGD women who had been incarcerated frequently tended to know people from the streets or prior prison stays and were able to leverage these social connections to survive the incarceration experience.[16,35] Conversely, transgender women who had only reported being incarcerated once for a limited time (i.e., less than 3 months) indicated that they felt very isolated in the prison environment and feared for their safety. In the same study, access to social support also varied according to whether there were other TGD people in a given facility. Some transgender women reported that

they had conflicts with other transgender people from the street, while others reported finding older transgender role models who helped them to navigate the prison environment.[16,35] Although TGD people may comprise a small overall proportion of incarcerated people, jails and prisons are increasingly recognizing the presence of this population and the need to support them. With the support of correctional administrators and health care professionals, many peer support groups have formed at local jails and prisons throughout the country. These peer-led groups enable incarcerated TGD people to come together and share information about how to navigate life on the inside as a TGD person and prepare for life after release. Although these groups have not been evaluated in correctional settings, current TGD clinical care guidelines highlight the potential for improved mental health among TGD people who participate in TGD support groups.[23]

For many TGD people incarcerated in nonprogressive or rural areas of the country, access to sources of social support from TGD peers is not possible because these inmates may be the only known TGD person in a given facility. Although correctional facilities prohibit incarcerated people from writing directly to one another, pen pal programs that enable incarcerated TGD people to correspond with one another can aid inmates in accessing sources of social support. Black and Pink is a nonprofit advocacy organization that supports incarcerated LGBTQIA+ people and those living with HIV. One of their primary initiatives is a nationwide pen pal program in which Black and Pink staff match incarcerated members with pen pals within and outside of the correctional environment. Pen pals correspond and build relationships with inmates and participate in harm reduction activities and affirmation. According to the 2015 LGBTQ Prisoner Survey Report, *Coming out of Concrete Closets,* incarcerated LGBTQ people reported that the pen pal program helped them to deal with the stress of being incarcerated and feel accepted in their gender identities and sexual orientations.[15] Further research is needed to empirically investigate the mental health benefits associated with social support gained through prison pen pal programs. However, increasing the number of incarcerated TGD people who have access to pen pal projects could increase access to social support and lead to positive psychological health outcomes.

Recommended Changes at the Individual Level

The following is a list of recommended institutional changes that are needed to support TGD people in navigating structural and interpersonal barriers to health and well-being while incarcerated. These recommendations are drawn from empirical research and dialog with criminal-justice–involved TGD people and activists, correctional health care professionals, and prior reviews and policy reports aimed at advancing the health of incarcerated TGD people in the United States and globally[15,16,29,49]:

- Allow access to clinician- or peer-led TGD community support groups within the correctional environment.

- Offer diverse sources of support, including access to pen-pal programs, resource lists, newspapers and books, and advocacy programs.

- Provide incarcerated TGD people with access to information regarding their legal rights and legal services to support them in responding to violations of their civil rights.

- Inform TGD people of the health care policies of the institution and clearly outline the steps and documentation required to access medically necessary care.

- Ensure case management for incarcerated TGD people is multidisciplinary and attended by all relevant people involved in the person's care.

- Safeguard continuity of care for TGD people between the community and incarceration to ensure that gender-affirming health service provision (e.g., access to hormones and dilators) is not interrupted.

▶ What Health Care Professionals Can Do to Address Individual-Level Factors That Influence the Health of Incarcerated TGD People

Correctional health care professionals are uniquely positioned to support incarcerated TGD people's efforts to manage victimization, gain access to sources of social support, and obtain medically necessary care. Many TGD people may struggle with the decision to conceal their gender identity and expression to avoid victimization. Correctional health care professionals can help incarcerated TGD people evaluate the physical and mental health risks or benefits of concealing their authentic selves within the correctional environment. This evaluation might include assessing the safety of, and options for changing, their current housing placement, as well as the benefits and risks of disclosing their TGD experience to one's cellmate. The assessment might also include processing the potential mental health harms of concealing their authentic self and potentially identifying strategies that enable the incarcerated person to minimize risks to their personal safety.

Many TGD people must confront restrictive policies to access gender-affirming medical care. Health care professionals should become familiar with all health care policies and help their patients to understand the limits of these policies as well as identify strategies to circumvent them. Health care professionals can also act as a go-between for patients and their community health care professionals by helping patients to secure documentation of their prior history of

gender dysphoria or gender-affirming hormone therapy as applicable. If gender-affirming care is not accessible, health care professionals could also recommend legal intervention and provide legal advocates with documentation of the health effects of restricted access to gender-affirming care, when applicable and appropriate.

Sources of social support are limited for incarcerated TGD people. Health care professionals can be a source of social support by treating their patients with respect and affirming their patient's gender in the context of care. They can also support access to peer support by advocating for or helping to put together peer or clinician-led support groups for incarcerated TGD people. Specifically, in facilities where there are several incarcerated TGD people, health care professionals can help incarcerated TGD people navigate administrative barriers and logistical challenges to aid TGD inmates come together via a supervised support group. In the case of peer-led groups, mental health professionals can provide oversight of the group and help TGD people develop the skills to facilitate the group. Mental health clinicians can also lead support groups in facilities that are not supportive of peer-led support groups or in situations where incarcerated TGD people are unable to run or not interested in running a peer group. Finally, health care professionals can inform their TGD patients about letter-writing programs (e.g., Black and Pink pen pal program) to gain access to external sources of social support.[15] Together, these strategies can help foster resilience among incarcerated TGD people and challenge structural and interpersonal sources of stigma that negatively impact the health of incarcerated TGD people. However, because little power is afforded to detainees, particularly those who are highly marginalized, TGD inmates' efforts to challenge institutional policies and practices could be met with further mistreatment. Consequently, before implementation, correctional health care professionals and their incarcerated TGD patients should consider the risks and benefits of interventions that encourage incarcerated TGD people to challenge institutional policies and practices.

SUMMARY

- Stigma within the U.S. jail and prison system works at multiple levels to negatively influence the health of incarcerated TGD people.

- Despite the existence of policies and practices that degrade TGD people and create inequitable access to medically necessary care and enacted forms of stigma that include verbal, physical, and sexual assault, many incarcerated TGD people are resilient and identify ways to survive the correctional environment.

- Significant changes are needed at each level of the correctional environment to ensure the safety and well-being of incarcerated TGD people, including revisions to restrictive housing and health care–related policies, the enforcement of antidiscrimination and violence policies, the promotion of gender-affirming practices on the part of correctional staff, and access to sources of social support for incarcerated TGD people.

- Although structural change may be slow to come for many correctional facilities, correctional health care professionals can do their part to help advance needed changes, while simultaneously helping TGD people navigate the correctional environment and achieve positive health outcomes even in the face of multiple, overlapping sources of stigma.

- Health care professionals should become educated on the institutional policies that impact the well-being of TGD people, educate TGD patients about these policies, and identify strategies to navigate harmful policies to improve the health of TGD patients.

- Health care professionals should also advocate for optimal housing placements for TGD patients, obtain TGD cultural responsiveness and clinical skills training to be better equipped to care for TGD patients, and support their TGD patients in accessing sources of social support.

- The implementation of recommended changes, together with the demonstrated efforts of correctional health care professionals to support their TGD patients in navigating the correctional environment, can help incarcerated TGD people achieve health equity and improved health outcomes.

CASE STUDY 1: TONY

Tony is a 31-year-old transgender man housed in a medium-security women's state prison in the Northeast. Upon incarceration, Tony was able to provide medical proof (i.e., prescription and physician letter) that he had been accessing medically monitored hormone therapy to masculinize his appearance for the 7 years prior to coming to prison. Thus, Tony was able to continue gender-affirming, masculinizing hormone therapy while incarcerated. At intake, a correctional health care professional noted in Tony's medical record that he was bald, had facial and chest hair, and presented with masculinized muscle tone. But because Tony had not had genital construction surgery, he was placed in a women's correctional facility. Due to Tony's masculine gender presentation, the prison warden determined that for the safety and comfort of the incarcerated cisgender women in the prison, Tony should be housed in a segregated housing unit, deemed "protective custody." In this unit, Tony had no access to the regular recreational or rehabilitative activities provided by the prison (e.g., literacy courses, recreational game time), and he was completely isolated from interacting with other inmates. Despite having no history of mental illness, after 1 month of being housed in protective custody, Tony exhibited a depressed mood, generalized anxiety, and

thoughts of suicide. The correctional psychiatrist prescribed Tony antidepressant medication to manage these symptoms. Tony was prescribed increasingly higher doses of antidepressant medication throughout his 8-month incarceration to manage his depression, anxiety, and suicidality. For the entirety of his incarceration, Tony was housed in protective custody. After being released from incarceration, Tony's mental health difficulties diminished, and he was weaned off all psychiatric medication within 4 months of release. This real-life case example demonstrates that genitalia-based housing assignments and the use of protective custody for housing transgender inmates can lead to poor mental health for incarcerated TGD people.

▶ Discussion Questions

1. Do you think that antidepressant medications were the right course of treatment for Tony? What, if any, other forms of treatment would you recommend for Tony?

2. What other housing options would you recommend for Tony, other than protective custody?

3. As a health care professional, what steps could you take to advocate for a more appropriate housing placement for Tony?

CASE STUDY 2: JAZMINE

Jazmine is a 20-year-old transgender woman housed in a medium-security men's state prison in the Northeast. Before incarceration, Jazmine had been taking oral estrogen and anti-androgens for 18 months to feminize her appearance. Since the death of her parents 2 years prior, Jazmine had been living between homeless shelters and on the street, and she accessed her hormones from friends, acquaintances, and a drop-in center for people engaged in sex work. Upon incarceration, Jazmine reported during her medical intake that she was taking 4 mg of estradiol and 200 mg of spironolactone by oral ingestion every day, a common hormone regimen and therapeutic dose for transgender women.[72] Intake examination by a correctional health care professional detailed in Jazmine's medical record that she had breasts, reduced facial and body hair, and feminine subcutaneous fat distribution. The correctional health care policy dictated that to continue hormone therapy while incarcerated, Jazmine was required to provide clinical documentation, including a prescription and letter from a physician. The following quote from Jazmine explains her response to this correctional health care policy:

I told them, "please, I need my hormones." Nope, no hormones. "You gotta get a letter from your doctor." How am I gonna get my letters? How am I gonna call my doctor? I don't have nobody to call. My parents are dead. I didn't have no information...no numbers...I didn't have nothing.[16]

A correctional health care professional explained what happened to Jazmine because of this correctional health care policy:

> We couldn't verify anything, and so [the hormones] weren't continued. It was devastating because [Jazmine] began to grow facial hair again, and they just were devastated. It impacts their depression and suicidality because they just feel so out of place.[49]

Because of her inability to provide medical documentation showing that she had been accessing hormones prior to incarceration, Jazmine's hormone therapy was ceased. As a result, Jazmine's features began to masculinize (e.g., facial hair growth, reduced breast development), which caused Jazmine significant gender dysphoria and mental distress, leading to depression and suicidality.

▶ Discussion Questions

1. What are some of the social factors that contributed to Jazmine lacking proper documentation of her prior hormone use?

2. Why do you think the cessation of hormone therapy led to poor mental health for Jazmine?

3. As a health care professional, what steps could you take to advocate for access to hormone therapy for Jazmine?

CASE STUDY 3: DR. BAUER

Dr. Cynthia Bauer is a correctional psychiatrist who has been working in a high-security men's prison in the Northeast for 4 years. Dr. Bauer received limited training on TGD mental health care during medical school and residency. Since being hired at the prison, her caseload has consistently included three or four transgender women. During her mental health intakes and bimonthly appointments with her transgender patients, Dr. Bauer noted that this group of inmates consistently reported more instances of abuse and violence than her other patients, causing fear, depressed mood, psychiatric distress, and suicidal thoughts and behaviors among her transgender patients. Her transgender patients also reported that the constant misgendering by correctional officers was particularly taxing on their mental health. Dr. Bauer decided that her office would be a "safe space" where she would affirm her transgender patients' gender identities and attempt to improve their mental health and comfort during their appointments. Dr. Bauer explained:

> In my office, I can call them he or she....Depending on what they want, I will either say "Miss or Mr. Williams"...I don't form a judgment or opinion. They are a person first and foremost.[49]

Because of the supportive clinical environment that Dr. Bauer was able to foster, even in a correctional setting that was otherwise stigmatizing, her transgender patients looked forward to their appointments in the "safe space" of her clinic office. Dr. Bauer's transgender patients trusted her as a clinician, leading to more open conversations about their mental health care and positive patient-clinician interactions.

▶ Discussion Questions

1. What are some of the social determinants of mental health inequities among Dr. Bauer's transgender patients? Consider both prison-based explanations and community-based determinants.

2. What types of counseling or treatment could Dr. Bauer provide to reduce mental health inequities experienced by her transgender patients?

3. How else could Dr. Bauer support change at the facility beyond a supportive clinical environment?

CASE STUDY 4: LONNI

Lonni is a genderqueer person whose pronouns are they/them. They are incarcerated in a minimum-security prison in the men's facility. Due to Lonni's gender-expansive expression, administrators did not know where to house them, so Lonni was placed in a single cell in the general population. After several months in a single cell, Lonni became very anxious and suffered from depression due to the social isolation. Lonni felt a strong desire to connect with other incarcerated people but was scared to reach out to the cisgender men in the general population for fear of victimization.

One day, Lonni saw a correctional officer transporting a transgender woman (whom they recognized from their hometown) from another cell block to the medical building. Lonni waved at the transgender inmate, and she waved back. It then occurred to Lonni that there may be other incarcerated TGD people on the prison campus that they might be able to connect with. The next day, Lonni had a visit with their social worker and proposed the idea of starting a peer-led, TGD support group at the prison. Lonni volunteered to lead the group and asked their social worker to help them get it started. The social worker was not sure that the administrators would support the formation of a TGD support group but was glad to see Lonni energized about the group and recognized that they were suffering from the social isolation of their solitary cell. The social worker told Lonni that she would work on it. She then proceeded to gather research on the benefits of peer support groups for TGD people and the mental health harms of social isolation, including reports of incarcerated TGD people who had died by suicide. Armed with data, the social worker made a case for the support group with the Director of Mental Health. The director was initially hesitant to allow such a group to be formed, but the social worker assured him that she would take full responsibility for the group and provide the necessary clinical oversight. After some thought, the director granted the social worker approval to create the TGD peer support group. Before starting the group, the social worker reached out to a local LGBTQIA+ health center to discuss the group and identify strategies she could use to support peer facilitators. Next, she provided Lonni with basic facilitation skills to support them in leading the group and worked with administrators to identify and invite the 10 known TGD inmates to join the group. The group met weekly for over a year, during which the social worker observed significant improvement in Lonni's mental health. Lonni felt pride in their ability to help other incarcerated TGD people navigate the correctional environment and began considering a career as a peer counselor once released from prison.

▶ Discussion Questions

1. What are the unique challenges that a genderqueer or nonbinary person like Lonni might face in a gender-binary prison?

2. Map the steps that the social worker took to help support Lonni in creating a peer support group.

3. What are some of the challenges that Lonni might experience in facilitating the group? How would you help Lonni navigate any group facilitation challenges?

REFERENCES

1. Glezer A, McNiel DE, Binder RL. Transgendered and incarcerated: a review of the literature, current policies and laws, and ethics. *J Am Acad Psychiatry Law.* 2013;41(4):551-559.
2. Flores AR, Herman JL, Gates GJ, Brown TNT. *How Many Adults Identify as Transgender in the United States?* Los Angeles, CA: The Williams Institute; 2016.
3. Grant JM, Mottet LA, Tanis LA, Harrison J, Herman JL, Keisling M. *Injustice at Every Turn: A Report of the National Transgender Discrimination Survey.* Washington, DC: National Center for Transgender Equality and National Gay and Lesbian Task Force; 2011.
4. Glaze L, Kaeble D. *Correctional Populations in the United States, 2013.* Washington, DC: US Department of Justice; 2014.
5. Reisner SL, Bailey Z, Sevelius J. Racial/ethnic disparities in history of incarceration, experiences of victimization, and associated health indicators among transgender women in the US. *Women Health.* 2014;54(8):750-767.
6. Garofalo R, Deleon J, Osmer E, Doll M, Harper GW. Overlooked, misunderstood and at-risk: exploring the lives and HIV risk of ethnic minority male-to-female transgender youth. *J Adolesc Health.* 2006;38(3):230-236.
7. Clements K, Katz M, Marx R. *The Transgender Community Health Project: Descriptive Results.* San Francisco, CA: San Francisco Department of Public Health; 1999.
8. Phelan JC, Link BG, Dovidio JF. Stigma and prejudice: one animal or two? *Social Sci Med.* 2008;67(3):358-367.
9. Link BG, Phelan JC. Conceptualizing stigma. *Annu Rev Sociol.* 2001:363-385.
10. Nemoto T, Bodeker B, Iwamoto M. Social support, exposure to violence and transphobia, and correlates of depression among male-to-female transgender women with a history of sex work. *Am J Public Health.* 2011;101(10):1980-1988.
11. Mizock L, Mueser KT. Employment, mental health, internalized stigma, and coping with transphobia among transgender individuals. *Psychol Sexual Orient Gender Diversity.* 2014;1(2):146-158.
12. Wolff KB, Cokely CL. "To protect and to serve?": an exploration of police conduct in relation to the gay, lesbian, bisexual, and transgender community. *Sexual Cult.* 2007;11(2):1-23.
13. James SE, Herman JL, Rankin S, Keisling M, Mottet L, Anafi M. *The Report of the 2015 U.S. Transgender Survey.* Washington, DC: National Center for Transgender Equality; 2016.
14. Reisner SL, White Hughto JM, Dunham EE, et al. Legal protections in public accommodations settings: a critical public health issue for transgender and gender-nonconforming people. *Milbank Q.* 2015 Jul 29;93(3):484-515.
15. Lydon J, Carrington K, Low H, Miller R, Yazdy M. *Coming Out of Concrete Closets: A Report on Black and Pink's LGBTQ Prisoner' Survey.* Boston, MA: Black and Pink; 2015.
16. White Hughto JM, Clark K, Altice FL, Reisner SL, Kershaw TS, Pachankis JE. Creating, reinforcing, and resisting the gender binary: a qualitative study of transgender women's healthcare experiences in sex-segregated jails and prisons. *Int J Prison Health.* 2018;14(2):1-20.
17. Jenness V, Maxson CL, Matsuda KN, Sumner JM. *Violence in California Correctional Facilities: An Empirical Examination of Sexual Assault.* Irvine, CA: University of California; 2007.
18. Rosenblum D. Trapped in sing sing: transgendered prisoners caught in the gender binarism. *Mich J Gender L.* 1999;6:499-571.
19. Reisner SL, White Hughto JM, Gamarel KE, Keuroghlian AS, Mizock L, Pachankis JE. Discriminatory experiences associated with post-traumatic stress disorder symptoms among transgender adults. *J Counsel Psychol.* 2016;63(5):509-519.
20. White Hughto JM, Reisner SL, Pachankis JE. Transgender stigma and health: a critical review of stigma determinants, mechanisms, and interventions. *Soc Sci Med.* 2015;147:222-231.
21. White Hughto JM, Pachankis JE, Willie TC, Reisner SL. Victimization and depressive symptomology in transgender adults: the mediating role of avoidant coping. *J Counsel Psychol.* 2017;64(1):41-51.
22. Neal T, Clements CB. Prison rape and psychological sequelae: a call for research. *Psychol Public Policy Law.* 2010;16(3):284-299.
23. Coleman E, Bockting W, Botzer M, et al. Standards of care for the health of transsexual, transgender, and gender-nonconforming people, version 7. *Int J Transgender.* 2012;13(4):165-232.
24. Link BG, Phelan J. Stigma power. *Soc Sci Med.* 2014;103:24-32.
25. Schilt K, Westbrook L. Doing gender, doing heteronormativity "gender normals," transgender people, and the social maintenance of heterosexuality. *Gender Soc.* 2009;23(4):440-464.
26. Brown GR, McDuffie E. Health care policies addressing transgender inmates in prison systems in the United States. *J Correctional Health Care.* 2009;15(4):280-291.
27. Routh D, Abess G, Makin D, Stohr MK, Hemmens C, Yoo J. Transgender inmates in prisons: a review of applicable statutes and policies. *Int J Offender Ther Compar Criminol.* 2015;61(6):645-666.
28. Sevelius J, Jenness V. Challenges and opportunities for gender-affirming healthcare for transgender women in prison. *Int J Prisoner Health.* 2017;13(1):32-40.

29. Bromdal A, Clark KA, Hughto JM, et al. Whole-incarceration-setting approaches to supporting and upholding the rights and health of incarcerated transgender people [Guest editorial]. *Int J Transgend.* 2019.

30. Clark K, White Hughto JM. "We are Guests in Their House": a qualitative analysis of correctional healthcare providers' knowledge, attitudes, and experiences caring for transgender inmates (Session: Experiences of LGBTQ and Female Inmates). Oral presentation at the American Society of Criminology Conference. New Orleans, LA; 2016.

31. Bassichis D, Spade D. *"It's War in Here": A Report on the Treatment of Transgender and Intersex People in New York State Men's Prisons.* New York: Sylvia Rivera Law Project; 2007.

32. Shay G. PREA's elusive promise: can DOJ regulations protect LGBT incarcerated people. *Loy J Pub Int L.* 2013;15:343.

33. Sumner J, Jenness V. Gender integration in sex-segregated US prisons: the paradox of transgender correctional policy. Handbook of LGBT Communities, Crime, and Justice. Springer; 2014, pp. 229-259.

34. Kaba F, Lewis A, Glowa-Kollisch S, et al. Solitary confinement and risk of self-harm among jail inmates. *Am J Public Health.* 2014;104(3):442-447.

35. Smoyer AB, White JM. *Separate but Equal? Contesting Transgender Prison Spaces.* Washington, DC: American Society of Criminology; 2015.

36. Sumner J, Sexton L. Lost in translation: looking for transgender identity in women's prisons and locating aggressors in prisoner culture. *Crit Criminol.* 2015;23(1):1-20.

37. Reisner SL, White JM, Bradford J, Mimiaga MJ. Transgender health disparities: comparing full cohort and nested matched-pair study designs in a community health center. *LGBT Health.* 2014;1(3):177-184.

38. Herbst JH, Jacobs ED, Finlayson TJ, et al. Estimating HIV prevalence and risk behaviors of transgender persons in the United States: a systematic review. *AIDS Behav.* 2008;12(1):1-17.

39. Lydon J, Carrington K, Low H, Miller R, Yazdy M. *Coming Out of Concrete Closets: A Report on Black and Pink's LGBTQ Prisoner' Survey.* Boston, MA: Black and Pink; 2015.

40. Tarzwell S. Gender liens are marked with razor wire: addressing state prison policies and practices for the management of transgender prisoners. *Colum Hum Rts L Rev.* 2006;38:167-219.

41. American Psychiatric Association. *Diagnostic and Statistical Manual of Mental Disorders, (DSM-5).* American Psychiatric Association; 2013.

42. American Medical Association. *Resolution 122: Removing Financial Barriers to Care for Transgender Patients.* Chicago, IL: American Medical Association; 2008.

43. White Hughto JM, Reisner SL. A systematic review of the effects of hormone therapy on psychological functioning and quality of life in transgender individuals. *Transgender Health.* 2016;1(1):21-31.

44. NCTE. LGBT People and the Prison Rape Elimination Act. Washington, DC: National Center for Transgender Equality; 2012.

45. Iyama K. We have tolled the bell for him: an analysis of the Prison Rape Elimination Act and California's compliance as it applies to transgender inmates. *Tul JL Sexual.* 2012;21:23.

46. Hastings A, Browne A, Kall K, diZerega M. *Keeping Vulnerable Populations Safe under PREA: Alternative Strategies to the Use of Segregation in Prisons and Jails.* Vera Institute of Justice; 2015.

47. American Psychological Association. *Transgender, Gender Identity, & Gender Expression Non-discrimination.* Washington, DC: American Psychological Association Council of Representatives; 2008.

48. Murad MH, Elamin MB, Garcia MZ, et al. Hormonal therapy and sex reassignment: a systematic review and meta-analysis of quality of life and psychosocial outcomes. *Clin Endocrinol (Oxf).* 2010 Feb;72(2):214-231.

49. Clark KA, White Hughto JM, Pachankis JE. "What's the right thing to do?": Correctional healthcare providers' knowledge, attitudes, and experiences caring for transgender inmates. *Soc Sci Med.* 2017;193:80-89.

50. Brown GR. Qualitative analysis of transgender inmates' correspondence implications for departments of correction. *J Correctional Health Care.* 2014;20(4):334-342.

51. White Hughto JM, Murchison G, Clark K, Pachankis JE, Reisner SL. Geographic and individual differences in healthcare access for U.S. transgender adults: a multilevel analysis. *LGBT Health.* 2016;3(6):424-433.

52. Clark KA, Fletcher JB, Holloway IW, Reback CJ. Structural inequities and social networks impact hormone use and misuse among transgender women in Los Angeles county. *Archiv Sexual Behav.* 2018:1-10.

53. Sanchez NF, Sanchez JP, Danoff A. Health care utilization, barriers to care, and hormone usage among male-to-female transgender persons in New York City. *Am J Public Health.* 2009;99(4):713-719.

54. Brown GR. Autocastration and autopenectomy as surgical self-treatment in incarcerated persons with gender identity disorder. *Int J Transgend.* 2010;12(1):31-39.

55. White Hughto JM, Clark KA, Altice FL, Reisner SL, Kershaw TS, Pachankis JE. Creating, reinforcing, and resisting the gender binary: a qualitative study of transgender women's healthcare experiences in sex-segregated jails and prisons. *Int J Prisoner Health.* 2018;14(2):69-88.

56. Clark KA, White Hughto JM, Pachankis JE. "What's the right thing to do?" Correctional healthcare providers' knowledge, attitudes and experiences caring for transgender inmates. *Soc Sci Med.* 2017;193:80-89.

57. Herek GM. Hate crimes and stigma-related experiences among sexual minority adults in the United States prevalence estimates from a national probability sample. *J Interpers Viol.* 2009;24(1):54-74.

58. Jenness V, Smyth M. The Passage of the Prison Rape Elimination Act: Discursive Politics and the Reconstitution of Prisoner Rape in a Culture of Control. Unpublished manuscript; 2007.

59. Edney R. To keep me safe from harm: transgender prisoners and the experience of imprisonment. *Deakin L Rev.* 2004;9:327.

60. Rosenblum D. Trapped in sing sing: transgendered prisoners caught in the gender binarism. *Mich J Gender L.* 1999;6:499.

61. Grant JM, Mottet LA, Tanis LA, Harrison J, Herman JL, Keisling M. *Injustice at every turn: A Report of the National Transgender Discrimination Survey.* Washington, DC: National Center for Transgender Equality and National Gay and Lesbian Task Force; 2011.

62. Stohr MK. The hundred years' war: the etiology and status of assaults on transgender women in men's prisons. *Women Criminal Justice.* 2015;25(1-2):120-129.

63. Beck A. *Sexual Victimization in Prisons and Jails Reported by Inmates, 2011–12.* Washington, DC: Bureau of Justice Statistics; 2013.

64. Okamura A. Equality behind bars: improving the legal protections of transgender inmates in the California Prison Systems. *Hastings Race Poverty LJ.* 2011;8:109.

65. Psaty BM, Koepsell TD, Lin D, et al. Assessment and control for confounding by indication in observational studies. *J Am Geriatr Soc.* 1999;47(6):749-754.

66. Jaffee KD, Shires DA, Stroumsa D. Discrimination and delayed health care among transgender women and men: implications for improving medical education and health care delivery. *Med Care.* 2016;54(11):1010-1016.

67. Blank TO, Descartes L, Asencio M. Cancer screening in gay and bisexual men and transgender people. Cancer and the LGBT Community. Springer; 2015, pp. 99-114.

68. The Fenway Institute. National LGBT Health Education Center; 2019. https://www.lgbthealtheducation.org/.

69. Center of Excellence for Transgender Health. Primary care protocol for transgender patient care. 2011. http://transhealth.ucsf.edu/protocols. Accessed November 15, 2015.

70. Edmiston EK, Donald CA, Sattler AR, Peebles JK, Ehrenfeld JM, Eckstrand KL. Opportunities and gaps in primary care preventative health services for transgender patients: a systematic review. *Transgender Health.* 2016;1(1):216-230.

71. Arkles G. Correcting race and gender: prison regulation of social hierarchy through dress. *New York University Law Review.* 2012;87(4):12-49.

72. Unger CA. Hormone therapy for transgender patients. *Transl Androl Urol.* 2016 Dec;5(6):877-884.

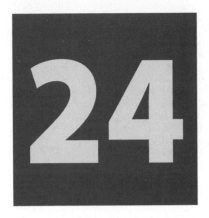

24

Caring for Transgender and Gender Diverse Veterans

Colleen A. Sloan

Michael R. Kauth

Jillian C. Shipherd

Transgender and gender diverse (TGD) people have likely served in the U.S. armed forces for as long as the nation has had a military, although their presence and experiences within the military did not gain substantial attention until much later. Unfortunately, this later attention was mainly negative and stigmatizing of TGD identities both within the military and the larger culture. While in recent years visibility and social attitudes regarding TGD people have become more affirming in the broader culture, military policy has gone back and forth. The long history of prohibiting open military service by TGD people makes it difficult to compile accurate estimates of the number of TGD military personnel and examine their military service. Moreover, the shifting, inconsistent military policy on TGD service has complicated the environment of service for TGD service members. These policies present unique challenges for TGD veterans, particularly within the Veterans Health Administration (VHA). This chapter first discusses U.S. military culture and history as it relates to the experiences of TGD service members. Next, health disparities for TGD veterans are reviewed, followed by a discussion of the VHA policies related to TGD health care. Finally, two case studies of TGD veterans are presented.

HISTORY OF THE U.S. MILITARY AND TGD SERVICE MEMBERS

In the all-volunteer U.S. armed forces, fewer than 10% of Americans serve in the military.[1] A disproportionate number of TGD Americans join the military. Although the exact population prevalence is unknown, researchers estimate that TGD people make up 0.3% (700,000) of the U.S. population, and yet 0.6% (149,800) of military veterans are estimated to be TGD people.[2,3] In the 2015 U.S. Transgender Survey, a large online survey of 27,715 TGD Americans, 18% of participants reported serving in the military.[4] These numbers suggest that TGD people have long served in the military

and served largely undetected (Figure 24-1). From the 2015 U.S. Transgender Survey, more than half (52%) of respondents said no one else knew about their TGD identity.[4] About one-third (34%) reported that a few or some people in the military knew about their TGD identity. Nearly 80% of survey respondents received an honorable discharge from the military. Of those who had left military service more than 10 years ago, about one-fifth (19%) believed their discharge was related to their TGD identity (Figure 24-1).

The military first issued a ban on service by TGD people in 1963, which was lifted briefly in June 2016. At first, the policy allowed TGD service members who were serving in secret to serve openly and receive transgender-related health care on military bases. This policy was then temporarily expanded to openly allow transgender people to join the military starting in January 2018. However, in July 2018, the military under the Trump Administration announced plans to reinstate the ban on TGD service members. The policy enacted in April 2019 requires that personnel serve under the requirements for their **sex assigned at birth** or receive a waiver to serve in their "preferred" gender if they can demonstrate medical stability for the past 18 months.[5] An exception was made for existing transgender service members who were receiving transition-related care to be allowed to complete their current service contracts and receive medical care. At the time of this writing, there are ongoing court cases that may influence future military policy on TGD service. The new Biden Administration may also change current policy on TGD service and make it more consistent with Obama-era Department of Defense (DoD) policy.

People join the military for a wide range of reasons. While it is not entirely clear why TGD people choose to join the service despite bans and discrimination, it is important to remember that young adults are still forming their personal identity and often looking for a place to belong. There are clear reasons why the military potentially

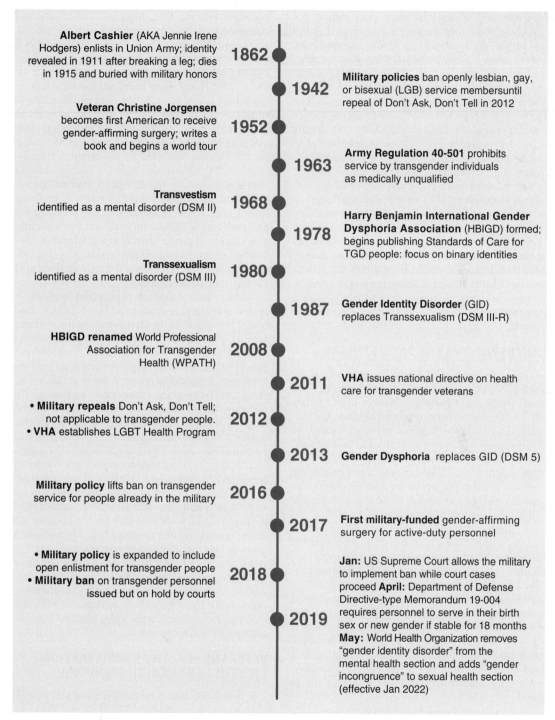

Albert Cashier (AKA Jennie Irene Hodgers) enlists in Union Army; identity revealed in 1911 after breaking a leg; dies in 1915 and buried with military honors

1862

1942 — **Military policies** ban openly lesbian, gay, or bisexual (LGB) service membersuntil repeal of Don't Ask, Don't Tell in 2012

Veteran Christine Jorgensen becomes first American to receive gender-affirming surgery; writes a book and begins a world tour

1952

1963 — **Army Regulation 40-501** prohibits service by transgender individuals as medically unqualified

Transvestism identified as a mental disorder (DSM II)

1968

1978 — **Harry Benjamin International Gender Dysphoria Association** (HBIGD) formed; begins publishing Standards of Care for TGD people: focus on binary identities

Transsexualism identified as a mental disorder (DSM III)

1980

1987 — **Gender Identity Disorder** (GID) replaces Transsexualism (DSM III-R)

HBIGD renamed World Professional Association for Transgender Health (WPATH)

2008

2011 — **VHA** issues national directive on health care for transgender veterans

• **Military repeals** Don't Ask, Don't Tell; not applicable to transgender people.
• **VHA** establishes LGBT Health Program

2012

2013 — **Gender Dysphoria** replaces GID (DSM 5)

Military policy lifts ban on transgender service for people already in the military

2016

2017 — **First military-funded** gender-affirming surgery for active-duty personnel

• **Military policy** is expanded to include open enlistment for transgender people
• **Military ban** on transgender personnel issued but on hold by courts

2018

2019 — **Jan:** US Supreme Court allows the military to implement ban while court cases proceed **April:** Department of Defense Directive-type Memorandum 19-004 requires personnel to serve in their birth sex or new gender if stable for 18 months **May:** World Health Organization removes "gender identity disorder" from the mental health section and adds "gender incongruence" to sexual health section (effective Jan 2022)

▲ **Figure 24–1.** A Timeline of TGD Military Veterans and Changes in Federal Policy and Healthcare would be appealing, at least for some TGD people. For TGD people who become estranged from their families of origin or become homeless with inadequate resources, the military offers a community and friendship, employment with benefits, and, in many cases, affordable housing. Moreover, the military offers an environment with clear rules about behavior, including hair and dress guidelines, and structure for advancement. This environment may be appealing for people who are struggling with their identity and are seeking guidance. For TGD people who served in secret in the past, those reasons also may have included the expectation of an environment with clear gender norms.[6] Clearly defined rules and a hypermasculine military culture may be attractive to TGD people who are struggling with how to manage their own internal distress regarding gender. Specifically, Brown[6] discussed testimonials from TGD veterans, specifically **trans women**, who described joining the military in attempts to prove their masculinity or to hide their true identities. In the traditionally masculine, heteronormative military culture, the gender rules are clear—avoid femininity and being perceived as gay—which, paradoxically, may make it easy to fit in but heighten fear of discovery.[7]

HEALTH DISPARITIES FOR TGD VETERANS

TGD military personnel who served in secret may have experienced chronic minority stress related to fear of being discovered, rejected, and discharged from the armed forces. *Minority stress* refers to chronic stigma, prejudice, and discrimination that creates a hostile social environment for LGBTQIA+ people and contributes to mental health conditions[8,9] (see Chapter 3, "Health Disparities").

A high proportion of TGD veterans have experienced sexual assault while in the service. In a nationwide online survey of 221 transgender veterans, 17.2% of participants reported having been sexually assaulted in the military. Of note, these findings were widely different for transgender women (15.2%) who had served as men and transgender men (30.0%) who had served as women.[10] These rates are much higher than the rates reported in the literature generally for sexual assault in the military, in which 20% of people presumed to be women and 1% of people presumed to be men report these experiences.[11-13] These statistics indicate that safety for transgender service members is an important concern. As would be expected, researchers have found that a history of military sexual assault predicted recent posttraumatic stress symptom severity, depressive symptom severity, and past-year drug use in transgender veterans.[10]

In addition to these mental health symptoms, one of the most striking health disparities for TGD veterans is related to suicide. VHA data indicate rates of suicidality, including ideation, plans, and attempts, between 4 and over 20 times

higher in veterans with diagnostic codes associated with transgender-related care compared with the general VHA population.[14,15] Lehavot, Simpson, and Shipherd[16] found that **gender minority stress** factors, including identity-specific **stigma** during military service, are associated with suicidality. A more recent study examined gender minority stress specifically related to military service and its relationship to suicidality in a sample of TGD veterans.[17] Results indicate that identity-based **discrimination** and rejection during the past year predicted frequency of past-year and past 2-week suicide ideation, mediated by self-reported identity-based shame during the past year. Likewise, findings related to military-specific gender minority stress indicate that military-related external gender minority stress (e.g., punishment or investigation related to gender identity) predicted past-year and past 2-week suicidal ideation and was associated with concealment of gender identity and gender identity–related fear and anxiety during military service. All of these findings suggest that gender minority stressors contribute to chronic suicidality in TGD veterans.[17]

Military service also places people at increased risk for several other health conditions. These include conditions related to physical injury, exposure to traumatic stressors like combat, and exposure to stressful living conditions during deployment and environmental toxins. Each of these experiences might result in long-term sequelae, with multiple exposures complicating recovery. Another factor that could complicate recovery from these experiences is simultaneous minority stress. Minority stress related to hiding one's gender identity and expression for fear of rejection, violence, or discharge from service is another potential stressor that TGD personnel may have experienced while in the military.[8,9,18] Health care providers need to assess for a history of military service, as well as both current and past minority stress. Current gender identity and **sex assigned at birth** are both relevant in health care settings, with gender identity being the predominant variable in care and sex assigned at birth a guide for some health screenings (e.g., prostate exams) and lab tests. Less than one-half of veterans, including TGD veterans, go to the VHA for health care,[19] so the unique needs of TGD veterans are important for all health care settings. The 2015 U.S. Transgender Survey found that among veteran respondents, only 40% had received care at VHA facilities.[4] Of those who received care at VHA, 72% said they are out as transgender to their providers.

VETERANS HEALTH ADMINISTRATION AND THE LGBT HEALTH PROGRAM

The patient population for the VHA comprises people who have served in the military. The DoD and VHA are separate federal entities, each with their own policies and procedures. VHA's Medical Benefits Package was established in the 1990s and can be found under Title 38 Code of Federal

Regulations (CFR) Section 17.38.[20] This policy details the types of care that are covered and lists six items that are explicitly excluded from coverage. One of these exclusions is "gender alterations," with no definition provided. As a result, the 152 VHA medical centers and roughly 1400 community-based outpatient clinics had different interpretations and policies about this exclusion and care for TGD veterans.

In 2011, to address these variations in policies, the nation-wide Directive on the Care for Transgender and Intersex Veterans was established to provide a standard interpretation of care (now Directive 1341).[21] In this more recent policy, the "gender alterations" exclusion became limited to surgi-cal gender-affirmation procedures. All other care, including gender identity counseling, hormone therapy, prosthetic support, vocal coaching, presurgical evaluations (and sup-port letters), long-term postoperative care, and treatment for complications, were included as benefits for TGD veterans. In addition, this VHA policy requires that staff treat veterans based on their self-identified gender identity, including for room assignments and pronoun use.

Dissemination of the VHA policy on transgender health began around the time that the DoD policy called "Don't Ask, Don't Tell (DADT)" was repealed. Even though DADT was never in place at VHA, questions began to arise about the treatment of sexual minority veterans. In order to offer consistent guidance to the field about culturally responsive care for veterans with **sexual and gender minority** identi-ties, an LGBT Health Program was formed in 2012 within the Office of Patient Care Services.[22] This program oversees both Directive 1341 on care for TGD veterans and VHA Directive 1340: Health Care for Veterans who Identify as Lesbian, Gay or Bisexual.[23] Together, these policies specify that VHA facil-ities are responsible for creating a welcoming environment that overcomes LGBTQIA+ veterans' expectations of rejec-tion due to their sexual and gender minority identities and the carryover of military culture to VHA (see more on rele-vant military history in this chapter). In addition, the policies specify that veterans with sexual and gender minority identi-ties must be treated with respect (e.g., name and pronoun use), and no attempts at conversion or changing their identi-ties (formal or informal) are allowed at VHA facilities. To support policy implementation, the LGBT Health Program has developed several training opportunities and clinical resources for VHA providers, some of which are also available to community providers through a free public health plat-form called VHA TRAIN (https://vha.train.org). Box 24-1 lists the VHA training modules relevant to TGD veteran health. Additionally, public websites relevant to LGBTQIA+ veteran health are available, such as https://www.mental-health.va.gov/LGBT/index.asp and https://www.patientcare.va.gov/LGBT/index.asp.

Changing a culture, however, takes more than the pas-sage of inclusive policies and training. Change is most likely when local champions can work within the existing

BOX 24–1 Available Trainings in the "Care For Transgender And Gender-Diverse Veterans in VHA" Program Series

Module Title
1. Diagnosing Gender Dysphoria
2. Assessment of Readiness and Consent for Hormone Therapy
3. Medical Evaluation for Feminizing Hormone Therapy
4. Medical Evaluation for Masculinizing Hormone Therapy
5. Feminizing Hormone Therapy
6. Masculinizing Hormone Therapy
7. Aging Transgender Veterans
8. Mental Health Evaluation for Gender Affirming Surgeries
9. Letters of Support
10. Gender Counseling
11. Care for Gender Non-binary Veterans

Free public access to these VHA trainings is available through VHA TRAIN: https://www.train.org/vha/welcome.

structures and address local needs. Thus, in 2016, VHA created a point-of-contact program with LGBT Veteran Care Coordinators (LGBT VCCs) at every facility who report to the VHA Medical Center Director and who are coordinated regionally by an LGBT regional lead. The local LGBT VCCs are responsible for the dissemination of inclusive signs and symbols throughout the facility, including "We Serve all Who Served" posters, rainbow lanyards, and other items. Importantly, the LGBT VCCs offer veterans a local person to turn to if they are unsure how to access affirmation-related care or if they encounter sexual and gender minority identity-related difficulties in the VHA facility. The LGBT VCCs work closely with the facility Patient Experience Coordinator (i.e., patient advo-cate) and other relevant offices when addressing patient concerns. The local LGBT VCC is a source of education for both veterans and VHA staff alike on unique aspects of care for sexual and gender minority veterans. These local champions also work with VHA and community resources to help create a healthy and healing environment where all veterans feel welcome and accepted. For more detail about the LGBT Health Program or to find a local LGBT VCC, see https://www.patientcare.va.gov/LGBT/index.asp. In addition to the resources and links listed within this chap-ter, important points and resources for non-VHA health care providers when treating TGD veterans can be found in Box 24-2.

1. All VHA facilities serve TGD Veterans. Most veterans, however, including TGD veterans, seek healthcare at non-VHA facilities. For additional information about enrollment in healthcare at VHA and other benefits: http://explore.va.gov or call 1-800-827-1000

2. TGD veterans may have been discharged from the military due to their identity. The type of discharge affects eligibility for services. If veterans have a history of military sexual trauma, they are eligible for military sexual trauma–related health care at no expense regardless of discharge status.

3. LGBT VCCs are available at every VA medical center. LGBT VCCs can assist TGD veterans with registration for VA health care and connection to relevant services.

4. Military service is a social determinant of health and cultural experience. Non-VA health care providers should educate themselves about military culture, especially as it relates to the individual experiences of their TGD veteran patients. For more information about military culture, please see https://www.mentalhealth.va.gov/communityproviders/military_culture.asp

SUMMARY

- TGD people have likely served in the U.S. armed forces for as long as the nation has had a military but have served largely undetected. It is difficult to compile accurate estimates of the number of TGD military personnel and examine their military service.

- The military's ban on service by TGD people was lifted briefly in 2016 before being reinstated in 2019. The new policy states that personnel serve under the requirements for their sex assigned at birth or receive a waiver to serve in their "preferred" gender if they can demonstrate medical stability for the past 18 months.

- TGD military personnel are at increased risk of mental health conditions likely related to chronic minority stress due to the fear of being discovered, rejected, and discharged from the armed forces. A high proportion of TGD veterans have experienced sexual assault while in the service. Suicidality is between 4 and 20 times higher in veterans, and for TGD personnel, gender minority stress contributes significantly to chronic suicidality.

- TGD veterans are at increased risk of several other health conditions, such as physical injury, exposure to traumatic stressors like combat, and exposure to stressful living conditions during deployment and environmental toxins.

- The Veteran's Health Administration excludes "gender alterations" from its medical benefits package. The 2011 Directive on the Care for Transgender and Intersex Veterans was established to provide a standard interpretation of care of the Veteran's Health Administrations medical benefits. Only surgical gender-affirmation procedures are excluded; all other care must be covered.

- An LGBT Health Program was formed in 2012. This program oversees both Directive 1341 on care for TGD veterans and VHA Directive 1340: Health Care for Veterans who Identify as Lesbian, Gay or Bisexual. In 2016, VHA created a point-of-contact program with LGBT Veteran Care Coordinators (LGBT VCCs) to address LGBTQIA+ patient concerns and educate both veterans and staff about sexual and gender minority veterans.

CASE STUDY 1: Veteran Smith

Veteran Smith is a 58-year-old White trans woman assigned male sex at birth whose pronouns are she/her/hers and who goes by the name Gloria. Gloria is a veteran from the post-Vietnam era, having served two decades in the U.S. Navy. She was married to a **cisgender** woman for almost 30 years. They separated after Gloria disclosed her transgender identity to her wife 2 years ago. They have two adult children together, one who no longer speaks to Gloria; her other child is "supportive," although Gloria notes that this child still calls her "dad." Gloria recalls having always been aware of "female tendencies" but perceived these experiences as indicating that "something was wrong." She reports feeling "sure" her father, a military veteran, would have punished her if she ever disclosed these feelings. As a result, Gloria joined the military at 18 years old to "correct" these feelings and help her with "being a man." Gloria served proudly for 20 years until she retired and then sought health care at a VHA facility.

While waiting for her appointment, Gloria saw a VHA poster in the waiting room that depicted rainbow-colored dog tags with the caption, "We Serve All Who Served" (https://www.patientcare.va.gov/LGBT/VA_LGBT_Outreach.asp), and this made Gloria feel that she might be safe in discussing her gender identity. The primary care provider met Gloria by introducing herself and stating her own gender pronouns. The provider then asked Gloria what name she uses. She also asked about Gloria's gender identity and pronouns. Gloria told her primary care provider that she needed to "talk to someone" but that she was afraid of "losing everything," including her VA health care and service-connected benefits. Her primary care provider referred Gloria to a mental health provider for counseling and support. In her first meeting with a mental health provider, Gloria reported, "I think I may be a woman…I have never acknowledged it." Over the course of several mental health visits with a trans-affirming provider, Gloria became more comfortable with her gender identity as a woman and decided to seek medical interventions for gender affirmation. Her mental health provider confirmed a diagnosis of Gender Dysphoria and referred her to an endocrinologist for medical evaluation and initiation of feminizing hormone therapy. She disclosed her gender identity to her wife, who was not supportive and opted to separate from Gloria. Gloria's VHA providers assisted her in connecting with trans-affirming social support, which was especially important as Gloria had always been well connected with other veterans who knew her by her presumed identity as a man. Gloria lost some veteran support but was able to maintain some relationships in her affirmed identity as a woman. She reported feeling more comfortable in public and at the VHA in particular, citing the importance of visual cues and signage, such as transgender flag posters and rainbow lanyards, and importantly the affirming nature of her providers. Gloria made effective use of **gender affirmation** services offered by the VHA, including hormone therapy and gender counseling, and she reports feeling more "authentic."

▶ Discussion Questions

1. How did the primary care provider know to ask about Gloria's preferred name and gender pronouns?

    Authors' response: Best practice is to approach all patients by introducing yourself with your name and pronouns then asking the patient what name they go by. This trans-affirming stance helps to shift toward a trans-inclusive culture with cisgender patients (while validating use of nicknames) and also creates an affirming environment where TGD patients feel safe disclosing their gender identity and using a name that is not their legal name.

2. Gloria describes a great deal of guilt regarding her decision to join the military, marry a woman, and have children, given that she "always knew" about her identity. How might you start to address these issues during Gloria's patient visit?

    Authors' response: Many veterans who are newly out about their gender identity judge themselves harshly for "not coming out sooner." However, it is important to understand that, at age 18 in the culture 30 years ago, this decision may not have been considered. One approach might be "So Gloria, can you tell me a little about yourself at age 18? What were you like then? Were you even

aware that people transitioned?" Socratic questioning about veterans' past choices that they are evaluating with today's knowledge can assist veterans in gaining more self-directed empathy.

3. Gloria embraces her veteran identity. As she becomes more involved in the trans* community, she describes feeling increasingly uncomfortable disclosing her veteran status for fear of judgment. How would you support Gloria with this challenge?

    Authors' response: Fortunately, many VHAs and LGBT health centers now have transgender veteran support groups that can help support veterans with the dual-minority stress of being both transgender and veterans. Additionally, when developing new friendships, it can be scary to consider losing support or being judged. That said, people in the transgender community understand how closing off a piece of one's identity can be harmful. Being willing to share oneself fully would be a new experience for Gloria. Practicing ways of revealing veteran identity and role-playing responding to concerns may be valuable.

CASE STUDY 2: VETERAN JOHNSON

Veteran Johnson is a 26-year-old Black nonbinary person assigned female sex at birth whose pronouns are they/them/theirs, and who goes by the name Shane. Shane is an Operation Enduring Freedom/Operation Iraqi Freedom (OEF/OIF) veteran of the Army who recently separated from the military and is presenting to VHA for the first time. They presented with trauma-related difficulties and substance use problems. During their first visit with an OEF/OIF case manager, Shane was misgendered and repeatedly referred to as a woman and with pronouns she/her/hers. The case manager proceeded to describe programs for women veterans. When Shane attempted to provide corrective feedback, the case manager looked puzzled and said, "What do you mean, miss?" Shane became frustrated and left the appointment.

On their way out of the VHA facility, they saw a rainbow-colored advertisement for the LGBT VCC, with direct contact information. Shane contacted the VCC, and they were offered a meeting that day. When Shane entered the office, the VCC, wearing a rainbow lanyard, greeted Shane stating, "Veteran Johnson, it's nice to meet you in person… what are your name and pronouns?" Shane immediately felt at ease and was able to describe their difficulty with the case manager during their recent visit. The VCC validated Shane's concerns and thanked them for their openness. The VCC informed Shane they would follow up with the clinician to provide education regarding the provision of care when working with TGD veterans. The VCC then oriented Shane to the mental health clinics that treat veterans with trauma-related problems, explaining that there is a clinic for women veterans and one for men veterans and that Shane would be welcome to use either clinic. Shane expressed a preference to be seen in the men's trauma clinic, and the VCC submitted a referral. The VCC asked Shane's permission to include Shane's name and pronouns in the referral, and Shane verbally consented to this. The VCC also accompanied Shane to the eligibility clerk, whom they asked for their preferred name to be listed on the cover sheet of their medical record. The VCC thanked Shane and explained how this would be helpful to the receiving provider, so they can affirm Shane when they speak to schedule an initial appointment. Shane expressed appreciation for the meeting with the VCC. Later, the VCC coordinated training in TGD health that included content related to nonbinary identities for the entire OEF/OIF case management team (including the case manager who had seen Shane previously). Shane eventually became reconnected with this important service, and they were treated with respect in their affirmed identity.

▶ **Discussion Questions**

1. Why might it be important for VHA staff to obtain verbal consent when documenting veterans' names and pronouns in their medical records?

   Authors' response: So documentation can be accurate and consistent. The current VA health record system has a preferred name field but not a gender pronoun field. In this case, the VCC included their pronouns in the consult so that providers would be aware.

2. Shane is connected to an affirming mental health provider in the trauma clinic. During a team meeting, a psychiatrist raises a concern about Shane, stating that their identity may be indicative of dissociative identity disorder (DID). What are some ways to address this comment and concern from the colleague within the team?

   Authors' response: In the description provided, there is no indication of DID. Clarify with the provider if additional assessments were conducted or if there is other information known. Absent those findings, this provider may be pathologizing normative gender identity development. TGD veterans may refer to prior timepoints as though they are referring to an alternate self, which is developmentally normal as a part of gender identity consolidation.

REFERENCES

1. Schultz J. Veterans by the numbers. The NCSL Blog 2019. https://www.ncsl.org/blog/2017/11/10/veterans-by-the-numbers.aspx.
2. Gates GJ. How many people are lesbian, gay, bisexual, and transgender? The Williams Institute, University of California at Los Angeles, April 2011. http://williamsinstitute.law.ucla.edu/wp-content/uploads/Gates-How-Many-People-LGBT-Apr-2011.pdf. Accessed December 15, 2020.
3. Gates GJ, Herman JL. Transgender military service in the United States. The Williams Institute, University of California at Los Angeles, May 2014. https://williamsinstitute.law.ucla.edu/wp-content/uploads/Transgender-Military-Service-May-2014.pdf. Accessed December 15, 2020.
4. James SE, Herman JL, Rankin S, Keisling M, Mottet L, Anafi M. *The Report of the 2015 US Transgender Survey*. Washington, DC: National Center for Transgender Equality; 2016.
5. Directive-type Memorandum (DTM)-19-004. Military Service by Transgender Persons and Persons with Gender Dysphoria. Department of Defense, March 12, 2019.
6. Brown GR. Transsexuals in the military: flight in hypermasculinity. *Arch Sex Behav.* 1988;17(6):527-537.
7. Poulin C, Gouliquer L, McCutcheon J. Violating gender norms in the Canadian military: the experiences of gay and lesbian soldiers. *Sex Res Social Policy.* 2018;15(1):60-73.
8. Hendricks ML, Testa RJ. A conceptual framework for clinical work with transgender and gender nonconforming clients: an adaptation of the minority stress model. *Prof Psychol Res Pr.* 2012;43(5):460-467.
9. Meyer IH. Prejudice, social stress, and mental health in lesbian, gay, and bisexual populations: conceptual issues and research evidence. *Psychol Bull.* 2003;129(5):674-697.
10. Beckman K, Shipherd J, Simpson T, Lehavot K. Military sexual assault in transgender veterans: results from a nationwide survey. *J Trauma Stress.* 2018;31(2):181-190.
11. Hoy T, Klosterman Rielage J, Williams LF. Military sexual trauma in men: a review of reported rates. *J Trauma Dissociation.* 2011;12(3):244-260.
12. Kimerling R, Gima K, Smith MW, Street A, Frayne S. The Veterans Health Administration and military sexual trauma. *Am J Public Health.* 2007;97(12):2160-2166.
13. Surís A, Lind L. Military sexual trauma: a review of prevalence and associated health consequences in veterans. *Trauma Violence Abuse.* 2008;9(4):250-269.
14. Blosnich JR, Brown GR, Shipherd JC, Kauth M, Piegari RI, Bossarte RM. Prevalence of gender identity disorder and suicide risk among transgender veterans utilizing Veterans Health Administration care. *Am J Public Health.* 2013;103(10):e27-e32.
15. Brown GR, Jones KT. Mental health and medical health disparities in 5135 transgender veterans receiving healthcare in the Veterans Health Administration: a case–control study. *LGBT Health.* 2016;3(2):122-131.
16. Lehavot K, Simpson TL, Shipherd JC. Factors associated with suicidality among a national sample of transgender veterans. *Suicide Life Threat Behav.* 2016;46(5):507-524.
17. Tucker RP, Testa RJ, Reger MA, Simpson TL, Shipherd JC, Lehavot K. Current and military-specific gender minority stress factors and their relationship with suicide ideation in transgender veterans. *Suicide Life Threat Behav.* 2019;49(1):155-166.
18. Livingston NA, Berke DB, Ruben MA, Matza AR, Shipherd JC. Experiences of trauma, discrimination, microaggressions, and minority stress among trauma-exposed LGBT veterans: unexpected findings and unresolved service gaps. *Psychol Trauma.* 2019;11(7):695-703.
19. Department of Veterans Affairs. VA utilization profile, FY 2016. National Center for Veterans Analysis and Statistics;2017.https://www.va.gov/vetdata/docs/QuickFacts/VA_Utilization_Profile.PDF. Accessed December 15, 2020.

20. 38 CFR 17.38 – Medical benefits package. https://www. govinfo.gov/app/details/CFR-2009-title38-vol1/CFR-2009-title38-vol1-sec17-38. Accessed December 15, 2020.

21. Directive 1341. Directive on the Care of Transgender and Intersex Veterans; 2011. https://www.va.gov/vhapublications/ViewPublication.asp?pub_ID=6431. Accessed December 15, 2020.

22. Kauth MR, Shipherd JC. Transforming a system: improving patient-centered care for sexual and gender minority veterans. *LGBT Health.* 2016;3(3):1-3.

23. VHA Directive 1340: Health Care for Veterans who Identify as Lesbian, Gay or Bisexual. https://www.va.gov/vhapublications/ViewPublication.asp?pub_ID=5438. Accessed December 15, 2020.

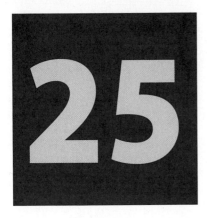

Affirming Care for People with Intersex Traits

Katharine B. Dalke

Niki S. Khanna

Frances W. Grimstad

INTRODUCTION

Intersex traits are a collective of congenital variations of **primary** and **secondary sex characteristics** that fall outside the usual binary medical definitions of female and male. Despite the use of the term "outside," intersex traits are a diverse, naturally occurring, and widely prevalent aspect of human sex and are thus within the expected range of human sex development. **Endosex** describes the alignment of sex traits within the usual binary definitions of female and male. To underscore that every person has a sex and that intersex traits are not inherently deviant, this text uses the term "endosex" in place of terms such as "normal" or "typical." The aim of this chapter is to outline a reparative, affirming, and trauma-informed approach to care for intersex persons, and it is written by an intersex psychiatrist, an intersex psychotherapist, and an endosex pediatric and adolescent gynecologist. Depathologizing and normalizing language is used wherever possible, and clinicians are encouraged to do the same in clinical care.

DEFINITIONS

Physical sex is far from binary: rather, human sex is influenced by multiple sex markers found in diverse configurations. Physical sex traits include sex chromosomes, sex hormones, internal genitalia, external genitalia, and secondary sex traits. Prenatal and pubertal sex developments are complex processes with multiple determinants and branch points. Before birth, all fetuses have the capacity to develop all primary sex traits. The development of primary sex traits involves a cascade of prenatal events in which sex chromosomes influence the development of gonads, which then produce sex hormones that lead to changes in the structure of internal and external genitalia. A similar process occurs at puberty, in which gonads begin to produce high levels of hormones that lead to changes in the shape and function of internal and external genitalia as well as secondary sex traits. Intersex traits are variations in these primary or secondary sex traits that do not align with the traditional binary configuration of endosex traits (Table 25-1). Because of the interrelated nature of sex development, a variation at one point often leads to variations at other points. These changes can include arrays of sex chromosomes, the structure and function of the gonads or internal genitals, production and action of sex hormones, shape of the external genitals, or the presence of secondary sex traits.

Because of the complexity of sex development, intersex traits are highly heterogeneous. Some are associated with specific genetic variations and known branch points in sex development. Because of this, these intersex traits are sometimes referred to medically as **differences of sex development (DSD),** although this term is not considered affirming by many in the intersex community. Other intersex traits, namely **hypospadias**, **Turner syndrome**, and **47,XXX karyotype,** are not consistently associated with other variations in sex development and are not consistently referred to as DSD.

A detailed discussion of the features of and medical approach to each intersex trait is beyond the scope of this chapter, and readers are encouraged to review the medical sources cited in this chapter for more details. Table 25-2 provides a brief overview of various intersex traits and associated conditions. However, there are several unifying principles that are essential for readers to know. Above all, most intersex traits pose no urgent physical risk to an individual. Some may be associated with variations in anorectal or urinary anatomy; these must be addressed to ensure that a person can pass stool or urine. **Congenital adrenal hyperplasia** (CAH), common among 46,XX people with intersex traits, may result in low levels of cortisol and aldosterone, which may be life threatening. In these individuals, levels of these hormones must be managed

Table 25–1. Intersex and Endosex Traits

Feature	Endosex Female	Intersex Traits	Endosex Male
Sex chromosomes	XX	XXY XO XY/XX mosaic	XY
Sex hormones	Estrogens	Variations in levels, action, or both	Androgens
Internal genitalia	Ovaries Fallopian tubes Uterus and cervix Upper vagina	Gonadal dysgenesis Ovotestes Müllerian variations	Testes Epididymis, ductus deferens, seminal vesicle, ejaculatory duct Prostate
External genitalia	Clitoris Vulva/labia	Glans length variations Labioscrotal variations Urethral variations	Penis Scrotum
Secondary sex traits	Breast development Menstruation Pubic and axillary hair	Gynecomastia Primary amenorrhea Sexual hair variations	Voice change Genital enlargement Pubic, axillary, and facial hair

Table 25–2. Intersex Traits and Associated Conditions

Sex Marker	Associated Conditions
Sex karyotype	47,XXY (Kleinfelter Syndrome) 45,XO (Turner Syndrome) 47,XXX 46,XX/XY mosaicism
Sex hormones	Congenital adrenal hyperplasia (classic or nonclassic) Androgen insensitivity syndrome 5-alpha reductase deficiency 117-beta hydroxysteroid dehydrogenase deficiency
Internal genitalia	Gonadal dysgenesis Müllerian agenesis Vaginal agenesis
External genitalia	Bladder or cloacal exstrophy Hypospadias

with steroid replacement. Fecal or urinary obstruction and salt-wasting CAH typically present at or shortly after birth. Later in life, some children and adults with specific and limited intersex traits may be at risk for gonadal cancers. Risk appears to correlate with the location and degree of cellular variation within the gonad, with the intra-abdominal gonads of people with **partial androgen insensitivity syndrome (PAIS)** or **gonadal dysgenesis** at highest risk.[4] Gonadal imaging and biopsy are sometimes used to help evaluate this risk.[4] Sometimes, even low-risk gonads are removed due to concerns for "mixed" feminine and masculine pubertal development, but increasing numbers of clinicians now consider the use of **pubertal suppressant agents** for this purpose instead. Over the long term, some intersex children and adults who have not had genital or gonadal surgery may benefit from attention to other nonurgent health concerns, such as diverse urinary voiding patterns and sexual function.[5]

The language of intersex traits is complex. Many people and health care professionals use the terms "intersex" and "DSD" interchangeably. Although no language is comfortable for all people, the terms "intersex" and "differences of sex development" were about equally acceptable to patients in one survey.[1] Community-led advocacy and support organizations in the United States tend to use intersex, differences of sex development, or the specific name of the intersex variation.[2,3] Terms like "hermaphroditism," "ambiguous genitalia," and "disorder of sex development" are widely considered offensive by intersex persons because they are stigmatizing, pathologizing, and objectifying. Clinicians caring for people with intersex traits must be exquisitely attuned to this language, in part because the medical approach to persons with intersex traits has itself been stigmatizing and traumatic.

PREVALENCE AND INTERSECTIONALITY

One of the challenges in identifying the prevalence of people with intersex traits in the United States is that, unlike for sexual orientation or gender identity, there is a lack of inclusion of questions to assess intersex status in population-based sampling.[6] Additionally, many people who were born with intersex traits may not know that they have these traits due to concealment of information by parents or health care professionals or may be reluctant to disclose their medical information due to external or internalized stigma.

In clinical samples, researchers and clinicians disagree about what constitutes an intersex trait. If the definition includes any variation in reproductive or sexual anatomy, then traits like hypospadias or 46,XXY karyotype increase the prevalence to 1.7% or 1 in 58. If limited to only those people with diversity of the external genitalia, the prevalence may be as low as 1 in 4500.

Scales are used clinically and academically to describe the appearance of primary and secondary sex characteristics along a continuum from endosex female to endosex male. These scales may aid in the description of sex traits and are often useful in clinical care, but they also have significant limitations. Most scales, including the Prader genital scoring system and the Ferriman Gallwey pubic hair distribution scale, were developed in predominantly White cohorts, which may inhibit generalizability.[7,8] For instance, while some studies have validated the Ferriman Gallwey scale among African American individuals, other studies have shown variations in hair pattern among other ethnicities.[9,10]

Crucially, there is no standard definition for the appearance of "normal" endosex genitalia. In fact, research suggests greater endosex genital diversity than clinically assumed. Lloyd and colleagues found a wide range of genital appearances among a cohort of women with endosex female genitalia, including persons who had a clitoral length up to 3.5 cm and labia majora length up to 12 cm.[11] None of the women in the study had any complaints about the appearance or function of their genitalia. Despite the elusive nature of ideal genitals, studies have suggested that physician bias about genital appearance influences surgical decision-making and approach for both endosex and intersex people. For instance, one study found that clinicians, especially those who identified as male or who were plastic surgeons (compared with gynecologists), were more likely to identify smaller labia as being considered normal and identify larger labia among endosex women as requiring surgical intervention.[12] Similarly, texts on intersex genital surgery often refer to moving anatomic features to their appropriate or "right" position and size, without defining what that is.[13] Another study found disparities in evaluation of the appearance of the genitals of 46,XX children with CAH: parents reported 30–50% satisfaction with their child's genital appearance, while 0% of surgeons did. In follow-up, 96% of families in the study decided to pursue genital surgery, highlighting the powerful impact that surgeons' impressions of what is "normal" can have on parents' decision-making.[14]

In clinical care, there are important intersections between intersex and queer experiences. Just as people of any sex may identify as lesbian, gay, bisexual, pansexual, or asexual, so too do intersex people, and some studies have suggested that intersex people may be more likely to be nonheterosexual than endosex people.[15] Intersex people may also be **transgender or gender diverse (TGD)**: up to 13% of people with some intersex traits do not identify with the sex that was assigned at birth.[15] Like endosex TGD people, intersex people who are **cisgender** may have body parts that do not align with their gender identity. Both TGD and intersex populations grapple with stigma, medical paternalism, and medical gatekeeping. But there are also key differences in these populations. While a priority of TGD advocacy is increasing access to desired medical care, a priority of intersex advocacy is educating the general population and medical community about unwanted medical interventions. In our experience, while some heterosexual, cisgender intersex people do identify as queer, many people who have intersex traits do not identify with queerness in any way, and are often more comfortable referring to themselves as having a biological variation or medical condition. Because of the similarities, there are aspects of care for queer and TGD people that are highly applicable to intersex care; because of the differences, there are core intersex-specific competencies that health care providers should acquire.

HISTORICAL APPROACHES AND TRAUMA

The traditional model of care for intersex people began in the 1950s, at a time when gender theory began to emerge and surgical techniques became more advanced. John Money remains the most visible representative of this approach, which was grounded in the theory that gender identity was determined by nurture rather than nature.[16] For intersex children, endonormative genitals were seen as essential to the treatment goals of achieving heterosexual and cisgender identities. Physicians undertook early medical and surgical interventions to align the child's anatomy with one side of the endosex genital binary paradigm and rear the child according to the surgically determined gender. Despite the lack of medical urgency for the majority of infants, so fraught was the birth of a healthy intersex child that decision-making around sex determination and surgery was deemed a "social emergency." Withholding of information from children, and often from parents, was also seen as essential, as any ambiguity in rearing might lead to gender ambivalence.

Since the 1990s, intersex advocates have increasingly brought to light the physical and emotional trauma of this model of care. People who received medical interventions for their intersex variations may have physical trauma from early, irreversible surgeries. These procedures can involve the reduction of the size of the glans or clitoris/penis, and in some cases, complete removal of the portion of the organ outside of the body. Other people may have had **vaginoplasty** or surgery to relocate the opening of the urethra from the underside to the tip of the glans. Some individuals may have had their internal reproductive organs, including gonadal tissue, removed. Surgeries can lead to scarring, loss of nerve sensation, urinary incontinence, and impaired sexual function. Some procedures, such as vaginoplasty and hypospadias repair, require postoperative maintenance and possible future revisions. Removal of gonadal tissue can result in a dependence on sex hormone replacement for the duration of one's life, as well as the loss of fertility.

Although many of these surgeries are presented to families of young children as urgent and medically necessary, the reality is more nuanced. There is little robust medical evidence to support making these decisions urgently. Most variations do not need to be addressed in a young child, unless urine or stool cannot leave the body safely, pelvic organs are exposed, or if tissue is actively cancerous. Unfortunately, clinicians continue to recommend surgery outside of these cases. In 2016, an international group of health care providers identified reasons for surgeries as including "functional genital anatomy to allow future penetrative intercourse (as a male or a female)," promoting development of "individual and 'social identities,'" averting genital stigma and mixed secondary sex trait development, and responding "to the parents' desire to bring up a child in the best possible conditions."[17] Clinicians working in transgender health will appreciate that these goals are driven by cisgender, heterosexual norms, and are based on the assumption that endonormative genitals are essential for a child and family to have "normal" psychosocial development. Clinicians should also be aware that elective genital surgeries have never been shown to be directly responsible for improving the health or well-being of intersex youth or adults, or their parents, over not having surgery at all.[18,19]

The circumstances in which medical care takes place can also be a source of psychological trauma for intersex people. Intersex people often describe confusion and pain caused by having a surgery that they did not fully understand, did not consent to, or were misled about, usually in areas of the body that are extremely vulnerable. Even without surgery, medical interventions, such as unnecessary examinations and hormonal therapies without the child's full knowledge or understanding, can cause confusion and distress in children.

Medical photography can also be distressing for intersex individuals. Often the subjects of these photographs are children, and the photographs themselves are typically close-up images of genitals. In some cases, adults are photographed. The process of being photographed in this manner is invasive, dehumanizing, and traumatic.[20] Children cannot consent to photography. Even when the parents or guardians of children or adult individuals themselves give consent, they may not be informed fully about how these photographs may be used, including that the images could be distributed extensively and available for years. We are aware of intersex people who found naked or close-up images of themselves in textbooks that pathologized their bodies. Some people had

this experience in a classroom of their peers, as their bodies or bodies similar to theirs were discussed in dehumanizing and othering ways. These events themselves can be traumatic and may also evoke memories of previous traumas. While medical imaging can have benefits to care (such as monitoring postoperative healing), the likelihood of psychological trauma must be taken into consideration when clinicians consider medical imaging as part of care for a patient with intersex traits. A clear rationale should be provided to the parents and patients regarding the necessity for the utilization of photography. The clinician should review the application, permanence, and distribution of the images, and the patient (and parents or guardians where applicable) must give full informed consent to medical photography without coercion.

Health care professionals who work with this population of patients must also be cognizant of how systemic oppression may impact the clinical care of an intersex person and their family. Language or cultural differences can prevent parents and children from communicating or fully appreciating the medical interventions, possible surgeries, and their outcomes or consequences. If clinicians do not hold a measure of cultural humility in working with patients with cultural or language needs different from their own, they might not provide the same level of consultation and care as they would to someone with a similar cultural or linguistic background.[21]

Because intersex variations are assumed to be very rare, many individuals are referred to research and teaching medical facilities for care. The benefits of these referrals are that patients and families have access to clinicians who may have advanced knowledge in intersex medicine, and that decisions are less likely to be made in isolation. This is why professional consensus groups often recommend care in specialized, multidisciplinary teams. Unfortunately, this also means that patients are seen in teaching settings, where they are studied by medical trainees. Families with lower socioeconomic status, those who do not possess medical insurance, or those whose documentation status is in question may not have any other choice, particularly if the intersex variation is co-occurring with a more serious issue. In these cases, the intersex person and their family may experience coercion to consent to medically unnecessary exams and tests, sometimes in the presence of several observers. Intersex people and their families may also feel pressured to undergo surgery and other interventions. Parents who do not provide consent for their child to undergo recommended exams, treatments, or surgery may be perceived as unsuitable or neglectful.

The experiences of Black, Indigenous, and People of Color with intersex traits are extremely understudied. The implicit biases that U.S. health care professionals have in particular toward Black patients, such as perceiving Black patients to have higher pain thresholds than other patients, or as having deviant sexualities or genders, could lead to more invasive and unnecessary treatment and surgeries on black and brown intersex children.[22] The legacy of historical medical experimentation and modern-day inequities in health care may heighten mistrust of clinicians by Black and Brown families. Importantly, the prominent faces of intersex advocacy are often White and gender-conforming, which has marginalized people of color even within support and advocacy spaces.

Notably absent from the health literature for intersex people are studies on the experience of medical trauma, and there is contention among health care providers regarding whether medical interventions on intersex variations are traumatic. Many health care providers interpret the lack of negative feedback from their patients as overall satisfaction, citing the so-called "silent majority" in support of current practices. In addition, satisfaction of the parents or caregivers can be conflated with the satisfaction of the child themselves, even in the absence of evidence of the child's satisfaction. Crucially, studies tracking outcomes of childhood surgeries into adulthood or even adolescence are woefully lacking.

Much anecdotal and qualitative information, however, has been reported to advocacy and support groups, with a common theme of medical trauma. Many such narratives were documented in a 2017 Human Rights Watch report, "I want to be like nature made me": Medically Unnecessary Surgeries on Intersex Children in the US."[23] While these stories are not often published in peer-reviewed journals, it is important to acknowledge their existence. Therefore, clinicians should approach intersex care from a trauma-informed perspective and be mindful that most intersex people start experiencing potentially traumatic medical interventions in childhood. As adults, intersex people may show an aversion to receiving medical care; distrust of health care professionals; dissociation, freezing, and muscle tension during medical exams; and anxiety and depression. An affirming, trauma-informed, and transparent approach to intersex care can help alleviate medical trauma responses, and potentially improve health care engagement.

IMPACT OF ENDONORMATIVITY AND TRAUMA ON HEALTH

Intersex people are included by the National Institutes for Health among **sexual and gender minority (SGM)** groups as an understudied health disparities population. This inclusion highlights the overlap between intersex and other SGM populations and draws attention to the relative lack of research on the health and health risks of people with intersex traits.[24] For instance, there are very little available data on the population health of people with intersex traits because, unlike for sexual orientation or gender identity, population surveys do not assess intersex status.[25] Because clinical studies tend to be granular in focus, evaluating the physical and mental health of intersex persons as an outcome of medical

or surgical treatment for a specific intersex trait or diagnosis, there is a dearth of naturalistic research evaluating clinical needs across intersex conditions.[26]

People with intersex traits appear to have increased rates of medical and mental health concerns relative to endosex people. For instance, dsd-LIFE, a multicenter study with aggregated survey data from a population of over 1000 intersex youth and adults across six European countries, found a lower physical quality of life for intersex respondents across intersex traits relative to the general population.[27] Intersex people were also more likely to report long-standing health problems and limiting health issues, as well as significantly higher rates of health concerns like diabetes, high cholesterol, cardiovascular disease, autoimmune disorders, and hearing and visual problems, than the general population.[28] There is insufficient evidence to clarify how much of these health problems are related to the physiology of the person's intersex condition, effects of hormones or surgery, experiences of stress or discrimination, or other unrelated health problems. Regardless, primary and specialty care providers serving intersex people must be aware of the spectrum of health risks that intersex patients may face, and avoid focusing on the person's genitalia or gender to the exclusion of general health concerns.

Research has yielded interesting but mixed findings regarding the mental health of intersex patients. For instance, in subgroup analyses of dsd-LIFE survey data, social relationship quality of life was significantly lower for intersex respondents than for the reference population, but mental health scores were comparable to or even higher than those within the reference population.[27] On the other hand, psychiatric disorders and suicide attempts among intersex people were reported at about four times the prevalence of the reference population.[29] In a follow-up analysis, there were mental health differences by gender, with all male-identified intersex respondents endorsing higher symptoms of depression and anxiety relative to the reference population. In contrast, only some female-identified persons with specific intersex traits reported the same.[7] Interestingly, the factors that appeared to correlate with depression and anxiety were levels of self-esteem, openness, and shame. These findings are in keeping with other studies confirming that intersex people, regardless of whether or not they have undergone genital surgery or have genital differences, often experience shame and stigma related to their intersex traits.[30–33]

A central aspect of intersex advocacy, since the founding of the Intersex Society of North America in 1993, has been the notion that societal stigma toward intersex traits, rather than the traits themselves, is responsible for mental health disparities experienced by intersex people. Unfortunately, research has only recently begun to explore the relationship between stigma and mental health among intersex populations, despite a growing literature illustrating this relationship among sexual and gender minorities.[34] Despite this lack of data, mental health clinicians must be attuned to how structural discrimination, interpersonal stigma, and internalized negativity may interact with a person's unique medical narrative and must seek to offer a normalizing and validating experience. Mental health clinicians should also be mindful that intersex adults may have difficulty forming strong interpersonal attachments and developing pride and positive self-regard due to their unique experiences. These include having information withheld from them by primary attachment figures, prolonged hospitalizations, and internalizing the belief that their bodies are shameful from interactions with their caregivers and clinicians. It is important to note that the lack of consent in early childhood, in this case regarding medical interventions, can lead to difficulty understanding and setting boundaries as an adult. Adults who were traumatized during previous medical encounters may also avoid future clinical care, dissociate during encounters and exams, choose not to follow treatment recommendations, and express anger toward their current care teams. Medical and mental health providers must appreciate that even "successful" elective genital surgery may compound shame and distress.[18]

FOUNDATIONS FOR AFFIRMING CARE

The intersex-affirming model (IAM) of care described in this section was developed in response to the legacy of medical trauma, erasure, and nonconsensual care and the impact of cisnormative, heteronormative, and endonormative bias on decision-making. It seeks to move away from the primary focus of an early "fix" in favor of a life-long process of support for the patient and family. Building on existing models of care as developed by consensus groups, IAM further shifts conversations that often involve reductive binary choices (such as full surgical intervention or none) to ones that disentangle various aspects of care, thereby offering segmented options that can be selected concomitantly, in sequence, or not at all.[35] The IAM for children, adolescents, and adults is based on the core principles that guide affirming care for TGD youth[36]:

1. The genders, sexualities, and bodies of intersex individuals are presumed to be normal aspects of human diversity.

2. A person's mental health symptoms are related to a combination of the society's reaction to their physical sex or gender identity, the experience of misalignment between the body and the self, or medical trauma.

Additionally, in recognition of the growing consensus from international organizations and groups of medical professionals that informed consent is a key aspect of preserving the human rights of intersex people, the IAM emphasizes that an individual is the best person to make decisions about their body for themselves, and care should be taken to ensure fully informed consent (Table 25-3).

IAM uses a systems framework and considers an individual's caregiving network and relationships between the individual and the care team. This type of approach can improve communication and comprehension, build tolerance for living with uncertainty, and allow for dynamic decision-making through the life cycle from infancy to adulthood. Intersectional awareness ensures that providers consider how an individual's social position impacts their medical care and experience. The IAM also centers on the patient and their experience of their identity and anatomy. By centering the patient, clinicians reframe their understanding of the common phrase "in the best interests of the patient," which can often be misconstrued as a paternalistic approach that involves the clinician and family thinking on behalf of the patient. Instead, clinicians afford the patient every opportunity to participate and declare their own interests and priorities. The model focuses on validating the patient's experience and supporting their autonomy, including their decisions surrounding gender, sexual pleasure, and fertility, and makes every attempt to avoid causing stigma surrounding intersex identity. The IAM also aims to reduce the likelihood of harm by deferring nonurgent, irreversible interventions until individuals reach an age at which they can actively participate in decision-making. Deferral of such interventions limits the potential for complications or misassignments (e.g., gender, sexual goals) that stem from decisions made without the person's involvement.

COMPONENTS OF INTERSEX-AFFIRMING CARE

Intersex-affirming care offers scaffolding on which a person's autonomy can be supported in decision-making. The model involves the following aspects:

Table 25–3. Comparison of Affirming and Traditional Models of Intersex Care

Traditional Model	Affirming Model
Sex defined by aligned hormones, gonads, and genitals	Sex defined by a balance of factors
Sex must be binary	Sex exists on a continuum
Intersex is a disorder	Intersex is a natural human variation
Gender is binary and predictable	Gender is flexible and exploratory
Genitals must be "normal" for parents	Parents can affirm genital diversity
Children will be harassed, ostracized, and distressed	Children can be prepared, nurtured, and supported
Only heterosexual, penovaginal intercourse is normal	A wide range of sexual activity is normal and enjoyable

1. *Multidisciplinary care:* The care of intersex persons should not occur in a vacuum; clinicians should not be siloed in the decisions they make. Given not only the medical and historic complexity of intersex health, multidisciplinary care is critical to ensuring that all aspects of care, including ethical, psychological, physical, and social components, are considered when determining the best plan of care. These perspectives are especially crucial when a person is too young to participate in decision-making.

2. *Psychological support:* Psychological support is critical to helping intersex persons and their families navigate a cisgender, endosex, and heteronormative world. Peer support normalizes, validates, and provides individuals and families with guidance about what to expect at different developmental moments. Professional psychological support should be provided to parents and caregivers who are navigating the complex care of their child. Despite evidence that families of babies and toddlers with intersex traits often experience distress, which can hinder their ability to give informed consent, many families do not have adequate support. Additionally, adopting a medicalized approach to decision-making can bias families toward medical interventions.[37-39] Therefore, even when patients and parents appear well-adjusted and deny acute psychological concerns, access to a health care provider experienced in caring for intersex people is still recommended. An experienced care provider can provide emotional support, demedicalizing language to facilitate decision-making, guidance for developmentally appropriate conversations about sex and gender, and space for the patient to explore their understanding of their identity and anatomy. Emotional barriers to decision-making or well-being can be addressed by exploring identity, addressing trauma, and identifying internalized stigma.

3. *A holistic approach to sex and gender:* All clinicians should be grounded in the understanding that sex and gender are **nonbinary,** that these two constructs do not predictably align with one another, and that gender can evolve over time, regardless of sex assigned at birth. Terminology such as "glans length variation" is depathologizing because it is gender-inclusive, embryologically accurate, and normalizing. Assumptions should not be made about an individual's gender identity or sexual orientation. Not all female people want an endonormative vagina, and not all people with a vagina desire penovaginal intercourse. Medical and surgical decision-making should be bolstered by discussions of the patient's gender and sexual goals.

4. *Cultural humility:* Clinicians must be honest with patients and families about the limits of their knowledge of the patient's variation. Additionally, clinicians should be mindful of their own endosex, cisgender, and heteronormative biases, especially as these intersect with or reflect Western, White norms that may not be values held by the patient or family. Clinicians should also be aware that children may not adhere to the cultural values in which they were raised once they reach adulthood and ensure that discussions with family members and young patients regarding decision-making are grounded in this possibility.

5. *Patient-collaborative care:* The patient is the person who must live with the results of any decisions made about their life, body, and identity. Whenever possible, the patient should be at the center of or leading these decisions. Any decisions prior to the patient developing the ability to participate should be based solely on whether the treatment is emergent; all others should be deferred. In time-sensitive, but not emergent, scenarios, strategies for decompressing urgency should be considered, as in pubertal suppressant medication for patients whose pubertal development or gender identity is uncertain. As patients mature and consider partly or fully irreversible interventions like hormones or surgery, they should be supported in balancing affirmation of their gender identity and sexual orientation with any known or potential risks of the variation or treatment. For example, a patient should understand how a persistent urogenital sinus can impact the ability to manage menstrual egress after someone with a uterus undergoes puberty.

6. *Informed consent/assent:* All care, including surgeries, testing, examinations, and photography, should be done with the fully informed consent of the patient when feasible. If a patient is very young or is not able to demonstrate the capacity to understand and appreciate the risks, benefits, alternatives, and impact of a procedure or exam, fully informed consent from their guardian should be provided, with additional steps taken to ensure fully informed assent of the patient.

7. *Disclosure of diagnosis:* In order for patients and their families to be fully aware of the care they are undertaking, medical information must be disclosed. Information regarding past medical interventions performed on intersex persons should not be withheld from them or their families, and clinicians who are approached by intersex persons who have newly accessed past medical records should make every effort to help them navigate their medical history. Behavioral health professionals can help families learn how to educate their children about their anatomical variation, and these professionals can support families and individuals in judiciously and sensitively sharing information with other people in their lives, such as daycare workers, extended family, friends, and romantic partners.

8. *Recognition of harms, human rights, and the unknown:* Clinicians should be able to understand and discuss the risks associated with both early and delayed medical and

BOX 25-1 Organizations That Support Delaying Nonemergent Procedures Until Patient Can Participate in Decision-Making

American Academy of Family Physicians
Amnesty International
Commissioners of Health and Human Rights of New York City
European Commission Bioethics Committee
Gay and Lesbian Advocates and Defenders
GLMA: Health Professionals for LGBTQ Equality
Human Rights Watch
Lambda Legal
Physicians for Human Rights
The American Civil Liberties Union
The United Nations
The World Health Organization

surgical therapies for intersex persons. This includes having open conversations about the limitations of existing data and the great deal of "unknown." Additionally, clinicians should be able to counsel families on how their present care fits with the most current standards of practice put forth by preeminent national and international medical and human rights organizations (Box 25-1) regarding the organizations that support delaying nonemergent interventions.

SUMMARY

- Intersex traits are variations in primary or secondary sex traits that do not align with the traditional binary configuration of endosex traits.

- An emerging body of research and growing consensus support the notion that intersex traits are a normal aspect of human diversity with which people can thrive if they receive support that centers their autonomy.

- In the past, intersex children often underwent early medical and surgical interventions to align the child's anatomy with one side of the endosex genital binary paradigm and rear the child according to the surgically determined gender. This model of care not only imposes permanent physical changes but also may result in psychological and emotional trauma.

- Research does not show any benefit or improvement in the health or well-being for intersex youth or adults who had elective genital surgeries compared with those who did not have surgery. In addition, disparities within the health care system may subject persons who belong to a racial or ethnic minority to differential treatment.

- The lack of longitudinal and naturalistic studies significantly hinders the development of evidence-based guidelines. Health care professionals are uniquely positioned to apply the art, evidence, and ethics of TGD health to promote the health of intersex persons.

- The intersex-affirming model of care focuses on validating the patient's experience and supporting their autonomy, including their decisions surrounding gender, sexual pleasure, and fertility, and makes every attempt to avoid causing stigma surrounding intersex identity. The IAM also aims to reduce the likelihood of harm by deferring nonurgent, irreversible interventions until individuals reach an age at which they can actively participate in decision-making.

CASE STUDY: N

N. is the first child of A. and B., who happily anticipated N's birth. In the delivery room, the midwife declares that N. is a healthy girl. The next day, the pediatrician examining N. identifies that N. has genital diversity: a longer glans and a palpable lump in the left groin. N. has otherwise been doing well. N is feeding without issue and has produced numerous wet and meconium diapers. A team of medical providers is consulted and perform an external exam later that day. They confirm the previous exam and an appropriately located anus. They recommend to N.'s parents that N should undergo more testing that day: an ultrasound of the lump, sex karyotype, and hormonal levels. A., who was trained as a physician in India before moving to the United States and now works in biomedical research, is confused about whether N is at immediate medical risk. She is informed by the doctors that "we don't know what your daughter's risk is until we do more testing." A. and B. agree to the testing, and the results are consistent with partial androgen insensitivity syndrome (PAIS). N.'s karyotype is 46,XY, the tissue in the groin could not be visualized, and the testosterone level is elevated. No rudimentary Mullerian structures are seen on the ultrasound. The new family is discharged home, with a follow-up appointment with urology for 3 months.

At the follow-up appointment, the surgeon, Dr. P, recommends that N. have two procedures. Dr. P recommends a biopsy of the gonads to determine how typical the gonads are, which will help predict the risk of cancer and the kind of puberty N. will experience, as well as whether or not N. can produce fertile gametes. Dr. P also mentions that the family could choose to have N.'s glans shortened while N is under anesthesia for the biopsy, "if you want her to look more female when people change her diaper." When B. asks about timing, he is told that "there are no real data to support doing it earlier or later, but most families choose before 18 months because the child is less likely to remember it, and healing may be easier."

▶ Discussion Questions

1. Using the IAM, what risks and benefits of gonadal biopsy and glans reduction can be understood by the family?

2. How can the surgeon bring the human rights context into the clinical discussion?

3. How would you encourage the family to think about their child's future gender identity?

4. How might the family's background inform the discussion or decision-making?

5. Who else should be involved in the patient's care?

Eleven years later, N. presents to the pediatric endocrinologist for follow-up care. N.'s parents had chosen for N. to have the gonadal biopsy, but not glans surgery. N.'s gonads were typically differentiated testes, with some surviving germ cells and no evidence of gonadal dysgenesis. N. is starting to show some signs of puberty, with the appearance of pubic hair and axillary hair. A. and B. tend to refer to N. with she/her pronouns, but N. discloses to the nurse that the pronouns they/them, which they use online and with friends, feel better. N. is not dating, and "isn't sure" about gender identity: "Sometimes I feel like a boy, sometimes I feel like a girl, and sometimes I feel like neither." N. is reluctant to talk about gender identity with their parents and has limited vocabulary to describe their situation: "They've only told me that my private parts are different from other kids. They don't say bad things about my body, but the church we go to says that being gay or transgender is a sin." N. hasn't been told about their chromosomes or gonads.

The endocrinologist informs the family that they "need to make a decision about N.'s puberty." If N. goes through endogenous puberty, N. will develop breasts but may also have glans and facial hair growth. The other option is gonadectomy and life-long estrogen hormone replacement therapy: "She'll never need them anyway, and we'll know exactly what pubertal changes she'll then get." Attempting to reassure the doctor, B. notes that the men in his Chinese-American family have relatively little facial hair.

▶ Discussion Questions

1. How can intersex- and gender-affirming models guide N and their family in considering gonadectomy or spontaneous puberty?

2. What other options might be available?

3. What additional resources might be useful in helping N identify their gender and body goals?

4. In what ways are A's, B's, and N's cultures important to consider in discussions and decision-making?

At age 17, N. is seen by the general pediatrician for a well visit. With the family, N. had chosen to start gonadotropin-releasing hormone agonists. After meeting with a psychologist and other families with PAIS through a support group, the family decided to stop medication and have N. go through endogenous puberty. During the social history, N. reports enjoying the soccer team and visiting colleges. N.'s pronouns are now she/her or they/them. She has also started dating and is interested in people of all genders. She does not have sex or masturbate. On physical exam, N. has breasts and signs of minimal androgen effect: sparse facial and pubic hair, and a 1-inch glans. She also has some fusion of the labioscrotal folds.

N. states that her mom has been encouraging her to talk with the pediatrician about seeing a surgeon for a vaginoplasty, "so I can have sex." When asked about this, N. reports that she does feel female and likes having a femme or androgynous gender expression. She's not sure whether she needs a vagina to feel like herself, or to have sex: she's interested in penetrative intercourse, but "there are other ways, too." She admits to leaning toward having vaginoplasty but acknowledges that "it might be because it would make it easier to date." N. is able to describe what PAIS is. She and her mother have consulted with multiple doctors, and she now understands that she is at moderately increased risk for testicular cancer. She wants to have her testes removed next summer and is thinking of trying either estrogen or estrogen/testosterone replacement. She understands a bit about vaginoplasty because a transgender girlfriend of hers recently had one.

▶ Discussion Questions

1. What types of nonsurgical and surgical options would be available to N. if she wants to have a vagina for penetrative intercourse?

2. How could intersex- and gender-affirming models guide N. in articulating her reasons to undergo or not undergo a vaginoplasty?

3. How can you best support N. in discussing the relationship between her anatomy and different forms of romance (emotional, physical, sexual)?

4. Who else can support her in approaching this decision?

5. At what stages of life might N. consider creating a vagina, and how might those stages impact N.'s decision-making?

REFERENCES

1. Johnson EK, Rosoklija I, Finlayson C, et al. Attitudes towards "disorders of sex development" nomenclature among affected individuals. *J Pediatr Urol.* 2017;13(6):608 e601-e608.

2. interACT. interACT Statement on Intersex Terminology. 2015. https://interactadvocates.org/interact-statement-on-intersex-terminology/. Accessed December 9, 2019.

3. Group A-DS. What is intersex and/or DSD? http://aisdsd.org/fact-check/. Accessed January 2, 2020.

4. Pyle LC, Nathanson KL. A practical guide for evaluating gonadal germ cell tumor predisposition in differences of sex development. *Am J Med Genet C Semin Med Genet.* 2017;175(2):304-314.

5. Kreukels BPC, Cohen-Kettenis PT, Roehle R, et al. Sexuality in adults with differences/disorders of sex development (DSD): findings from the dsd-LIFE Study. *J Sex Marital Ther.* 2019;45(8):688-705.

6. Tamar-Mattis S, Gamarel KE, Kantor A, Baratz A, Tamar-Mattis A, Operario D. Identifying and counting individuals with differences of sex development conditions in population health research. *LGBT Health.* 2018;5(5):320-324.

7. Prader A. Genital findings in the female pseudo-hermaphroditism of the congenital adrenogenital syndrome; morphology, frequency, development and heredity of the different genital forms. *Helv Paediatr Acta.* 1954;9(3):231-248.

8. Ferriman D, Gallwey JD. Clinical assessment of body hair growth in women. *J Clin Endocrinol Metab.* 1961;21:1440-1447.

9. Yildiz BO, Bolour S, Woods K, Moore A, Azziz R. Visually scoring hirsutism. *Hum Reprod Update.* 2010;16(1):51-64.

10. Wolf WM, Wattick RA, Kinkade ON, Olfert MD. Geographical prevalence of polycystic ovary syndrome as determined by region and race/ethnicity. *Int J Environ Res Public Health.* 2018;15(11).

11. Lloyd J, Crouch NS, Minto CL, Liao LM, Creighton SM. Female genital appearance: "normality" unfolds. *BJOG.* 2005;112(5):643-646.

12. Reitsma W, Mourits MJ, Koning M, Pascal A, van der Lei B. No (wo)man is an island—the influence of physicians' personal predisposition to labia minora appearance on their clinical decision making: a cross-sectional survey. *J Sex Med.* 2011;8(8):2377-2385.

13. Hutson JM. Surgical treatment in infancy. In: Hutson JMW, Garry L, Grover SR, eds. *Disorders of Sex Development: An Integrated Approach to Management.* Berlin, Heidelberg: Springer; 2012.

14. Nokoff NJ, et al. Prospective assessment of cosmesis before and after genital surgery. *J Pediatr Urol.* 2017;13(1):28 e1-28 e6.

15. Almasri J, Zaiem F, Rodriguez-Gutierrez R, et al. Genital reconstructive surgery in females with congenital adrenal hyperplasia: a systematic review and meta-analysis. *J Clin Endocrinol Metab.* 2018;103(11):4089-4096.

16. Money J, Hampson JG, Hampson JL. Hermaphroditism: recommendations concerning assignment of sex, change of sex and psychologic management. *Bull Johns Hopkins Hosp.* 1955;97(4):284-300.

17. Mouriquand PD, Gorduza DB, Gay CL, et al. Surgery in disorders of sex development (DSD) with a gender issue: If (why), when, and how? *J Pediatr Urol.* 2016;12(3):139-149.

18. Roen K. Intersex or diverse sex development: critical review of psychosocial health care research and indications for practice. *J Sex Res.* 2019;56(4-5):511-528.

19. Elders J, Sacher D, Armona R. *Re-thinking Genital Surgeries on Intersex Infants.* Palm Center; 2017.

20. Creighton S, Alderson J, Brown S, Minto CL. Medical photography: ethics, consent and the intersex patient. *BJU Int.* 2002;89(1):67-71; discussion 71-62.

21. Dogra N, Reitmanova S, Carter-Pokras O. Teaching cultural diversity: current status in U.K., U.S., and Canadian medical schools. *J Gen Intern Med.* 2010;25(suppl 2):S164-168.

22. Hoffman KM, Trawalter S, Axt JR, Oliver MN. Racial bias in pain assessment and treatment recommendations, and false beliefs about biological differences between blacks and whites. *Proc Natl Acad Sci U S A.* 2016;113(16):4296-4301.

23. Watch HR. "I want to be like nature made me": medically unnecessary surgeries on intersex children in the US. In: *Youth IAfI: Human Rights Watch*; 2017.

24. Committee NIoHSaGMRC. NIH FY 2016-2020 Strategic Plan to Advance Research on the Health and Well-being of Sexual and Gender Minorities. 2015. https://dpcpsi.nih.gov/sites/default/files/sgmStrategicPlan.pdf. Accessed December 12, 2019.

25. Tamar-Mattis S, Gamarel KE, Kantor A, Baratz A, Tamar-Mattis A, Operario D. Identifying and counting individuals with differences of sex development conditions in population health research. *LGBT Health.* 2018;5(5):320-324.

26. Sandberg DE, Gardner M, Cohen-Kettenis PT. Psychological aspects of the treatment of patients with disorders of sex development. *Semin Reprod Med.* 2012;30(5):443-452.

27. Rapp M, Mueller-Godeffroy E, Lee P, et al. Multicentre cross-sectional clinical evaluation study about quality of life in adults with disorders/differences of sex development (DSD) compared to country specific reference populations (dsd-LIFE). *Health Qual Life Outcomes.* 2018;16(1):54.

28. Falhammar H, Claahsen-van der Grinten H, Reisch N, et al. Health status in 1040 adults with disorders of sex development (DSD): a European multicenter study. *Endocr Connect.* 2018;7(3):466-478.

29. de Vries ALC, Roehle R, Marshall L, et al. Mental health of a large group of adults with disorders of sex development in six European countries. *Psychosom Med.* 2019;81(7):629-640.

30. Meyer-Bahlburg HFL, Khuri J, Reyes-Portillo J, New MI. Stigma in medical settings as reported retrospectively by women with congenital adrenal hyperplasia (CAH) for their childhood and adolescence. *J Pediatr Psychol.* 2017;42(5):496-503.

31. Meyer-Bahlburg HF, Reyes-Portillo JA, Khuri J, Ehrhardt AA, New MI. Syndrome-related stigma in the general social environment as reported by women with classical congenital adrenal hyperplasia. *Arch Sex Behav.* 2017;46(2):341-351.

32. Meyer-Bahlburg HFL, Khuri J, Reyes-Portillo J, Ehrhardt AA, New MI. Stigma associated with classical congenital adrenal hyperplasia in women's sexual lives. *Arch Sex Behav.* 2018;47(4):943-951.

33. Ediati A, Juniarto AZ, Birnie E, et al. Social stigmatisation in late identified patients with disorders of sex development in Indonesia. *BMJ Paediatr Open.* 2017;1(1):e000130.

34. Hatzenbuehler ML, Pachankis JE. Stigma and minority stress as social determinants of health among lesbian, gay, bisexual, and transgender youth: research evidence and clinical implications. *Pediatr Clin North Am.* 2016;63(6):985-997.

35. Krege S, Eckoldt F, Richter-Unruh A, et al. Variations of sex development: the first German interdisciplinary consensus paper. *J Pediatr Urol.* 2019;15(2):114-123.

36. Rafferty J, Committee on Psychosocial Aspects of Child and Family Health; Committee on Adolescence; Section on Lesbian, Gay, Bisexual, and Transgender Health and Wellness. Ensuring comprehensive care and support for transgender and gender-diverse children and adolescents. *Pediatrics.* 2018;142(4).

37. Wisniewski AB. Psychosocial implications of disorders of sex development treatment for parents. *Curr Opin Urol.* 2017;27(1):11-13.

38. Tamar-Mattis A, Baratz A, Baratz Dalke K, Karkazis K. Emotionally and cognitively informed consent for clinical care for differences of sex development. *Psychol Sexual.* 2014;5(1):44-55.

39. Timmermans S, Yang A, Gardner M, et al. Does patient-centered care change genital surgery decisions? The strategic use of clinical uncertainty in disorders of sex development clinics. *J Health Soc Behav.* 2018;59(4):520-535.

Community-Building, Advocacy, and Partnership

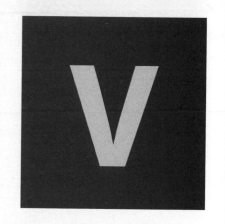

Community Engagement and Outreach

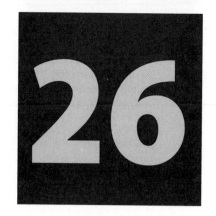

Cei Lambert

INTRODUCTION

In order to successfully engage **transgender and gender diverse (TGD)** patients in care, clinicians and the health care institutions in which they work must first prove that their facilities are safe and welcoming places to be. A double bind exists for many TGD patients wherein they seek, in an ostensibly free market, to be able to choose the health care professional and location that provides the best services for their needs. Regardless of a patient's privilege, the reality is that between insurance, geographic limitations, and a declining number of primary care clinicians, many people have little choice over whom they have as their clinician and where they see that person. Therefore, it is incumbent on health care professionals and their practice settings to educate themselves about and institute best practices to ensure that TGD patients receive sensitive and appropriate care.

Epidemiological data show that TGD patients are probably part of every clinician's practice. With a reported 3% or more of the population identifying as gender diverse in some way,[1] it is a matter of *when* a clinician sees someone who is gender diverse, not *if*. As part of the commitment to optimize care for all patients, to serve patients with the utmost fidelity, to provide autonomy and choices, and above all, to do no harm, gender-affirming care is a requirement. It is not enough for clinicians to know how to prescribe hormone therapy, make a referral for gender-affirming surgery, or write letters supporting a person's desire to update the legal documentation of their **gender identity**. It is necessary to understand and respond to the social and cultural factors affecting gender minority people in a clinical context to provide the best possible care. After all, gender is a social and cultural construct, and without this context, it is not possible to appropriately understand why gender affirmation is important or how many nonclinical factors are critical to making someone feel included in society.[2]

How can clinicians find out the social and cultural constructs faced by TGD people? The answer is by engaging TGD people themselves in conversations and decision making about practice transformation and care. In short, clinicians and administrative leaders of their practice environments must engage in outreach with gender diverse communities to understand how to provide holistic, gender-affirming care. Although not all community outreach and engagement personnel need to share the identity of the groups they seek to serve, it is crucial to have some people who do share those identities, and for those people to be in positions of influence.[3] After all, as promoted by leaders in the disability rights movement, "nothing about us, without us."[4]

This chapter discusses how to build and reach out to networks of TGD people, identify and combat implicit biases against TGD people, understand and address intersections of identities when engaging community members, and use these networks to liaise effectively with the community. The chapter explores how to build enduring systems that perpetuate community involvement throughout the lifetime of a health care facility and how to address barriers to outreach with TGD people. By the end of this chapter, readers should have a good sense of what health care professionals and the institutions in which they work can do to bring the voices of gender diverse people into the decision-making process, and what to do with the information gathered. The guidance provided here is grounded in community health center work and is applicable across all health care organizations and affiliates.

BUILDING REACH AND NETWORKS

Before researching how to contact TGD people to gather their input and begin reaching out, clinicians should first take stock of their current clinical context as well as their individual and colleagues' feelings toward TGD patients and understanding of TGD people's life experiences. Is the clinic seeing TGD patients? If so, are clinicians providing gender-affirming care? If the practice is providing care, does it also provide behavioral health care? If the practice provides both medical and behavioral health care, is it expected that all of the health care professionals see and work with TGD patients? This short assessment can reveal: (1) whether or not the health care staff know about the TGD people who come into the clinic (these people are there, even if they are not identified); (2) if the practice provides the services necessary to support gender affirmation; (3) if the practice responsively serves TGD people for all of the other medical and behavioral health reasons they may come to the clinic; and (4) whether or not the staff can identify where and why they are or are not serving TGD people appropriately. This last point refers largely to the presence of implicit (or unconscious) bias, and how these biases affect one's practice.

Once this self-assessment of the current clinical practice and services for TGD people is complete, it is important to take stock of the practice's capacity to cultivate and support community outreach efforts. Outreach and social/community programs are frequently considered ancillary or optional, under- or unfunded, and staffed by volunteers whose ability to provide consistent engagement may vary widely.[5]

▶ A Word on Implicit Bias

Implicit bias happens when subconscious messages that a certain group is "bad," "lazy," "wrong," "imaginary," or any number of other stereotypes begin to influence a person's actions toward members of that group.[6] All of us have implicit biases that are learned via exposure to family, friends, schools, mentors, media, and other influences that teach—overtly or covertly—that certain people are inherently less worthy than others simply because of their identities. Actions based on these biases translate into marginalization, **stigma**, **discrimination**, and violence, and a world in which people are divided and divisive. Individuals who are stigmatized are typically members of a subordinate group, and often (although certainly not always), the stigmatization is carried out by a person in a dominant social position who enacts bias into discrimination (Figure 26-1). It is critical to building trust and engagement with *any* community to identify, acknowledge, and combat implicit bias.[7-13]

Dominant Groups

- Greater access to power and resources
- Make the rules
- Define what is "normal", "right", and "true"
- Assumed to be leaders, smart, competent
- Given the benefit of the doubt
- Often unaware of dominant group memership or privilege
- Are more comfortable with members of subordinated groups who model their behavior on the dominant group

Subordinate Groups

- Less access to power and resources
- Often seen as less-than, inferior, deficient
- Often assimilate, collude, abide by the rules set by dominant group, and try to "fit in"
- Track the daily indignities they experience and are usually very aware of oppression
- Have their truth and experiences questioned and often invalidated
- Know more about dominant group members than dominant group members know about them
- Often struggle to find their voice

Key concepts of dominant/subordinate group dynamics

- Not always about numbers
- Visible and invisible
- Innate and chosen (horizontal and vertical identity)
- Multiple group memberships

- Code switching
- Not always about individual behaviors or feelings
- You didn't ask for it and you can't give it back

▲ **Figure 26–1.** Dominant and subordinate group patterns and examples. (Data from Collins PH, Bilge S: Intersectionality. Cambridge, UK: Polity, Press; 2016.)

In her book *Men, Women, and Worthiness*, author and psychologist Brené Brown suggests that we must learn to separate a person's inherent worth from their identities and that all people, regardless of their identities, are worthy of kindness, justice, self-determination, and care.[14] It can be helpful when working to create buy-in for community engagement and outreach to acknowledge the inherent *worthiness* of all people, the validity of their identities, and the diversity of opinion around whom one likes and agrees with. It is also critical to bring awareness, acknowledgment, and a stated commitment to working on one's own bias. Caring professions are uniquely positioned to promote inclusivity because a basic ethical tenet of these vocations is to provide care for all people in need.

NUTS AND BOLTS: WHAT DOES A COMMUNITY OUTREACH PROGRAM FOR TRANSGENDER AND GENDER DIVERSE PEOPLE LOOK LIKE?

Three main strategies can be used to build a community outreach and engagement network: (1) the internet; (2) in-person/meet-space networking (any kind of social engagement that happens in a physical location rather than online); and (3) professional affiliation groups (such as a TGD Engineers meet-up or TGD community advisory board within a company). For many TGD people, the internet is a safer space than in-person community spaces, and so it is not unreasonable to go online to find gender diverse people to provide insight and guidance for clinical practice. Several studies in recent years have sought the opinion and recommendations of gender diverse people using internet surveys and questionnaire portals. For example, the 2015 U.S. Transgender Survey was conducted largely (but not entirely) using internet recruitment and web-based surveys. This survey, conducted by The National Center for Transgender Equality, is the largest survey to date of gender diverse people in the world.[15] The survey yielded an enormous amount of information about the discrimination faced by TGD communities and the scale of the negative health sequelae caused by these social determinants of health. Clinical practices can conduct similar surveys within their existing patient population and in the surrounding geographic community to better understand the health care needs of current and future TGD patients.

Another idea is for a practice to consider creating a dedicated online "space" or developing a presence within an existing "space." Creating a chatroom hosted by a single health care organization is probably not always feasible. However, existing social media platforms can be used to create a "space" and to post advertisements for in-person meet-ups and other opportunities to get involved. These include Instagram, Facebook, Snapchat, and dating apps used by TGD people, such as Grindr (a dating app geared toward gay men) and Scruff (another app for men seeking sex with men, which is more inclusive of TGD masculine people). Because the internet is rapidly evolving, it is important to have flexibility in any internet outreach strategy. Focus on creating content and engagement tools that have permanence, but which can be translated into many different online communication platforms (image-heavy for Instagram, text-focused on Facebook groups, etc.).

The internet is an imperfect tool, and for many people, it is inaccessible. Although most people in the United States assume that the internet is universally available, the truth is that internet access and literacy are still available mainly to the financially privileged, those in urban and suburban settings, and those with stable housing. Because of the interacting minority stressors faced by many TGD people, an internet-only outreach campaign would likely reach only a particular segment of the population a health care facility seeks to serve. TGD people face disproportionate rates of homelessness (one in five TGD people report being discriminated in housing and 20–40% of homeless youth are TGD identified[16]) and financial hardship (TGD adults are four times more likely to have a household income of less than $10,000 per year compared with the general population[17,18]), which can compromise their ability to access the internet consistently if at all. For this reason, in-person and other networking strategies are needed.

Having a meet-space can be very helpful in achieving community outreach goals with TGD people. Many TGD people do not have a place where they can express their gender identity and also feel safe; a physical location staffed by culturally responsive and confident employees can fill this role. Depending on geographic location, it may be challenging for TGD people to find community. In rural areas, people are more spread out and specific regions may be sparsely populated, so that connecting online is the most practical option. In urban areas, it may feel unsafe for TGD people to congregate for fear of being identified and targeted as a group. Despite its usefulness, it is important not to assume that the internet is a cure-all for people in isolation who seek community. Internet access is far more of a luxury than most people appreciate, and regardless of location, there may be many barriers to access. Even if someone does have internet access, this is no guarantee that the communities available—particularly in rural settings—will be able to meet their needs. It is not sufficient to counsel TGD people in rural locations to "find online support/social groups"; rather, a community health center can often act as a safe social hub, provided the staff are trained and engaged. A physical space can be used for support groups, educational seminars, and other programming related to the needs of TGD people. The secondary focus of such groups and spaces can be to provide insight into the health care needs of the community that can be used to improve policies, practices, and both the content and delivery of care.

There are also many existing physical spaces that serve as gathering hubs for TGD people, and community outreach workers can network in clubs, bars, and other locations in which casual socializing occurs. However, it is important to identify the reasons why a community outreach worker is entering a space to avoid overt or inadvertent voyeurism and to allow TGD people to have privacy and safety while socializing. Many spaces used by TGD people are considered safe by the people there, and if a community outreach worker does not understand the culture, norms, and expectations of the space, they may be asked to leave or, worse, can compromise the safety of the space for all. Fidelity is key, and if a community outreach worker is going to seek to engage TGD people in groups or clubs or other spaces, they must be transparent about who they are and why they are there in the space. For example, if a community outreach worker seeks to provide information about HIV, STI testing, and rapid-HIV saliva testing, the worker should communicate first with the person running the space (owner, organizer) to ask permission and establish ground rules. Ideally, the worker, preferably a person who is themselves TGD, should spend time in the space before doing any outreach to understand the culture, needs, and demographics of the people it serves. If it seems inappropriate for a community outreach worker to be physically present in a particular space, a flier with contact information can be effective in reaching people in that space while preserving safety and privacy.

People who hold TGD identities are frequently asked to take on duties outside their usual job description as community liaisons and outreach staff but without additional compensation or time. As part of a practice's overall community outreach and engagement strategy, it is critical to provide more time and compensation when more work is asked of a member of any underrepresented group. As stated previously, it is necessary to have staff who hold TGD identities as part of the team who create an effective community outreach and engagement program, and it is necessary to build in appropriate financial and logistical assumptions for this purpose.

THE ROLE OF COMMUNITY OUTREACH AND ENGAGEMENT AS A PATHWAY TO TRANSFORMATIVE SOCIAL CHANGE

Typically, a community outreach and engagement program that is provided by a health center has a two-part focus: (1) to provide a community social/support space and (2) to find individuals willing and able to speak to the needs of their community or communities such that the health center can integrate such feedback into their strategy and service. A third focal point is needed: to cultivate lasting social change for TGD people on a variety of scales. Social change is progressive, with wholesale cultural shift being slow and generally resulting from steady and consistent pressure on systemic factors that cause marginalization. Figure 26-2 presents a staged approach to cultivating social change. The stages build toward an eventual goal of lasting transformative change, but in daily work, several stages of the process are likely to be engaged depending on the context, availability of resources, and the particular need of the person.

At the most basic level, a health center can provide resources (stage 1) for TGD people. Resources can include those provided by the center itself, such as gender-affirming hormone therapy and surgery referral, as well as resources in the community (e.g., support groups, safe shelters, and other holistic supports). Provision of resources can often be accomplished passively via signage, posters, web announcements, and resource lists. The second stage of cultivating

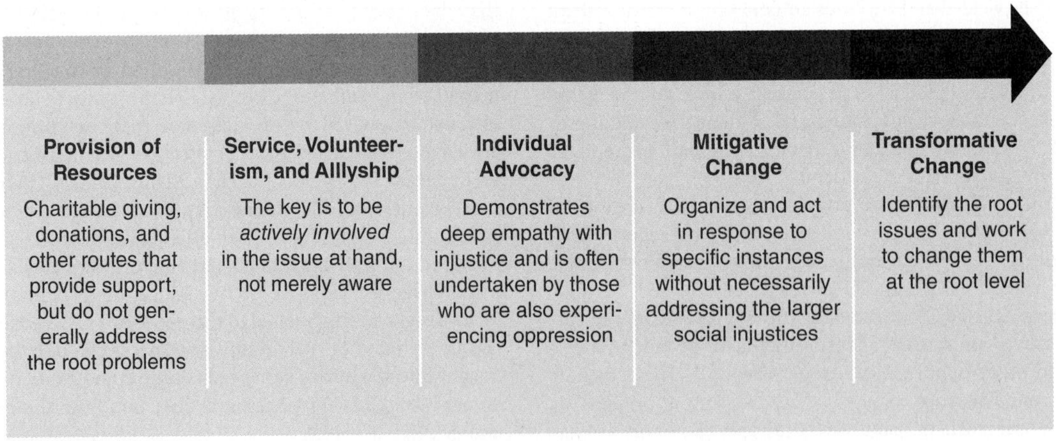

Provision of Resources	Service, Volunteerism, and Alllyship	Individual Advocacy	Mitigative Change	Transformative Change
Charitable giving, donations, and other routes that provide support, but do not generally address the root problems	The key is to be *actively involved* in the issue at hand, not merely aware	Demonstrates deep empathy with injustice and is often undertaken by those who are also experiencing oppression	Organize and act in response to specific instances without necessarily addressing the larger social injustices	Identify the root issues and work to change them at the root level

▲ **Figure 26–2.** The progression of social change. (Data from Gorski P: Approaches to Cultivating Social Change. EdChange and the Equity Literacy Institute. Revised December 21, 2017. http://www.edchange.org/handouts/approaches-activism.pdf.)

change occurs when a health care professional or health center becomes actively involved (stage 2) in advocating for the needs of TGD people beyond the clinic. The staff may volunteer at TGD events like Transgender Day of Remembrance, act as allies to give TGD people voice (and learn how to provide better care in the bargain), and engage in service to the TGD communities. Simultaneously, clinicians and other staff may be engaged in individual advocacy (stage 3), in which the needs of a particular TGD patient are addressed, and strategies are employed to assist the person in overcoming barriers and getting their needs met. Providing gender-affirming care is just the beginning of this stage of social change: it is also important to incorporate social advocacy into clinical care.

The final two stages are often challenging, whether they are being addressed by the health center or by external stakeholder groups focused exclusively on creating social change. Mitigative change (stage 4) happens when there is an organized response to a particular element of oppression, such as laws limiting access to gender-affirming care. Health center and health center staff can engage in mitigative change by providing testimony and resources to lawmakers about the importance of gender affirmation to combat negative health outcomes, by writing letters in support of patients seeking to update their documentation to reflect their gender (this is also individual advocacy), and by ensuring that internal health center policies do not contribute to social injustice. Transformative change (stage 5) occurs when the underlying issues that create discrimination and marginalization are identified, addressed, and removed. For example, it would be transformative change for society to accept that gender is a social construct and that gender is far more expansive than the binary of man and woman. If there were widespread social acceptance of gender diversity, it would become anathema to discriminate against TGD people and, in fact, "gender diverse" people would be able to live as individuals who simply have gender, as all humans have gender identities.

TRANSGENDER AND GENDER DIVERSE PEOPLE AS COMMUNITY OUTREACH AND ENGAGEMENT WORKERS FOR TRANSGENDER AND GENDER DIVERSE PEOPLE

When someone is doing community outreach and engagement for people with whom they share identities, the work can be tiring, triggering, and also exceptionally fulfilling. To retain community outreach workers who are TGD, an employer must provide trauma-informed supports to help the person reduce and manage triggering experiences and prevent burnout. Many TGD people seek to work in a role that allows them to uplift the TGD communities. This approach can be a wonderful synergy for a health center seeking to create a robust community outreach and engagement program for TGD patients.

It is critical that organizations not take advantage of employees who derive personal satisfaction from serving a community or communities of which they are a member. Personal satisfaction is not a paycheck, stable job on a career trajectory, or retirement account. Community outreach workers must be compensated appropriately, given access to benefits, and helped to advance in a way that aligns with their skills and interests, just like any other employee. People will not stay in positions where they are undercompensated and un/underappreciated, even if they are very committed to the mission of the employer. To create a lasting community outreach program for TGD people, employees who are TGD must be given reasons to stay beyond "you're lucky to be helping people like you." It's also in the best interest of the health center to decrease turnover and create sustainable internal career ladders for employees. The retention of institutional knowledge and supporting people in their advancement into management and leadership increases the likelihood that a health care organization can make meaningful and lasting change, and part of this process is managing burnout and preventing uncompensated work asks.

INTERSECTIONALITY AND COMMUNITY OUTREACH

A more expansive dialogue on the social determinants of health affecting TGD people is explored elsewhere in this book, and an understanding of these factors is important for creating buy-in to grow a network of TGD people to help guide a health care organization's strategy. People who are TGD hold many other identities in addition to a minority gender identity; unique experiences of stigma and discrimination can occur at the intersection of these identities (Figure 26-3). An understanding of how these other identities interact with a person's gender identity can help to provide a foundation for the development of trust in the clinic and the practice's staff.

For people with multiple marginalized identities, community outreach can play a key role in linking people to care and using community connection to combat negative health outcomes created by oppressive social structures. Always consider how someone's social circumstances and identities influence their access to health care and health care decision making, particularly when building and implementing outreach and engagement practices. While community outreach programs that offer simultaneous safe social spaces and linkage-to-care can be effective in engaging TGD people who also hold other marginalized identities, it is important to remember that they do not meet all of their constituents' social needs. Therefore, particularly for individuals who hold multiple marginalized identities, community outreach programs that do not address: (1) the need for food/shelter; (2) the need for unstructured socialization and community; (3) the need for a *consistently* safe space; and (4) the needs of

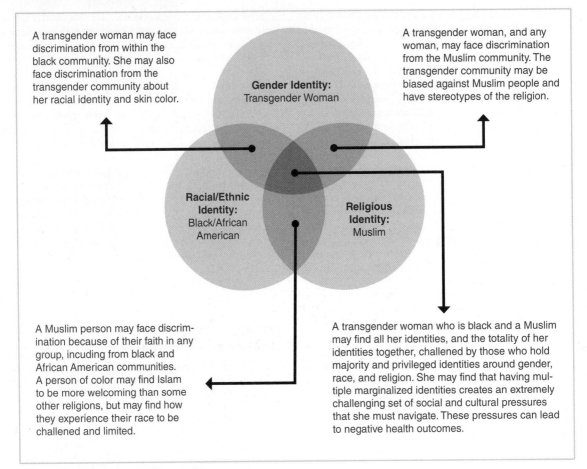

A transgender woman may face discrimination from within the black community. She may also face discrimination from the transgender community about her racial identity and skin color.

A transgender woman, and any woman, may face discrimination from the Muslim community. The transgender community may be biased against Muslim people and have stereotypes of the religion.

Gender Identity:
Transgender Woman

Racial/Ethnic Identity:
Black/African American

Religious Identity:
Muslim

A Muslim person may face discrimination because of their faith in any group, incuding from black and African American communities. A person of color may find Islam to be more welcoming than some other religions, but may find how they experience their race to be challened and limited.

A transgender woman who is black and a Muslim may find all her identities, and the totality of her identities together, challened by those who hold majority and privileged identities around gender, race, and religion. She may find that having multiple marginalized identities creates an extremely challenging set of social and cultural pressures that she must navigate. These pressures can lead to negative health outcomes.

▲ **Figure 26–3.** Intersectionality: an example.

affinities and identities beyond gender identity, are unlikely to be successful in the long term.

As previously discussed, it is crucial to include people who hold diverse TGD identities as members of the team doing the outreach work. In some communities, there are different expectations and access abilities around education, work norms, and more. Mentorship plays a key role in building a community outreach workforce that is representative of individuals who have histories of discrimination and stigmatization. To successfully recruit community outreach workers who will be able to holistically engage the TGD communities and its intersections with race, socioeconomic status, linguistic background, homelessness, and more, it is important to ask:

- What are the goals for this program, and are the goals clearly stated in my job postings and employee asks?

- What are the measurement tools for success, and do these tools fit the needs of the community with which we

are seeking to engage and employees who are doing this engagement?

- For example, it may be necessary to provide job skills training and mentorship to people who have not had the privilege of a "traditional" education that includes telephony, writing, and other components often taken for granted by employers.

- What characteristics are we seeking in employees, and are we focused on finding a person who will effectively reflect the TGD and intersectional communities we wish to serve?

Job descriptions seeking community outreach and engagement staff should carefully consider what credentials and expertise are asked for. An ideal candidate may have uncontested expertise and insight into the needs of the community but may not look like an "ideal candidate" on paper. The core of any community outreach effort must be the community itself, and efforts that prioritize ease or speed above the needs of the group in question are unlikely to be successful.

PROGRAMMING FOR COMMUNITY OUTREACH AND ENGAGEMENT FOR TRANSGENDER AND GENDER DIVERSE PEOPLE

Before developing community activities or programming either within the health care organization or at a site in the community (see Figure 26-2), ground rules should be cocreated with community members. The health center can start by creating a draft of ground rules that align with its mission and ask the community to do the same. All written ground rules should be treated as living documents that can be easily updated and shared. Table 26-1 provides some ideas for programming in these two arenas.

Developing a robust and persistent community outreach and engagement strategy takes time, and it is helpful to look for low-lift and high-return activities, like attending and participating in community-led and focused events, especially at

the beginning of outreach efforts. As trust with the community increases and buy-in from leadership is obtained, higher lift activities can be taken on.

EXECUTIVE AND LEADERSHIP BUY-IN AND PARTICIPATION: A PREREQUISITE AND AN EXPECTATION

According to a recent publication by The National LGBT Health Education Center, "to achieve a safe and supportive workplace for LGBTQ staff, leadership must set the tone for the entire health center by clearly communicating that the health care organization's commitment to diversity includes patients and staff of all sexual orientations and gender identities."[3] A good way to think about a sustained community and outreach engagement strategy is that it must have "bookends": the front-line staff must be trained and bought-in so that when TGD people engage with the clinic they are supported, and the executive/C-suite/board-level staff must be trained and bought-in so that they can prioritize

Table 26–1. Community Outreach and Engagement Programming Ideas

Programming Inside the Clinic	Cross-Walk to Provision of Care	Arena(s) of Activating Social Change[a]	Estimated Level of Challenge/ Lift for the Organization
A Clinical Support Group (depression/ anxiety, substance use, smoking cessation, etc., specifically for the gender diverse community)	High	1,2,3,4	Medium
A Peer-Led/Social Support Group	Medium	1,2,3,4	Medium
In-Services on Gender-Affirming Care	High	1	Low
In-Services on Cultural/Social Aspects of Gender Diversity	Medium/Low	1	Low
Support Groups for families, partners, friends, and supporters of gender diverse people	Medium/High	1,2,3,4,5	Medium
Film Screening and other facilitated access to cultural content relating to gender diversity	Low	1,4	Low
Community creative activity (art project, talent show, etc.)	Low	1,2,3,4	Low
Connecting activity for nonmedical gender affirmation (clothing exchange, binder swap, etc.)	Medium	1,2,4	Low
Hosting a speaker/thought leader within the gender diverse community	Low	1,2,4	Medium
Creating and hosting a community advisory board	High	1,2,4,5	High

(Continued)

Table 26–1. Community Outreach and Engagement Programming Ideas *(Continued)*

Programming Outside the Clinic	Cross-Walk to Provision of Care	Arena(s) of Activating Social Change[a]	Estimated Level of Challenge/Lift for the Organization
Speaking to an existing group about clinic offerings	High	1,2,3	Medium
Tabling at an event	High	1,2,3	Medium
Sponsoring and working a community event (pride parade, transgender day of remembrance, etc.)	Medium	1,2,4	High
Staffing a walk-in clinic at a community space	High	1,2,3,4	High
Providing clinical and structural guidance for spaces with clinical functions (schools, prisons, shelters, etc.)	High	1,2,4,5	Medium
Attending and participating in community-led and focused conferences and fora	High	1,2,3,4,5	Low
Surveying gender diverse people about what they need from the clinic—can be online or in-person	High	2,3,4,5	Low
Attending programming/activities about and for people with intersecting identities including gender diversity	Medium	2,3,4,5	Low
Providing transportation to community events	Medium	1,2,3	Medium
Creating or providing sponsorship for the creation of materials relating to gender affirmation/identity (ideally in several languages)	High	1,2,3,4,5	Medium

[a]These numbers refer to the stages that effect change shown in Figure 26-2. 1: Provision of services; 2: Service, volunteerism, and allyship; 3: Individual advocacy; 4: Mitigative change; 5: Transformative change.

gender identity support in strategic planning, allocation of resources, and clinic goals.

Ideally, TGD people should be recruited into positions across the health center, including in executive leadership and at the board level. Because of systematic discrimination faced by many TGD people, however, leadership positions are often not occupied by TGD people or even individuals with other minority identities. A positive feedback loop can be created when a health center actively seeks out TGD people for leadership roles and prioritizes advancing deserving TGD candidates. It is important that all internal policies and structures reflect the ethics and values reflected in patient care. A holistically integrated organization committed to the needs of TGD people includes coverage for gender-affirming medical services in employee medical insurance policies, streamlined and effective ways for employees to note their

name and pronouns at work, nonexploitative engagement of TGD employees in conversations about how to best serve the TGD communities, and paid time off for gender diverse employees to recover from gender-affirming surgeries and other procedures.

Whether for TGD people or for other marginalized groups, community outreach and engagement efforts are often subordinated to seemingly more pressing needs within a health center. In addition to a commitment to serve the needs of TGD people, there must also be a commitment from the executive level to participate in community outreach and engagement. Because of the long history of mistreatment that TGD people have experienced in medical settings, it is uniquely important for this group to be given opportunities to build trust with the health clinic and clinic staff before, during, and after the clinic visit.

SUMMARY

- At the most basic level, advocacy for TGD people is part of a larger ethos that promotes and celebrates diversity across all identities and for all people. Cultural and social stigma have placed TGD people in marginalized positions in most aspects of daily life, and so it is critical to actively combat bias and discrimination based on gender identity.

- For health centers, part of combating this bias involves building trust with TGD communities, particularly because of the harm inflicted on TGD people by the medical profession. Community outreach and engagement are key strategies to build this trust and enable health centers to enhance care for TGD people in expansive and holistic way.

- Creating and sustaining a community outreach and engagement program requires a health center to first identify networks and connections that can facilitate culturally sensitive outreach to TGD communities. Once this is accomplished, the health center can offer resources while seeking information from the community on what is needed.

- When the needs of the community are understood, the health center can use its own or other existing platforms to create programming that engages and supports TGD people. As the health center provides this programming, it can continue to elicit feedback from TGD patients and use it to improve both clinical care and the outreach and engagement programming.

- Ultimately, community outreach and engagement should be integrated into all levels of clinical strategy, from basic service provision to the creation of formal community advisory boards and the presence of TGD people at the highest levels of clinic management.

- Eventually, transformative change practices will make such targeted engagement unnecessary, but until there are massive social shifts in addressing bias and accepting difference, it will be necessary to proactively engage marginalized communities like TGD people.

CASE STUDY: ENHANCING OUTREACH AND ENGAGEMENT EFFORTS

After reading this chapter, you feel inspired to enhance outreach and engagement efforts of your (health professional school)(practice)(hospital) to TGD communities and have a sense of how to begin this work.

▶ Discussion Questions

1. How would you assess the current responsiveness of your (school)(practice)(hospital) to the health care needs of TGD patients? For example, do you feel your team is culturally competent, but not yet able to provide concrete services or resources? Do you have advertised services but struggle with team members who need more cultural context and inclusion training?

2. How would you determine your (school's)(practice's)(hospital's) capacity to cultivate and support community outreach efforts? Describe a concrete tool that would help you measure your capacity, such as a survey, community open forum, etc.

3. What steps would you take to develop a comprehensive community outreach program?

4. What resources could you provide to TGD patients within your (school)(practice)(hospital)? What resources can you direct TGD patients to outside your (school) (practice)(hospital)?

5. How would you go about increasing the number and visibility of TGD employees at your (school)(practice) (hospital)?"

REFERENCES

1. Flores AR, Herman JL, Gates GJ, Brown TNT. *How Many Adults Identify as Transgender in the United States?* The Williams Institute, UCLA School of Law; 2016.
2. Saha S, Beach MC, Cooper LA. Patient centeredness, cultural competence and healthcare quality. *J Natl Med Assoc.* 2008;100(11):1275-1285.
3. National LGBT Health Education Center. Recruiting, Training, and Retaining LGBTQ-Proficient Clinical Providers: A Workforce Development Toolkit. 2019. https://www.lgbtqia healtheducation.org/wp-content/uploads/2019/05/Recruiting-and-Retaining-LGBTQ-proficient-providers.pdf. Accessed November 28, 2020.
4. Nothing About Us Without Us: The Shared Goals of the Harm Reduction and Sex Worker Rights Movements. August 2, 2010. Archived from the original on September 20, 2010. https://web.archive.org/web/20100920194907/http:/www.sexworkaware ness.org/nothing-about-us-without-us-the-shared-goals-of-the-harm-reduction-and-sex-worker-rights-movements/. Accessed November 28, 2020.
5. The National LGBT Health Education Center. Creating a Transgender Health Program at Your Health Center: From Planning to Implementation. 2018. https://www.lgbtqiaheal theducation.org/wp-content/uploads/2018/10/Creating-a-Transgender-Health-Program.pdf. Accessed November 28, 2020.
6. Gonzalez CM, Deno ML, Kintzer E, Marantz PR, Lypson ML, McKee MD. Patient perspectives on racial and ethnic implicit bias in clinical encounters: Implications for curriculum development. *Patient Educ Couns.* 2018;101:1669-1675.
7. Burgess DJ, Beach MC, Saha S. Mindfulness practice: a promising approach to reducing the effects of clinician implicit bias on patients. *Patient Educ Couns.* 2017;100:372-376.
8. Gonzalez CM, Deno ML, Kintzer E, Marantz PR, Lypson ML, McKee MD. Patient perspectives on racial and ethnic implicit bias in clinical encounters: implications for curriculum development. *Patient Educ Couns.* 2018;101:1669-1675.
9. Burgess DJ, Beach MC, Saha S. Mindfulness practice: a promising approach to reducing the effects of clinician implicit bias on patients. *Patient Educ Couns.* 2017;100:372-376.

10. Maina IW, Belton TD, Ginzberg S, Singh A, Johnson TJ. A decade of studying implicit racial/ethnic bias in healthcare providers using the implicit association test. *Soc Sci Med.* 2018;199:219-229.

11. Sabin JA, Riskind RG, Nosek BA. Health care providers' implicit and explicit attitudes toward lesbian women and gay men. *Am J Public Health.* 2015;105:1831-1841.

12. Zestcott CA, Blair IV, Stone J. Examining the presence, consequences, and reduction of implicit bias in health care: a narrative review. *Group Process Intergroup Relat GPIR.* 2016;19:528-542.

13. McDowell MJ, Goldhammer H, Potter JE, Keuroghlian AS. Strategies to mitigate clinician implicit bias against sexual and gender minority patients. *Psychosomatics.* 2020;61(6):655-661.

14. Brown B. *Men, Women, and Worthiness: The Experience of Shame and the Power of Being Enough.* Audiobook. SoundsTrue; 2012.

15. James SE, Herman JL, Rankin S, Keisling M, Mottet L, Anafi M. *The Report of the 2015 U.S. Transgender Survey.* Washington, DC: National Center for Transgender Equality; 2016.

16. Housing and homelessness. In The National Center for Transgender Equality. *Blueprint for Equality: A Transgender Federal Agenda.* 2019. https://www.transequality.org/sites/default/files/docs/resources/NCTE%20Federal %20Blueprint%20 2016%20web_0.pdf. Accessed November 28, 2020.

17. Badgett MVL, Durso L, Schneebaum A. New Patterns of Poverty in the Lesbian, Gay, and Bisexual Community. 2013. https://williamsinstitute.law.ucla.edu/publications/lgb-patterns-of-poverty/. Accessed November 28, 2020.

18. Grant JM, Mottet LA, Tanis J. Injustice At Every Turn: A Report of the National Transgender Discrimination Survey. 2011. The National Gay and Lesbian Task Force and the National Center for Transgender Equality. https://www.transequality.org/sites/default/files/docs/resources/NTDS_Report.pdf. Accessed November 28, 2020.

Advocacy for Transgender and Gender Diverse Patients

27

Sean Cahill

INTRODUCTION

As outlined elsewhere in this book, **transgender and gender diverse (TGD)** patients experience striking health disparities that correlate with structural inequality, including social **discrimination** and violent victimization. Health care professionals can play a key role in advocating for TGD patients within their health care institutions, with insurance companies, and with local, state, and federal governments. This chapter presents data on the discrimination TGD Americans face, how it affects their health and well-being, and how it functions as a barrier to accessing health care. It then outlines actions that health care professionals can take to support their TGD patients and help them access the health care they need and deserve.

ANTITRANSGENDER DISCRIMINATION, HARASSMENT, AND VIOLENT VICTIMIZATION

It is important for health care professionals to understand the wide prevalence of anti-TGD discrimination, how it affects TGD people's health and well-being, and how it prevents TGD patients from accessing care.

PREVALENCE

Anti-TGD discrimination, harassment, and violent victimization are widespread and occur across the life course. The 2015 GLSEN School Climate Survey found that 82%* of students said their school engaged in LGBT-related

discriminatory policies or practices.[1] Sixty-six percent of respondents said that they had personally experienced anti-LGBT discrimination in their school. Twenty-two percent reported being prevented from wearing clothes considered inappropriate based on their "legal sex." Fifty-one percent of transgender students had been prevented from using their chosen name or pronouns, and 60% of transgender students had been required to use a bathroom or locker room based on their **sex assigned at birth** and not based on their current **gender identity**. Approximately 20% of all LGBTQ students reported being physically harassed for their gender identity, while 55% were verbally harassed for their gender identity.

Large population-based datasets also show that, compared with **cisgender** youth, transgender youth are more likely to experience violent victimization, including being threatened or injured with a weapon at school, being forced to have sexual intercourse, and experiencing dating violence. They also experience higher rates of substance use, suicide risk, and sexual risk behaviors.[2]

Victimization often continues into adulthood. The 2015 U.S. Transgender Survey found that, in the past year, 30% of those who had a job reported workplace discrimination, 46% were verbally harassed, 9% were physically attacked, 10% were sexually assaulted, and 12% experienced homelessness.[3]

Transgender people are more likely than the general population to be incarcerated.[4] Transgender prisoners are especially vulnerable to sexual victimization in prison: they report sexual abuse at about ten times the rate of heterosexual, cisgender male prisoners and about 2.5 times the rate of heterosexual cisgender female prisoners.[5]

▶ Impact of Discrimination on Transgender Health

Anti-TGD discrimination is widespread. It affects TGD patients' health and well-being and prevents transgender patients from accessing care. It is important for health care

---

* Percentages are rounded. Data reported in report were to one-tenth of 1%. The GLSEN 2015 School Climate Survey surveys LGBTQ youth about pro- and anti-LGBT policies and actions that their school administration implements. Although this textbook uses the terms "LGBTQIA+" and "transgender and gender diverse (TGD)," many research studies use other language. When citing this research, the terminology used in the study is used for accuracy's sake.

professionals to understand these dynamics so that they can take action to intervene and support transgender patients who are experiencing discrimination.

Discrimination is a barrier to seeking routine preventive care as well as emergency care. Transgender youth report a lack of access to health care services and a fear of discrimination at the hands of health care professionals.[6] Transgender adults in the U.S. Transgender Survey reported widespread discrimination in health care. Thirty-three percent of those surveyed said they have had a negative experience with a health care provider in the past year; 23% avoided care due to fear of being mistreated; and 33% avoided health care because they could not afford it.[3]

Anti-LGBT discrimination itself can worsen health outcomes. In a 2017 study, 69% of LGBT people who reported sexual orientation- or gender identity-based discrimination in the past year reported that it negatively affected their psychological well-being, and 44% reported that it negatively affected their physical well-being.[7]

A study of Massachusetts transgender residents found that one in four (24%) reported experiencing discrimination in a health care setting in the past year. Those who reported experiencing discrimination in public accommodations were about twice as likely to report adverse emotional and physical symptoms, such as headache, upset stomach, and pounding heart, and feeling angry, sad, or frustrated related to that experience of discrimination. Of those reporting discrimination in health care, 19% did not seek care when they were sick or injured after experiencing discrimination, and 24% did not seek subsequent preventive or routine care.[8]

▶ Socioeconomic Effects of Discrimination and Marginalization on Access to Care

Discrimination, harassment, victimization, and **stigma** contribute to higher rates of poverty, homelessness, sex work, and incarceration among TGD people, especially transgender women. These experiences affect the ability of TGD people to access health insurance. Exclusionary policies and lack of culturally responsive, gender-affirming care also prevent TGD people from accessing the care that they need.

▶ Poverty

Transgender people experience twice the poverty rate as the general U.S. population (29% vs. 14%), and three times the unemployment rate (15% vs. 5%), according to the 2015 U.S. Transgender Survey.[3] A Williams Institute analysis of poverty data from state Behavioral Risk Factor Surveillance System surveys (2014–2017) found that 29.4% of transgender respondents were poor. Black transgender people had more than twice the rate of poverty than white transgender people (38.5% vs. 18.6%), while Hispanic transgender people were nearly three times as poor (48.4%).[9]

Insurance Coverage

There are limited data on insurance rates among TGD people, but it is likely that, given other evidence of economic hardship, TGD people are less likely than the general population to be insured. The 2015 U.S. Transgender Survey found a slightly lower percentage of insurance coverage among transgender people: 86% compared to 89% for the general adult population, according to the American Community Survey.[3] The uninsured rate among low-income transgender people dropped from 59% in 2013 to 35% in 2014 during the implementation of key aspects of the Affordable Care Act.[10] Whether or not insurance plans cover transgender health care needs is a related issue that is addressed later in this chapter.

Lack of Culturally Responsive, Affirming Care

Transgender people experience widespread discrimination in health care, including being refused needed care; health care professionals refusing to touch them; using excessive precautions (plastic gloves); being blamed for their health status, such as HIV or other STIs; and health care professionals being rough or abusive.[11]

Transgender people of color seek out LGBTQIA+-friendly health care professionals, but often worry about experiencing racism in such contexts. Some also worry about experiencing transphobic care from clinicians of color.[12] It can be very challenging for TGD people of color to find clinicians who are able to provide affirming care that is respectful of their intersectional identities.

The training of health care professionals in standards of health care for TGD people is key to ensuring clinically competent and culturally responsive care for TGD patients. Cultural humility training helps reduce health disparities by developing provider proficiency in understanding the unique issues gender minority people face. Until recently, medical schools devoted little time to teaching LGBT-related content.[13] Thankfully, this is changing. A recent study of rural Midwestern health care professionals found that those who received education specific to LGBT health as part of their professional degree program had more favorable attitudes toward LGBT patients.[14]

NONDISCRIMINATION POLICIES AT THE STATE AND FEDERAL LEVELS

Clearly TGD people experience a great deal of trauma in their lives. It is important for clinicians to understand not only how to address trauma, but also how to engage in advocacy efforts on behalf of their TGD patients. This advocacy can take place internally, within a health care organization, or externally via advocacy efforts with insurance companies, or to promote TGD-supportive policies with governmental bodies and agencies. This section describes state- and municipal-level policies that prohibit discrimination against TGD people, as well as policies adopted by professional organizations such as the Joint Commission. It then describes rollback of federal nondiscrimination regulations by the Trump Administration and their implications for transgender health care.

State and Municipal Nondiscrimination Laws

Gender Identity Nondiscrimination Laws (Municipal and State)

Twenty-one states and the District of Columbia have outlawed antitransgender discrimination in employment and housing, and 20 states plus DC have outlawed discrimination in public accommodations (Figure 27-1).[15] Hundreds of municipalities also prohibit gender identity-based discrimination. Research has shown that the existence of statewide transgender nondiscrimination policies and protransgender policies related to identity documents and other areas correlates with better health outcomes for transgender people in three domains; transgender people living in states with protransgender policies had fewer recent poor mental health days, fewer average alcoholic drinks per day, and a shorter length of time since their last health care checkup (Figure 27-2).[16]

Many states prohibit transgender exclusions in health insurance. These policies prevent insurers from explicitly refusing to cover transgender health care needs such as hormone replacement therapy or gender affirmation surgery. Some also prohibit blanket exclusions of transgender health care coverage. Some of these policies are statutes passed by state legislatures, while others are letters of determination issued by state insurance regulators and agencies. According to the Movement Advancement Project, as of February 2020, 22 states and the District of Columbia banned explicit exclusions of transgender health care needs.[17]

Many states also prohibit gender identity discrimination in insurance, which can take the form of insurers refusing to cover transgender people, canceling an individual's plan following the receipt of transgender-related health care, or charging them higher premiums. These laws are usually statutory, but are sometimes issued by state agencies (Naomi Goldberg and Logan Casey, Movement Advancement Project, written communication, February 7 and February 27, 2020).

Gender Identity Nondiscrimination Policies by Health Care Organizations

Since 2011, the Joint Commission has required hospitals, long-term care facilities, and other health care organizations that it accredits to prohibit discrimination on the basis of gender identity and sexual orientation as a criterion for accreditation.[18] Most major health professional

organizations, such as the American Medical Association, the American Nursing Association, and the Association of American Medical Colleges, support and advocate for sexual orientation and gender identity nondiscrimination policies.[19] According to the Healthcare Equality Index, a project of the Human Rights Campaign, 99% of HEI participants (673 out of 680 health care facilities) documented that they explicitly prohibited gender identity- and sexual orientation-based discrimination in their patient nondiscrimination policy. HEI also researched the publicly available policies of 952 other health care facilities that did not participate in the HEI and found that only 634, or 67%, explicitly prohibited gender identity- and sexual orientation-based discrimination.[20]

Rollback at the State and Federal Levels

State Antitransgender Bills

Since the mid-2010s, municipalities and states have passed laws making it harder for transgender people to access public restrooms and other public accommodations and expanding the ability of religious conservatives to refuse to provider health care and other services to LGBTQIA+ people based on religious or moral objection.[21,22] In 2020, at least eight states considered bills that would criminalize the provision of gender-affirming care to minors.[23]

Gender Identity Nondiscrimination Language in Federal Policy

Gender identity nondiscrimination language was included by the Obama Administration in implementing regulations for the Affordable Care Act's subsidized private insurance exchanges as well as regulations governing Medicaid and the Program of All-Inclusive Care for the Elderly.[24] The 2016 Section 1557 rule explicitly prohibits gender identity-based discrimination, including discrimination against intersex and nonbinary people, in health care facilities and programs receiving federal funding. The 2016 Section 1557 rule also prohibits discriminatory coverage exclusions for transgender people in health insurance plans, expanding access to medically necessary gender-affirming services for transgender people. In 2020, the Trump Administration reversed this nondiscrimination, as well as transgender nondiscrimination protections governing public and private insurance coverage, and elder services.[24] This repeal effort is now caught up in the federal courts. As of 2020, at least 18 state Medicaid programs cover gender-affirming hormone therapy and surgery.[25,26] Depending on what happens with the federal nondiscrimination regulations, the number of state Medicaid departments covering transgender care may decrease, which would be devastating for transgender people, who are more likely to rely on Medicaid for their health care due to higher rates of poverty and disability.

KEY

● **LGB**
Law covers sexual orientation

✓ **LGBT**
Law covers sexual orientation and gender identity/ expression

State	Employment	Housing	Pub. Accomm.	Credit	State Employees
Alabama					
Alaska					● LGB
American Samoa					
Arizona					● LGB
Arkansas					
California	✓ LGBT	✓ LGBT	✓ LGBT		✓ LGBT
Colorado	✓ LGBT	✓ LGBT	✓ LGBT	✓ LGBT	✓ LGBT
Connecticut	✓ LGBT	✓ LGBT	✓ LGBT	✓ LGBT	✓ LGBT
Delaware	✓ LGBT	✓ LGBT	✓ LGBT		✓ LGBT
D.C.	✓ LGBT	✓ LGBT	✓ LGBT		✓ LGBT
Florida					
Georgia					
Guam	✓ LGBT				✓ LGBT
Hawaii	✓ LGBT	✓ LGBT	✓ LGBT		✓ LGBT
Idaho					
Illinois	✓ LGBT	✓ LGBT	✓ LGBT	✓ LGBT	✓ LGBT
Indiana					✓ LGBT
Iowa	✓ LGBT	✓ LGBT	✓ LGBT	✓ LGBT	✓ LGBT
Kansas					✓ LGBT
Kentucky					✓ LGBT
Louisiana					
Maine	✓ LGBT	✓ LGBT	✓ LGBT	✓ LGBT	✓ LGBT
Maryland	✓ LGBT	✓ LGBT	✓ LGBT		✓ LGBT
Massachusetts	✓ LGBT	✓ LGBT	✓ LGBT	✓ LGBT	✓ LGBT
Michigan					✓ LGBT
Minnesota	✓ LGBT	✓ LGBT	✓ LGBT	✓ LGBT	✓ LGBT
Mississippi					
Missouri					● LGB
Montana					✓ LGBT
Nebraska					
Nevada	✓ LGBT	✓ LGBT	✓ LGBT	✓ LGBT	✓ LGBT
New Hampshire	✓ LGBT	✓ LGBT	✓ LGBT		✓ LGBT
New Jersey	✓ LGBT	✓ LGBT	✓ LGBT	✓ LGBT	✓ LGBT
New Mexico	✓ LGBT	✓ LGBT	✓ LGBT	✓ LGBT	✓ LGBT
New York	✓ LGBT	✓ LGBT	✓ LGBT	✓ LGBT	✓ LGBT
North Carolina					✓ LGBT
North Dakota					
N. Mariana Islands					● LGB
Ohio					✓ LGBT
Oklahoma					
Oregon	✓ LGBT	✓ LGBT	✓ LGBT	✓ LGBT	✓ LGBT
Pennsylvania					✓ LGBT
Puerto Rico	✓ LGBT				✓ LGBT
Rhode Island	✓ LGBT	✓ LGBT	✓ LGBT	✓ LGBT	✓ LGBT
South Carolina					
South Dakota					
Tennessee					
Texas					
U.S. Virgin Islands					✓ LGBT
Utah	✓ LGBT	✓ LGBT			✓ LGBT
Vermont	✓ LGBT	✓ LGBT	✓ LGBT	✓ LGBT	✓ LGBT
Virginia	✓ LGBT	✓ LGBT	✓ LGBT	✓ LGBT	✓ LGBT
Washington	✓ LGBT	✓ LGBT	✓ LGBT	✓ LGBT	✓ LGBT
West Virginia					
Wisconsin	● LGB	● LGB	● LGB		✓ LGBT
Wyoming					

▲ **Figure 27–1.** LGBT nondiscrimination laws in the United States. (Reproduced with permission from Movement Advancement Project. https://www.lgbtmap.org/equality-maps/non_discrimination_laws.)

KEY

● T
Law covers gender identity

✓ LGBT
Law covers sexual orientation and gender identity/ expression

✓
Policy includes transgender health care

x
Policy excludes transgender health care

★
Bans exclusions on transgender health care

State	Priv. Insurance Nondiscrimination	Medicaid	Trans Inclusive Health Benefits for State Employees
Alabama			
Alaska		x	
American Samoa			
Arizona		x	x
Arkansas			x
California	✓ LGBT ★	✓	✓
Colorado	✓ LGBT ★	✓	
Connecticut	● T ★	✓	✓
Delaware	✓ LGBT ★	✓	✓
D.C.	✓ LGBT ★	✓	✓
Florida			x
Georgia		x	
Guam			x
Hawaii	✓ LGBT ★	✓	✓
Idaho			x
Illinois	✓ LGBT ★	✓	
Indiana			✓
Iowa			
Kansas			
Kentucky			✓
Louisiana			x
Maine	✓ LGBT ★	✓	
Maryland	★	✓	✓
Massachusetts	● T ★	✓	✓
Michigan	✓ LGBT ★	✓	
Minnesota	✓ LGBT ★	✓	✓
Mississippi			x
Missouri		x	
Montana	★	✓	✓
Nebraska		x	x
Nevada	✓ LGBT ★	✓	✓
New Hampshire	✓ LGBT ★	✓	✓
New Jersey	● T ★	✓	
New Mexico	● T ★		
New York	✓ LGBT ★	✓	
North Carolina			x
North Dakota			x
N. Mariana Islands			
Ohio		x	x
Oklahoma			
Oregon	✓ LGBT ★	✓	✓
Pennsylvania	● T ★	✓	✓
Puerto Rico	✓ LGBT	✓	
Rhode Island	✓ LGBT ★	✓	✓
South Carolina			
South Dakota			
Tennessee		x	x
Texas		x	
U.S. Virgin Islands			
Utah			
Vermont	✓ LGBT ★	✓	
Virginia	● T ★		
Washington	✓ LGBT ★	✓	✓
West Virginia		x	x
Wisconsin	✓ LGBT ★	✓	✓
Wyoming		x	

▲ **Figure 27–2.** LGBT health care laws and policies in the United States. (Reproduced with permission from Movement Advancement Project. https://www.lgbtmap.org/equality-maps/healthcare_laws_and_policies/medicaid.)

The Trump Administration pursued a number of other policies that discriminate against transgender people or enable discrimination against them, including policies that allow a refusal of services, including health care, based on religious or moral belief, a ban on military service, housing prisoners based on "biological sex" and not gender identity, and allowing religious homeless service providers to refuse to house transgender people.[27-31] The Trump Administration also promoted religious refusal policies and dismantled gender identity and sexual orientation nondiscrimination policies.[22]

In June 2020, the U.S. Supreme Court ruled that anti-transgender and antigay employment discrimination violates Title VII of the 1964 Civil Rights Act, which prohibits sex discrimination.[32] The Trump Administration argued, however, in a brief to the U.S. Supreme Court related to the transgender discrimination case, that Title VII of the 1964 Civil Rights Act does not cover gender identity-based discrimination.[33] A 6-3 majority on the U.S. Supreme Court rejected this argument.

However, the Trump Administration also appointed many federal judges who oppose legal equality for transgender people. For example, U.S. Supreme Court Justice Amy Coney Barrett, appointed in October 2020, expressed opposition in 2016 to interpreting Title IX's prohibition of sex discrimination to include antitransgender people. Discussing the 2015 North Carolina law that prohibited transgender people from using bathrooms consistent with their gender identity, Judge Coney Barrett told an audience at the Jacksonville University Public Policy Institute:

> …people will feel passionately on either side about whether physiological males who identify as female should be permitted in bathrooms, especially where there are young girls present…It does seem to strain the text of the statute to say that Title IX demands it.

THE ROLE OF THE HEALTH CARE PROFESSIONAL IN ADVOCACY FOR TGD PATIENTS

Health care professionals can take a number of steps to support and advocate for TGD patients. First, if a TGD patient experiences discriminatory treatment in any aspect of life, including health care and insurance coverage, the provider can refer the patient to an impact litigation organization like the Transgender Law Center (https://transgenderlawcenter.org/), Lambda Legal (www.lambdalegal.org), the ACLU LGBT Rights Project (https://www.aclu.org/issues/lgbt-rights), and GLBTQ Legal Advocates and Defenders (www.glad.org). These organizations defend TGD people experiencing discrimination who have a case that could help effect a change in policy or practice. If the individual situation that the TGD person is experiencing does not constitute a case

with impact potential, these groups should be able to refer the individual to a public interest lawyer who could help. Individuals experiencing discrimination should also report their situation to their state Attorney General and their statewide Commission Against Discrimination, and to TGD advocacy groups like the National Center for Transgender Equality (NCTE).

According to the NCTE, 19 states and the District of Columbia require private insurers to cover gender-affirming hormone therapy and surgery. Nineteen states and DC (an overlapping but different group) require Medicaid to cover these elements of transgender health care.[26] According to the NCTE and Transcend Legal, most large private insurers cover transgender health care needs. If they do not, both organizations offer resources to connect transgender patients with legal assistance (www.transequality.org, https://transcendlegal.org/resources).

The Center for American Progress has analyzed discrimination complaints filed under the ACA's nondiscrimination provision. There were many examples of transgender people being denied care because of their gender identity or transgender status. For example, a transgender woman was denied a mammogram because she was a transgender woman, and transgender people were denied sexual assault medical forensic examinations.[34] Other examples of antitransgender discrimination experienced in health care and reported to the federal government under Section 1557 of the ACA include the following:

- A transgender woman went to the hospital with cold symptoms, but her care was delayed because of repeated questions about her gender identity and inappropriate questions about her anatomy at intake.

- A transgender woman with a disability was repeatedly harassed by the driver of a medical transport service that took her to and from her doctor's appointments.

- A transgender woman was separated from her wife during an emergency room visit and her wife was not permitted to enter her room for more than two hours.

- While recovering from an appendectomy, the doctor treating a transgender woman refused to call her by the correct pronouns and said the doctor does not deal with "these kinds" of patients.[35]

Clinicians can play a key role in minimizing the likelihood that TGD patients will experience discrimination in health care. First, they can make sure that they and their staff are trained in how to provide affirming, culturally responsive care for TGD patients (see Chapter 11, "Basic Principles of Trauma-Informed and Gender-Affirming Care"). Many free online trainings and resources are available at the National LGBTQIA+ Health Education Center at www.lgbtqiahealtheducation.org.

Second, health care professionals can ensure that their practice or institution has policies in place that support TGD patients, including nondiscrimination policies. Information on model policies is available at www.lgbtqiahealtheducation.org. The Joint Commission also published a field guide to improving care for LGBT patients.[35]

Third, clinicians can support local and state coalitions that advocate for insurance coverage of medically necessary transgender health care. The Massachusetts Transgender Health Coalition is one such network of advocates and health care professionals. It has engaged the state Division of Insurance, which regulates private insurance plans, and MassHealth, the state's Medicaid program. The coalition has encouraged regulators to require private and public insurance coverage of health care services beyond gender-affirming hormones and surgery, including hair removal, chest reconstruction, and facial feminization and masculinization surgery. The coalition has also raised concerns about age of majority restrictions, the exclusion of coverage of voice modification therapy and surgery, and burdensome requirements related to medical documentation, prior authorization, and appeals processes. State regulators are especially receptive to clinicians' testimony in support of insurance coverage of these medically necessary health services.

Fourth, health care professionals can also ensure that any professional associations that they are members of have gender identity nondiscrimination policies and have issued statements supportive of TGD people's access to medically necessary care. GLMA: Health Professionals Advancing LGBTQ Equality has a list of supportive professional associations and positions that they have adopted that you can use to advocate within your professional association.[36]

Fifth, health care professionals can partner with or refer patients to legal services to address social and structural issues that impede quality health care for TGD people. A number of LGBTQIA+-focused health centers around the country—including Whitman-Walker Health in Washington, DC and the Los Angeles LGBT Center's Transgender Health Program—offer name and gender marker updates, health insurance eligibility and coverage appeals, advanced directive preparation, immigration support, and help fighting discrimination and harassment in employment, housing, and public accommodations.[37] In Massachusetts, the statewide LGBTQ Youth Commission offers assistance with identity documents, including for homeless TGD people who may lack legal documents like birth certificates or Social Security cards. Health Law Advocates and the Massachusetts Transgender Political Caucus can also help TGD patients address their medical-legal partnership needs.

Sixth, health care professionals can support TGD rights activists working at the local, state, and federal level to promote supportive, inclusive policies and fight back against state-sponsored discrimination. NCTE has a State Action Center that can help health care professionals connect with people advocating for TGD equality in their state (https://transequality.org/2020-state-action-center). It is often helpful to advocates to have

medical professionals testify at legislative hearings or state division of insurance hearings. By doing so, health care professionals can help effect change that makes it easier for TGD people to access the care they need and reduces the social prejudice and victimization that correlates with health disparities, addressing upstream causes of poor health outcomes.

SUMMARY

- In addition to providing affirming and culturally humble care, health care professionals can take a variety of actions to support their TGD patients and help address the social determinants of health that contribute to their increased vulnerability. These activities include:

  - Play key role in advocating for TGD patients within their health care facility. This can take the form of advocating for changes on forms and in clinic policies.

  - Advocate for systemic change with colleagues through professional associations, for example by securing a primary care association's statement of support for gender identity nondiscrimination legislation.

  - Support efforts to promote TGD supportive public policies and resist efforts to remove legal protections for TGD people and criminalize TGD health care.

- Health care professionals should know that their opinions are highly valued by policy makers. They can cite research linking discrimination to poorer health and well-being and restricted access to care. They can also provide testimony about TGD patients for whom they care and how public policy issues affect them both positively and negatively.

- In addition to providing formal testimony, health care professionals can advocate for their TGD patients through discussions with elected officials, letters to the editor of local newspapers, and other methods. The testimony and opinions of health care providers carry a lot of weight with policy makers and members of society, and can help advance legal equality for TGD individuals.

CASE STUDY 1: BRENDAN JONES

Brendan Jones is a transgender male patient of Dr. Lydia Sanchez who uses "he/him" and "they/them" pronouns. Brendan lives in a small town in the hills and travels 2 hours to access gender-affirming care. They are a generally healthy 32-year-old. While in for their annual physical, Dr. Sanchez sensed that there was something different about Brendan. Brendan confided in Dr. Sanchez that they were experiencing discrimination in some public accommodation settings, in particular at their bank and in stores. A bank teller insisted on calling Brendan "ma'am," and when Brendan explained that they did not identify as a woman and used "he, him" and "they, them" pronouns, the teller turned to another teller and said, "I'm dealing with an 'it,' apparently." Brendan indicated that they had had similar experiences in other retail settings. Dr. Sanchez expressed support for Brendan and said that they shouldn't be treated that way. She also told Brendan that they should file a complaint with the state Attorney General. "What good would that do?" Brendan asked. "It's legal to discriminate on the basis of gender identity in South Carolina."

That night after work Dr. Sanchez researched the issue and connected with GLMA: Health Professionals Advancing LGBTQ Equality and South Carolina Equality. Several months later, Dr. Sanchez testified in support of a bill before the state legislature to ban discrimination on the basis of sexual orientation and gender identity in employment, housing, and public accommodations. In her testimony, Dr. Sanchez cited research indicating that antitransgender discrimination hurt the health and well-being of TGD individuals and constituted a barrier to accessing care. While the bill did not pass in the legislature, Dr. Sanchez helped convince her state primary care association to take a stance in support of legal protections for LGBTQ patients. Dr. Sanchez also followed up with Brendan and connected them to support services at an LGBTQ-friendly community center, and offered them a referral to counseling to address the trauma that they experienced due to the discrimination. She also told Brendan about her advocacy with the state legislature and PCA. Brendan thanked her and said, "You're my hero!" As a result of this interaction, Brendan got more involved with efforts to pass a nondiscrimination law as well. In so doing, they met other people who had had similar experiences of discrimination and developed a support network of TGD friends and activist colleagues.

▶ Discussion Questions

1. Did Dr. Sanchez provide affirming and supportive care to Brendan?
2. Did she take steps to address structural drivers of vulnerability for Brendan and other TGD patients?
3. Did Dr. Sanchez educate her professional colleagues and local elected officials of a social problem that affected the health and well-being of her patients?
4. Should Dr. Sanchez not have shared news of her activism with Brendan? Did this information help Brendan in any way?

CASE STUDY 2: D.J.

Dr. Lydia Sanchez provides care to D.J., a new gender **nonbinary** patient who uses "they/them" pronouns. D.J. was referred to Dr. Sanchez by a friend due to her skill in providing gender-affirming and culturally humble care. When D.J. arrived at the clinic, they were asked to complete a new patient registration form. The form did not ask about gender identity or sex assigned at birth. It just asked a sex question

with the options "male" and "female." The form did not ask the patient for pronouns or name used if it doesn't match the name on the patient's insurance. During the clinical encounter, D.J. expressed concern about the registration form's method of asking or not asking about sex and gender identity. Dr. Sanchez acknowledged D.J.'s concerns, and assured them that she would address the issue and get back to D.J. about a resolution. After the visit, Dr. Sanchez spoke with the administrative director for the clinic, John Richards, and asked him to find a way to ask the questions in a more affirming way for nonbinary and other gender diverse patients. Richards researched the issue and found recommendations on the website of the National LGBTQIA+ Health Education Center. He added these to the registration form, replacing the existing sex question.

▶ Gender Identity

What is your current gender identity? (Check one):

- Female
- Male
- Transgender Woman/Transgender Female
- Transgender Man/Transgender Male
- Other* (e.g., nonbinary, genderqueer, gender diverse, or gender fluid). Please specify _____.
- Choose not to disclose

What sex were you assigned at birth? (Check one):

- Male
- Female

Dr. Sanchez shared the proposed changes with D.J. through the patient portal, and D.J. responded with their support for the changes. When D.J. returned 6 months later for another visit, they completed the form and thanked Dr. Sanchez for the changes that the clinic had made to the registration form.

▶ Discussion Questions

1. Did Dr. Sanchez's actions support the quality of clinical care that patients like D.J. receive?
2. Was Dr. Sanchez responsive to D.J.'s concerns?
3. Do the questions that the clinic added to their registration form allow for nonbinary patients to self-identify?

REFERENCES

1. Kosciw JG, Greytak EA, Giga NM, et al. *The 2015 National School Climate Survey: The Experiences of Lesbian, Gay, Bisexual, Transgender, and Queer Youth in Our Nation's Schools.* New York: Gay, Lesbian and Straight Education Network; 2016.

2. Johns MM, Lowry R, Andrzejewski J, et al. Transgender identity and experiences of violence victimization, substance use, suicide risk, and sexual risk behaviors among high school students—19 states and large urban school districts, 2017. *MMWR Morb Mortal Wkly Rep.* 2019;68:67-71.

3. James SE, Herman JL, Rankin S, et al. *The Report of the 2015 U.S. Transgender Survey.* Washington, DC: National Center for Transgender Equality; 2016.

4. Grant J, Mottet L, Tanis J. *Injustice at Every Turn: A Report of the National Transgender Discrimination Survey.* Washington, DC: National Center for Transgender Equality and National Gay and Lesbian Task Force; 2011. https://transequality.org/sites/default/files/docs/resources/NTDS_Report.pdf.

5. Beck AJ, Berzofsky M, Krebs C. Sexual Victimization in Prisons and Jails Reported by Inmates, 2011–12 National Inmate Survey, 2011–2012. Supplemental tables: Prevalence of sexual victimization among transgender adult inmates. U.S. Department of Justice, Office of Justice Programs, Bureau of Justice Statistics; 2013. https://www.bjs.gov/content/pub/pdf/svpjri1112.pdf.

6. Grossman AH, D'Augelli AR. Transgender youth: invisible and vulnerable. *J Homosex.* 2006;51(1):111-128.

7. Singh S, Durso L. *Widespread Discrimination Continues to Shape LGBT People's Lives in Both Subtle and Significant Ways.* Center for American Progress; 2017.

8. Reisner SL, White Hughto JM, Dunham E, et al. Legal protections in public accommodations settings: a critical public health issue for transgender and gender nonconforming people. *Milbank Q.* 2015;93(3):484-515.

9. Badgett MVL, Choi SK, Wilson BDM. *LGBT Poverty in the United States: A Study of Differences between Sexual Orientation and Gender Identity Groups.* Los Angeles: UCLA School of Law, Williams Institute; 2019.

10. Baker K, Durso LE, Cray A. Moving the needle: the impact of the Affordable Care Act on LGBT communities. 2014. https://cdn.americanprogress.org/wp-content/uploads/2014/11/LGBTandACA-report.pdf.

11. Lambda Legal. *When Health Care Isn't Caring: Lambda Legal's Survey of Discrimination against LGBT People and People with HIV.* New York: Lambda Legal; 2010.

12. Howard SD, Lee KL, Nathan AG, et al. Healthcare experiences of transgender people of color. *J Gen Intern Med.* 2019;34(10):2068-2074.

13. Obedin-Maliver J, Goldsmith ES, Stewart L, et al. Lesbian, gay, bisexual and transgender-related content in undergraduate medical education. *JAMA.* 2011;306:971-977.

14. Sharma A, Shaver JC, Stephenson RB. Rural primary care providers' attitudes towards sexual and gender minorities in a midwestern state in the USA. *Rural Remote Health.* 2019;19(4):5476.

15. Human Rights Campaign. Maps. Employment, Public Accommodations. file:///C:/Users/scahill/Downloads/hrc-map.pdf.

16. DuBois SN, Yoder W, Guy AA, Manser K, Ramos S. Examining associations between state-level transgender policies and transgender health. *Transgender Health.* 2018;3(1):220-224.

17. Movement Advancement Project. Healthcare Laws and Policies. https://www.lgbtmap.org/equality-maps/healthcare_laws_and_policies. Accessed February 20, 2020.

18. The Joint Commission. *Advancing Effective Communication, Cultural Competence, and Patient- and Family-Centered Care: A Roadmap for Hospitals.* Oak Brook, IL: Joint Commission Resources; 2010. http://www.jointcommission.org/assets/1/6/ARoadmapforHospitalsfinalversion727.pdf.

19. GLMA. Compendium of Health Profession Association LGBT Policy and Position Statements. 2013. http://www.glma.org/_data/n_0001/resources/live/GLMA%20Compendium%20of%20Health%20Profession%20Association%20LGBT%20Policy%20and%20Position%20Statements.pdf.

20. Human Rights Campaign. Healthcare Equality Index 2019: Promoting equitable and inclusive care for lesbian, gay, bisexual, transgender and queer patients and their families. 2019. https://assets2.hrc.org/files/assets/resources/HEI-2019-FinalReport.pdf?_ga=2.215456983.1378384808.1582810498-1322667838.1578596372. Accessed February 20, 2020.

21. Wang T, Cahill S. Anti-transgender political backlash threatens health and access to care. *Am J Public Health.* 2018;108(5):609-610.

22. Cahill S. Trump shreds LGBT health protections. *Public Health Post,* June 28, 2019.

23. Lam K. National firestorm on horizon as states consider criminalizing transgender treatments for youths. *USA Today,* February 6, 2020.

24. Keith K. Court vacates new 1557 rule that would roll back antidiscrimination protections for LGBT individuals. *Health Affairs,* August 18, 2020. https://www.healthaffairs.org/do/10.1377/hblog20200818.468025/full/.

25. Movement Advancement Project. *Healthcare Laws and Policies: Medicaid Coverage for Transition-Related Care.* 2019. https://www.lgbtmap.org/img/maps/citations-medicaid.pdf.

26. National Center for Transgender Equality. *Know Your Rights—Health Care.* https://transequality.org/know-your-rights/health-care.

27. Department of Housing and Urban Development. Revised Requirements Under Community Planning and Development Housing Programs (FR-6152), 2019. https://www.reginfo.gov/public/do/eAgendaViewRule?pubId=201904&RIN=2506-AC53.

28. Jan T. Proposed Rule HUD Would Strip Transgender Protections at Homeless Shelters. *The Washington Post,* May 22, 2019. https://www.washingtonpost.com/business/2019/05/22/proposed-hud-rule-would-strip-transgender-protections-homeless-shelters/.

29. U.S. Department of Justice, Federal Bureau of Prisons. Change Notice. *Transgender Offender Manual,* May 11, 2018. https://www.documentcloud.org/documents/4459297-BOP-Change-Order-Transgender-Offender-Manual-5.html.

30. Simmons-Duffin S. Trump administration plans to roll back anti-discrimination rules tied to HHS funding. National Public Radio, All Things Considered, November 5, 2019. https://www.npr.org/2019/11/05/776496146/trump-administration-plans-to-roll-back-anti-discrimination-rules-tied-to-hhs-fu.

31. Simonoff C, Wang T, Cahill S. In its third year in office, the Trump Administration dramatically expanded discriminatory anti-LGBT policies. Boston: The Fenway Institute; January 2020. https://fenwayhealth.org/wp-content/uploads/Trump-Administration-Year-3-Brief.pdf.

32. Supreme Court of the United States. *Bostock v. Clayton County, Georgia.* Certiorari to the United States Court of Appeals for The Eleventh Circuit. No. 17–1618. June 15, 2020. https://www.supremecourt.gov/opinions/19pdf/17-1618_hfci.pdf. Accessed July 6, 2020.

33. Law T. Trump administration asks Supreme Court to permit employment discrimination against transgender workers.

Time, August 17, 2019. https://time.com/5654844/title-vii-trump-transgender-department-of-justice-supreme-court/.

34. Gruberg S, Bewkes FJ. The ACA's LGBTQ nondiscrimination regulations prove crucial. March 7, 2018. https://www.american progress.org/issues/lgbtq-rights/reports/2018/03/07/447414/acas-lgbtq-nondiscrimination-regulations-prove-crucial/.

35. Joint Commission. *Advancing Effective Communication, Cultural Competence, and Patient- and Family-Centered Care for the Lesbian, Gay, Bisexual, and Transgender (LGBT) Community: A Field Guide.* Oak Brook, IL: Joint Commission Resources; 2011. http://www.jointcommission.org/assets/1/18/LGBTFieldGuide.pdf.

36. GLMA: Health Professionals Advancing LGBTQ Equality. Compendium of Health Profession Association LGBT Policy & Position Statements. (No date). http://www.glma.org/_data/n_0001/resources/live/GLMA%20Compendium%20of%20Health%20Profession%20Association%20LGBT%20Policy%20and%20Position%20Statements.pdf.

37. National Center for Medical-Legal Partnership at George Washington University, National LGBT Health Education Center. Transgender Health and Medical-Legal Partnerships. (No date). https://www.lgbthealtheducation.org/wp-content/uploads/2018/08/Transgender-Health-and-Medical-Legal-Partnership-1.pdf.

Glossary

47, XXX karyotype: A chromosomal disorder in which there are three X chromosomes; it is associated with an increased risk of learning disabilities, delayed motor development, weak muscle tone, and behavioral problems, although these effects vary widely in affected individuals.

Administrative sex: The sex recorded in the patient demographic section of the electronic health record; it may differ from the sex assigned at birth and current gender identity.

Adverse childhood experiences (ACEs): Specific types of trauma experienced before age 18 years; includes abuse (physical, emotional, or sexual), neglect (physical or emotional), and household dysfunction (exposure to divorce; a member of the household with mental illness, a substance use disorder, or who is incarcerated; or witnessing violence in the home).

Anatomical inventory: A record of a patient's current organs; in some cases, the anatomical inventory also records a patient's body modifications.

Anorexia nervosa: An eating disorder characterized by restrictive eating patterns; weight loss (or lack of appropriate weight gain in children); difficulty maintaining a suitable body weight for height, age, and stature; and often a distorted body image.

Antiandrogen therapy: The use of medications that suppress the body's production or response to testosterone and allow the effects of estrogen to be more apparent.

Anticipated stigma: Having an expectation of experiencing stigma.

Assigned female sex at birth/Assigned male sex at birth: Refers to the sex that is assigned to an infant, most often based on the infant's visible anatomical (e.g., genital) and other biological characteristics. Commonly abbreviated as AFAB (assigned female at birth) or AMAB (assigned male at birth).

Avoidant/restrictive food intake disorder (ARFID): An eating disorder characterized by highly selective eating.

BDSM: An initialism that stands for bondage/discipline, dominance/submission, and sadism/masochism describing an array of erotic behaviors that center interpersonal power dynamics.

Binary: In contrast to the term "nonbinary," this term describes a personal characteristic (or social structure or system) with only two possible options; could describe designations for sex (e.g., female or male), binary gender (e.g., girl/woman/feminine or boy/man/masculine), or sexual orientation (e.g., gay or straight).

Binge-eating disorder: An eating disorder characterized by eating large quantities of food (often quickly and to the point of physical discomfort); feeling a loss of control during the binge; experiencing shame, distress, or guilt afterward; and not regularly using compensatory measures to counter the binging.

Body image: An experience of physical self that affects self-concept, self-esteem, and one's sense of autonomy in the world.

Bulimia: An eating disorder characterized by a cycle of binging and compensatory behaviors such as self-induced vomiting, laxative or diuretic use, or compulsive exercise that are designed to undo or compensate for the effects of binge eating.

Cisgender: A person whose gender identity aligns with society's expectations based on their sex assigned at birth; for example, a person assigned female sex at birth whose gender identity is woman/female. The term "cisgender" comes from the Latin prefix cis, meaning "on the same side of."

Cognitive behavioral therapy: A time-limited, problem-focused therapeutic approach emphasizing manualized or standardized interventions that implement empirically supported techniques in an individualized manner.

Congenital adrenal hyperplasia (CAH): A group of disorders affecting the adrenal glands that can cause a variety of effects, including differences in the external genitalia in girls and early puberty. The most common type can be life-threatening due to abnormal levels of adrenal hormones.

Cycle of violence: A model that explains the patterns of behavior in an abusive relationship.

Dialectical behavioral therapy: An evidence-based manualized psychotherapy that promotes validation and self-acceptance alongside strategies to increase emotion regulation and change problematic thoughts and behaviors.

Differences of sex development (DSD): Medical term for intersex traits.

Discrimination: Unjust or prejudicial treatment of a person or group based on race, sex, age, or gender identity.

Disordered eating: A range of irregular eating behaviors that do not meet *Diagnostic and Statistical Manual of Mental Disorders, 5th edition* criteria for a specific eating disorder.

Distal stressors: Stress-inducing events that occur due to an individual's gender minority identity; examples include gender-related discrimination, rejection, victimization, and identity nonaffirmation.

Double-incision mastectomy: Surgery to create a flat chest that utilizes longer incisions under the pectoral shadow.

Eating disorders (noun): Clinical presentations that meet *Diagnostic and Statistical Manual of Mental Disorders, 5th edition* clinical criteria for specific eating disorders.

Ecological (or ecosocial) framework/model: The use of multilevel interventions that address individual, institutional, organizational, and societal/public policy issues to reduce inequities and barriers to health and well-being for TGD populations.

Electrolysis: Hair-removal intervention that treats each follicle individually by inserting a needle to deliver electrocautery.

Electronic health record (EHR): Electronic version of a patient's medical chart that includes key elements, such as demographics, insurance, appointments, diagnoses, medications, laboratory values, and visit notes; required to meet a minimum set of expectations to receive certification through the Office of the National Coordinator for Health Information Technology (ONC).

Enacted stigma: The experience of being stigmatized.

Endogenous hormone: A hormone produced in the body.

Endosex traits: Primary and secondary sex characteristics that align with binary notions of female and male bodies.

Estrogen: A group of hormones that produce female secondary sex characteristics and control reproductive function.

Exogenous hormone: A hormone produced outside the body given in the form of a medication.

Facial gender-affirming surgery: A group of surgical procedures that can be utilized to alter gendered dimensions of the face. Often called "facial feminization surgery," it can also be used to "masculinize" facial features and for people of all genders, including nonbinary people. Procedures include craniofacial reconstruction of the bones (forehead, jaw, chin) as well as changing the soft tissue.

Financial toxicity: Hardship occurring as a result of the financial burden of surgical and medical care.

Gaff: An undergarment designed to hide the external genital bulge in order to attain a flatter, gender-affirmed appearance.

Gender (noun): The characteristics and roles of individuals according to social norms, with aspects that are psychological, social, and behavioral. While sex is often described as female, male, and intersex, gender may be described as woman, feminine, man, masculine, androgynous, and much more.

Gender affirmation (noun): Psychological, social, legal, medical and/or surgical processes changes to recognize, accept, and express one's gender identity. Psychological affirmation may involve gender exploration through psychotherapy. Social changes can include changing one's pronouns, name, clothing, and hairstyle. Legal changes can include changing one's name, sex designation, and gender markers on official government-issued documents. Medical changes can include receiving gender-affirming hormones and/or surgeries. Although this process is sometimes referred to as *transition*, the term *gender affirmation* is recommended.

Gender-affirming hormone therapy (GAHT): The use of hormones (e.g., **testosterone** or **estrogen**) and other hormone-modulating medications that produce or enhance secondary sex characteristics to promote physical affirmation and reduce gender dysphoria.

Gender dysphoria: Distress experienced by some people whose gender identity does not align with society's expectations' based on their sex assigned at birth. *The Diagnostic and Statistical Manual of Mental Disorders* (DSM-5) includes gender dysphoria as a diagnosis for people whose distress is clinically significant and impairs social, occupational, or other important areas of functioning. The degree and severity of gender dysphoria is highly variable among transgender and gender diverse people.

Gender emergence: The process of identifying and accepting one's own gender identity, and the process of sharing one's gender identity with others (i.e., disclosing one's gender identity to friends, family, etc.). Also may be called "coming out."

Gender expression (noun): The way a person communicates their gender to the world through mannerisms, clothing, speech, behavior, etc. Gender expression varies depending on culture, context, and historical period.

Genderfluid: Describes a person whose gender identity is not fixed. A person who is genderfluid may always feel like a mix of more than one gender, but may feel more aligned with a certain gender some of the time, another gender at other times, multiple genders sometimes, and sometimes no gender at all.

Gender identity: A person's inner sense of themselves as girl/woman/feminine, boy/man/masculine, combinations of or beyond girl/woman/feminine or boy/man/masculine (such as having a **nonbinary** gender identity), or having no gender.

Gender identity change effort: Psychological approaches that aim to change a person's gender identity to align with societal expectations based on their sex assigned at birth. Sometimes referred to as "conversion therapy," a term that falsely implies that these efforts constitute a legitimate clinical practice instead of harmful discrimination rooted in societal stigma and transphobia.

Gender marker: The gender designated on a person's official government-issued documents, such as a passport, driver's license, or birth certificate.

Gender minority stress: Chronic stress unique to the experience of transgender and gender diverse individuals caused by lifetime experiences of stigma, discrimination, and violence that has a social basis in structural, institutional, and policy-level conditions.

Gender narrative: An individual's history of experienced gender awareness that includes the development, exploration, acceptance or rejection, identification, and persistence of one's gender, as well as any symptoms of gender dysphoria.

Genderqueer: An umbrella term that describes a person whose gender identity is beyond traditional binary notions of girl/woman/feminine or boy/man/masculine. Some people may also use terms such as gender expansive or nonbinary.

Gonadal dysgenesis: Any congenital disorder that causes impaired development of the gonads.

Gonadectomy: General term for removal of the gonads, including testicles (orchiectomy) and ovaries (oophorectomy).

Harm reduction: An approach that aims to minimize negative health, social, or legal impacts of a potential high-risk behavior without requiring the individual to stop the behavior or blaming them for engaging in the behavior.

Health information technology (HIT): The use of electronic and computer technology in the collection, recording, storage, processing, and exchange of health information.

Hypospadias: A congenital condition usually affecting males in which the urethra opens on the underside of the penis or in the perineum.

Hysterectomy: Surgical removal of the uterus only, although the term is often used colloquially to include removal of the ovaries. Hysterectomy can be subtotal, leaving the cervix, or total, in which the cervix is removed while preserving maximal vaginal tissue. When performing gender-affirming hysterectomy, salpingectomy or removal of the fallopian tubes is almost always performed with hysterectomy.

Implicit bias: Unconscious attitudes or stereotypes that affect one's assessment of, interactions with, or decisions about people or situations based on background, cultural environment, or personal experiences.

Informed consent: The process in which a health care professional and patient discuss the benefits and risks of and realistic expectations for the full range of treatment options available for that patient. It also includes the process of assessing the patient's capacity to understand this explanation.

Internalized stigma: Adoption of stigmatized attitudes toward the self.

Intersectionality: A theoretical framework that explores how systems of oppression and privilege, as well as the power relations associated with these systems, construct our perspectives and experiences; this framework seeks to inform the empowerment of individuals and groups of people negatively impacted by those power relations.

Intersex traits: Congenital variations of primary and secondary sex characteristics that are beyond traditional binary medical and societal notions of female and male bodies.

Intimate partner violence (IPV): A systematic pattern of behaviors where one person tries to control the thoughts, beliefs, and/or actions of their partner, someone they are dating, or someone with whom they have an intimate relationship; also called partner abuse, domestic violence, battering, and dating abuse.

Kink: An umbrella term for non-normative and alternative sexual practices.

Laser hair removal: Hair-removal intervention that uses a light beam to remove hair. Different laser types are used for different skin and hair colors.

LGBTQIA+: An initialism that stands for lesbian, gay, bisexual, transgender, queer (or questioning), intersex, asexual, and any and all gender and sexual minority people.

Medical trauma: Ongoing negative psychological consequences resulting from events in which a patient experienced abuse in a medical setting. It can also result from events that involved interaction with the medical system.

Metoidioplasty: Creation of a penis using the **natal phallus,** or clitoris, which has usually undergone hormone-responsive hypertrophy in patients taking testosterone. The resulting penis is 4–7 cm in length.

Military sexual trauma (MST): Trauma caused by sexual assault or harassment experienced during military service.

Misgender: To refer to a person by a pronoun or other gendered term (*e.g., Ms./Mr.*) that incorrectly indicates that person's gender identity or is otherwise inappropriate for or offensive to them.

Name used: The name a person goes by and wants others to use in personal communication, even if it is different from the name on that person's insurance or identification documents (e.g., birth certificate, driver's license, and passport). *Chosen name* is recommended over *preferred name*. The terms *Chosen name* or *Name used* can be put on patient health care forms alongside *Name on your insurance (if different)* and *Name on your legal identification documents* *(if different).* In conversation with patients, health care staff can ask, "What name do you want us to use when speaking with you?" or "What is your chosen name?"

Neopronouns: A group of new pronouns that are gender-inclusive. Examples include ze pronouns, e pronouns, and ey pronouns.

Nonbinary: Describes a person whose gender identity is a combination of or beyond the traditional girl/woman/feminine and boy/man/masculine binary identities. Sometimes abbreviated as NB or enby.

Orthorexia: A preoccupation with "healthful" eating and an inability to eat foods that do not meet the person's definition of healthful.

Other specified food and eating disorder (OSFED): A disordered pattern of eating behavior that causes significant clinical distress or negatively impacts social or occupational functioning but does not meet the full clinical criteria for an eating disorder or is of limited duration. OSFED may be followed by a description of the disordered eating behavior (e.g., OSFED: bulimia nervosa of low frequency).

Outing: The act of exposing an individual's sexual orientation and/or gender identity.

Packer: A prosthetic device that creates the appearance of a penis and testicles or the shape of external genitalia.

Partial androgen insensitivity syndrome (PAIS): A condition in which an individual with XY chromosomes is partially resistant to male hormones. Affected persons have testis development (although the testes may not descend into the scrotum) and differences in the external genitalia.

Pedicle graft: A way to move tissue that leaves the blood and nerve supply attached.

Pelvic floor physical therapy: Specialty care provided by allied health professionals with a doctorate of physical therapy. This care assists patients with voiding and other disorders that can involve dysfunction of the pelvic floor, including difficulty with vaginal dilation after vaginoplasty.

Penile prosthesis: A device surgically implanted within the new penis following phalloplasty to allow for erections.

Periareolar mastectomy: Surgery to create a flat chest that involves incisions around the nipple-areolar complex.

Perineal urethrostomy: A procedure that results in a urethral meatus in the perineum. It can be performed in cisgender men or TGD people experiencing urinary complications. Sitting to void, or using a stand-to-pee device, would be the result of this surgery.

Phalloplasty: A procedure that uses tissue from another part of the body to construct a penis. Locations with independent nerve and blood supply include the forearm (radial forearm phalloplasty [RFF]), thigh (anterolateral thigh phalloplasty [ALT]), and back (musculocutaneous latissimus dorsi [MLD]). Abdominal flap phalloplasty does not have an independent nerve and blood supply.

Posttraumatic stress disorder (PTSD) (noun): A disorder characterized by persistent intrusive symptoms, avoidance behaviors, mood and cognitive alterations, and heightened arousal and reactivity after experiencing a traumatic event or acute stressor.

Preexposure prophylaxis (PrEP): Use of antiviral medication to prevent acquisition of HIV infection by people without HIV who are at risk of being exposed to HIV through sexual contact or injection drug use.

Primary sex characteristics: The sex organs that are present at birth (gonads and external genitalia) that are traditionally used as the basis for designating female and male sex.

Pronouns: Words used when referring to an individual but not using the individual's name. Examples of pronouns are she/her/hers, he/him/his, and they/them/theirs. The appropriate phrasing is "What are your pronouns?" when seeking this information.

Proximal stressors: Gender-minority individuals' internal reactions to distal stressors, including expectations of violence or discrimination and nondisclosure of one's gender identity to prevent mistreatment.

Pubertal suppressant agents: Agents that desensitize the pituitary gland to the effects of gonadotropin-releasing hormone, thereby decreasing the release of hormones that stimulate puberty. Use of these agents is reversible.

Resilience: The use of adaptive coping strategies that enable individuals and communities to thrive despite adversity.

Revision surgery: Surgery performed to correct functional or visual sequelae from a previous surgery, ranging from a minor office procedure to improve soft tissue contour or remove scarring to operations that are more intensive than the initial procedure.

Scrotoplasty: A procedure that uses the labia majora to create a scrotum.

Secondary sex characteristics: The physical characteristics that appear at puberty and are controlled by the production of the sex hormones estrogen and testosterone.

Secondary traumatization: Trauma, often experienced by health care workers, that occurs when an individual hears about or is exposed to aversive details of a traumatic event; may present with PTSD-like signs and symptoms, including intrusive symptoms like nightmares and distressing thoughts, avoidance behaviors, changes to mood and cognition, and heightened arousal or reactivity.

Sex assigned at birth (SAAB) (noun): The sex (usually female or male) assigned to an infant, most often based on the infant's visible anatomical (e.g., genital) and other biological characteristics. Sometimes referred to as birth sex, natal sex, biological sex, or sex; however, sex assigned at birth is the recommended term.

Sex steroids: Hormones that control sexual development, secondary sex characteristics, and reproductive function.

Sexual and gender minorities (SGM): A term that describes a broad group of people with sexual orientations, gender identities, gender expressions, and sex development that do not align with societal expectations or norms, including but not limited to people who identify as lesbian, gay, bisexual, transgender, nonbinary, queer, intersex, asexual, and Two Spirit.

Sexual history (noun): A history of a patient's sexual practices, concerns, illnesses, partners, preventive actions, and risk factors.

Sexual orientation (noun): How a person characterizes their physical, emotional, and romantic attachments to other people.

Social determinants of health: Social conditions that are necessary for optimal health, including economics, environment, education, food, social context, and health care.

Stand-To-Pee device (STP) (noun): A device used to facilitate standing urination.

Stigma: Negative beliefs about a person or group based on perceived beliefs, identities, or behaviors.

Structural violence (noun): Social structures that stop individuals, groups, and societies from reaching their full potential.

Testicular prostheses: Implants used to fill the scrotum.

Testosterone: Sex steroids that produce secondary sex characteristics traditionally associated with males and that control reproductive function.

Trans feminine: Describes a person who was assigned a male sex at birth and identifies with femininity to a greater extent than with masculinity.

Transgender and gender diverse (TGD): Describes people whose gender identity and sex assigned at birth do not align based on traditional expectations; for example, a person assigned a female sex at birth who identifies as a man; or a person assigned a male sex at birth who identifies as a woman. Include gender diverse people with gender identities that may be a combination of or beyond identities in the traditional girl/woman/feminine and boy/man/masculine binary gender paradigm; for example, people who are genderfluid or nonbinary. The term "transgender" is sometimes abbreviated as *trans*.

Trans masculine: Describes a person who was assigned a female sex at birth and identifies with masculinity to a greater extent than with femininity.

Transphobia: Discrimination toward, or fear, marginalization, and hatred of, transgender people or those perceived as transgender. Individuals, communities, policies, and institutions can be transphobic.

Trauma: An event, series of events, or set of circumstances that are perceived by an individual as physically or emotionally harmful or life-threatening and overwhelm ordinary human stress responses; these experiences have a lasting adverse effect on an individual's functioning and mental, physical, social, emotional, or spiritual well-being.

Trauma-informed care: An organizational structure and treatment framework that centers on understanding, recognizing, and responding to the effects of all types of trauma.

Tucking: The practice of tucking the testicles into the inguinal canals and securing the phallus backward between the legs to create a flatter genital region.

Turner syndrome: A disorder caused by the absence of the second X chromosome (45, X, or X0); individuals are phenotypically female and may have short stature, webbed neck, undifferentiated gonads, and heart defects.

Unspecified feeding and eating disorder (UFED): A category of eating disorder that is typically used for brief contacts when a clinician is uncertain about the clinical presentation, such as in an emergency room setting, or when there is not sufficient information to make a specific diagnosis.

Urethral fistula: A leak or communication of the urethra with the skin in a location other than the urethral meatus.

Urethral lengthening: Surgical extension of the urine channel through the new penis created during metoidioplasty or phalloplasty.

Urethral stricture: Narrowing of the urethra resulting from scarring.

Vaginoplasty: Surgery in which vulvar subunits (clitoris, urethral meatus, labia minora, and labia majora) and the vaginal canal are created.

Vicarious traumatization: Trauma, often experienced by health care workers, that occurs when an individual hears about or is exposed to aversive details of a traumatic event; may present with PTSD symptoms that resemble those of patients with direct trauma histories.

Vulvoplasty: Surgery in which vulvar subunits (clitoris, urethral meatus, labia minora, and labia majora) and introitus are created, but no vaginal canal. Sometimes called zero- or limited-depth vaginoplasty.

Window of tolerance: A term coined by Daniel Siegel to describe the zone of arousal in which an individual is able to effectively manage a range of emotions without becoming physiologically hyperaroused (e.g., high energy, anxious, angry, overwhelmed, hypervigilant, or in fight-or-flight mode) or hypoaroused (e.g., shut down, numb, depressed, passive, withdrawn, ashamed, or in freeze mode).

Index

Note: Page numbers followed by f and t indicate figures and tables.